Handbook of
Health Behavior Research I
Personal and Social Determinants

Handbook of
Health Behavior Research I
Personal and Social Determinants

Edited by

David S. Gochman

University of Louisville
Louisville, Kentucky

Plenum Press • New York and London

Library of Congress Cataloging-in-Publication Data

Handbook of health behavior research / edited by David S. Gochman.
      p.   cm.
    Includes bibliographical references and indexes.
    Contents: I. Personal and social determinants -- II. Provider
determinants -- III. Demography, development, and diversity --
IV. Relevance for professionals and issues for the future.
    ISBN 0-306-45443-2 (I). -- ISBN 0-306-45444-0 (II). -- ISBN
0-306-45445-9 (III). -- ISBN 0-306-45446-7 (IV)
    1. Health behavior. 2. Health behavior--Research.   I. Gochman,
David S.
    [DNLM: 1. Health Behavior--handbooks. 2. Research--handbooks.   W
49 H236 1997]
RA776.9.H363   1997
613--dc21
DNLM/DLC
for Library of Congress   97-14565
                                                           CIP

ISBN 0-306-45443-2

© 1997 Plenum Press, New York
A Division of Plenum Publishing Corporation
233 Spring Street, New York, N. Y. 10013

http://www.plenum.com

Printed in the United States of America

DEDICATION

Throughout my career I have been helped and encouraged by many persons. There are a few whose help was so special that my debt to them is enormous. It is in recognition of what I owe them that this *Handbook* is dedicated to Zelda S. Ackerman, O. J. Harvey, and D. Eldridge McBride, and to the memories of John H. Russel, William A. Scott, and John P. Kirscht. Mrs. Ackerman, my advisor in New York City's High School of Music and Art (now LaGuardia High School), facilitated my early entrance into academia. "Mac" McBride and John Russel, inspired and committed teachers, advisors, and counselors during my formative years at Shimer College, served as role models and continued as my friends over the decades. Bill Scott and O. J. Harvey were encouraging and supportive advisors during my graduate training at the University of Colorado. Bill taught me methodological rigor and innovation, and O. J. encouraged me to think in new and divergent ways. Both of them maintained high standards for their own performance, and demanded no less from me and others.

Jack Kirscht was a pioneer in health behavior research, a community activist, and a person of great wit, humor, and charm. In 1967 he convinced me to come to the University of Michigan's School of Public Health and to bring my research interests in cognitive development and structure to the area of health behavior. He was also a contributor to my 1988 book. Health behavior research lost a giant with his untimely death. He is very much missed by many as a friend and colleague and as a teacher and scholar.

Contributors

Lu Ann Aday, School of Public Health, University of Texas at Houston, Houston, Texas 77225

William C. Awe, School of Public Health, University of Texas at Houston, Houston, Texas 77225

Tom Baranowski, Department of Behavioral Sciences, M.D. Anderson Cancer Center, University of Texas at Houston, Houston, Texas 77030

Victoria L. Champion, School of Nursing, Indiana University, Indianapolis, Indiana 46202-5117

William C. Cockerham, Department of Sociology, University of Alabama at Birmingham, Birmingham, Alabama 35294-3350

William W. Dressler, Department of Anthropology, University of Alabama, Tuscaloosa, Alabama 35487-0210

Kimberley A. DuCharme, Department of Physical Education, Wilfrid-Laurier University, Waterloo, Ontario N2L 3C5, Canada

Joan M. Eakin, Department of Behavioural Science, Faculty of Medicine, University of Toronto, Toronto, Ontario M5S 1A8, Canada

Kristi J. Erdal, Department of Psychology, Arizona State University, Tempe, Arizona 85287-1104

Horacio Fabrega, Jr., Western Psychiatric Institute and Clinic, University of Pittsburgh School of Medicine, Pittsburgh, Pennsylvania 15213

Reed Geertsen, Department of Sociology, Utah State University, Logan, Utah 84322-0730

David S. Gochman, Kent School of Social Work, University of Louisville, Louisville, Kentucky 40292

Richard R. Lau, Institute for Health, Health Care Policy, and Aging Research, Rutgers University, New Brunswick, New Jersey 08903

James E. Maddux, Department of Psychology, George Mason University, Fairfax, Virginia 22030-4444

Kathryn S. Oths, Department of Anthropology, University of Alabama, Tuscaloosa, Alabama 35487-0210

Steven Prentice-Dunn, Department of Psychology, University of Alabama, Tuscaloosa, Alabama 35487-0348

John W. Reich, Department of Psychology, Arizona State University, Tempe, Arizona 85287-1104

Ronald W. Rogers, Department of Psychology, University of Alabama, Tuscaloosa, Alabama 35487-0348

Irwin M. Rosenstock, College of Health and Human Services, California State University (Emeritus), Long Beach, California 90801

Alexander Segall, Department of Sociology, University of Manitoba, Winnipeg, Manitoba R3T 2N2, Canada

Victor J. Strecher, University of Michigan Comprehensive Cancer Center, University of Michigan, Ann Arbor, Michigan 48109

Barbara J. Tinsley, Department of Psychology, University of California, Riverside, California 92521

Ingrid Waldron, Department of Biology, University of Pennsylvania, Philadelphia, Pennsylvania 19104-6018

Alex J. Zautra, Department of Psychology, Arizona State University, Tempe, Arizona 85287-1104

Preface to All Volumes

THE STATE OF THE ART

The *primary* objective of this *Handbook* is to provide statements about health behavior research as a basic body of knowledge moving into the 21st century. It is expected that the *Handbook* will remain in use and current through 2005, at least. The *Handbook* presents a broad and representative selection of mid-1990s health behavior findings and concepts in a single work. While texts and books of readings are available in related areas, such as health psychology (e.g., DiMatteo, 1991; Stone et al., 1987), medical anthropology (e.g., McElroy & Townsend, 1989; Nichter, 1992), medical sociology (e.g., Cockerham, 1995; Helman, 1990; Wolinsky, 1988), behavioral health (e.g., Matarazzo, Weiss, Herd, Miller, & Weiss, 1984), behavioral risk factors (e.g., Hamburg, Elliott, & Parron, 1982), and changing health behaviors (Shumaker et al., 1990), none of these works was intended to address basic research-generated knowledge of health behavior, and none was intended to transcend individual disciplines. Accordingly, none of these works presents a broad and representative spectrum of basic health behavior research reflecting multidisciplinary activities. One work with a title identical to this one but for one word, the *Handbook of Health Behavior Change* (Shumaker et al., 1990), deals almost exclusively with applications. This *Handbook* thus presents the reader with the "state of the art" in health behavior research, something not found elsewhere.

In the context of this primary objective, it was not intended that the chapters be journal articles. Authors were encouraged to provide extensive coverage of their topics and to provide original findings to the degree that such findings were relevant. They were not encouraged to write research reports, and the reader should not expect the chapters to read as though they were journal articles.

HEALTH BEHAVIOR AS BASIC RESEARCH

Health behavior is not a long-established, traditional area of inquiry, comparable to chemistry or psychology, but a newly emerging interdisciplinary and multidisciplinary one. Health behavior is still establishing its identity as a domain of scientific research.

Although the earlier work (Gochman, 1988) that helped define it is now nearly a decade old, there are still relatively few institutional or organizational structures, i.e., departments and programs, that reflect the field, and few books and no journals are directed at it.

A *second* objective of the *Handbook* is to reaffirm the identity of health behavior and help secure its position as an important area of basic research, worthy of being studied in its own right. In the context of their discussion of the emergence of medical anthropology, Foster and Anderson (1978, pp. 2–3) stated: "When a sufficient number of researchers focus on the same, or related, topics, and as significant new data begin to appear, the stage is set for the emergence of a new discipline or subdiscipline. But some spark is essential to coalesce these emerging interests around a common focus; usually, it seems, an appropriate name supplies this spark." It is hoped that this *Handbook* will provide such a spark.

LEVELS OF ANALYSIS

Personal, Social, and Provider Determinants

A *third* objective, very much related to the first two, is to view health behavior research as transcending particular behaviors, specific illnesses or health problems or strategies for intervention, or single sets of determinants. One major way of achieving this objective is to look at health behavior in transaction with a range of personal, social systems: as an outcome or product, as well as a factor that affects these systems (in this context, the term *system* is often used interchangeably with *unit* or *entity*), rather than primarily as a set of risk factors or as targets for interventions directed at behavioral change. Volumes I and II of this *Handbook* thus deal largely with characteristics of the system of concern, and focus on specific health behaviors, or specific health problems or conditions, as ways of demonstrating the impact of these systems.

Volume I begins with conceptualizations of health and health behavior and then moves from smaller to larger systems, demonstrating how health behavior is determined by—and often in transaction with—personal, family, social, institutional and community, and cultural factors. These levels of analysis cannot be neatly differentiated, and at times the distinctions between them are arbitrary: Families, organizations, and institutions are all social systems. Moreover, although all individuals differ in their responses to and interpretations of family, social, and cultural norms, personalities and cognitive structures nonetheless reflect family, social, and cultural factors; additionally, families, social groupings, and organizations all reflect elements of the culture in which they exist. Furthermore, the categorizing and sequencing of sections and chapters in no way reflect an attempt to exclude material that deals with other levels of determinants; they serve primarily to facilitate focusing more on one of these determinants than on others. Volume I concludes with an integration that relates categories of health behaviors to characteristics of personal and social systems, identifies common themes, and suggests future research directions.

Since so much of health behavior is determined by providers—the health professionals and institutions that comprise the care delivery system—Volume II examines the way encounters with health providers determine health behaviors, and how health behaviors and the providers reciprocally affect one another. Volume II begins with an overview section on communication, continues with a section on interactional and structural determinants, i.e., professional characteristics, perceptions, power, and role relations, and organizational, locational, and environmental factors; and then presents major sections on the impact of provider characteristics on adherence to and acceptance of both disease-focused and lifestyle regimens.

Populations and Professional Applications

Volume III begins with an overview section on the demography of health behavior and continues with an examination of health behaviors in a range of populations selected on the basis either of the life-span continuum; of a health status risk due to an existing condition, a socially constructed label, or restrictive economic and environmental conditions; or of membership in defined communities. Volume IV examines the relevance of knowledge generated by health behavior research for the training and clinical (and other) practice activities of health professionals; for health services management and health policy; and for planned applications in school, family, community and workplace settings, and the media. Volume IV aims to position health behavior research in the 21st century through a discussion of the four major disciplines that inform health behavior research: health psychology, medical anthropology, medical geography, and medical sociology. Volume IV also presents a working draft of a taxonomy of health behavior and of a matrix framework for organizing health behavior knowledge.

Glossary and Index

Each of the volumes concludes with a glossary of health behavior concepts and definitions, and an index. Both of these reflect the contents of the entire *Handbook*.

A FRAMEWORK FOR ORGANIZING HEALTH BEHAVIOR KNOWLEDGE: A WORK IN PROGRESS

A Taxonomy for Health Behavior

Reviewing the contributed chapters in a volume with the editorial objective of integration led to the development of a "work in progress" taxonomy of health behaviors that became a primary organizing principle for the final chapter of each of the first three volumes. The taxonomy continued to evolve from Volume I to Volume III. The integration of Volume I would have been modified and organized slightly differently had it been written *after* those for Volumes II and III, but the fundamentals remained the same. Virtually all of the health behavior findings reported could be subsumed under one of six categories: health cognitions; care seeking; risk behaviors; lifestyle; responses to illness, including adherence; and preventive, protective, and safety behaviors.

A Matrix Framework

The working taxonomy appears in a different way in Volume IV. With one minor modification—the distinction between nonaddictive and addictive risk behaviors—it combines with the range of personal and social systems used as organizing principles in Volumes I and II, and in the integration chapters for Volumes I through III, to become part of a matrix framework for organizing health behavior knowledge. This framework is presented in Chapter 20 of Volume IV, entitled "Health Behavior Research, Cognate Disciplines, Future Identity, and an Organizing Matrix: An Integration of Perspectives."

DIVERSITY OF PERSPECTIVES

A *fourth* objective is to assure that the reader is exposed to varied perspectives in conceptual models, disciplines, populations, and methods, as well as to nonmedical frames of reference. The *Handbook* exposes the reader to a range of theories and models. The contributors bring expertise from their training or professional involvements in varied disciplines, including (in alphabetical order) anthropology, biology, communications, dentistry, education, engineering, ethics, geography, health management and policy, health promotion and health education, medicine, nursing, psychiatry, psychology, public health, social work, and sociology.

DIVERSITY OF READERS

A *fifth* objective is to assure the relevance of the *Handbook* for persons in a number of fields who are interested in issues related to research in health behavior. The potential readership includes researchers in the social and behavioral sciences who want to know more about health behavior in general, or particular aspects of it, or who want to develop their own health behavior research; students in courses that integrate social and behavioral science and health, in disciplines such as anthropology, psychology, and sociology, and in professional programs in dentistry, medicine (including psychiatry), nursing, public health, and social work; professionals who provide, plan, implement, and evaluate health services and programs: fitness and exercise physiologists; family planners; health educators and promoters; health managers; health planners; hospital administrators; nutritionists; pharmacists; physicians in community and family practice; physiatrists; public health dentists, nurses, physicians; rehabilitation therapists; social workers; and so forth.

THE PRACTICAL RELEVANCE OF HEALTH BEHAVIOR RESEARCH

The practical value of increasing knowledge and understanding of health behavior through rigorous, systematic research is implicit in the grave concern with health status in many contemporary societies. Solutions to an appreciable number of health problems require large-scale efforts at local, regional, and national levels to develop and enforce policies to control, minimize, and ultimately reduce air, land, and water pollution; the hazards of transportation; and the risks of the workplace environment. Many of these solutions transcend individual health behaviors. Solutions to other health problems, however, involve policies, programs, and processes that interact with the personal health behavior of individuals and the population at large, in their family, social, workplace, institutional, and community milieus.

As material in Volume IV demonstrates, attempts to change individual health behaviors, either through individual therapeutic interventions or through larger-scale health promotion or health education programs, have been less than impressive. Many attempts are purely programmatic, hastily conceived, and lacking in theoretical rationale or empirical foundation. A major reason for this is the lack of *basic* knowledge about the target behaviors, about the contexts in which they occur, and about the factors that determine and stabilize them. Basic research in health behavior, aside from being worthy of study in its own right, may very well increase the effectiveness of interventions and programs designed to bring about behavioral change.

DELIBERATE OMISSIONS

Notably absent from the *Handbook* are chapters devoted to topics such as "Type A" personality, psychosomatics, and stress. While these considerations may be linked to health status, and sometimes to health behavior, they have been omitted because they are more generally models for understanding the etiology of disease and illnesses. Furthermore, while "holism" has become a catchword among many who disavow the traditional medical model, the term has come to include charlatanism and cultism, as well as some impressive approaches to treatment. At present, it remains more a statement of faith suggesting future research alternatives than a body of well-thought-through, rigorously conducted research. Moreover, caution against a reverse "ethnocentrism" and overly romanticized views of non-high-technological medicine is cogently provided by Eisenberg and Kleinman (1981). In their words (Eisenberg & Kleinman, 1981, p. 10): "Healing ceremonies can be efficacious, but hardly substitute for antibiotics or surgery." Accordingly, there is no section on "holism" or "holistic medicine" or "holistic health" in the *Handbook*.

REFERENCES

Cockerham, W. C. (1995). *Medical sociology* (6th ed.). Englewood Cliffs, NJ: Simon & Schuster.

DiMatteo, M. R. (1991). *The psychology of health, illness, and medical care: An individual perspective.* Belmont, CA: Brooks/Cole.

Eisenberg, L., & Kleinman, A. (Eds.). (1981). *The relevance of social science for medicine.* Dordrecht, Netherlands: Reidel.

Foster, G. M., & Anderson, B. G. (1978). *Medical anthropology.* New York: Wiley.

Gochman, D. S. (Ed.). (1988). *Health behavior: Emerging research perspectives.* New York: Plenum Press.

Hamburg, D. A., Elliott, G. R., & Parron, D. L. (Eds.). (1982). *Health and behavior: Frontiers of research in the biobehavioral sciences.* Washington, DC: National Academy Press.

Helman, C. G. (1990). *Culture, health and illness* (2nd ed.). London: Wright/Butterworth.

Matarazzo, J. D., Weiss, S. M., Herd, J. A., Miller, N. E., & Weiss, S. M. (Eds.). (1984). *Behavioral health: A handbook of health enhancement and disease prevention.* New York: Wiley.

McElroy, A., & Townsend, P. K. (1989). *Medical anthropology in ecological perspective* (2nd ed.). Boulder, CO: Westview.

Nichter, M. (Ed.). (1992). *Anthropological approaches to the study of ethnomedicine*. Amsterdam, Netherlands: Gordon and Breach Science Publishers.

Shumaker, S.A., Schron, E. B., Ockene, J. K., Parker, C. T., Probstfield, J. L., & Wolle, J. M. (Eds.). (1990). *The handbook of health behavior change*. New York: Springer.

Stone, G. C., Weiss, S. M., Matarazzo, J. D., Miller, N. E., Rodin, J., Belar, C. D., Follick, M. J., & Singer, J. E. (Eds.). (1987). *Health psychology: A discipline and a profession*. Chicago: University of Chicago Press.

Wolinsky, F. D. (1988). *The sociology of health: Principles, practitioners, and issues* (2nd ed.). Belmont, CA: Wadsworth.

Preface to Volume I

PERSONAL AND SOCIAL DETERMINANTS OF HEALTH BEHAVIOR

The content and organization of Volume I flow from the *Handbook*'s objective of viewing health behavior research as transcending particular behaviors, specific illnesses or health problems, programs or strategies for intervention, or single sets of determinants. One major way of achieving this objective is to look at health behavior in transaction with a range of personal, social systems: as an outcome or product, as well as a factor that affects these systems (in this context, the term "system" is often used interchangeably with "unit" or "entity"), rather than primarily as a set of risk factors or as targets for interventions directed at behavioral change. The volume thus deals with characteristics of several levels of social systems, and focuses on specific health behaviors, or specific health problems or conditions, as ways of demonstrating the impact of these systems.

This volume begins with a working definition of health behavior and health behavior research; discussions of varied ways of constructing meanings of health, illness, and related terms; and analyses of the cultural, political, and economic contexts of these constructions through selected periods of human history. Then, moving from smaller to larger systems, Volume I demonstrates how health behavior is determined by—and is often in transaction with—personal, family, social, institutional and community, and cultural factors. These units of analysis cannot be neatly differentiated, and at times the distinctions between them are arbitrary: families, organizations, and institutions are all *social* systems. Moreover, although all individuals differ in their responses to and interpretations of family, social, and cultural norms, personalities and cognitive structures nonetheless reflect family, social, and cultural factors; and families, social groupings, and organizations all reflect elements of the culture in which they exist. Furthermore, the categorizing and sequencing of parts and chapters in no way reflect an attempt to exclude material that deals with other levels of determinants; they serve primarily to facilitate focusing more on one of these determinants rather than on others. This volume's integrating chapter, in addition to identifying common themes and making suggestions for future research, relates six categories of health behaviors to a range of personal and social systems, thus introducing a matrix organizing framework for health behavior knowledge.

Acknowledgments

Many persons provided greatly valued assistance during the nearly four years from the time the *Handbook of Health Behavior Research* was conceptualized until its publication, and I owe all of them my thanks. The substantial help I received from some of them merits special recognition. Among the support staff at the Raymond A. Kent School, I especially wish to thank Shannon R. Daniels and Kelley E. Davis for their expeditious and careful photocopying of what must have seemed like tons of manuscripts, Jane Isert for her dedication in assuring that calls and mail from contributors and from the publisher reached me in a timely way, and Sally Montreuil-Palmarini for expediting mailings of material to contributors.

Among the highly professional and committed staff at the University of Louisville's Ekstrom Library, special thanks go to all of the reference librarians, and particularly to Carmen Embry (now at Barrier Islands Art Center) for some insightful content suggestions; Sharon Edge for her expediting access to materials; and S. Kay Womack (now at the University of Oklahoma) for her astute and knowledgeable guidance through computer and other literature searches, particularly in areas in which little had been written that was adequately indexed.

Thomas R. Lawson, Director of the Kent School, deserves recognition for his continued encouragement of my scholarly activities, his efforts in securing a sabbatical leave for me to assure the *Handbook*'s timely completion, and his generosity in providing necessary supplies and personnel resources.

A great debt is owed to all of the authors whose scholarly chapters grace the *Handbook*, and add immeasurably to its value, for the care they devoted to their work, and for their receptivity and constructive responses to the high density of editorial suggestions made throughout the *Handbook*'s progress. A number of authors and others also provided suggestions about potential contributors for several topics. Among those whose help in this quest was exceptional were M. Robin DiMatteo, Eugene B. Gallagher, Russell E. Glasgow, Michael R. Kauth, Jeffrey Kelley, James E. Maddux, Lillian C. Milanof, R. Prasaad Steiner, and David P. Willis.

Gene Gallagher, along with Zeev Ben-Sira (whose untimely death occurred prior to the final revision of his chapter), John G. Bruhn, Patricia J. Bush, Henry P. Cole, Reed Geertsen, Marie R. Haug, Richard R. Lau, Alexander Segall, and Ingrid Waldron had all contributed to the 1988 book. Their willingness to contribute anew to this one is most appreciated.

Finally, Richard Millikan merits special recognition for the excellence of his copyediting work, his ability to perceive issues that cross-cut the four volumes, and for his skill in helping me clarify my own thinking; and Eliot Werner, Executive Editor at Plenum Publishing Corporation, deserves special thanks for his vision and encouragement in the area of health behavior research, for his faith in the value of the *Handbook*, and for being laid back and calming in the face of my "overfunctioning" and obsessive-compulsivity.

Contents

Chapter 4.   The Health Belief Model and Health Behavior 71

Victor J. Strecher, Victoria L. Champion, and Irwin M. Rosenstock

Chapter 5.   Beliefs about Control and Health Behaviors 93

John W. Reich, Kristi J. Erdal, and Alex J. Zautra

I

CONCEPTIONS OF HEALTH BEHAVIOR

1

Health Behavior Research

Definitions and Diversity

David S. Gochman

What "health behavior" means and how it is treated in this *Handbook* provide a framework for the first part of this introductory chapter. The chapter begins with a working definition of health behavior, discusses key related terms, and provides a definition of "health behavior research." The chapter continues with a discussion of conceptions of health, disease, illness, and sickness and concludes by identifying some research issues that relate to these conceptions.

HEALTH BEHAVIOR

A Working Definition

Although the domain of health behavior has not been rigidly bounded, a *working definition* emerging from earlier tasks (Gochman, 1981, 1982, 1988) establishes health behavior as (Gochman, 1982, p. 169; 1988, p. 3):

David S. Gochman • Kent School of Social Work, University of Louisville, Louisville, Kentucky 40292.

Handbook of Health Behavior Research I: Personal and Social Determinants, edited by David S. Gochman. Plenum Press, New York, 1997.

those personal attributes such as beliefs, expectations, motives, values, perceptions, and other cognitive elements; personality characteristics, including affective and emotional states and traits; and overt behavior patterns, actions and habits that relate to health maintenance, to health restoration and to health improvement.

This definition, accepted by others (e.g., Glanz, Lewis, & Rimer, 1990), provides the focus of this *Handbook*. "Behavior," moreover, denotes something that people *do* or *refrain from doing*, although not always consciously or voluntarily. It is not something *done to them*. A treatment is not a behavior. Furthermore, mending of broken bones, healing of wounds, immunity against disease, resistance to infection, and the like, are not behaviors. They are, rather, physiological functions. Health behavior thus does not mean clinical improvement or physiological recovery as such, but it does include analyses of specific actions—e.g., taking medication in an appropriate fashion or remaining in a difficult and challenging rehabilitation program—that affect improvement or recovery.

A person's health status or health condition is not a behavior, but a person's perceptions of health status or of its deterioration or improvement, or of recovery or nonrecovery from an illness or accident, or other changes in health status *are* health behaviors. Finally, the definition's broad construction of behavior explicitly includes not only directly observable, overt actions, but also those mental events and feeling states that are "observed" or measured indirectly. Since, as Steuart notes, virtually all human activities are linked in some manner to health and illness, "there is no such thing as 'health behavior' … separable from other behaviors" (Steuart, 1993, p. S116). Some behaviors, however, seem more cogently linked to health and illness than others.

This definition of health behavior also recognizes that these personal attributes are influenced by, and otherwise reflect, family, social, societal, institutional, and cultural determinants (Gochman, 1982, p. 169).

Preventive and Protective Behavior, Illness Behavior, and Sick Role Behavior

The working definition comprises several other definitions, including those set forth by Kasl and Cobb (1966a,b) in their seminal articles defining specific categories of health-related behavior, and affirmed more than a quarter of century later by Alonzo (1993). Among these categories are *preventive, protective, illness, and sick role behaviors*.

Preventive and Protective Behavior. For Kasl and Cobb (1966a), the term *health behavior* denotes those actions undertaken by persons who believe they are well—and who are not experiencing any signs or symptoms of illness—for the purpose of remaining well. This usage confines health behavior to preventive actions, and for Kasl and Cobb the terms are synonymous. Langlie (1977) defines a preventive behavior as "any medically recommended action, voluntarily undertaken by a person who believes himself to be healthy, that tends to prevent disease or disability and/or detect disease in an asymptomatic stage" (Langlie, 1977, p. 247).

Both Kasl and Cobb and Langlie define health behavior as being geared toward prevent-

ing and detecting disease in healthy, asymptomatic persons by the use of medically recommended actions (Alonzo, 1993). Medical or technological behaviors with decisive, definitive preventive value include accepting immunizations against infectious diseases such as diphtheria, infantile paralysis, pertussis, tetanus, and typhoid fever, and consuming foods that contain Vitamins A, C, and D to prevent pellagra, scurvy, and rickets. Such actions are termed *primary prevention*, as opposed to those that involve early detection.

Preventive behaviors, however, also include *nonmedical* activities. Breslow and his colleagues (e.g., Belloc & Breslow, 1972) were among the pioneers in identifying a specific list of nonmedical, mundane preventive behaviors, which include duration of sleep; eating habits, including regularity, frequency, amount eaten, and eating breakfast; weight management; physical recreational activity, including active sports, swimming or walking, working in the garden, doing exercises, taking weekend trips, and hunting or fishing; consumption of alcoholic beverages, including frequency and amount; and not smoking. Other everyday primary preventive behaviors include wearing seat belts and motorcycle helmets; obeying traffic laws; adherence to health and safety regulations at work; and engaging only in *safe* sex activities.

A survey of physicians (Sobal, Valente, Muncie, Levine, & DeForge, 1985) found strong professional consensus about the preventive importance of these everyday behaviors, particularly about eliminating smoking and using protective equipment and clothing. It must be made clear, however, that these behaviors are less decisively preventive than are immunizations.

Primary preventive behaviors have been conceptualized in several ways. Kirscht (1983), for example, commented on the variability in the diffusion of preventive behaviors, noting that some, e.g., regular tooth brushing, were adopted widely, while others were never widely established on a voluntary basis, e.g., use of automobile seat belts before legislation mandating their use was enacted. Gauff and Miller (1986) distinguished between passive prevention—

which does not involve individual behaviors but relies on societal public health activities such as chlorination of water, sewage treatment, and highway design—and active prevention—which reflects specific individual activities such as flossing, engaging in exercise, and eating a balanced diet. Langlie (1977, 1979) distinguished between direct risk preventive behaviors, such as pedestrian and driver activities, and indirect risk preventive behaviors, such as use of seat belts, exercise, and nutrition.

(3) Other health behaviors have *secondary* preventive value; i.e., they do not decisively prevent a condition from occuring, but they facilitate the early detection of a condition and thus minimize its impact. Such behaviors include—but certainly are not limited to—undergoing periodic examinations to detect the early signs of cancer, heart disease or, dental conditions. Gauff and Miller (1986) refer to these as "physician-generated prevention."

Complementing these primary and secondary preventive behaviors that have empirical linkages to health status are what Harris and Guten (1979) term "health protective behaviors." These are actions that people engage in to protect, promote, or maintain health, whether the actions are medically approved or not (Harris & Guten, 1979), and are embraced under the concept of health behavior independently of their objective effectiveness. Such health protective behaviors might include praying, telling beads, or saying "mantras"; taking laxatives, emetics, enemas, cold showers, and hot baths; consuming megadoses of vitamins; eating an abundance of garlic and onions; wearing copper bracelets as a treatment for arthritis or amulets with sassafras around the neck to ward off colds; and following fad diets. Other protective behaviors are actions that are taken to reduce the likelihood of disease, defect, injury, and disability from the environmental dangers inherent in transportation systems; from food, air, and water supplies; and from workplaces (Alonzo, 1993).

Illness Behavior. For Kasl and Cobb (1966a), illness behavior denotes those actions under-

taken by persons who are uncertain about whether they are well, who are troubled or puzzled by bodily sensations or feelings they believe are signs or symptoms of illness, who want to clarify the meaning of these experiences and thus determine whether they are well, and who want to know what to do if they are not. Mechanic (1966/1972, 1978, chap. 9) and Suchman (1965/1972) provided seminal analyses of such "care-seeking" or "help-seeking" behavior that have guided decades of illness behavior research.

Mechanic's (1966/1972) model of illness behavior embraces "an individual's recognition that he needs advice, his decision whether to seek it, his choice of counsellor" (p. 128). Suchman's phrasings are different, but the behaviors are similar. Both models examine the personal determinants of these illness behaviors, as well as how these behaviors are socially and culturally conditioned. Illness behaviors include—but are not limited to—responses to bodily signs and symptoms; seeking opinions and advice from persons who are believed to have health expertise, whether these persons are officially recognized by the larger society (allopathically trained physicians, state-licensed health care professionals) or not (folk practitioners, healers, lay therapists); and seeking opinions and advice from relatives, friends, neighbors, and colleagues; as well as doing nothing but waiting to see whether the unusual signs or symptoms go away. Denton (1978, pp. 108–109) (citing Saunders & Hewes, 1969) provided a colorful list of care-seeking behaviors that attests to the richness of the alternative resources available: electrotherapists, naturopaths, gymnasia, Turkish baths, elastic stockings, Lydia Pinkham's Vegetable Compound, Carter's Liver Pills, bicarbonate of soda, oil of cloves, and the *Reader's Digest*, all of which lie beyond scientific medicine.

Sick Role Behavior. For Kasl and Cobb (1966b) and others (e.g., Parsons, 1951), sick role behavior denotes those actions undertaken by persons who have already been designated as being sick, either by others or by themselves. Such behaviors include—but again are not limited to—the medically normative ones of acceptance of a prescribed regimen; returning for medical appointments; limitation of activity and of personal, family, and social responsibilities; and actions related to recovery and rehabilitation. Yet they may also include seeking out alternative practitioners or healers, prayer, and visiting shrines.

The critical distinctions that Kasl and Cobb and others make between various types of health behaviors are nonetheless important and should not be minimized. For example, although Williams and Wechsler (1972) observed only modest linkages between selected preventive behaviors in a pilot study and raised the question of whether it made sense to talk about preventive behavior as a unitary construct, it remains for future research to determine empirically whether there are commonalities or underlying unities among the behaviors embraced within each of the categories of "health behaviors" or whether the categories are uniformly and differentially related to diverse levels of determinants. It is their common presumed relationship to health, however, that brings the several categories together.

Societal Health Behavior. Alonzo's (1993) cutting edge conceptualization adds a fourth category: societal health behavior. This category reflects "what society does for the collectivity," in contrast to what individuals can do for themselves. This definition includes those societal acts that foster health education, ensure food safety, license professional providers, and monitor the environment.

A Work-in-Progress Taxonomy

The integrating chapters of Volumes I through III of this *Handbook* use a six-category taxonomy for health behavior that emerged from reviewing all of the contributions to each volume. These categories are: health cognitions; care seeking; risk behaviors; lifestyle; responses to illness, including adherence; and preventive, protective, and safety behaviors. This work-in-progress taxonomy is further defined and elaborated in Chap-

ter 20 of Volume IV, which adds a seventh category by distinguishing between addictive and nonaddictive risk behaviors. This taxonomy, which builds upon the essential foundations established by Kasl and Cobb (1966a,b), Harris and Guten (1979), Langlie (1977,1979), and others, is then proposed as one axis in a matrix for organizing health behavior research knowledge.

HEALTH BEHAVIOR RESEARCH

Health behavior research is an emerging interdisciplinary, systematic examination of these health behaviors and their determinants. Health behaviors can be analyzed in at least three ways: as risk behaviors, as targets for change, or as interesting in their own right.

Antecedent or Consequent; Input or Outcome

As *risk behaviors*, health behaviors are examined as antecedents or causes of diseases, illnesses, and health status (e.g., Belloc & Breslow, 1972). Such an approach is taken by social epidemiologists. As *targets for change*, health behaviors are viewed as objectives for systematic interventions directed at producing behavioral changes and ultimately at generating changes in health status (e.g., Breslow, 1978/1980). Such an approach is taken by health educators, by health promotion campaigns, and by public health programs. As subjects of scientific study because of their *own intrinsic interest*, health behaviors are analyzed as consequences or outcomes, as well as correlates and concomitants, of personal and social factors that embrace the family as well as societal institutions and cultural influences. Moreover, health behaviors are viewed as being in continual dynamic interrelationships with these personal and social factors.

Although this *Handbook* considers health behavior in all three ways, the third way is intended as the major focus. Understanding these personal and social contexts, the causes and anchorings of health behaviors, as well as their effects upon these contexts, should increase the likelihood of successfully modifying health behaviors and of developing effective services, programs, and policies related to prevention and health promotion. A perspective that considers health behaviors as phenomena worthy of being understood on their own terms, and not to be studied simply because they affect health or because they can be modified to improve health, is more likely to generate basic, conceptually derived, rigorous, systematic scientific investigations, and thus is more likely to lead to greater understanding of these behaviors, than are perspectives that place health behaviors in an ancillary position.

What Health Behavior Research *Is Not*

A good definition should state not only what something *is*, but also what it *is not*. Health behavior is conceptually distinct from treatment and from physiological/biological/pharmacological responses to treatment. It is also conceptually distinct from health care and from the organization or structure of the health care delivery system. Health behavior as an area of research is thus *not primarily* concerned with the technology of health care, with medical procedures, with psychotherapy, or with other interventions. Further, it is *not primarily* concerned with the delivery of health care or services or with the organization of the health care delivery system. Yet it touches profoundly upon all of these. Health behavior research *is* concerned with the way such interventions and institutional structures affect the health behavior of individuals. Health behavior research *is not primarily* concerned with health status. Yet a person's perceptions of health status and social and cultural definitions of health and health status are assuredly important health behaviors.

*Health Behavior Research **Is Not** Behavioral Medicine.* Health behavior research *is not identical* with behavioral medicine, which has been defined as the "field concerned with the development of behavior science knowledge and techniques relevant to the understanding of physical health and illness and the application of this knowledge and these techniques to prevention, treatment and rehabilitation" (Schwartz & Weiss, 1978, p. 4). Although some areas within behavioral medicine are also contained by health behavior, the basic paradigm proposed for behavioral medicine (Schwartz & Weiss, 1978, p. 7) reflects the medical model's systematic concern with the prevention, etiology, pathology, diagnosis, treatment, and rehabilitation of specific disorders, rather than with a broader range of health-relevant actions that do not relate to specific diseases or problems. In contrast, health behavior is defined independently of pathology, diagnosis, and treatment of specific disorders. It includes a concern for general health maintenance and improvement in addition to behaviors that are problem-specific.

Moreover, health behavior research does not automatically begin with a medical framework and its assumptions. It does not accept uncritically the basic premises of the medical model, in which physicians and other societally sanctioned health care practitioners establish and reify implicit norms of function and dysfunction. Health behavior embraces both mental and nonmental disorders and recognizes the interaction between them. It questions the traditional philosophical mind–body dualism that had led to separation and fragmentation of research in the health area, to say nothing of the separation and fragmentation of training and delivery of care and services.

*Health Behavior Research **Is Not** Behavioral Health.* Health behavior research *is not* "behavioral health," which Matarazzo (1980, p. 813) defines as

an interdisciplinary field dedicated to promoting a philosophy of health that stresses *individual responsibility* in the application of behavioral and biomedical science knowledge and techniques to the *maintenance* of health and the *prevention* of illness and dysfunction by a variety of self-initiated individual or shared activities.

As can be inferred from Matarazzo's definition, "behavioral health" is committed to the *application* of knowledge, rather than to developing basic knowledge. Furthermore, behavioral health (Matarazzo, 1984) emphasizes an ideology aimed at improving health status by the combination of applied knowledge and individual responsibility. While health behavior research accepts the importance of increasing knowledge, as an area of basic inquiry it must remain value-free about how persons ought to behave and thus must pursue neutrality about individual responsibility. Furthermore, the knowledge it generates calls attention to larger system factors that mediate health behaviors, that often present barriers to individual action, and that present greater health risk factors than personal habits. More important, it is the *nonmedical* and *basic science* perspective of health behavior research that will be most likely to generate this knowledge.

HEALTH, DISEASE, ILLNESS, AND SICKNESS

This discussion begs the question "What is health?" and the corollary questions "What is disease?," "What is illness?," and "What is sickness?" The definitions, perceptions, and conceptualizations of these questions are important areas of health behavior research. Wylie (1970, p. 100) cautioned years ago: "Any attempt to define what health means lays the definer open to attack by critics armed with heavy reference books. Fortunately, this phenomenon has not prevented many groups and individuals from suggesting definitions...." Dines and Cribb (1993) warn that "health is an abstract idea that is constantly alluded to in our conversations, but once we try to capture and define it, it melts to nothing like candyfloss on our tongue" (p. 3), and "health may be a concept that can be defined in a number of different ways—all of which have equal validity" (p. 8).

Diaz-Guerrero (1984), addressing the issue of whether there is a universal conception of health, analyzed the Semantic Differential responses of large samples representing 30 different cultures. The data revealed that health is looked at similarly across cultures in many ways. There is apparently cross-cultural agreement that health is characterized as "good," "potent," and "active," but Diaz-Guerrero recognizes that the meanings of these adjectives vary from one culture to another.

"Disease" allows a narrower meaning. For example, Mechanic (1978, p. 25) defined it as "a medical hypothesis that implies particular pathological processes underlying a specific clinical syndrome" usually involving specific agents, nutritional deficiency, or biological inadequacy. DiMatteo (1991, p. 7), in concurrent fashion, viewed disease as "the collection of physical findings and symptoms that, when taken together, form a definable entity." Yet even "disease," with its more focused meaning, is increasingly used to refer to behavioral and social processes for which no such specificity can be demonstrated (e.g., conditions such as anorexia, or antisocial behaviors).

"Illness, by contrast, can be depicted as the social and psychological phenomena that accompany these putative physiological problems" (Conrad, 1990, p. 1259). "Illness" is usually defined independently of disease and refers to the *experiencing* of appreciable departures from some normative "healthy" state (e.g., Denton, 1978, pp. 15–25; DiMatteo, 1991, p. 121). "Illness" is a subjective experience, in contrast to the "objectivity" of a diagnosed disease, and is highly determined by social and cultural contexts. It is a "profoundly social phenomenon that may or may not rest on disease as a foundation" (Conrad, 1990, p. 1259).

"Wellness" is a corollary term that has captured the imagination of health behavior theorists (e.g., Bruhn & Cordova, 1977, 1978) and is "defined as a philosophy that views individuals as having some influence on their degree of healthiness ... that individuals are actively engaged in the process of enhancing their healthiness, not just maintaining it" (Bruhn, 1988, p. 73). Cowen

(1991), noting the absence of "wellness" from Webster's unabridged dictionary, suggested that the English language needs it as a word and that the term embraces earthy indicators such as eating, sleeping, and doing one's tasks well; it also embraces more ethereal indicators such as having a sense of control, feelings of purpose and belonging, and satisfaction with one's existence; and involves competence, resilience, supportive social institutions, and empowerment. Abstracting from a number of definitions, Conrad (1994) suggests that "wellness is usually defined in terms of changing one's lifestyle and adopting health promoting behaviors" (p. 385) and notes that it has increasingly become a moral issue, viewed as something that people ought to be seeking.

Works that define health, disease, and illness often do not provide definitions for "sickness" (although they elaborate on "sick role"). Sickness can be considered as the social side of the illness experience, the way other persons and society define and respond to an illness episode (e.g., Kurtz & Chalfant, 1991, chap. 4).

It is apparent that these definitions generate paradoxes and inconsistencies. For example, persons may have a diagnosable disease, but if they do not experience or perceive the disease, they are not ill (DiMatteo, 1991, chap. 5); others may be free of disease yet not be enjoying a healthy existence (Dines & Cribb, 1993, p. 6). Synthesizing the work of others, Dines and Cribb (1993, p. 5) comment that "it is easier to specify departures from the norm than it is to specify the norm itself."

Lewis cautions that it is virtually impossible "to recognize disease, or health, as an absolute" (Lewis, 1953/1980, p. 115), and Wolinsky's observation that there is a lack of consensus in defining health and illness remains true (Wolinsky, 1988, chap. 4). It is beyond the scope of this chapter to discuss health, illness, sickness, and disease in depth, or to provide simple, categorical definitions for them. But it is important to show the pluralism of perspectives that are applied to them. Moreover, such pluralism, or diversity, is itself an important domain of health behavior research. There is thus an intellectual paradox

inherent in the definitional process: The *process* of defining these terms has an impact on the *substance* of the definition. Eight elements, at least, contribute to the complexity and difficulty of definition.

Lay versus Professional or Scientific Definitions

The *first* element is the simultaneous existence of lay and professional or scientific definitions. While lay and professional or scientific definitions overlap appreciably, they are nonetheless different, and their differences have important implications for health behavior and health behavior research. Although differences between lay and professional definitions exist in relation to other phenomena (e.g., the chemical and physical universes, human nature, religion), the disparities between the two types of definitions have greater life-or-death relevance for the human condition in the area of health. To extend Hayes-Bautista's (1978) sociology of knowledge paradigm, professional definitions, like other aspects of professional knowledge, are more formal, i.e., are more likely to be produced by specific acknowledged sources and to be explicit and recorded in identifiable documents; emerge from a greater depth of knowledge; are acquired in a more structured, uniform way; and have fewer contradictions and greater clarity than lay definitions.

While other abstractions such as love and justice are also freely used by both professionals and laypersons, Dines and Cribb (1993, p. 8) note the definitional problems unique to the concept of health, observing that few other terms enjoy both narrow and broad definitions without challenge. The widening gap between professional (medical) and lay perspectives contributes further to the difficulty (e.g., Helman, 1991).

Multiple Professional or Scientific Definitions

A *second* element that contributes to the difficulty of definition is the existence of multiple

10

PART I • CONCEPTIONS OF HEALTH BEHAVIOR

professional or scientific definitions. Physicians, sociologists, anthropologists, and psychologists offer different definitions of health and illness. For example, physicians generally offer medical definitions that emphasize the presence or absence of "pathology." Psychological definitions emphasize perceptions, feelings of well-being, and equilibrium. Sociological definitions emphasize ability to perform roles and tasks or adherence to some norm of expected behavior. Anthropological definitions emphasize cultural meanings of symptoms and responses to them.

Pluralism of Definitions within a Discipline

A *third* element is the existence of plural definitions within the various disciplines and professions. Depending on theoretical or ideological commitments, persons working in the same field may view the terms differently. For example, Alonzo (1984) points out that within sociology, the structural–functional perspective views health in terms of the equilibrium of society and disease as dysfunctional because it disrupts social equilibrium by impairing the expected performance of individuals. Alternatively, according to Alonzo, the ideational or interactional perspective in sociology views disease independently of—or as not inherent in—specific behaviors or performances, and emphasizes instead the importance of the social labeling of disease. Twaddle (1973, 1979) views health and disease within a sociological framework of deviance. Gerhardt (1989a,b) elaborates on these definitions and adds definitions that reflect a phenomenological paradigm in which health is viewed as the social proficiency of an indisputably competent member of a society, as attributed by others; and a conflict model that views health as a somewhat idealized state induced through discrepancies and deficiencies in social realities—the unsatisfactory prevalence of political and economic inequities.

Different perspectives also exist within medical anthropology. Illness can be viewed alternatively as a means of release from unbearable pressure, of accounting for personal failure, of gaining attention, of expiating sinfull feelings, and of social control (Foster & Anderson, 1978, chap. 8; Landrine & Klonoff, 1992).

Multiple Definitions on the Part of Individuals

A *fourth* element that contributes to the difficulty of defining these terms is that lay individuals themselves often entertain multiple definitions either simultaneously (e.g., Dines & Cribb, 1993, pp. 7–8) or at different times in their life cycles. For example, younger persons might view as health or as a natural state in older persons a condition that they might view as illness in themselves.

Multidimensionality

A *fifth* element that contributes to the difficulty of defining these terms is the acknowledgment that health must include at least three dimensions. As Levine and Sorenson (1984, p. 224) note, there is consensus among varied cultural groups that both professional and lay definitions of health include an absence of symptoms or signs of illness, a sense or feeling of well-being, and the capacity to perform. For convenience, these elements can be thought of as biomedical, personal, and sociocultural components. "Biomedical" subsumes a host of biological, biochemical, and physiological processes; "personal," a variety of affective, perceptual, behavioral, and other psychological components; and "sociocultural," myriad performance, interactional, social structural, and cultural components.

For example, the common-denominator definition of the World Health Organization (WHO), "Health is a state of complete physical, mental and social well-being and is not merely the absence of disease or infirmity" (WHO, 1948, p. 100), recognizes that health is multifaceted in nature and involves these three components. Furthermore, while health and disease may have some linkages, this definition acknowledges that health has a reality that is independent of disease. A person may have a disease and yet be healthy (Dines & Cribb, 1993). This consensual definition, however, does not say much about what health is or about what is meant by "well-being."

Analyses of health, illness, and disease as dramatic parts of the human experience have continued through recorded history. Herzlich's (1973) thoughtful yet concise narrative of the history of medicine stresses that thinking about health and illness has always reflected a mixture of biological or medical components with components that are personal, social, and cultural. Despite what might be termed the emerging dominance of the "body orientation" (p. 2; Herzlich's quotation marks), which was facilitated and reinforced by advances in anatomy, physiology, and the other sciences, there has always been an appreciation of the personal, social, and environmental factors that generate disease and support its absence. Herzlich points out (p. 2) that Hippocrates, who is regarded as the founder of medicine because of his systematic concern for the body and its symptoms, also recognized the effect of environmental factors in disease. A strictly "medical" definition of health, or a totally biomedical perspective on illness and disease, thus has no productive place in this discussion.

Diversity of Focal Phenomena

Granting the importance of considering these three interacting dimensions, a *sixth* element that contributes to the complexity of defining these basic terms is the diversity of phenomena that have been used as focal points. Different definitions of health and illness present varying degrees of juxtaposition, conflict, and equilibrium among the medical, personal, and social perspectives. Some common themes in the analyses leading to these definitions are these: whether health and disease exist along a continuum, or whether they reflect a dichotomy; whether health is just the absence of some pathology, or whether it is something positive—what Herzlich con-

trasts as "health-in-a-vacuum" versus "health in reserve (Herzlich, 1973, p. 56). Others use terms such as "wellness" to denote health as something more than just the absence of disease (e.g., Bruhn & Cordova, 1977, 1978; Conrad, 1994; Cowen, 1991). Other themes involve the comparative validity of scientific/professional/medical definitions in relation to folk/layperson/phenomenological definitions; the role of equilibrium and homeostasis concepts in defining health and illness; the use of "normative" standards (and, if they are to be used, which ones); how health and illness are related to various types of social conflict; and whether health is an asymptotic, elastic, or open-ended concept (Polgar, 1968; Wylie, 1970).

Health: State or Process?

A *seventh* contributing element is the lack of agreement on whether health is a state or a process. Most definitions, particularly biomedical ones and that of the WHO, consider it as a state or condition of being, as an end or goal to be sought. An extreme of this approach, as Dines and Cribb (1993, chap. 1) suggest, ends up defining health as the end result of socioeconomic status and/or what one has achieved in life, both of which are intermingled. Dines and Cribb suggest, alternatively, that health can be considered as a means to the achievement of personal potential.

A few atypical approaches raise the question of whether it makes more sense to think of health as a process. Within the context of Kierkegaardian psychology, health is viewed as the ability to deal with paradox or contradiction (Schneider, 1991), such as tendencies to expand or constrict thoughts, feelings, and sensations, and to attach or separate.

Medical Pluralism

Finally, an *eighth* element that contributes to the difficulty is the simultaneous existence of several different health practice systems. Analyses of the organization of a society's health care practices provide a context in which these plural perspectives can be observed. Kennedy (1973) demonstrated, for example, that perceptions of health and illness vary with the mixture in any culture of "scientific" medicine, religious or "primitive" medicine, public health practice, folk medicine, and public safety practice. Gran (1979) also showed similar mixtures of health practice systems in preindustrial Arabic societies.

CONCEPTUAL MODELS

There are many useful conceptual models for examining, comparing, and integrating the diverse perspectives on health and illness. Wolinsky's (1988, chap. 4) tridimensional conception is a good illustration of these perspectives. Wolinsky first identifies the medical model perspective, which emphasizes physiological malfunctioning, germ theory, and clinical signs and symptoms of malfunctioning as indicators of illness, and the absence of these characters as a definition of "what is not disease" rather than of "what is health." Wolinsky examines the history of this model and critically evaluates its assumptions and its implications. A second perspective, the sociocultural approach, emphasizes an individual's capacity to perform expected roles and tasks and to function socially. Health in these terms is defined relative to a person's role enactments and participation in social processes. Persons who do not perform roles and tasks as expected, and who do not participate in expected ways in social processes, are considered as deviant (e.g., Twaddle, 1973). Illness and "sick role" behavior become ways of accounting for, explaining, and controlling such deviance. The third perspective, the psychological approach, considers health as the personal experience of general well-being. Persons who "feel" well are considered healthy; those who "feel" distressed or impaired or not at ease are considered ill.

For the purposes of this chapter, the diverse perspectives of health and illness are considered as examples of two broad approaches: the personal and the sociocultural. *Personal perspectives* are those that focus *primarily* on the person existing within a social environment; *sociocultural perspectives* are those that focus *primarily* on the social, societal, and cultural influences upon the individual.

Personal Perspectives

For convenience, representative examples of personal perspectives are grouped under three headings: functioning and equilibrium; breakdown; and personal construction.

Functioning and Equilibrium. When functioning is smooth and unimpaired, then equilibrium or homeostasis exists. Health has often been identified with such equilibria, with an organism functioning smoothly within its environment, continually adapting to it, and readily restoring equilibrium when it has been disrupted. Elkes (1981) has identified the historical importance of equilibrium or homeostatic concepts to the field of medicine and the importance of self-regulation as a component of health and well-being. Polgar's (1968) scholarly analysis shows that contemporary equilibrium concepts have their origins in the Indo-European historical past, predating the Galenian concepts of "four fluids," and that the concept of equilibrium was inherent in the ancient Oriental notion of yin and yang. Closely related to equilibrium conceptions is Seeman's (1989) position that health is "organismic lawfulness and regulation in all parts of the human system" (p. 1107).

Engel (1962/1975) urges a movement away from considering disease in terms of cell pathology and toward considering it in terms of "failures or disturbances in the growth, development, functions and adjustments of the organism as a whole or of any of its systems" (1975, p. 185), and argues that "there is no sharp dividing line between health and disease" (p. 191), that they "are relative concepts which do not easily lend themselves to simple definition" (p. 185). Health is defined as a state in which the organism is "functioning effectively, fulfilling needs, successfully responding to the requirements or demands of the environment, whether internal or external, and pursuing its biological destiny, including growth and reproduction" (p. 185). Wylie (1970, p. 103) suggests that "health is the perfect, *continuing* adjustment of an organism to its environment" and that "disease would be an imperfect continuing adjustment."

Patrick, Bush, and Chen (1973), recognizing the functional dimensions of health as well as the social norms that define these functions, developed a complex and comprehensive formula for operationalizing health in mathematical terms. Their formula includes the performance of social and physical activities and mobility in relation to age, and the value or preference that society attaches to these activities, together with physical symptoms and prognoses.

Blaxter and Paterson's analyses of lay models of disease in three generations of working-class Scottish women (Blaxter, 1983; Blaxter & Paterson, 1982) showed clearly that the women defined health not so much in terms of the presence or absence of specific structural or anatomical conditions (Blaxter & Paterson, 1982, p. 27) as in terms of being able to carry out normal work, household, and social functions. "Good health was being able to work, being healthy enough 'for all practical purposes' " (p. 28). Moreover, the respondents clearly distinguished between illness and disease, acknowledging that persons could have a disease without being ill, that disease and health could exist simultaneously (p. 34). Additional support for defining health as the absence of disease symptoms and as functional capacity—the ability to do what one has to do—is found in the responses of lower working-class women in South Wales (Pill & Stott, 1987).

Reflecting wisdom in popular culture, Kaplan (1994) advances the Ziggy theorem to declare that health needs to be viewed as "doin' stuff." Ziggy, the cartoon character, recognizes the unassailable fundamental that "life is doin' stuff" ... as opposed to death, which is *not* "doin'

stuff" (Kaplan, 1994, p. 451). Health thus becomes the basis for "doin' stuff."

Breakdown. Disequilibrium exists (by definition) when functioning is more than casually or routinely disrupted and equilibrium is not readily reestablished. Such imbalances or disequilibria are presumed to be stressful to the organism and are considered to lead eventually to disease and illness (e.g., Bahnson, 1974; Borysenko, 1984; Cassel, 1974). Serious questions have been raised, however, about the causal linkages between stress and illness (e.g., Kobasa, Maddi, & Kahn, 1982). Moreover, there is accumulating evidence (e.g., Wiebe & McCallum, 1986) that part of the relationship between stress and health status may be attributed to health behaviors.

Breakdown is the failure of functioning and equilibrium. Polgar's (1968) historical analysis revealed that such departures from harmony were thought to result from becoming "civilized," a function of the way people lived, of their moving away from nature. Antonovsky's (1973) innovative thinking about the failure of functioning and equilibrium moved in the direction of a generic disease model, the "breakdown concept," and away from conceptions of specific diseases. The breakdown concept avoids dichotomizing persons as sick or well, but considers them along a continuum.

The breakdown concept assumes that it is possible to classify any condition along four dimensions: degree of pain, prevention of role and task performance, threat to life, and external recognition that the condition requires care. The degree to which persons are located along these four dimensions is a measure of the degree of their "breakdown." For example, regardless of the specific nature of a condition, a person who is not experiencing pain, whose role and task performance is only mildly impaired, whose condition is in no way life-threatening, and who is not readily recognized by others as needing professional care has a much lower degree of breakdown than a person in great pain, who cannot perform social tasks and roles, whose condition—

if not life-threatening—is "urgent," and who is readily recognized by others as needing professional care.

Antonovsky's scale for measuring breakdown demonstrated not only that a small number of breakdown profiles could accommodate the health status of a large sample of Israeli women, but also that some degree of breakdown, rather than complete health, was normative for this sample. Moreover, different ethnic groups had characteristically different breakdown profiles.

Antonovsky (1987) also noted that illness is not a rare phenomenon and that researchers, rather than search for the cause of illness, should look instead for the causes of health, what Antonovsky referred to as the "salutogenic perspective." Antonovsky proposed that organisms display heterostasis and disorder more readily than they display regulatory, homeostatic processes. Whether disequilibrium is normative or pathological remains open to question. Nicholas and Gobble (1990), accepting part of Seeman's position that health is defined in terms of integration and organization, urged at the same time that conceptualizations of health and illness pay more attention to disequilibrium, particularly as human life moves through its developmental phases, and is characterized as increasing in disregulation over time.

Personal Construction. Researchers moving away from scientifically and medically correct descriptions of the disease process and toward increasing understanding of personal or phenomenological definitions or conceptions of the disease process are beginning to explore "commonsense" views or schemata of disease (Bishop & Converse, 1987; Cameron, Leventhal, & Leventhal, 1993; Kirchgässler, 1990; Lacroix, Martin, Avendano, & Goldstein, 1991; Lau & Hartman, 1983). Lau and Hartman, for example, explored the variability of lay conceptions of common illnesses. Their observations revealed that the simple "germ" model of disease—in which people uniformly and sequentially experience unusual or unpleasant symptoms, define themselves

as sick, are thus motivated to visit a physician, and are cured by virtue of the physician's killing the germs with drugs or medicine—is an inadequate representation of how diseases are personally experienced. Lau and Hartman found that commonsense representations of diseases vary considerably and that this variability reflects five different dimensions: the condition's identity, its short- or long-term consequences, the timing of its course, its cause(s), and its cure. Lau and Hartman reasoned that when these commonsense individual "lay schemes" for evaluating or interpreting signs and symptoms no longer provide an adequate "fit," i.e., when they no longer can account for what persons are experiencing, then persons are inclined to believe they have something serious and take appropriate action.

Closely related to such representations is the concept of attribution of illness (e.g., Campbell, 1975a,b; Mechanic, 1978, pp. 254–255). Mechanic pointed out that persons vary in how they make sense out of their bodily experiences, how they attribute illness to events that disrupt their functioning, and how they define health in relation to total functioning as well as to experiences of specific symptoms (p. 254). They also vary in how they attribute causes to their conditions.

Moreover, personal constructions of health-related definitions have been shown to vary developmentally and with the life cycle (e.g., Gochman, 1985). Campbell (1975a,b) showed both similarities and differences between youngsters' and parents' definitions of health and illness. While youngsters and their mothers showed strong consensus about the relative importance of specific signs and symptoms as indicators of illness (e.g., fever, vomiting), mothers were more likely to attribute these signs and symptoms to illness when they occurred in their children than when they occurred in themselves.

Furthermore, as might be expected from developmental theories, youngsters' health-related definitions and health-related concepts are more concrete, more egocentric, and less abstract than those of adults, and demonstrate developmental changes that are congruent with

Piagetian as well as Lewinian models (e.g., Burbach & Peterson, 1986; Gellert, 1962, 1978; Gochman, 1985; Natapoff, 1982; Rashkis, 1965; Simeonsson, Buckley, & Monson, 1979).

Finally, the linkage of health and illness representations to the person must be noted. Charmaz (1990), urging that investigations of cognitive representations begin with the phenomenal rather than with preconceived categories, suggested that the illness schemata developed by persons living with chronic conditions be seen as integral to their identities, with their restored or reconstructed self-concepts.

Sociocultural Perspectives

Representative examples of social, societal, and cultural perspectives on health, illness, and disease can similarly be grouped under three parallel headings: functioning and equilibrium in social contexts, social breakdown, and social constructions of health and illness.

Social Functioning and Equilibrium. Smooth social functioning and societal equilibrium presume that individual members will actively participate in the society's processes and activities and will satisfactorily perform the roles and tasks required of them (e.g., Parsons, 1951; Twaddle, 1979). Alonzo's (1984) analyses bridge the gap between the personal and sociocultural perspectives. Avoiding some of the rigidity of the "structural" view of homeostasis in which society rather than the person attempts to maintain equilibrium, and in which disease is viewed as dysfunctional because it disturbs expected social behavior and thus threatens social equilibrium, Alonzo (1984) proposes an interactional or situational–adaptation model that recognizes that social situations vary in the degree to which they permit "adaptation." Alonzo's framework envisions persons as generally active and continually striving for equilibrium within an environment that is constantly in flux. He reasons that it is necessary to examine the way in which bodily experiences (biophysical sensations) that have

the potential to be signs and symptoms of illness are continually evaluated in relation to social "objectification," or labeling. Moreover, adaptation is defined in terms of how well people can "contain" or limit the impact of such signs and symptoms so that their social functioning remains unaffected. Such containment may involve minor modifications or compromises of role performance in order that the persons may continue to be active in their social situations. Containment of such signs and symptoms is a major theoretical construct for Alonzo.

Most daily situations allow for the easy containment of everyday signs and symptoms and do not routinely produce such signs and symptoms. But some situations themselve produce such signs and symptoms or do not permit their ready containment. Health and illness are then viewed in terms of how readily signs and symptoms are containable within any situation or context.

Social construction can also be observed in accounts provided by medical anthropologists. In many societies, illness is perceived in terms of violating religious norms, breaking taboos, angering spirits, being cursed, or being victimized by sorcery.

Social Breakdown. Societal breakdown occurs when individual members do not behave or perform as the norms of the society require. To prevent breakdown from occurring, societies attempt to place limits on, or otherwise control, such departures from expected behaviors. As Parsons (1951, p. 430) noted, "Health is intimately involved in the functional prerequisites of the social system," and disease and illness are considered to be conditions that may impair individual members' abilities to perform as expected. While it was recognized that illness in many instances was "something which merely 'happened to people' " (Parsons, 1951, p. 430) and was not something they could control, in other instances disease and illness could be considered to reflect personal and motivational determinants. To the degree that this latter view is valid, society provides and institutionalizes mechanisms of social control to avoid breakdown and thus assures continuity of normative functioning. One such mechanism involves the conditional granting of sick role and release from role and task responsibilities (Parsons, 1951, pp. 312–313), which not only insulates the "deviant" person from society but also has the further function of reintegrating the deviant through therapeutic intervention and cure. Thus, concepts of health and illness are used as mechanisms of control to reestablish the normative "healthy" state and prevent social breakdown.

Another perspective related to social breakdown is found in Shuval, Antonovsky, and Davies's (1973) analysis of illness as a mechanism for coping with failure. Although failure to perform as expected is recognized as existing in all societies, if such failure can be attributed to illness, then illness can become a legitimate rationale for a person's not behaving in a socially expected way, i.e., not succeeding or achieving.

Social Construction.   Herzlich's anthropological–sociological investigation in France revealed that lay definitions of health consistently demonstrated a "social construction," involving an interplay between personal experiences and social and cultural norms and values. A predominant social or cultural "theme" observed among Herzlich's respondents is that the "way of life," such as living in a large, urban setting, is the primary source of illness, while the major intrapersonal pathogenic factor is whether the person is or is not a "defender" against illness, i.e., whether the person does or does not exhibit a variety of mechanisms and skills to ward off the pathogenic effect of the environment and the way of life. These observations are parallel to the historical view that Polgar (1968) mentions, in which illness is ascribed to moving away from nature.

Herzlich (1973) further demonstrated that medical definitions of health and illness also involve "social construction" in that they often reflect the effects of prevailing social and cultural values upon what is considered "scientifically known" about biology and physiology. This was affirmed in Nichter's (1992) proposal "that disease is a construct created and reproduced by any/all medical systems on the basis of some generally agreed upon criteria" (p. xii) and that these criteria do not necessarily coincide with observable facts. Moreover, Herzlich noted consistencies and regularities in these "social constructions" of health and illness, as well as in the lay beliefs about causality of illness and disease. Paradoxically, Herzlich (1973, chap. 8) noted, illness, at times, is viewed positively—as a liberator that enables a person to get away from the demands of everyday life and be free to pursue reading or other intellectual activities!

CONSENSUS AND CONFUSION

Remaining amid and underlying this diversity is a strong consensus among both professionals—physicians and scientists—and laypersons that health and the related concepts of illness and disease involve—in varying degrees—biomedical, personal, and sociocultural dimensions. Confusion, or lack of convergence, exists primarily in relation to the relative importance of each of these dimensions and which of the many facets of each should be incorporated in any definition. Although lack of consensus on precise definitions is an important issue wherein attempts are made to evaluate the success of health interventions, programs, or systems of care (e.g., Wylie, 1970), it is not a barrier to conducting health behavior research.

Furthermore, any present or future research findings that might show increased consensus or unanimity in how professionals believe these terms should be defined would not by itself establish the validity or acceptability of such definitions. Wylie (1970) cautioned that such definitions are tentative and evolutionary in character. It is *not* a goal for health behavior research to define these terms "definitively," but rather to determine what definitions exist in populations. The value for health behavior research of increased consensus, however, would lie in the greater precision that would be afforded when such professional beliefs and definitions are compared with lay beliefs and definitions in studies of such issues as professional–client interactions, compliance, and responsiveness to health promotion programs. It follows that additional investigation of lay definitions and of how these definitions either resemble or differ from those held by professionals forms an agenda for future health behavior research.

Both the consensus and the confusion provide incentives and impetus for a future research agenda. Among the important issues to be resolved in the future are those related to the confounding of method, discipline, and perspective; to generalizability; to population diversity; and to the search for meaning.

Confounding Effects. Available findings reflect a diversity of methods, from the systematic questionnaire techniques and self-reports of psychology (e.g., Bishop & Converse, 1987), to the focused, structured interviews of sociology (e.g., Blaxter, 1983), to the open, fluid, field observations of anthropology (e.g., Herzlich, 1973). Behind these diverse methods are a range of theoretical perspectives, ideologies, purposes, and rationales. Although the reported findings make sense intuitively, and the divergences are not difficult to accept, it remains impossible to separate the diversity of observations from the diversity of the research process. It is thus difficult to determine whether the lack of consensus about what health means is genuine or an artifact. One challenge for future health behavior research would be to bring diverse methods and frames of reference together in a systematic, interdisciplinary way in order to determine more rigorously what these lay definitions are.

Generalizability. The findings reported in this chapter represent the literature available through standard searches (e.g., systematic reviews of selected journals, computer searches, awareness of what others are doing, use of relevant bibliographical material). It is hard to escape the conclusion that definitions of health and illness have not been systematically examined in a large number of diverse populations. Questions thus arise about whether one can generalize beyond the limited national samples alluded to in this chapter (e.g., Canadian, French, German, Israeli, Scottish, American, and Welsh). Diaz-Guerrero's (1984) findings represent one attempt at a cross-national, cross-cultural effort, but conducting the interdisciplinary research identified in the previous section on a large number of randomly selected populations would be a second important task for future health behavior research. Helman (1991, p. 1081) asks: "Why are some conditions regarded as "diseases" in one culture but not in another?"

An additional generalizability issue arises from questions about the validity of models proposed to measure health and illness, e.g., Antonovsky's (1973) breakdown model and Alonzo's (1984) containment model, for populations at large and for demographic groups within such populations. Health behavior research into these promising and intellectually stimulating models, using varied populations, is a third important task for the future.

Population Diversity. The other side of the consensus coin is the existence of consistent, coherent differences within demographic segments of a population. A fourth task for future health behavior research is the determination of how various groups within a population differ from one another in their definitions, as well as how much diversity in definitions exists within any such group. Systematic study of diverse samples of persons with different ethnic, educational, socioeconomic, or age characteristics might reveal levels of demographic diversity or consensus that would have important practical value in, for example, increasing the success of programs and improving communication between professionals and clients.

Search for Meaning. Most of the research on definitions of health, illness, and disease has dealt with the denotative aspects of a definition. Ben-Sira's (1977) conception of "involvement with a disease" is one of the few studies that have dealt with connotative aspects: the personal impact or salience of health, illness, and disease. Determining the "effective meaning" of these phenomena for populations and population subgroups, in contrast to their "intellectual" meaning, is yet a fifth task for future health behavior research.

SUMMARY

This chapter has developed some definitions for health behavior and several of its categories, and for health behavior research and health, disease, and illness. The chapter identifies a work-in-progress taxonomy of health behavior that will be used elsewhere in the *Handbook*. The chapter considers issues that create difficulty in establishing such definitions, as well as personal and sociocultural perspectives that are generally part of such definitions. It concludes with an agenda for future research.

REFERENCES

Alonzo, A. A. (1984). An illness behavior paradigm: A conceptual exploration of a situational–adaptation perspective. *Social Science and Medicine, 19,* 499–510.

Alonzo, A. A. (1993). Health behavior: Issues, contradictions and dilemmas. *Social Science and Medicine, 37,* 1019–1034.

Antonovsky, A. (1973). The utility of the breakdown concept. *Social Science and Medicine, 7,* 605–612.

Antonovsky, A. (1987). The salutogenic perspective: Toward a new view of health and illness. *Advances, 4*(1), 47–55.

Bahnson, C. B. (1974). Epistomological perspectives of physical disease from the psychodynamic point of view. *American Journal of Public Health, 64,* 1034–1039.

Belloc, N. B., & Breslow, L. (1972). Relationship of physical health status and health practices. *Preventive Medicine, 1,* 409–421.

Ben-Sira, Z. (1977). Involvement with a disease and health-promoting behavior. *Social Science and Medicine, 11,* 165–173.

Bishop, G. D., & Converse, S. A. (1987). Illness representations: A prototype approach. *Health Psychology, 5,* 95–114.

Blaxter, M. (1983). The causes of disease: Women talking. *Social Science and Medicine, 17,* 59–69.

Blaxter, M., & Paterson, E. (1983). *Mothers and daughters: A three-generational study of health attitudes and behaviour.* London: Heinemann.

Borysenko, J. (1984). Stress, coping, and the immune system. In J. D. Matarazzo, S. M. Weiss, J. A. Herd, N. E. Miller, & S. M. Weiss (Eds.), *Behavioral health: A handbook of health enhancement and disease prevention.* New York: Wiley.

Breslow, L. (1978/1980). Risk factor intervention for health maintenance. In D. Mechanic (Ed.), *Readings in medical sociology* (pp. 68–79). New York: Free Press. [Reprinted from *Science,* 1978, *200,* 908–912.]

Bruhn, J. G. (1988). Life-style and health behavior. In D. S. Gochman (Ed.), *Health behavior: Emerging research perspectives* (pp. 71–86). New York: Plenum Press.

Bruhn, J. G., & Cordova, F. D. (1977). A developmental approach to learning wellness behavior. Part 1. Infancy to early adolescence. *Health Values, 1,* 246–254.

Bruhn, J. G., & Cordova, F. D. (1978). A developmental approach to learning wellness behavior. Part II. Adolescence to maturity. *Health Values, 2,* 16–21.

Burbach, D. J., & Peterson, L. (1986). Children's concepts of physical illness: A review and critique of the cognitive-developmental literature. *Health Psychology, 5,* 307–325.

Cameron, L., Leventhal, E. A., & Leventhal, H. (1993). Symptom representations and affect as determinants of care seeking in a community-dwelling, adult sample population. *Health Psychology, 12,* 171–179.

Campbell, J. D. (1975a). Attribution of illness: Another double standard. *Journal of Health and Social Behavior, 16,* 114–126.

Campbell, J. D. (1975b). Illness is a point of view: The development of children's concepts of illness. *Child Development, 46,* 92–100.

Cassel, J. (1974). An epidemiological perspective of psychological factors in disease etiology. *American Journal of Public Health, 64,* 1040–1043.

Charmaz, K. (1990). "Discovering" chronic illness: Using grounded theory. *Social Science and Medicine, 30,* 1161–1172.

Conrad, P. (1990). Qualitative research on chronic illness: A commentary on method and conceptual development. *Social Science and Medicine, 30,* 1257–1263.

Conrad, P. (1994). Wellness as virtue: Morality and the pursuit of health. *Culture, Medicine and Psychiatry, 18,* 385–401.

Cowen, E. J. (1991). In pursuit of wellness. *American Psychologist, 46,* 404–408.

Denton, J. A. (1978). *Medical sociology.* Boston: Houghton MIfflin.

Diaz-Guerrero, R. (1984). Behavioral health across cultures. In J. D. Matarazzo, S. M. Weiss, J. A. Herd, N. E. Miller, & S. M. Weiss (Eds.), *Behavioral health: A handbook of health enhancement and disease prevention* (pp. 164–180). New York: Wiley.

DiMatteo, M. R. (1991). *The psychology of health, illness, and medical care: An individual perspective.* Belmont, CA: Brooks/Cole.

Dines, A., & Cribb, A. (Eds.). (1993). *Health promotion concepts and practice.* Oxford, England: Blackwell.

Elkes, J. (1981). Self-regulation and behavioral medicine: The early beginnings. *Psychiatric Annals, 11,* 48–57.

Engel, G. L. (1962/1975). A unified concept of health and disease. In T. Millon (Ed.), *Medical behavioral science* (pp. 185–200). Philadelphia: W. B. Saunders. [Reprinted from G. L. Engel. (1962). *Psychological development in health and disease.* Philadelphia: W. B. Saunders.]

Foster, G. M., & Anderson, B. G. (1978). *Medical anthropology.* New York: Wiley.

Gauff, J. F., & Miller, G. L. (1986). A prospectus for a conceptualization of preventive health behavior theory. *Health Marketing Quarterly, 3*(4[Summer]), 97–105.

Gellert, E. (1962). Children's conceptions of the content and functions of the human body. *Genetic Psychology Monographs, 61,* 293–405.

Gellert, E. (1978). What do I have inside me? How children view their bodies. In E. Gellert (Ed.), *Psychosocial aspects of pediatric care* (pp. 19–35). New York: Grune & Stratton.

Gerhardt, U. (1989a). *Ideas about illness: An intellectual and political history of medical sociology.* New York: New York University Press.

Gerhardt, U. (1989b). The sociological image of medicine and the patient. *Social Science and Medicine, 29,* 721–728.

Glanz, K., Lewis, F. M., & Rimer, B. K. (Eds.). (1990). *Health behavior and health education.* San Francisco: Jossey-Bass.

Gochman, D. S. (1981). On labels, systems, and motives: Some perspectives on children's health behavior. In *Self-management educational programs for childhood asthma: 2. Conference manuscripts* (pp. 3–20). Sponsored jointly by Center for Interdisciplinary Research in Immunologic Diseases, University of California at Los Angeles National Institute of Allergy and Infectious Diseases and Asthma and Allergy Foundation of America. Bethesda, MD: NIAID.

Gochman, D. S. (1982). Labels, systems and motives: Some perspectives for future research. In D. S. Gochman & G. S. Parcel (Eds.), Children's health beliefs and health behaviors. *Health Education Quarterly, 9,* 167–174.

Gochman, D. S. (1985). Family determinants of children's concepts of health and illness. In D. C. Turk & R. D. Kerns (Eds.), *Health, illness, and families: A life-span perspective* (pp. 23–50). New York: Wiley.

Gochman, D. S. (1988). Health behavior: Plural perspectives. In D. S. Gochman (Ed.), *Health behavior: Emerging research perspectives* (pp. 3–17). New York: Plenum Press.

Gran, P. (1979). Medical pluralism in Arab and Egyptian history: An overview of class structures and philosophies of the main phases. *Social Science and Medicine, 13B,* 339–348.

Harris, D. M., & Guten, S. (1979). Health protective behavior: An exploratory study. *Journal of Health and Social Behavior, 20,* 17–29.

Hayes-Bautista, D. E. (1978). Chicano patients and medical practitioners: A sociology of knowledges paradigm of lay-professional interaction. *Social Science and Medicine, 12,* 83–90.

Helman, C. G. (1991). Limits of biomedical explanation. *Lancet, 337,* 1080–1083.

Herzlich, C. (1973). *European Monographs in Social Psychology. Health and illness: A social psychological analysis* (D. Graham, trans., No. 5). London: Academic Press.

Kaplan, R. M. (1994). The Ziggy theorem: Toward an outcomes-focused health psychology. *Health Psychology, 13,* 451–460.

Kasl, S. V., & Cobb, S. (1966a). Health behavior, illness behavior, and sick-role behavior. I. Health and illness behavior. *Archives of Environmental Health, 12,* 246–266.

Kasl, S. V., & Cobb, S. (1966b). Health behavior, illness behavior, and sick-role behavior. II. Sick-role behavior. *Archives of Environmental Health, 12,* 531–541.

Kennedy, D. A. (1973). Perceptions of illness and healing. *Social Science and Medicine, 7,* 787–805.

Kirchgässler, K. U. (1990). Change and continuity in patient theories of illness. The case of epilepsy. *Social Science and Medicine, 30,* 1313–1318.

Kirsch, J. P. (1983). Preventive health behavior: A review of research and issues. *Health Psychology, 2,* 277–301.

Kobasa, S. C., Maddi, S. R., & Kahn, S. (1982). Hardiness and health: A prospective study. *Journal of Personality and Social Psychology, 42,* 168–177.

Kurtz, R. A., & Chalfant, H. P. (1991). *The sociology of medicine and illness* (2nd ed.). Needham Heights, MA: Allyn & Bacon.

Lacroix, J. M., Martin, B., Avendano, M., & Goldstein, R. (1991). Symptom schemata in chronic respiratory patients. *Health Psychology, 10,* 268–273.

Landrine, H., & Klonoff, E. A. (1992). Culture and health-related schemas: A review and proposal for interdisciplinary integration. *Health Psychology, 11,* 267–276.

Langlie, J. K. (1977). Social networks, health beliefs, and preventive health behavior. *Journal of Health and Social Behavior, 18,* 244–260.

Langlie, J. K. (1979). Interrelationships among preventive health behaviors: A test of competing hypotheses. *Public Health Reports, 94,* 216–225.

Lau, R. R., & Hartman, K. A. (1983). Common sense representations of common illnesses. *Health Psychology, 2,* 167–185.

Levine, S., & Sorenson, J. R. (1984). Social and cultural factors in health promotion. In J. D. Matarazzo, S. M. Weiss, J. A. Herd, N. E. Miller, & S. M. Weiss (Eds.), *Behavioral health: A handbook of health enhancement and disease prevention* (pp. 222–229). New York: Wiley.

Lewis, A. (1953/1980). Health as a social concept. In D. Mechanic (Ed.), *Readings in medical sociology* (pp. 113–127). New York: Free Press. [Reprinted from British Journal of Sociology, 1953, *2*, 109–124.]

Matarazzo, J. D. (1980). Behavioral health and behavioral medicine: Frontiers for a new health psychology. *American Psychologist*, *35*, 807–817.

Matarazzo, J. D. (1984). Behavioral health: A 1990 challenge for the health sciences professions. In J. D. Matarazzo, S. M. Weiss, J. A. Herd, N. E. Miller, & S. M. Weiss (Eds.), *Behavioral health: A handbook of health enhancement and disease prevention* (pp. 3–40). New York: Wiley.

Mechanic, D. (1966/1972). Response factors in illness: The study of illness behavior. In E. G. Jaco (Ed.), *Patients, physicians and illness: A sourcebook in behavioral science and health* (2nd ed.) (pp. 128–140). New York: Free Press. [Reprinted from *Social Psychiatry*, 1966, *1*, 11–20.]

Mechanic, D. (1978). *Medical sociology: A comprehensive text (2nd ed.)*. New York: Free Press.

Natapoff, J. N. (1982). A developmental analysis of children's ideas of health. In D. S. Gochman & G. S. Parcel (Eds.), Children's health beliefs and health behaviors. *Health Education Quarterly*, *9*, 34–45.

Nicholas, D. R., & Gobble, D. C. (1990). On the importance of disregulatory processes in models of health. *American Psychologist*, *45*, 981–982.

Nichter, M. (Ed.). (1992). *Anthropological approaches to the study of ethnomedicine*. Amsterdam, Netherlands: Gordon & Breach.

Parsons, T. (1951). *The social system*. Glencoe, IL: Free Press.

Patrick, D. L., Bush, J. W., & Chen, M. M. (1973). Toward an operational definition of health. *Journal of Health and Social Behavior*, *14*, 6–23.

Pill, R. M., & Stott, N. C. H. (1987). The stereotype of "working-class fatalism" and the challenge for primary care health promotion. *Health Education Research: Theory and Practice*, *2*(2), 105–114.

Polgar, S. (1968). Health. In D. L. Sills (Ed.), *International encyclopedia of the social sciences*. New York: Macmillan and Free Press.

Rashkis, S. R. (1965). Children's understanding of health. *Archives of General Psychiatry*, *12*, 10–17.

Saunders, L., & Hewes, G. W. (1969). Folk medicine and medical practice. In L. R. Lynch (Ed.), *The cross-cultural approach to health behavior*. Rutherford, NJ: Fairleigh Dickinson University Press.

Schneider, K. J. (1991). Paradox and health. *Humanistic Psychologist*, *19*(1), 68–81.

Schwartz, G. E., & Weiss, S. M. (1978). (Eds.), *Proceedings of the Yale conference on behavioral medicine*. Department of Health, Education and Welfare Publication No. (NIH) 78-1424. Washington, DC: U.S. Government Printing Office.

Seeman, J. (1989). Toward a model of positive health. *American Psychologist*, *44*, 1099–1109.

Shuval, J. T., Antonovsky, A., & Davies, A. M. (1973). Illness: A mechanism for coping with failure. *Social Science and Medicine*, *7*, 259–265.

Simeonsson, R. J., Buckley, L., & Monson, L. (1979). Conceptions of illness causality in hospitalized children. *Journal of Pediatric Psychology*, *4*, 77–84.

Sobal, J., Valente, C. M., Muncie, H. L., Levine, D. M., & DeForge, B. R. (1985). Physicians' beliefs about the importance of 25 health promoting behaviors. *American Journal of Public Health*, *75*, 1427–1428.

Steuart, G. (1993). Social and behavioral change strategies. *Health Eduction Quarterly*, Supplement 1, S113–S135.

Suchman, E. A. (1965/1972). Stages of illness and medical care. In E. G. Jaco (Ed.), Patients, physicians and illness: A sourcebook in behavioral science and health (2nd ed.) (pp. 155–171). New York: Free Press. [Reprinted from *Journal of Health and Human Behavior*, 1965, *6*, 114–128.]

Twaddle, A. C. (1973). Illness and deviance. *Social Science and Medicine*, *7*, 751–762.

Twaddle, A. C. (1979). *Sickness behavior and the sick role*. Boston: G. K. Hall.

Wiebe, D. J., & McCallum, D. M. (1986). Health practices and hardiness as mediators in the stress–illness relationship. *Health Psychology*, *5*, 425–438.

Williams, A. F., & Wechsler, H. (1972). Interrelationships of preventive actions in health and other areas. *Health Services Reports*, *87*, 969–976.

Wolinsky, F. D. (1988). *The sociology of health: Principles, practitioners, and issues* (2nd ed.). Belmont, CA: Wadsworth.

WHO (World Health Organization). (1948). *Official records of the World Health Organization. No. 2. Proceedings and final acts of the international health conference held in New York from 19 June to 22 July 1946*. United Nations: WHO Interim Commission.

Wylie, C. M. (1970). The definition and measurement of health and disease. *Public Health Reports*, *85*, 100–104.

2

Historical and Cultural Foundations of Health Behavior

A Comparative Approach

Horacio Fabrega, Jr.

Concerns about health and well-being and ways of explaining and handling its perturbations are universal to human societies. Each society's culture articulates what health and illness mean and how they are to be dealt with and promoted. In preindustrial societies, illness often has sacred implications, symbolizing—if not constituting—actual social, moral, or spiritual failures. In such societies, the explanatory models and idioms of distress and the associated practices of healing lead to the inference that an illness or disease is a social, religious, or political condition of individuals and their families. By contrast, in modern, secular, and "profane" societies, illness or disease usually signifies a mechanical or organic failure of the body or its component parts and systems, with no such social, religious, or political implications.

Horacio Fabrega, Jr. • Western Psychiatric Institute and Clinic, University of Pittsburgh School of Medicine, Pittsburgh, Pennsylvania 15213.

Handbook of Health Behavior Research I: Personal and Social Determinants, edited by David S. Gochman. Plenum Press, New York, 1997.

In industrial societies, the meanings of health and health behavior are almost separate from and opposed to those of disease and medical treatment and thus cannot be easily employed to formulate a comparative frame of reference. The perspective in such societies reflects an assumption of an *individualistic* and *separate* person who pursues health of "himself" or "herself" and of "his" or "her" body through concrete and specific actions dictated by a highly secular rationale about mind and body. To make sense of similar concerns in societies governed by different beliefs and orientations about self, the behavioral world, and its significant objects and phenomena pertaining to medicine necessitates a more general approach and a different set of orienting concepts. In "sociocentric" societies that are more governed by holism and integration of body and mind (also referred to as "primitive," "pre-industrial," or "non-Western" societies) and in which individuals seem to orient to the group and not to an autonomous self, social practices in relation to health and well-being reflect a spiritual, moral, and political concern. For this reason and related reasons pertaining to cultural factors, a concentration solely on health and health behavior in this discussion would not be as useful as one centered on sickness and healing.

Given the availability of a considerable body of knowledge about social and cultural aspects of medicine in many differing societies, it is surprising that little or no effort has been devoted to developing a comparative theoretical formulation of social and cultural approaches to health and disease—a conceptual system for explaining how societies respond to the challenge of disease. The essence of the theoretical problem is to (1) describe how concerns about disease and injury are patterned in different types of societies; (2) describe the social characteristics of how these societies deal with the effects of disease and injury on health and well-being; and (3) explain in a logically consistent and empirically satisfying way how changes in these social aspects of medicine are related to historical transformations that affect the organization of society.

The purpose of this chapter is to provide an outline for such a conceptual system or theory. It provides a scientific understanding of social and medical characteristics of societies, including transformations in approaches to sickness and healing, that appear to have occurred during prehistory and past historical epochs. First, the chapter defines the basic concepts needed to describe societies that differ in size and complexity and particularly in social interpretations and responses to disease and injury. Second, assumptions needed to conceptualize change and variation in the cultural features and social organization of a society's institution of medicine are discussed. Third, a more descriptive review of how social aspects of medicine may be conceptualized from a biological and social evolutionary standpoint is provided. Finally, a summary outline of how sickness and healing are experienced and carried out in different types of societies is presented.

No attempt is made to document all the vast and complex literature on which the theory is based (Fabrega, 1974, 1997). The conceptual approach constitutes an interpretation of and perspective on social–cultural aspects of medicine viewed from an evolutionary standpoint based on studies in the social sciences and biology. Details and specifics of the theory are less important than the overall formulation of and approach to the problem.

EVOLUTIONARY PERSPECTIVE ON SICKNESS AND HEALING

By way of establishing a common language, the nonmedical and medical concepts used in this discussion are to be understood as having the meanings defined below. Concepts and principles relating to social evolutionism are discussed in Sanderson (1988, 1990).

Nonmedical Concepts

The *individual* is the person who constitutes the population unit of a society or social formation (the terms *society* and *social formation* are used interchangeably in this chapter).

A *gene* is one of the units of genetic information that constitutes an individual's genome or genetic structure.

A *social formation* is a historically specific group, system, or unit comprised of individuals and described in terms of culture, political economy, and level of social organization.

The *culture* is the system of symbols and their meanings of a particular social formation.

A *meme* is one of the units of symbolic information that comprise the culture of a social formation (Dawkins, 1976, 1982).

The *political economy* is the social practices and power arrangements that collectively govern subsistence and economic production, including the relations and means of production.

The *social organization* is the way in which a society's population is organized, including in particular its degree of complexity with respect to ethnic/religious groups, social classes, occupations, and the like.

The *social type* is the specific kind of social formation characterized in terms of size, social complexity, and usually a distinctive type of political economy. Six social types are conceptualized (Johnson & Earle, 1987; Sanderson, 1988, 1990): family-level societies (nomadic groups, hunter-gatherers), village-level societies (simple horticultural), pre-states and chiefdoms (intensive horticultural), states and civilizations (agrarian states, empires), modern industrial societies (19th to mid-20th century); postindustrial (sometimes called postmodern) European societies (late 20th century).

Medical Concepts

Illness denotes a state of perceived ill health that is subjectively experienced and defined and socially validated in the immediate family or group.

Disease denotes a pathological condition associated with disturbances in the physiological systems of the body; it is ordinarily describable in terms of a society's official medical tradition.

Sickness refers to the social construction of an episode of illness—the way illness is handled as a social entity and the way it is dealt with in the society. It reflects the cultural presuppositions that provide meaning and organize action with respect to an illness as well as the ideology associated with the political economy of the society and its medical tradition; it takes into account ideas and efforts associated with healing (Frankenberg, 1980; Kleinman, 1980).

Healing, as a concept, incorporates basic concerns about health and well-being and pursuits aimed at bring about these desirable states. It takes into account the social processes and actions brought to bear in the attempt to prevent or counteract a condition of disease or illness. Since healing reflects cultural and political economic factors of the society, it constitutes the therapeutic complement of sickness; it includes actions and dispositions of family and group members, including persons/agents/resources used in curing (e.g., healers, folk practitioners, physicians, medicines, surgical techniques, social practices, and conventions). *How to talk about*

A *healmeme* is one of the units of cultural information that give meaning to the domain of health, well-being, sickness, and healing. Healmemes underlie and constitute the habits, beliefs, and behaviors related to health, sickness, and healing. The set of healmemes of a specific society provides the meanings of and guides the actions directed toward health, sickness, and healing in that society. (See Fabrega, 1997, for further elaboration of this concept.)

The *parameters of sickness and healing* are the social and cultural characteristics of a society's medicine. They determine how sickness and healing are envisioned and conducted in a society as a result of the enactment of healmemes and establish the pattern of a society's medical institutions (Fabrega, 1997).

GENERAL ASSUMPTIONS AND PRINCIPLES

This historical and cultural assessment of the development of the medical constructs in various types of societies proceeds on the basis of the following assumptions:

1. Individuals change over time in their organization and functioning, and such changes can be explained theoretically using the theory of biological evolution (i.e., involving genetic variation, mutation, physiological and psychological adaptations, and natural selection) (Barkow, 1991; Barkow, Cosmides, & Tooby, 1992; Dawkins, 1986; Williams, 1966).

2. Across time, social formations undergo historical transformation that can be explained using the research strategy and accompanying theories of evolutionary materialism (Sanderson, 1990).

3. Social types are prototypical forms of societies that differ with respect to political economy and differentiation or complexity. Such social types can be conceptualized as constituting stages in social evolution (Chirot, 1994; John-

son & Earle, 1987; Maryauski & Turner, 1992; Sanderson, 1988, 1990).

4. Societies show general and repeatable patterns of social evolution that conform to the processes of parallel and convergent evolution (Sanderson, 1990).

5. Social transformation or evolution is a change in the structure and complexity of a social formation. It comes about as a result of individuals deliberately and purposively selecting new and improved ways of coping with social conflicts and problems. This process involves social selection of memes. For this reason, acts of individuals are adaptive and reflect changes in habitual ways of thinking and feeling (Barkow, 1991; Dawkins, 1976, 1982; Johnson & Earle, 1987; Sanderson, 1988, 1990).

6. Natural selection of genes, the ultimate cause of biological evolution, operates on a much longer time scale than social evolution. Natural selection can be a consequence of a particular social transformation or phase of social evolution. Societies can evolve socially and culturally, however, but the individuals who comprise them need not necessarily evolve in a biological sense (i.e., genetically).

7. Illness, disease, and the pursuit of health are recurrent phenomena in social formations that bring about behaviors to promote well-being and healing. The interpretation and handling of illness as a social fact, and the specific characteristics of sickness and healing that are determined by the society's set of healmemes, reflect the society's culture, level of social organization, and political economy.

8. Characteristics of sickness and healing are often products of nonmedical factors. These factors include, for example, the society's ecology, demography, social organization, level of social differentiation, and location in a nexus of societies that share cultural, political, economic, and medical factors such as epidemiology and morbidity and mortality levels.

9. The parameters of health, sickness, and healing differ in different societies.

MEDICAL EVOLUTIONARY ASSUMPTIONS AND PRINCIPLES

In conjunction with the aforementioned general assumptions, the following more specific assumptions are implicit in this discussion:

1. Health and wellness are universally valued conditions. Conversely, the condition of illness is psychologically and socially undesirable and prompts a natural response to heal (i.e., to self-heal or "other heal," depending on who is ill) In short, illness gives rise to a need for corrective action, through the use and refinement of old healmemes and the development or invention of new healmemes. Sickness and healing (which can be given the genetic designation *SH*) are thus biologically based phenomena in the sense that an individual's capacity to show organized and meaningful responses during illness, and of others to interpret these responses as meaningful and to respond accordingly, are based on traits that are a product of biological evolution. The use of and search for healmemes are natural concomitants of illness and hence are intrinsic to human biology and human societies, given the ubiquity of disease (Cockburn, 1971; Fabrega, 1997).

2. Healmemes constitute adaptations of individuals, who search for and develop healmemes (i.e., new information about sickness and healing) that are believed to promote health and heal illness. Since the function of healmemes is to lessen the negative effects of illness or disease and to facilitate prevention and treatment of disease, application of these new healmemes can lead to decreases in the levels of morbidity and mortality.

3. Sickness and healing evolve. A society's beliefs, attitudes, and social practices related to problems of disease and health pursuits change in systematic ways in association with changes in the content of healmemes and in social structure and political economy.

4. In addition to medical and epidemiological factors, changes in the ecology, demography, culture, and social structure of a social for-

mation are associated with (indeed usually cause) changes in pictures of morbidity and mortality.

5.   Changes in the level and character of morbidity and mortality, such as new disease entities or epidemics or an augmentation in the level of old diseases, create human crises that compel the refinement of old healmemes and the search for and invention of new healmemes.

6.   The invention and learning of specific new healmemes constitute the more proximal, immediate factors that promote the evolution of sickness and healing. Healmemes are what directly affect how sickness and healing evolve and are configured.

7.   These factors and others that lead to the production of new healmemes and the rejection of old ones are complex and originate at different levels of the individual/social/intersocietal nexus.

8.   Different social types and different stages in the evolution of social formations display different parameters of sickness and healing. The contents of the healmemes of a given social type or stage of social evolution differ in systematic ways from those of other social types and stages (Cockburn, 1971; Fabrega, 1974, 1976, 1979a,b, 1997).

9.   Healmemes are readily learned and imitated by members of a society. If they are judged effective in the short run, they are learned by others of the same generation and passed on to succeeding generations. If they are judged ineffective in the short run, they are discarded or rejected.

10.   Individuals constitute adaptive units. In inventing new healmemes, learning old healmemes, and passing on healmemes, they promote the propagation and inheritance of healmemes. As a result of the temporal and spatial summation of a society's healmemes, the parameters of sickness and healing change and evolve in systematic ways.

11.   In the long run, healmemes can bring about a state of adaptedness or maladaptedness (which includes aspects of morbidity and mortal-

ity of disease) in some or all of the individuals of a social formation.

12.   Healmemes create and underlie parameters of sickness and healing, and these parameters undergo stasis, devolution, and extinction, as well as progressive evolution. Some healmemes are universal (e.g., the desire to be rid of the pain of illness, the desire to relieve a comember's pain associated with illness) and some are culturally specific (e.g., choice of suitable healer, use of specific medication).

13.   At different levels of social complexity or differentiation, and at different stages of social evolution, the distal and proximal causes of the social evolution of sickness and healing differ.

14.   The ultimate causes of the evolution of sickness and healing are biological. In other words, psychological and physiological adaptations of individuals encoded in genetic information promote the search for new and better ways of coping with environmental contingencies, and this search underlies social evolution. Such adaptations also underlie and account for the search for and use of healmemes. The degree of connectedness between genetic and cultural changes associated with the development and implementation of healmemes is difficult to establish (and is much contested).

CONCEPTUALIZING THE EVOLUTION OF MEDICAL SYSTEMS

Viewed in abstract terms, an evolutionary process implies three elements. The first element is an entity or system that changes. In the context of this chapter, this element is a medical system or institution that comprises social practices related to the pursuit of health and well-being, the prevention of sickness, and the treatment of sickness through healing practices. The second element is agencies, forces, or processes that perturb or change the system—in particular, changes in the way sickness and healing are structured and carried out in a society. The third element is the production, variation, selection, and retention of units of the system. The information that underlies the beliefs and actions related to sickness and healing is seen to consist of "units" that vary, are selected by agents of some sort, and are differentially "passed on" to subsequent generations as a consequence of their adaptive value or their use or utility.

Nature of Healmemes

It is obvious that in the evolution of medical systems, treatment factors have played extremely important roles in transforming society's structuring of sickness and the carrying out of healing. Given their importance, the cultural information units of the medical system have been termed *healmemes* (i.e., healing units). They could as well have been termed *sickmemes*, however, to emphasize that units of the medical system are also relevant to the programming of ill persons concerning what to expect from sickness and what to demand and seek in the way of healing during a condition of illness, including the definition of illness, the threshold for sickness (which determines adoption of the "sick role"), and standards of restoration of "health."

That healmemes might just as aptly be thought of as sickmemes underscores the reciprocal nature of sickness and healing in the social construction of a medical event as sickness. What evolves in the domain of sickness and what evolves in the domain of healing each affects the other when the focus is symbolic material reflected in medically relevant social behavior, habits, and routines. To put it differently, sick persons and healers share and make use of a body of cultural information about health and well-being, sickness and healing, and they orient to each other in a given medical context accordingly. This view of sickness and healing as being symbolically complementary in terms of cultural information enables one to conceptualize the sets of traits pertaining to the medical system as biologically (i.e., genetically) based and to handle them as homogeneous and unitary (and designated *SH*) (Fabrega, 1997).

Processes that Affect Healmemes

Medical units of information, the healmemes, are affected by evolutionary processes in two respects. First, the production and invention of healmemes of a society are consequences of changes in the prevalence, morbidity, and mortality of disease. Outbreaks of disease and patterns of morbidity and mortality motivate individuals to search for healmemes. The level of disease in a society is influenced, in turn, by social, ecological, biological, and cultural factors. Second, evolution of the medical system implies that these same types of factors affect the rejection or retention of healmemes. Viewed in the larger context, in other words, it is the effects of healmemes on health, morbidity, social functioning, and mortality of the population that determine whether the healmemes will be retained or rejected. By "larger context" is meant the impact of epidemiological factors of disease on social organization and complexity and the resulting fit of the population in the ecological setting.

Contrasts in the Biological and Social Evolution of Medical Systems

The selection of healmemes can be conceptualized as taking place by means of two processes. The most fundamental process is biological evolution, in which individuals, or perhaps genes or clusters of genes, constitute the units of selection. In other words, individuals learn and invent healmemes. The capacity for this symbolic activity is based on biologically evolved factors, and it is also possible that some healmemes may be more directly governed by genes. In the long run, the effectiveness of healmemes (i.e., as medical adaptations), whether linked directly and tightly or indirectly and loosely to genes (*SH*), determines what genetic units and healmemes are selected and retained. The connection between genes and behavior could be conceptualized as involving what have been termed *epigenetic rules*, but the nature of this connection is complex, poorly understood, and highly contested. Ultimately, the genes that make up *SH* are selected in relation to other genes that influence inclusive fitness.

The second process by which the selection of healmemes takes place is social and cultural evolution. To clarify this process, it is useful to keep in mind that the units of information that condition ways of thinking and behaving with respect to illness and healing (i.e., the healmemes) can also be termed *institutions* (Hodgson, 1993). Hodgson defined institutions as patterns of behavior and habits of thought of a relatively enduring nature that are intrinsic to and shared by persons interacting in human communities or societies. Institutions vary as to content and serve to pattern, organize, and provide meaning to behavior in different areas. Medical institutions impose ordered behavior in the areas pertaining to illness and in this way constitute social conditions of sickness and healing.

The healmemes of a collectivity or society are widely shared, transmitted, and played out behaviorally among the members of that society and may be held to constitute its medical institution.

Connection of the Medical with the Social

Healmemes held by individual members of a society as well as those that constitute its medical institutions interact and mix with other memes and social institutions. As an example, a variety of economic, political, and religious institutions operate in a society to regulate individual behavior and social action more generally. Institutions are internalized cognitively by people and serve to standardize behavior in different social spheres and within social organizations (which themselves are forms that institutions can take in complex societies). Varieties of these institutions,

and perhaps ordered clusters of them, can be held to be subject to processes of social and cultural evolution as adumbrated by social scientists.

In social–cultural evolution, institutions compete with one another and, depending on their value, utility, or function, are differentially selected. They are learned by direct communication or imitation and so are disseminated in the society. Provided they contribute to adaptation in the short run, they may be passed on to succeeding generations. Medical institutions undergo selection along with other types of institutions, e.g., political, economic, and religious institutions. Thus, healmemes may conflict and compete with each other and with other types of cultural information and institutions (i.e., other memes).

It is not difficult to visualize the process by which institutions that pertain to the medical system are selected, a process that complements biological/genetic evolution. As an example, in postindustrial societies, a number of different types of institutions compete with medical ones. Culinary and leisure-related institutions (i.e., widely shared patterns of thought, feeling, and action that pertain to pleasurable eating and relaxing) frequently compete with healmemes involving appropriate foods and lifestyles that have evolved in the healing of certain diseases as well as in general health maintenance and disease prevention. Institutions that pertain to choice of occupation and the attainment of success or prestige can compete with healmemes or medical institutions that enjoin rest, relaxation, and leisure.

The healmeme that pertains to dyadic healing (i.e., that enjoins an exclusive reliance on a doctor–patient relationship) is now competing with newly developed healmemes that involve managed care and group medical practices. The escalating cost of malpractice insurance and the increase in disability and negligence litigation make plain that the healmemes that structure a doctor–patient relationship (e.g., those that enjoin trust, goodwill, commitment, and faithfulness) compete (unfavorably, it would seem) with political institutions that pertain to civil liberties, property violation, and freedom in the pursuit of one's self-interest.

In the area of preserving life, it is obvious that healmemes or medical institutions conflict with economic institutions that pertain to savings, income, property, and the like, as when individuals or families are forced to consider making trade-offs pertaining to treatment of a chronic or terminal disease.

Levels of Selection of Healmemes

In order to formulate the process and consequences of social–cultural evolution more elaborately and precisely, one would have to specify such things as, for example, which types of institutions compete with healmemes (i.e., the medical institutions), the level of organization at which institutions that influence sickness and healing are selected, and how all of this takes place. In other words, some social selection is limited to individual institutions and healmemes, whereas other forms of selection would seem to involve sets of these healmemes, as when indigenous medical traditions compete with biomedicine during the process of modernization (Wilson & Sober, 1989).

In small-scale societies, a different type of complexity is found in attempts to visualize and formulate the social–cultural evolution of the medical system. For example, in these types of societies, it is often difficult to determine whether a particular healmeme is a "pure" medical institution or a religious institution; in enacting a particular type of ritual, a person in a family-level society may be seeking medical treatment *and* spiritual/religious "healing."

Similarly, in seeking to restore a split in group relations, a people of an agricultural society may follow simultaneously what one could term both a political institution and a medical one, since doing so may be thought to neutralize the ritual poisons that cause the sickness and to promote political and economic security in the

group. In these types of societies, fewer institutions that possess symbolically multivalent meanings (i.e., meanings that extend across the medical into the political, religious, or other arena) appear to order and regulate social action. Consequently, it would be difficult to determine whether competition and selection take place between truly distinct *types of institutions*.

Selection among genetic and symbolic units of information occurs in various ways and for varied reasons. At the level of genes or individuals, selection and retention of information takes place by "natural means" (i.e., by the physical and social environment) provided the information so selected contributes to the evolutionary process. At this level, evolution of sickness and healing by selection of healmemes operates on an extended, biological time line.

At the cultural and social level, items of information that individuals originate or learn about that affect thought and behavior are selected on a shorter time line in terms of their consequences. These items of information are by definition adaptations in that they are purposively and deliberately selected because they are thought to enhance well-being and satisfaction, at least in the short run.

At higher levels still, selection may favor larger units of organization (i.e., group selection). A particular healmeme can be selected because it constitutes a better way for the person or *for the collectivity* to carry out healing, organize medical care, or promote well-being and health. One might expect complementarity between sickness and healing at these higher levels such as that at the individual level, but it does not occur, given the character of human societies.

Sickness and healing can also be affected as a consequence of selection of other types of memes or institutions. Selection of political "memes" or institutions, for example, can have positive or negative effects on patterns of sickness and healing, which in turn can have negative or positive effects on the overall fitness of individuals or their genes or both.

In summary, in an evolutionary frame of reference, the medical system is seen as a hierarchical structure that describes how genes, individuals, institutions, and societies operate and function. From the standpoint of demography and epidemiology, this medical system explains patterns of morbidity, mortality, disease incidence/prevalence, and age and gender distribution. By powerfully influencing the selection, use, invention, and eventual retention of healmemes, this more material, "infrastructural" level plays a determinate role in the way sickness and healing are structured and carried out.

From the standpoint of symbolic, culturally ordered behavior—the medical "superstructure"—one sees sickness and healing experienced and carried out among persons and groups of persons. At this level, it is possible that whole sets of healmemes can be selected for the benefit of the collectivity as a result of social and political economic policies that most individuals of the society have little to say about. Finally, to the extent that societies can be classified and ordered as to level of complexity and social organization, so too, in theory, can their medical structures and parameters of sickness and healing.

Feedback in the Medical Evolutionary Process

Not only can the evolution of sickness and healing be conceptualized as taking place at every level of the medical structure, but also the effects of selection at one level can affect selection at another level. For example, changes in the genes that affect vulnerability to disease and physiological adaptability will cause sickness and healing to be patterned differently as a result of genetic selection ("strict" biological evolution). A significant change in this pattern could affect how a society's medical system functions as a whole, which might in turn affect adaptation and selection at higher levels of (social and cultural) evolution.

Conversely, it is possible to conceive of changes taking place largely at the level of institutions (e.g., religious practices, marital prefer-

ences, leisure pursuits) that will affect how sickness and healing are thought of and implemented. In time, changes initiated at the level of nonmedical institutions could influence, through complex "superstructural" feedback, the configuration of genes that undergird the medical structure.

The degree of autonomy or amount of feedback in the events that occur at different levels of evolution of the medical structure is obviously complex, problematic, and likely to be hotly debated. The controversy arises because the subject involves matters pertaining to atomism versus holism, or organicism versus reductionism, as they affect evolution, concerning which social and biological scientists and philosophers of science have strong differences of opinion.

HEALMEMES IN SELECTED SOCIAL TYPES

This section summarizes the ways in which concerns and behaviors related to health, sickness, and healing are structured and executed in different social types. Several caveats pertaining to the discussion that follows seem warranted. First of all, the discussion deals with *exemplar instances of illness and healing* that disrupt the normal flow of awareness and adaptation in hypothetical individuals. Excluded, then, are minor ailments and, more important, the sickness conflagrations associated with major epidemics that by their nature necessarily stamp medical concerns in special ways.

Second, it should be emphasized that the cultural characteristics of a particular social type differ significantly across geographic–ecological bounds and historical periods. Such differences will necessarily impart to medical concerns and behaviors distinct features that cannot be expected to be included in what are treated here as *generic properties* of health, illness, and healing. As an example of this last point, and as will be described subsequently, in summarizing the ways in which medical concerns in states and civilizations are structured and dealt with, this chapter brings under one rubric the constructs of health and the health behaviors, sickness behaviors, and practices of healing in many different social formations, including such diverse social formations as those of ancient China, India, Babylonia, Greece, Rome, and also Islamic societies, as well as late Medieval and so-called "Renaissance Western" societies.

That this approach is taken means, and this is the third caveat, that of necessity medical concerns are depicted from an *abstract* point of view. In other words, specific cultural and "scientific" details of the academic and lay/folk beliefs pertaining to health, sickness, and healing are sacrificed in favor of more generic and structural features of the way members of the populations oriented and behaved.

Furthermore, and this is the fourth caveat, in such social types, there is good reason to believe that the state exerted different degrees of influence in arranging for the medical care of poor people. Such differences cannot easily be incorporated in a general frame of reference.

A related consideration, and the fifth caveat, is that the degree to which what one can term a medical *profession* controlled healing in these social formations varied greatly and is not at present clearly understood.

There is reason to believe that in Italian city states, as an example (Park, 1991), during the late Medieval period, magistrates and officials of different social groups and formal organizations paid "respectable" physicians to intervene in the care of the poor generally and during epidemics, more specifically. Not well known, however, is the extent to which the state controlled medical practitioners in India, China, and Babylonia. Nor is it clear whether *one group* of healers operated in such a dominant fashion as did the physicians of the Italian city states and also the physicians of England (Cook, 1986).

All types of states and civilizations seem to have developed a more "respectable" and "academic" physician group that in fact can be identified with a corpus of medical ethics. It is unclear, however, whether these more highly respected physicians were formally favored by the state and to some extent even regulated or controlled, as they seem to have been in the Italian peninsula and also to some extent in England. Differences in the degree of dominance, visibility, and state support would obviously have made differences in the way concerns pertaining to health, sickness, and healing were conceived of and dealt with, but these differences also cannot be expected to be realistically portrayed in the general frame of reference of this chapter.

Finally, the health, sickness, and healing concerns of social types are *singular*, *specific*, and also *more mundane* than those brought into focus during the major epidemics to which social types such as states and civilizations (and possibly also chiefdoms and pre-states) were vulnerable. Although of paramount importance in causing morbidity and mortality and in transforming orientations and policies pertaining to health and medicine, at the level of individuals and families, the concerns and reactions evoked by major epidemics cannot be regarded as typical because of the terror and the pervasive sense of vulnerability to contagion they engendered and the group-related actions they precipitated, which often were regulated by administrators and magistrates of the salient governing bodies.

Instead, the focus is on conditions of sickness that arose, persisted, and increasingly disabled an individual in an otherwise relatively healthy family. Emphasis is placed on the properties of these sicknesses as social episodes and the experiences and actions aimed at healing and restoring health that they set in motion. A basic assumption is that the character of sickness and healing differs across social types because the social organization and political economy of social types differ significantly (Cockburn, 1971; Fabrega, 1974, 1976, 1979a,b, 1997).

Family-Level Societies

Family-level societies demonstrate the following characteristics or healmemes:

1. The individual's awareness (or the per-

ception by another) of a high sense of physical distress, weakness, lassitude, fatigue, pain, and physiological disturbances constitutes a necessary and sufficient condition for illness and signals need for healing.

2. Sickness and healing are associated with a high sense of discouragement, sociomoral disarticulation, existential crisis, and despair.

3. Sickness is a condition that entails or requires abstention from ordinary, everyday responsibilities.

4. The sick person is the final arbiter of sickness and wellness.

5. Sickness has a holistic (psychosomatic, somatopsychic, and spiritual) identity, and no part of the sickness picture is overvalued or disvalued.

6. A sense of victimization associated with sickness and healing is total and global: Self/others/ancestors/spirits are held to be at fault.

7. Self, group members, spirits, ancestors, and environment are implicated in the cause and fate of sickness.

8. A sense of crisis, threat, mystery, fearfulness, and the possibility of impending termination is a necessary, private, and public component of sickness (illness requiring healing).

9. Dependence, passivity, and a sense of helplessness with consequent anticipation of group intervention and support are "natural" components of sickness.

10. Resignation to a possibly uncertain short-term future marked by worldly nonexistence or anticipation of full integration into the group with restoration of well-being is intrinsic to the state of sickness and the pursuit of healing.

11. A high sense of group/communal burden, obligation, and responsibility in the immediate group is associated with sickness and healing.

12. Sickness and healing are confined to the home environment.

13. The possibility of sickness is always high, as is the sense of powerlessness to prevent or undo it (i.e., low optimism).

14. Options and resources associated with healing are limited and finite.

Village-Level Societies

In village-level societies, the 14 healmemes identified for family-level societies continue to operate. In addition, the following healmemes are observed:

15. The sense of being victimized by another person from outside the group becomes relevant and in some instances dominant.

16. There is some heightening and narrowing of dependence on immediate family and expectation that it will support and heal, with consequent lessening of dependence on the group as a whole.

17. There is some awareness that persons in the group and intragroup happenings may be causal in a condition of sickness.

18. The potential for intragroup blame is present in a state of sickness.

19. One finds some dependence on and expectation of help from a special person, a protohealer, for relief of symptoms and for the resolution of the social/moral and existential ambiguities associated with sickness; options and resources of healing are thus enhanced.

20. The group/communal obligation and responsibilities are lessened and negotiated by healer and family.

21. Some healing is moved to special locations, but the home setting retains primacy.

Chiefdoms and Pre-States

In chiefdoms and pre-states, healmemes 1–3 observed in family-level societies continue to be important, but are less binding. For example, the first two may be modified as follows: (1) A high sense of physical distress and malaise may be sufficient but not always necessary for perception of illness and (2) sickness is associated with more optimism. Then, continuing from 1–3:

4. Family members and healers gain some influence over the course and social definition of sickness.

5. The sense of victimization linked to the condition of sickness is less global and total and is

more differentiated. The sense of existential despair and annihilation is less dominant. There is less resignation to a possible termination (greater optimism, less pessimism).

6. Members of the group become important sources for explaining and accounting for illness. Conflicts in intragroup relations begin to play a more significant role in constituting sickness.

7. The person becomes more important as a specific object or target of illness. A sense of personal vulnerability/responsibility becomes more integral to the condition of illness as a result of possible actions of others in the group. As a result, sickness is more sociological.

8. The condition of illness and its social construction as sickness becomes a more deliberate, singular phenomenon — more contingent on situational factors connecting to self, less contingent on purely physiological failures, and less contingent on global preternatural factors.

9. Sickness retains holistic identity and valorization, but discrete (somatic/behavior) manifestations begin to acquire importance to self and family as clues of causation, social typification, and possible stigmatization. Semantics and vocabularies of illness and sickness expand.

10. Options and resources of healing are enhanced significantly. The role of healer is well defined, and one finds the beginnings of differentiation as to type, emphasis, mode of diagnosis, and treatment.

11. The characteristics of the condition of illness, including in particular its physiological manifestations, become important in choices of healing.

12. Exploitation of sickness (i.e., of the sick role) for personal and social gains becomes an important contingency or possibility of illness and healing.

13. There is high dependence on healers for the outcome of sickness.

14. Competition among healers begins.

15. Healers acquire responsibility for cure and play a crucial role in negotiating (validating) sickness.

16. Greater power and autonomy are ascribed to healers.

17. Healers begin to be compensated for efforts and blamed for failures.

18. The sick person often frequents the healer's quarters or special locations during ceremonies or rituals of treatment.

States and Civilizations

In states and civilizations:

1. Illness is still constructed as holistic with a high spiritual component, but mystery, danger, and existential nihilism and despair are less frequent concomitants; there is more optimism.

2. Illness comes to be seen as a common phenomenon and is thought of and experienced as more commonplace and quotidian; it becomes more secularized. The aforementioned physiological failures (intense weakness, fatigue, pain, physical symptoms) constitute sufficient but not necessary conditions for illness.

3. The sociological dimension of sickness (i.e., the link of illness and healing to intergroup relations and situations) remains important.

4. The expectation of a healer's intervention is high; the healer plays a dominant role in shaping, validating, explaining, and resolving the condition of illness.

5. Chronic sickness problems and the qualities of the illness are crucial in determining the labeling of illness and the choice of healer.

6. Knowledge structures pertaining to illness and healing are very elaborate, influential, and diversified. They become literate, complex, and intricate — a "functional" theory of illness. The model of illness is thus multifactorial and personalized. Specialist healers treat and prevent illness.

7. The person becomes a more active, self-conscious consumer of health care and healing, although the family retains an important role in selecting, seeking, and monitoring the healer.

8. The options and resources for healing are greatly expanded and diversified. The greater

number and variety of healers allow differentiated choices by self and family. Fellow members of social, religious, and ethnic groups are very influential in the choices, forms, and quality of healing.

9. There is a hierarchy of healers, ranked as to repute, knowledge, competence, and modality of healing; there is high competition among healers.

10. The healer is still seen as "curer," but also assumes an important role as an advisor on health and a "preventer" of illness. The sick person is not just a sick person, but becomes a "patient." The (sick or well) person's partnership with a healer is crucial in monitoring the planning and promoting of health and in preventing or eliminating illness. Sicknesses acquire concrete identity as illness types, although they are explained functionally (i.e., not ontologically), and these types are significantly shaped by the healer; i.e., they are partially commercialized (as described in 13 below). Sickness begins to be defined as a longitudinal entity (i.e., it acquires a temporal dimension).

11. Unregulated exploitation of sickness by the self is possible and frequent through sanctions of the healer, use of a variety of healers, awareness of differences and the personalized nature of sickness, and availability of different ways of healing.

12. Organizations, corporations, and other social institutions establish places for the housing of the ill and settings of healing.

13. Despite functional and personalized theories of illness (as compared to ontological theories), health, well-being, and states of sickness (named/explained in terms of illness terminologies and narratives) become more materialized, almost objectified, and, like commodities that are willfully sought, pursued, purchased, negotiated over, modified, and shortened or lengthened. The healer plays a crucial role in constructing sickness, but the self is the ultimate "gold standard" arbiter of the condition of illness.

14. Sickness and healing activities constitute a dominant economic enterprise in a society.

Healing becomes a full-time occupation. The institution of medicine is virtually industrialized.

15. Sick persons and families are responsible for paying for healing among the well-to-do. Corporations and the like, religious institutions, lay organizations, and in rare instances the state sponsor, support, and defray the costs of healing the socially needy and marginal.

16. Healers become organized into professional associations and stipulate ethical codes that articulate formal responsibilities and obligations.

17. Mental illness as madness or insanity becomes a more visible and prominent form of illness in the society.

18. Stigmatization of mental illness is prominent in most societies.

19. There is comprehensive holistic interpretation of illness and sickness, with the beginnings of higher valorization of the somatic sphere. Somatization and psycholigization become differentiated bases for labeling and valuing sickness and illness.

20. Sickness is made a more commercial object, its manifestations shaped and regulated by healers, and its valorization influenced by type of physiological and behavioral manifestations.

21. Sickness can be a product of or caused by any number of special factors that implicate the person's biography and life habits as well as ethical/moral and spiritual status.

Modern Industrial Societies

The healmemes of modern industrial societies are characterized as follows:

1. The knowledge structures of biomedicine operate as powerful scripts that program illness and healing, constituting sickness as a physically altered condition of the person brought about by objective, mechanical, ontologically separated disease objects that alter or disturb physiology. The condition of sickness as disease is thus rendered a discrete entity, concrete in its properties—knowable, explainable, and curable naturalistically.

2. Biomedicine becomes the dominant ideology or tradition in society and is sponsored, certified, and regulated by the state. Principles of biomedicine are implemented as social policy and biomedical principles regulate social life.

3. The options and resources for healing are greatly expanded by the creation of medical specialties based on physiological systems and types of disease under the governance of biomedical sciences.

4. Sickness and healing become fully secularized. The spiritual component of sickness and healing is disallowed. Sickness is rationalized, objectified, and materialized in concrete terms.

5. Sickness is transformed into expressions of disease objects having defined natural histories and standardized treatment protocols under the control of physicians.

6. Full control, prediction, and elimination of disease are thought of as a possible social reality. The burden, suffering, and outcome of sickness are balanced by great optimism regarding the scope and possibilities of biomedicine.

7. The existential nihilism and despair linked to a condition of sickness become meliorated and blurred. Great optimism is associated with individual states of sickness.

8. The causes and experiences associated with sickness become focused on and limited to the individual, and in this sense sickness can be said to be fully individualized. The conduct of healing also becomes more fully individualized; the "doctor–patient" relationship becomes exclusive, determinate, and contractual.

9. Physicians are defined as technical or scientific experts and acquire full autonomy and power as arbiters (i.e., validators) of sickness. They dominate dialogues of sickness and healing and are accorded full responsibility for the outcome of sickness. Their role as advisors on health and well-being diminishes.

10. Sick persons become dependent "patients," full "consumers" of physicians' services and of medical products; in theory, they begin to acquire the formal, socially validated, and legal right to blame physicians in the event of failures.

11. The cost of sickness and healing is transferred to third-party organizations including the state.

12. Sickness and the "sick role" become the object of social regulation, with the state an important and influential agency operating through the surveillance of physicians who determine what constitutes illness and wellness. Motivations for illness become possible options that are identifiable as disvalued features of the self that are defended, denied, and rendered transparent or opaque depending on the specifics of the doctor–patient relationship; motivations for illness and sickness as well as wellness become negotiable via the intercession of physicians.

13. The concept of mind–body dualism is crucial in identifying the type of illness.

14. The construction of mental illness as insanity or madness is important, but there is significant broadening of the meaning of mental illness, with development and expansion of the discipline or specialty of psychiatry. The somatization component of sickness becomes highly valorized and the psychologization component denigrated. Psychosomatic illnesses and diseases become distinct entities, objects of psychiatric intervention.

Postindustrial Societies

In postindustrial societies:

1. Persons are highly informed of technical advances in medicine as biomedical knowledge becomes public knowledge through expansion of communications and health promotion industries.

2. Persons and families have a plethora of options pertaining to health and well-being. Physician specialty types expand, holistic physicians and practitioners of alternative systems proliferate, and health extension industries create options and promote new opportunities for self-healing.

3. State and economic institutions reinforce the centrality of health and personal responsibility for the causation of illness; sickness

is thus constituted partially as self-victimization, and hence self can be and is blamed for conditions of illness and impaired health.

4. Passivity, dependence, and helplessness associated with sickness are blunted, discouraged, and eschewed as sick persons are held more accountable for their state of health. Failures and limitations of physicians are magnified and rendered objects of condemnation; trust in physicians diminishes. Litigation surrounding unsuccessful ministrations of physicians and negative consequences of healing becomes a prominent recourse of action.

5. Persons become aware that illness (as biomedically validated) must have a disease state to explain it. State and economic institutions, using knowledge structures of biomedicine, begin to stipulate the valid configurations of illness (what will count as a legitimate and reimbursable sickness picture). Thus, the self or the immediate social group no longer can fully validate states of sickness; only the physician and ultimately the state acquire this power. Paradoxically, the person is a more knowledgeable, more active consumer, but is judged to be less truthful by the official institution of medicine (as personified by physicians and third-party and state operatives).

6. Biomedical knowledge structures pertaining to health, sickness, and healing become highly elaborated, easily communicated and learned, and highly influential in regulating social life.

7. The pursuit of health, the avoidance of illness, and the resort to healing become elements of self-definition and self-regulation and, in the society at large, come to approximate personal civic religions.

8. Individual states of illness are less common and less feared and the self feels more empowered about their prevention and control. The experience of sickness becomes naturalized, yet, paradoxically, sickness becomes defined as inherent in the human condition, universal, inevitable, immanent, uncontrollable.

9. Sickness and healing, like health and well-being, are experienced as material or mechanical conditions and processeses that the self has more control over and hence are more fully commercialized.

10. The limits of the biomedical enterprise in controlling and eliminating disease are widely appreciated.

11. The domain of sickness and healing expands to include attributes of physical appearance, personality, and behavior.

12. The benefits and possibilities of medical care are defined as limited and finite, and the cost of healing becomes a dominant component of the experience of sickness. There is growing skepticism and pessimism about the power of biomedicine and the scope of its capacity to control sickness and health.

13. Persons seek new ways to validate illness and sickness, and the capitalist health/medical industry correspondingly expands as alternative medical traditions, wellness pursuits, and life extension programs become important industries and sought-after enterprises that compete with biomedicine in the medical market. These developments contribute to the undermining of biomedicine as the official ideology pertaining to sickness. Thus, as physicians and the state begin to constrain the (valid) boundaries of sickness, alternative medical industries capitalize on individuals' awareness of illness and need for validation, providing new options and opportunities for sickness in a dialectical process that affects individual health needs and profit (societally/culturally determined) imperatives.

14. The health/wellness industry interprets more conditions as sickness and provides more alternatives for treating them. The possibilities for sickness also increase as the boundaries of sickness and healing become blurred and inchoate: Cosmetic surgery, elective treatments, and lifestyle parameters are medicalized; physiologies become programmable; personalities and lifestyles become manipulable.

15. The proliferation of "official" biomedical knowledge and knowledge structures of alternative medical/wellness traditions profoundly increases the items of relevant medical information

(the number of potentially relevant healmemes). The validity of items of medical information becomes subject to variation and change and is highly contested. The maintenance of health, prevention of disease, and pursuit of healing become highly problematized.

16. Bioethical implications of "healing" pertaining to the materialization of body parts and functions and alteration of states of sickness loom as social and psychological dilemmas that confuse and create ambiguities about the meaning of sickness, health, and well-being, and the valid and ethically justifiable beginning and end of life.

17. The script of official biomedical healing becomes public and visible as state, professional, and private/lay organizations begin to sponsor efforts aimed at standardizing medical practice and defining the boundaries, limits, and rationing of biomedicine.

18. Persons become highly rational and challenge the authority of physicians. The health/wellness industry actively competes with and challenges the biomedical industry.

19. Persons who are mentally ill experience and anticipate less social stigma, as mental illnesses and mental health problems become more naturalized and regularized components of sickness and healing. Many emotional problems associated with medical diseases and the mental illnesses become increasingly medicalized, and more strictly controlled by the medical professions; psychiatry as a medical specialty narrows and contracts to a neurobiological emphasis. Paradoxically, there occurs an expansion in lay support groups and alternative mental/emotional therapies for help with psychological problems associated with medical illnesses, eating/alcohol disorders, and specific disease support groups.

20. In official biomedicine, the doctor–patient relationship becomes less exclusive. The "quality of doctoring" becomes identified as a determinate feature of medical practice that is desirable and important but interpreted in terms of officially stipulated standards of treatment protocols and minimal competencies of practice.

The patient's relationship with a specific physician becomes less central, and groups of affiliated physicians become identified as units of healing.

SUMMARY AND CONCLUSIONS

A comparative theoretical approach toward health and health behavior with an emphasis on sickness and healing has been proposed. It is conceptualized from a biocultural frame of reference in which the societal problems of disease that are manifested as sickness and healing have been analyzed as biological and cultural phenomena and the transformations in the way sickness and healing are structured and enacted are explained in terms of the complementary processes of biological and social evolution.

The salient characteristics of health pursuits, sickness, and healing have changed during the course of evolution. The changes have included, for example, changes in what constitutes the social composition of a medical event. Thus, the group, the family, or the individual may bear the principal burden of and responsibility for sickness and healing. There have also been systematic changes in the role played by social relations that pertain to the ill person, and by aspects of his or her morality and spirituality, in the interpretation of sickness and healing. An individual's interpersonal relations and conflicts may constitute an explicit focus in some social types but not in others; sickness and healing may be construed as scared and holy in some, as secular and natural phenomena in others. An associated factor that changes is whether sickness as compared to wellness is held to be under the control of the individual or whether other persons or even impersonal agencies (e.g., the state, political or economic groups) are held to exert an influential role. The social or official position of the healer in society and the structure of the healing relationship clearly constitute parameters that have also changed systematically in relation to social evolution. Finally, attention was given to the role played by mental illness in the interpretation of a society's medical problems and to potential differences in the way the (bodily as compared to mental) manifestations of illness were evaluated.

Each social type is conceptualized as constructing both sickness and the conduct of healing differently. The impact of the biological sciences on medicine in modern industrialized societies constitutes an obvious watershed or evolutionary breakthrough in the way sickness and healing have evolved. It has been implied, however, that in the sweep of evolution, many such evolutionary breakthroughs in the configuration of sickness and healing have occurred and that such major transition points are not in fact always clearly demarcated. For example, it can be contended, as illustrated, that some of the changes in the patterning of sickness and healing associated with biomedicine and industrial societies were already found in (ancient) states and civilizations. Moreover, it would appear that developments in what was termed postindustrial society, although governed by the biological sciences as was the preceding stage, may also constitute a possible transition point having important evolutionary implications for the conceptualization of sickness and the conduct of healing.

The analysis in this chapter identifies by implication, but leaves open and unexplored, the mechanisms and specific evolutionary developments that clothe and give content to the major transformations of sickness and healing in societies. In other words, the analysis (1) provides an initial framework for conceptualizing sickness and healing in evolutionary terms and (2) makes evident the need for in-depth and focused studies that systematically explain how evolutionary transformations have occurred. Such studies should specify the kinds of forces or developments in a society that change its disease pictures, how these factors lead to specific changes in the interpretation of illness as sickness, how these changes in turn affect the development and invention of specific healmemes, and how each of these changes the structure of healing and healing; what effects healmemes have in the short run on health and well-being and on soci-

etal events; which healmemes are selectively retained and why; and what effects, if any, these changes might have in the long run with respect to social organization and political economy and, eventually, at the level of the genome. Analyses of this kind have been undertaken, but there is a need for more studies cast, one hopes, in a logically explanatory way that accords with evolutionary theories.

RESEARCH ISSUES AND IMPLICATIONS

An evolutionary conceptualization of health, sickness, and healing provides a way of organizing and understanding medical phenomena in human societies of different types. By clarifying the universal and the culturally variable in social aspects of medicine, it also provides a more thorough understanding of how individuals and societies are likely to respond to the inevitable social changes that will continue to affect pictures of disease and injury in future epochs. Ultimately, an evolutionary conceptualization of medicine promises to clarify the direction in which postindustrial health policies and developments seem to be headed.

A truly comprehensive and inclusive formulation would require that issues pertaining to health, sickness, and healing also be examined in early human groups, before the emergence of modern *Homo sapiens*—which is, of course, impossible. Related medical themes can be studied, however, in primate groups that are judged as evolutionarily closely related to modern humans. Observations of ethologists and comparative psychologists have concentrated for the most part on aspects of social and affective communication, forms of social organization, emotional bonding and distress, and cognition, self-awareness, and theory of mind. Clearly, controlled and naturalistic studies of ill, debilitated, and disabled primates could help clarify whether—and if they are, how—such states are expressed, communicated, and dealt with among closely related as well as unrelated conspecifics. Many of the psychological themes that are important to primatologists could and should be examined in the setting of disease and injury with great profit to the comparative study of health, sickness, and healing.

Matters of health, sickness, and healing can also no longer be studied in social types that constituted earlier stages of cultural evolution. Moreover, in existing underdeveloped societies in which many of the approaches to health, sickness, and healing appear to retain traditional, indigenous emphases, the presence of the competing biomedical tradition, because of its social power and political/economic state support, has strongly modified orientations to and ways of formulating health and coping with sickness. Thus, there are but limited means and resources available to anyone hoping to better delineate the way health is conceptualized and sickness and healing are dealt with in earlier social types. Field studies among nonliterate and other preindustrial societies and archival studies of documents pertaining to health policies and medical practice in earlier historical epochs, and in societies governed by different cultural interpretations of medical issues, provide clues from which inferences can be drawn about the evolution of health, sickness, and healing. The formulation presented in this chapter in fact constitutes a preliminary synthesis and distillation of contemporary anthropological and social historical studies of medicine in both the Western and the non-Western tradition.

Some of the topics that are important for a comprehensive, evolutionary account of medicine and that could be further clarified through research studies are summarized below. Because of space limitations, only selected themes and issues pertaining to certain societies can be covered. Additional issues can readily be appreciated.

Nonhuman Groups. What are the effects of disease and injury in groups of chimpanzees (regarded as the closest relatives to man among animals)? Is sickness as a social state recognized and acknowledged among related individuals?

What behavioral changes seem to occur in the context of terminal diseases and severe injury?

Hunter-Gatherer Societies. Does a mother behave differently toward a male as compared to a female child who is sick? Is the concern shown sick children different depending on the seeming seriousness or duration of sickness? Do group members resent the condition of persistent illness in a group member? What are the similarities and differences in the way group members handle the weakness and fatigue of chronic sickness as compared to their handling of advanced pregnancy? To what extent do individuals conceptualize health as a specific, desired state as compared to merely the absence of disease and injury?

Sedentary, Agricultural Societies. What aspects of an episode of illness determine or predict that a healer will be sought? In the event that more than one type of specialist healer is available in a group, how are actual choices made and what regimen of those proffered is actually followed? What are the factors that determine or predict that an adult of advanced age will or will not be given less care and support in the event of disease and injury? Do group members recognize sickness pictures that are feigned, and how do they deal with such "conditions" in the event that they do? What aspects of general behavior and social functioning are most valued as indicators of health and well-being?

States and Civilizations. What aspects of behavior and adaptation constitute directives for good health in all the "great," ancient traditions of medicine (i.e., the Ayurvedic, Chinese, European-Galenic, and Islamic)? What are the commonalities and differences in the conceptualization of food intake, diet, sexuality, physical activity/hygiene, and bodily size and shape as indicators of health in these traditions? What kinds of sicknesses were stigmatizing in ancient societies, and how were such biases played out in behavior and social policy? What aspects of social behavior, separate from those that indicated insanity or madness, were viewed as pathological and medical in the ancient traditions? In traditional societies that retain ancient orientations and practices of medicine, how are the agonies of protracted and painful sicknesses dealt with? Was a form of euthanasia practiced in ancient societies, and are such practices implemented in contemporary traditional, preindustrial societies?

REFERENCES

Barkow, J. H. (1991). *Darwin, culture and genes.* Toronto, Canada: Toronto University Press.

Barkow, J., Cosmides, L., & Tooby, J. (Eds.) (1992). *The adapted mind: Evolutionary psychology and the generation of culture.* London: Oxford University Press.

Chirot, D. (1994). *How societies change.* Thousand Oaks, CA: Pine Forge Press.

Cockburn, T. A. (1971). Infectious diseases in ancient populations. *Current Anthropology, 12,* 45–62.

Cook, H. J. (1986). *The beehive of the old medical regime in old Stuart London.* Ithaca, NY: Cornell University Press.

Dawkins, R. (1976). *The selfish gene.* New York: Oxford University Press.

Dawkins, R. (1982). *The extended phenotype.* San Francisco: W. H. Freeman.

Dawkins, R. (1986). *The blind watchmaker.* New York: Norton.

Douglas, M. (1986). *How institutions think.* Syracuse, NY: Syracuse University Press.

Fabrega, H., Jr. (1974). *Disease and social behavior: An interdisciplinary perspective.* Cambridge: Massachusetts Institute of Technology Press.

Fabrega, H., Jr. (1976). The function of medical-care systems: A logical analysis. *Perspectives of Biology and Medicine, 20,* 108–119.

Fabrega, H., Jr. (1979a). The scientific usefulness of the idea of illness. *Perspectives of Biology and Medicine, 22,* 545–558.

Fabrega, H., Jr. (1979b). Elementary systems of medicine. *Culture, Medicine and Psychiatry, 23,* 167–198.

Fabrega, H., Jr. (1997). *Evolution of sickness and healing.* Berkeley, CA: University of California Press.

Frankenberg, R. (1980). Medical anthropology: A theoretical perspective. *Social Science and Medicine, 14B*(4), 197–207.

Hodgson, G. M. (1993). *Economics and evolution.* Ann Arbor: University of Michigan Press.

Johnson, A. W., & Earle, T. (1987). *The evolution of human societies.* Stanford, CA: Stanford University Press.

Kleinman, A. (1980). *Patients and healers in the context of culture.* Berkeley: University of California Press.

Maryauski, A., & Turner, J. H. (1992). *The social cage.* Stanford, CA: Stanford University Press.

Park, K. (1991). Healing the poor: Hospitals and medical assistance in Renaissance Florence. In J. Barry & C. Jones (Eds.), *Medicine and charity before the welfare state* (pp. 26–45). New York: Routledge, Chapman & Hall.

Sanderson, S. K. (1988). *Macrosociology.* New York: Harper & Row.

Sanderson, S. K. (1990). *Social evolutionism.* Cambridge, MA: Blackwell.

Schotter, A. (1981). *The economics theory of institutions.* Cambridge, England: Cambridge University Press.

Ullmann-Margalit, E. (1977). *The emergence of norms.* Oxford, England: Oxford at the Clarendon Press.

Williams, G. C. (1966). *Adaptation and natural selection: A critique of some current evolutionary thought.* Princeton, NJ: Princeton University Press.

Wilson, D. S., & Sober, E. (1989). Reviving the superorganism. *Journal of Theoretical Biology, 136,* 337–356.

II

PERSONAL DETERMINANTS

COGNITIVE DETERMINANTS

The personal, social, and cultural constructions of beliefs about health and illness discussed in Chapters 1 and 2 are further elaborated in cognitive research on personal determinants of health behavior. By far the largest share of research on personal determinants has been cognitively driven. The term *cognition* denotes "those personal thought processes that serve as frames of reference for organizing and evaluating experiences. Beliefs, expectations, perceptions, values, motives, and attitudes all provide the person with ways of filtering, interpreting, understanding, and predicting events" (Gochman, 1988, p. 21). The term *health cognitions* refers to beliefs, expectations, perceptions, values, motives, and attitudes that provide frames of reference for organizing and evaluating health, illness, disease, and sickness regardless of whether those cognitions have demonstrable empirical linkages with health status and regardless of whether they are objectively valid.

Cognitive approaches to human behavior emphasize phenomenology: events as they are psychologically experienced, the world as it is perceived by the person in contrast to the world of physical "reality." Important cognitive approaches in health behavior research include those that deal with how health and illness are represented or organized within the individual's cognitive structure, the health belief model, locus of control models, protection motivation theory, behavioral intention theory, and stage of adoption models. Health as a motive or value, and those motives that are relevant to health behavior, represent another important cognitive determinant. For convenience, cognitive determinants can be considered under three broad categories: representations, predictive models, and motivation.

Representations

Cognitive representations refer to mental images or personal schemata related to health, illness, or disease. To use Tolman's term, they are *cognitive maps* of the health domain (Tolman, 1948/1961). Bishop and Converse (1986) use the term *prototype model* to describe the way in which personal beliefs form a schema with which to interpret physical symptoms. Commonsense or laypersons' views of epidemiology have been shown to be related to personal illness histories (e.g., Jemmott, Croyle, & Ditto, 1988) and to critical and meaningful events in the person's life (e.g., Hunt, Jordon, & Irwin, 1989). Personal schemata have also been found relevant to the area of exercise (Kendzierski, 1990), treatments (Furnham, 1989), patients' perceptions of epilepsy (Kirchgässler, 1990), symptom perceptions in chronic respiratory patients (Lacroix, Martin, Avenado, & Goldstein, 1991), beliefs about contagion and germs (Nemeroff, 1995), and care-seeking behavior (Cameron, Leventhal, & Leventhal, 1993).

In Chapter 3, Lau reviews the research literature on cognitive representations of health and illness and provides a detailed account of some relevant investigations and data.

Predictive Models

In the 1950s and 1960s, the health belief model and models derived from the concept of locus of control were the major predictive models in health behavior research. The 1970s through the mid-1990s and 1980s witnessed the emergence of research driven by protection motivation theory, behavioral intention theory (eventually termed the "theory of reasoned action" or the "theory of planned behavior"), and stage theories (sometimes referred to as "transtheoretical models"). A comparison of major cognitive theories showing their similarities, differences, strengths, and weaknesses is provided by Weinstein (1993).

Health Belief Model. The health belief model, long considered to be the major frame of reference in health behavior research, and at one time referred to "in virtually every dissertation related to health behavior" (Green, 1974, p. 324), has been generating health behavior research since the middle 1950s. It was originally developed to explain why persons engage in and predict when they will engage in specific preventive behaviors such as accepting a vaccine or participating in a tuberculosis screening procedure (e.g., Rosenstock, Derryberry, & Carriger, 1959), but has been expanded to predict illness and sick role behaviors. Basic components of the model are perceived susceptibility to an illness, perceived severity or seriousness of that illness, perceived benefits of taking a specified action, and perceived barriers to taking that action.

Reviews of research generated by the model, together with critical analyses, have been provided by Becker (1974), Janz and Becker (1984), and Kirscht (1988). Janz and Becker (1984), for example, have used a "significance ratio" (p. 36) to compare the predictive value of the several variables encompassed by the model and to show historical changes in the way the variables

were conceptualized and measured and in their relative effectiveness. For studies published prior to 1974, "perceived susceptibility" was the best overall predictor. For studies published during the 10-year period 1974–1984, "perceived barriers" was the best predictor, followed by "perceived benefits" and "perceived susceptibility." "Perceived seriousness" was far less valuable as a predictor. Yet, in a prospective study, Eckert and Goldstein (1983) observed that perceived severity played a role as a trigger to seeking medical care, as well as a role in the choice of source of care. The magnitude of its importance, however, was influenced by income level. Janz and Becker's observations are congruent with the increased attention paid to conceptualizing and measuring perceived benefits and perceived barriers since 1980, particularly in studies that attempted to develop measures of benefits and barriers that were congruent with the phenomenological world of respondents (e.g., Eisen, Zellman, & McAlister, 1985), in contrast to the presumptive reality of medical technology.

Kirscht (1988) demonstrated the model's value as a predictor of a variety of health actions and provided insights into its complexity and status. He also showed how the model has become less involved in the prediction of "medically" determined or medically specified behaviors and more involved in the prediction of a broad spectrum of health-relevant but non-medically specified behaviors. Moreover, his discussion of ways of dimensionalizing behaviors (e.g., habitual or nonhabitual; repetitive or one-time; initiating or stopping) and how differences along these dimensions have important implications for the predictive value of the model was a critically important conceptual contribution.

In Chapter 4, Strecher, Champion, and Rosenstock provide a mid-1990s assessment of the health belief model.

Locus of Control Models. A second major cognitive predictive model stems from Rotter's (1966) conception of locus of control. The degree to which persons perceive themselves as being in control over events in their lives (internal locus of control), in contrast to perceiving that events or outcomes in their lives are capricious or subject to control by others (external locus of control), has been found to be related to the likelihood that they will engage in selected health behaviors, although the evidence is not uniformly conclusive. Wallston and Wallston (1978) provided one of the earliest systematic reviews of this literature, and Seeman and Seeman's (1983) longitudinal analysis showed that persons who believe that they are more "in control" in relation to health and illness are more likely to engage in health-promoting behaviors than persons who believe that they are less "in control."

Lau (1988) identified a diverse group of health behaviors that were successfully predicted by locus of control and in addition provided a critical assessment of the model. Lau also identified a number of issues related to the measurement of locus of control, which is one of the few cognitive dimensions related to health that have been widely studied from a psychometric or instrument-construction perspective. Lau showed that such beliefs were multidimensional. In addition to the scales discussed by Lau, a children's health locus of control scale has been developed by Parcel and Meyer (1978) for use with young populations.

At the mid-1990s, locus of control by itself has less of a presence in the research literature, but its content appears in important ways in the concept of "self-efficacy," the belief that one has the skills to perform a behavior or to accomplish something.

In Chapter 5, on beliefs about control, Reich, Erdal, and Zautra review the more recent literature and provides empirical data showing the complex interplay between beliefs about control, social interactions, and perceptions about health status.

Protection Motivation Theory. The initial formulation of protection motivation theory appeared in the late 1970s, and the theory emerged as a major conceptual framework by the mid-1980s (e.g., Wurtele & Maddux, 1987). This third cognitive predictive model integrates elements of the health belief model such as perceived susceptibility and perceived severity with concepts related to cognitive responses to fear arousal, such as appraisals of threat and of ability to cope with the threat (e.g., Wurtele & Maddux, 1987). Findings emphasize the need for caution in using fear arousal and in estimating perceptions of threat. Millar and Millar (1995) observed that thinking about disease detection, which is presumed to be threatening, resulted in negative affective responses and negative mood change, with potentially negative implications for coping and problem solving. Kulik and Mahler (1987) and Kreuter and Strecher (1995) observed that risk perceptions are often inaccurate and that patients are likely to show optimistic biases in their expectations of negative events. Questions about the role of threat are raised by Blalock, DeVellis, Afifi, and Sandler (1990) in the context of their study of risk perception and participation in colorectal screening for cancer.

In Chapter 6, Rogers and Prentice-Dunn review the history of the theory, providing evidence that supports the theory and comparisons with other related models.

Behavioral Intention Theory. The theory of behavioral intentions (e.g., Fishbein & Ajzen, 1975), a fourth cognitive predictive model with implications for health behavior, also emerged in the late 1970s. According to behavioral intention theory, a person's attitude toward some act, moral beliefs related to the act, and perceptions of social norms relevant to the act determine the person's intention to engage in the act. The concept of "specificity of intention" is critical to this theory. General attitudes toward an object appear less powerful as predictors of behavior in relation to that object than does an intention to engage in a specific behavior. Moreover, unlike the health belief, locus of control, or protection motivation models, behavioral intention theory routinely includes normative pressures and factors that facilitate or deter the specified behavior.

In Chapter 7, on theories of planned behavior (TPB) and reasoned action (TRA), Maddux and DuCharme deal with the evolution of behavioral intention theory, its mid-1990s status, and how it integrates critical elements of all of the other cognitive models.

Stage Models and Transtheoretical Models. Stage models recognize that behavior change often involves a temporal sequence of different processes, with implications that successful intervention strategies must acknowledge these processes and be stage-specific. The precaution adoption process suggested by Weinstein (e.g., Weinstein & Sandman, 1992) identifies five distinct stages between ignorance and the completion of a preventive or precautionary behavior: (1) unawareness, (2) awareness but no personal engagement, (3) engaged but deciding on a course of action, (4) planning to act but not yet doing so, and (5) acting. Two additional stages are (6) not acting (if the result of the decision process is that action is not needed) and (7) maintenance.

The transtheoretical model (e.g., Prochaska, 1994; Prochaska & DiClemente, 1992; Prochaska et al., 1994) identifies five stages of change as (1) precontemplation, a period when change is not even being considered; (2) contemplation, a period of time in which serious thought about change in the near future is begun; (3) preparation, a period of time in which serious thought is given to changing in the immediate future; (4) action, a period of time in which overt change is made; and (5) maintenance, a period of time during which action has started and has been continued. The transtheoretical model also incorporates critical components of decisional balance theory and has been shown to have value for a range of health behaviors, such as smoking cessation, fat intake, and mammography (Prochaska et al., 1994).

Other Predictive Models. Other cognitive predictive models include decisional balance theory and subjective expected utility theory. Decisional balance theory refers to the way the positive and negative aspects of taking action are evaluated in the process of behavioral change (e.g., Marcus, Rakowski, & Rossi, 1992; Rakow-

ski, Fulton, & Feldman, 1993). The transtheoretical model subsumes the components of decisional balance theory (e.g., Prochaska et al., 1994).

Subjective expected utility theory makes use of a simple mathematical model to account for the way people evaluate the probabilities and desirabilities of alternative behaviors and choose the one with the highest product of the two (e.g., Ronis, 1992). Subjective expected utility theory has been integrated with the health belief model to predict dental flossing behavior (Ronis, 1992).

Health as a Value or Motive

The importance of another type of cognition, health as a motive or value, has received little systematic research attention, although it relates to these cognitive models. Although the original health belief model assumed that high levels of perceived susceptibility and perceived severity were themselves motivational, subsequent research showed that health as a motive is independent of perceived susceptibility (Gochman, 1977) and that health motivation is a factor in organizing health-related beliefs and intentions (Gochman, 1972). Lau, Hartman, and Ware (1986) provided a careful analysis of health as a value, devised a way of measuring it, and successfully incorporated that measure in predictions derived from the locus of control model.

The question of the role of health as a value in the prediction of health behaviors can be transformed into asking what values are relevant to health behavior. Research (Gochman, 1975) has shown that health may be less salient in the population than is presumed, and less salient than other values, such as concern for appearance. Kristiansen (1984) observed that health as a value contributed to the prediction of preventive health behaviors, but that other values contributed as well. On the other hand, Smith, Wallston, Wallston, Forsberg, and King (1984) observed that value of control in relation to health care processes was not a significant predictor of health-related behaviors among those facing terminal illness.

The relative strength of health and appearance motivation in West German and American samples was demonstrated by Cockerham, Kunz, and Lueschen (1988). West German eating behaviors were less driven by appearance than were the eating behaviors of Americans, but in neither population was health itself a significant factor in eating behaviors.

Appearance motivation was also found to be negatively linked to safe-sun practices (Jones & Leary, 1994). Furthermore, it is related to impression management, or people's concerns about how they present themselves socially. Such concerns may increase a range of health risks from skin cancer to HIV, since concern about the presentation of self may be a barrier to skin protection and to the purchase and use of condoms (Leary, Tchividjian, & Kraxberger, 1994).

The very name of the Health Motivation Assessment Inventory (McEwen, 1993), derived from the health belief model, gives promise of a relevant instrument to measure such motivation. Examination of its content reveals, however, that it measures a number of perceptual and belief variables that are presumed to be motivating, but does not measure health motivation—or motivation germane to health—at all.

Other Cognitive Approaches

Other approaches not identified with any of the major cognitive models are reflected in the following studies: Minkler's (1978) examination of health-relevant beliefs and attitudes in the elderly and the incongruity between their cognitions and behaviors and that between their cognitions and "reality"; McKee's (1975) observation of large attitudinal differences between users and nonusers of nonprescription or "recreational" drugs; Kahn, Anderson, and Perkoff's (1973) analysis of the perceptions of need for care held by users of emergency rooms; Mburu, Smith, and Sharpe's (1978) report of how attitudes toward modern medicine determine use of health services among the Matungulu people of Kenya; Crandall and Duncan's (1981) comparison of attitudinal and situational factors as predictors of physician use, as well as their observations that attitudes and beliefs about physicians, personal health, and health care were better predictors of physician use among low-income persons than were financial resources; Stacy, Bentler, and Flay's (1994) observations that attitudes were inconsistent in predicting risk behaviors; Selstad, Evans, and Welcher's (1975) observations that females who had undergone an abortion and who a year later were not regular users of contraception were more likely than regular users to believe that premarital sex activity was wrong; and Wagenfeld, Vissing, Markle, and Petersen's (1979) observations of attitudinal and ideological differences between participants in the laetrile movement and the general population. Those in the laetrile movement, for example, were less likely to be convinced of the importance of regular physical examinations and more likely to use chiropractors and other alternatives to "orthodox" medical care.

NONCOGNITIVE PERSONALITY DETERMINANTS

Although a number of personal variables have also been linked conceptually and empirically to health behavior, no personality models, factors, theories, or concepts have had as great and as pervasive an impact on health behavior research as have the models derived from cognitive theories. Helsing and Comstock's (1977) observation that "psycho-social characteristics have not been studied as thoroughly as demographic factors" (p. 1044) remains as true of the larger area of health-related behaviors in the mid-1990s as it was 20 years before in relation to seat belt use.

Discussion of research on personal characteristics can be considered under three headings, depending on the *primary* focus: discrete personal characteristics, trigger factors, and integrations of these two.

Discrete Personal Characteristics

Discrete personal characteristics include not only traditional concepts of personality variables, such as anxiety or dependency, but also demographic characteristics, such as educational and income levels—which are often (usually inappropriately) considered as "social" or as components of socioeconomic status—and health status.

Personality Variables.   A large portion of the research on personality variables was conducted to increase understanding of smoking and other risk-taking behavior and to evaluate the impact of antismoking and other risk reduction campaigns. (Some of these studies also examined demographic and other characteristics in addition to personality variables.) Attempts have been made to relate smoking to extraversion (e.g., Cherry & Kiernan, 1976), to stimulation seeking (e.g., Eysenck, 1965), and to seeking positive affect (e.g., Leventhal & Avis, 1976; Tomkins, 1968), but the conclusions have been unclear. In summarizing the literature on personal determinants of smoking behavior in youngsters, for example, Flay, d'Avernas, Best, Kersell, and Ryan (1983) stated that there are "few personality variables that discriminate consistently between adolescents who will begin to smoke regularly and those who will remain nonsmokers" (p. 138), a finding that remains valid in the mid-1990s.

Radelet (1981) observed that nonusers of tranquilizers were less reluctant to admit to having unpleasant feelings and were less likely to have friends who used tranquilizers than were tranquilizer users. Duckitt and Broll (1983) were unable to find consistent or appreciable personality differences—i.e., anxiety, extraversion, critical independence, sensitivity, shrewd pragmatism, inhibition—in illness behaviors such as days spent in bed.

Murphy's (1978) analysis of differential use of a symptom checklist by two groups of Montreal women revealed that although the group that had higher scores were very similar to the group with lower scores on most personality dimensions, as a group they had higher ego ideals and higher levels of awareness of their own needs beyond basic security, and that the score differences could be accounted for in terms of differences in "self-actualization."

The concepts of attachment style and affect regulation have emerged in relation to perception and reporting of symptoms and to visits to health professionals. Negative emotionality—feelings of nervousness, irritation, and emotional lability—were observed to be related to increased reporting of symptoms (Feeney & Ryan, 1994).

Helsing and Comstock's (1977) analysis of nonuse of seat belts revealed that nonusers were more likely than users to have more aggressiveness and greater feelings of depressed mood, alienation, and general stress and unhappiness. Nonuse was also associated with infrequency of church attendance, but not consistently related to aspects of preventive behaviors other than to a longer time since their last dental visit and (for females) since their last Pap smear. Nonusers were also more likely to be female rather than male and to have fewer years of education and lower income.

Magarey, Todd, and Blizard's (1977) concise study of factors associated with breast self-examination and delay in reporting breast symptoms demonstrated that conscious factors such as fear of breast loss, disease, or dying were of little relevance in contrast to the greater predictive value of unconscious uses of denial and other defense mechanisms.

Income, Education, Occupation, and Age. Lave, Lave, Leinhardt, and Nagin (1979) found that low-income, unmarried males who are new to their communities and who are in good health are less likely to have a regular source of health care than women, or married persons, who have resided in their communities for some time, who have higher incomes, or who may be in poorer health. Okada and Wan (1979) showed that when economic barriers to care are removed, poor persons still do not seek out dental care to the degree that the nonpoor do.

Luft, Hershey, and Morrell (1976) observed that use of physician services in a rural community is better predicted by health status and by having a regular source of care than by income and insurance coverage. Monteiro (1973) showed that income was increasingly less important as a determinant of care-seeking behavior than other factors. Christie and Lawrence (1978) observed that attitudes toward hospitalization were negatively correlated with age among men and positively correlated with age among women.

Swigar, Quinlan, and Wexler (1977) observed that among women who applied for abortion, those who chose eventually not to have an abortion did not differ in age, race, marital status, occupation, partner's age, and partner's occupation from those who did have the abortion. The only distinguishing characteristics were the woman's and partner's educational levels. Those who had the abortion, and their partners, had more years of education. Smoking and smoking cessation were found to be related to age and health status (Salive et al., 1992) and to occupational status (Covey, Zang, & Wynder, 1992).

Okafor's (1983) report of hospitalization among rural Nigerians showed the impact of education in conjunction with perceptions of need. Finally, Titkow's (1983) analysis of illness behavior in Warsaw showed that educational level was a determinant of utilization of sources of care beyond the district clinics, of selectivity in use of certain hospitals, and of seeking nongovernmental laboratory tests.

Health Status. The role of health status as a determinant of health behavior was examined by Kulik and Mahler (1987), who observed that acutely ill college students believed themselves to be more vulnerable to health problems in the future (even if these problems were unrelated to their present condition) and were more interested in receiving preventive materials, than apparently healthy students. Garrity, Somes, and Marx (1978) observed that perceived health status was primarily a function of recent life changes. Wan's (1976) discriminant analysis showed that perceived health status was a function of employment status; the severity of physical disability, including the need for assistance in mobility; and psychological well-being. Moreover, Wan concluded that measures of personal and social functioning are more valuable as predictors of perceived health than socioeconomic status or psychological well-being. The discrepancies between the findings of Garrity, Somes, and Marx and those of Wan are attributable largely to the differences in the data they were analyzing.

Trigger Factors

Trigger factors, those events that seem to precipitate health behavior—particularly use of a health service—were dramatically described by Zola (1973), who elaborated on how stressful events or experiences of personal or social disequilibrium "triggered" a medical care visit for symptoms that had existed for some time. Among the major triggers, Zola identified interpersonal crises and perceptions of interference with social or personal relations or with vocational or physical activity. Mechanic and his colleagues have documented the trigger role of psychological stress in determining perceptions of health status (Tessler & Mechanic, 1978) and in the seeking of care (Tessler, Mechanic, & Dimond, 1976).

Building on Zola's work, Bloor (1985) noted that care seeking, in a sample of boarding house residents in Scotland, was likely to occur when there was a break in the everyday accommodation that characterizes the way most people adapt to symptoms, at the same time that there was also a relevant external cue encouraging the seeking of care. Bloor suggests that work often promotes accommodation to symptoms and illness and allows persons suffering to temporize and postpone seeking care. Verbrugge (1985) provided documentation of how daily events, in conjunction with bad moods, trigger medical drug use, medical and dental care seeking, lay referral behaviors, and restricted activities.

Integrative Approaches

Andersen (e.g., Andersen, 1968, cited in Andersen, 1995) proposed a basic model that integrates personal characteristics and triggering factors. Andersen's "behavioral model" initially identified three categories of factors to be taken into account in predicting a number of health behaviors: predisposing, enabling, and need factors. The model has served as the basis for numerous path analyses to predict or account for use of health services, but has implications for other health behaviors as well. Wan and Soifer (1974) were able to demonstrate, for example, that need variables—health status and responsiveness to illness—were the most important predictors of physician visits, more so than the enabling factors of insurance coverage, costs of visits, and income (which had no effect at all). Selwyn (1978) used this model to discriminate between users and nonusers of child health services among poor residents of a *barrio* in Colombia. A path analysis by Bush and Osterweis (1978) demonstrated that perceived morbidity—a need factor—is the best predictor of use of prescription medicine, although age, race, and gender—predisposing factors—contribute appreciably, as does perceived availability of care, an enabling factor. Bush and Iannotti (1988) demonstrated how path analysis as a statistical tool could be used to compare and contrast the predictive value of different levels of personal factors.

In Chapter 8, Aday and Awe provide a mid-1990s critical analysis of the development and status of the health services utilization model, showing its increasing complexity and how it has incorporated larger systems such as government and health agencies.

REFERENCES

Andersen, R. M. (1968). *Behavioral model of families' use of health services*. Research Series No. 25. Chicago, IL: Center for Health Administration Studies, University of Chicago.

Andersen, R. M. (1995). Revisiting the behavioral model and access to medical care: Does it matter? *Journal of Health and Social Behavior, 36*, 1–10.

Becker, M. H. (1974). The health belief model and personal health behavior. *Health Education Monographs, 2* (entire issue).

Bishop, G. D., & Converse, S. A. (1986). Illness representations: A prototype approach. *Health Psychology, 5*, 95–114.

Blalock, S. J., DeVellis, B. M., Afifi, R. A., & Sandler, R. S. (1990). Risk perceptions and participation in colorectal cancer screening. *Health Psychology, 9*, 792–806.

Bloor, M. J. (1985). Observations of abortive illness behavior. *Urban Life, 14*, 300–316.

Bush, P. J., & Ianotti, R. J. (1988). Pathways to health behavior. In D. S. Gochman (Ed.), *Health behavior: Emerging research perspectives* (pp. 87–102). New York: Plenum Press.

Bush, P. J., & Osterweis, M. (1978). Pathways to medicine use. *Journal of Health and Social Behavior, 19*, 179–189.

Cameron, L., Leventhal, E. A., & Leventhal, H. (1993). Symptom representations and affect as determinants of care seeking in a community-dwelling, adult sample population. *Health Psychology, 12*, 171–179.

Cherry, M., & Kiernan, K. (1976). Personality scores and smoking behaviour: A longitudinal study. *British Journal of Preventive and Social Medicine, 30*, 123–131.

Christie, D., & Lawrence, L. (1978). Patients and hospitals: A study of the attitudes of stroke patients. *Social Science and Medicine, 12*, 49–51.

Cockerham, W. C., Kunz, G., & Lueschen, G. (1988). On concern with appearance, health beliefs, and eating habits: A reappraisal comparing Americans and West Germans. *Journal of Health and Social Behavior, 29*, 265–270.

Covey, L. S., Zang, E. A., & Wynder, E. L. (1992). Cigarette smoking and occupational status. *American Journal of Public Health, 82*, 1230–1234.

Crandall, L. A., & Duncan, R. P. (1981). Attitudinal and situational factors in the use of physician services by low-income persons. *Journal of Health and Social Behavior, 22*, 64–77.

Duckitt, J., & Broll, T. (1983). Life stress, personality and illness behavior: A prospective study. *Psychological Reports, 53*, 51–57.

Eckert, J. K., & Goldstein, M. C. (1983). An anthropological approach to the study of illness behavior in an urban community. *Urban Anthropology, 12*, 125–139.

Eisen, M., Zellman, G. L., & McAlister, A. L. (1985). A health belief model approach to adolescents' fertility control: Some pilot program findings. *Health Education Quarterly, 12*, 185–210.

Eysenck, H. J. (1965). *Smoking, health and personality*. New York: Basic Books.

Feeney, J. A., & Ryan, S. M. (1994). Attachment style and affect regulation: Relationships with health behavior and family experiences of illness in a student sample. *Health Psychology, 13*, 334–345.

Fishbein, M., & Ajzen, I. (1975). *Belief, attitude, intention and behavior: An introduction to theory and research.* Reading, PA: Addison-Wesley.

Flay, B. R., Avernas, J. R., Best, J. A., Kersell, M. W., & Ryan, K. B. (1983). Cigarette smoking: Why young people do it and ways of preventing it. In P. J. McGrath & P. Firestone (Eds.), *Pediatric and adolescent behavioral medicine.* (pp. 131-183). New York: Springer-Verlag.

Furnham, A. (1989). Overcoming "psychosomatic" illness: Lay attributions of cure for five possible psychosomatic illnesses. *Social Science and Medicine, 29*, 61-67.

Garrity, T. F., Somes, G. W., & Marx, M.B. (1978). Factors influencing self-assessment of health. *Social Science and Medicine, 12*, 77-81.

Gochman, D. S. (1972). The organizing role of motivation in health beliefs and intentions. *Journal of Health and Social Behavior, 13*, 285-293.

Gochman, D. S. (1975). The measurement and development of dentally relevant motives. *Journal of Public Health Dentistry, 35*, 160-164.

Gochman, D. S. (1977). Perceived vulnerability and its psychosocial context. *Social Science and Medicine, 11*, 115-120.

Gochman, D. S. (1988). Personal determinants: Cognitive determinants. In D. S. Gochman (Ed.), *Health behavior: Emerging research perspectives.* (pp. 65-70). New York: Plenum Press.

Green, L. W. (1974). Editorial. In M. H. Becker (Ed.), The health belief model and personal health behavior. *Health Education Monographs, 2*, 324-325.

Helsing, K. J., & Comstock, G. W. (1977). What kinds of people do not use seat belts? *American Journal of Public Health, 67*, 1043-1050.

Hunt, L. M., Jordan, B., & Irwin, S. (1989). Views of what's wrong: Diagnosis and patients' concepts of illness. *Social Science and Medicine, 28*, 945-956.

Janz, N. K., & Becker, M. H. (1984). The health belief model: A decade later. *Health Education Quarterly, 11*, 1-47.

Jemmott, J. B., III, Croyle, R. T., & Ditto, P. H. (1988). Commonsense epidemiology: Self-based judgments from laypersons and physicians. *Health Psychology, 7*, 55-73.

Jones, J. L., & Leary, M. R. (1994). Effects of appearance-based admonitions against sun exposure on tanning intentions in young adults. *Health Psychology, 13*, 86-90.

Kahn, L., Anderson, M., & Perkoff, G. T. (1973). Patients' perceptions and uses of a pediatric emergency room. *Social Science and Medicine, 7*, 155-160.

Kendzierski, D. (1990). Exercise self-schemata: Cognitive and behavioral correlates. *Health Psychology, 9*, 69-82.

Kirchgässler, K. U. (1990). Change and continuity in patient theories of illness: The case of epilepsy. *Social Science and Medicine, 30*, 1313-1318.

Kirscht, J. P. (1988). The health belief model and predictions of health actions. In D. S. Gochman (Ed.), *Health behavior: Emerging research perspectives* (pp. 27-41). New York: Plenum Press.

Kreuter, M. W., & Strecher, V. J. (1995). Changing inaccurate perceptions of health risk: Results from a randomized trial. *Health Psychology, 14*, 56-63.

Kristiansen, C. M. (1984, August). *Using the value of health to predict health behavior.* Paper presented at the 92nd annual convention of the American Psychological Association, Toronto.

Kulik, J. A., & Mahler, H. I. M. (1987). Health status, perceptions of risk, and prevention interest for health and nonhealth problems. *Health Psychology, 6*, 15-27.

Lacroix, J. M., Martin, B., Avendano, M., & Goldstein, R. (1991). Symptom schemata in chronic respiratory patients. *Health Psychology, 10*, 268-273.

Lau, R. R. (1988). Beliefs about control and health behavior. In D. S. Gochman (Ed.), *Health behavior: Emerging research perspectives* (pp. 43-63). New York: Plenum Press.

Lau, R. R., Hartman, K. A., & Ware, J. E., Jr. (1986). Health as a value: Methodological and theoretical considerations. *Health Psychology, 5*, 25-43.

Lave, J. R., Lave, L. B., Leinhardt, S., & Nagin, D. (1979). Characteristics of individuals who identify a regular source of medical care. *American Journal of Public Health, 69*, 261-267.

Leary, M. R., Tchividjian, L. R., & Kraxberger, B. E. (1994). Self-presentation can be hazardous to your health: Impression management and health risk. *Health Psychology, 13*, 461-470.

Leventhal, H., & Avis, N. (1976). Pleasure, addiction, and habit: Factors in verbal report or factors in smoking behavior. *Journal of Abnormal Psychology, 85*, 478-488.

Luft, H. S., Hershey, J. C., & Morrell, J. (1976). Factors affecting the use of physician services in a rural community. *American Journal of Public Health, 66*, 865-871.

Magarey, C. J., Todd, P. B., & Blizard, P. J. (1977). Psycho-social factors influencing delay and breast self-examination in women with symptoms of breast cancer. *Social Science and Medicine, 11*, 229-232.

Marcus, B. H., Rakowski, W., & Rossi, J. S. (1992). Assessing motivational readiness and decision making for exercise. *Health Psychology, 11*, 257-261.

Mburu, F. M., Smith, M. C., & Sharpe, T. R. (1978). The determinants of health services utilization in a rural community in Kenya. *Social Science and Medicine, 12*, 211-217.

McEwen, M. (1993). The Health Motivation Assessment Inventory. *Western Journal of Nursing Research, 15*, 770-779.

McKee, M. R. (1975). Drug abuse knowledge and attitudes in "Middle America." *American Journal of Public Health, 65*, 584-591.

Millar, M. G., & Millar, K. (1995). Negative affective consequences of thinking about disease detection behaviors. *Health Psychology, 14*, 141-146.

Minkler, M. (1978). Health attitudes and beliefs of the urban elderly. *Public Health Reports, 93*, 426-432.

Monteiro, L. (1973). Expense is no object …: Income and physician visits reconsidered. *Journal of Health and Social Behavior, 14*, 99-115.

Murphy, H. B. M. (1978). The meaning of symptom-check-list

scores in mental health surveys: A testing of multiple hypotheses. *Social Science and Medicine, 12,* 67–75.

Nemeroff, C. J. (1995). Magical thinking about illness virulence: Conceptions of germs from "safe" versus "dangerous" others. *Health Psychology, 14,* 147–151.

Okada, L. M., & Wan, T. T. H. (1979). Factors associated with increased dental care utilization in five urban, low-income areas. *American Journal of Public Health, 69,* 1001–1009.

Okafor, S. I. (1983). Factors affecting the frequency of hospital trips among a predominantly rural population. *Social Science and Medicine, 17,* 591–595.

Parcel, G. S., & Meyer, M. P. (1978). Development of an instrument to measure children's health locus of control. *Health Education Monographs, 6,* 149–159.

Prochaska, J. O. (1994). Strong and weak principles for progressing from precontemplation to action on the basis of twelve problem behaviors. *Health Psychology, 13,* 47–51.

Prochaska, J. O., & DiClemente, C. C. (1992). Stages of change in the modification of problem behaviors. In M. Hersen, R. M. Eisler, & P. M. Miller (Eds.), *Progress in behavior modification: Vol. 28* (pp. 184–218). Sycamore, IL: Sycamore Publishing.

Prochaska, J. O., Velicer, W. F., Rossi, J. S., Goldstein, M. G., Marcus, B. H., Rakowski, W., Fiore, C., Harlow, L. L., Redding, C. A., Rosenbloom, D., & Rossi, S. R. (1994). Stages of change and decisional balance for 12 problem behaviors. *Health Psychology, 13,* 39–46.

Radelet, M. J. (1981). Health beliefs, social networks, and tranquilizer use. *Journal of Health and Social Behavior, 22,* 165–173.

Rakowski, W., Fulton, J. P., & Feldman, J. P. (1993). Women's decision making about mammography: A replication of the relationships between stages of adoption and decisional balance. *Health Psychology, 12,* 209–214.

Ronis, D. L. (1992). Conditional health threats: Health beliefs, decisions, and behaviors among adults. *Health Psychology, 11,* 127–134.

Rosenstock, I. M., Derryberry, M., & Carriger, C. K. (1959). Why people fail to seek poliomyelitis vaccination. *Public Health Reports, 74,* 98–103.

Rotter, J. B. (1966). Generalized expectancies for internal versus external control of reinforcement. *Psychological Monographs, 80*(1), No. 609 (entire issue).

Salive, M. E., Cornoni-Huntley, J., LaCroix, A. Z., Ostfeld, A. M., Wallace, R. B., & Hennekens, C. H. (1992). Predictors of smoking cessation and relapse in older adults. *American Journal of Public Health, 82,* 1268–1271.

Seeman, M., & Seeman, T. E. (1983). Health behavior and personal autonomy: A longitudinal study of the sense of control in illness. *Journal of Health and Social Behavior, 24,* 144–160.

Selstad, G. M., Evans, J. R., & Welcher, W. H. (1975). Predicting contraceptive use in postabortion patients. *American Journal of Public Health, 65,* 708–713.

Selwyn, B. J. (1978). An epidemiological approach to the

study of users and nonusers of child health services. *American Journal of Public Health, 68,* 231–235.

Smith, R. A., Wallston, B. S., Wallston, K. A., Forsberg, P. R., & King, J. E. (1984). Measuring desire for control of health care processes. *Journal of Personality and Social Psychology, 47,* 415–426.

Stacy, A. W., Bentler, P. M., & Flay, B. R. (1994). Attitudes and health behavior in diverse populations: Drunk driving, alcohol use, binge eating, marijuana use, and cigarette use. *Health Psychology, 13,* 73–85.

Swigar, M. E., Quinlan, D. M., & Wexler, S. D. (1977). Abortion applicants: Characteristics distinguishing dropouts remaining pregnant and those having abortion. *American Journal of Public Health, 67,* 142–146.

Tessler, R., & Mechanic, D. (1978). Psychological distress and perceived health status. *Journal of Health and Social Behavior, 19,* 254–262.

Tessler, R., Mechanic, D., & Dimond, M. (1976). The effect of psychological distress on physical utilization: A prospective study. *Journal of Health and Social Behavior, 17,* 353–364.

Titkow, A. (1983). Illness behaviour and action: The patient role. *Social Science and Medicine, 17,* 637–646.

Tolman, E. C. (1948/1961). Cognitive maps in rats and men. In E. C. Tolman, *Behavior and psychological man* (1st paperbound ed.) (pp. 241–264). Berkeley: University of California Press. (Reprinted from *Psychological Review, 1948, 55,* 189–208.)

Tomkins, S. (1968). A modified model of smoking behavior. In E. F. Borgatta & R. R. Evans (Eds.), *Smoking, health, and behavior.* Chicago: Aldine.

Verbrugge, L. M. (1985). Triggers of symptoms and health care. *Social Science and Medicine, 20,* 855–876.

Wagenfeld, M. O., Vissing, Y. M., Markle, G. E., & Petersen, J. C. (1979). Notes from the cancer underground: Health attitudes and practices of participants in the laetrile movement. *Social Science and Medicine, 13A,* 483–485.

Wallston, K. A., & Wallston, B. S. (1978). Health locus of control. *Health Education Monographs, 6,* No. 2 (entire issue).

Wan, T. T. H. (1976). Predicting self-assessed health status: A multivariate approach. *Health Services Research, 11,* 464–477.

Wan, T. T. H., & Soifer, S. J. (1974). Determinants of physician utilization: A causal analysis. *Journal of Health and Social Behavior, 15,* 100–108.

Weinstein, N. D. (1993). Testing four competing theories of health-protective behavior. *Health Psychology, 12,* 324–333.

Weinstein, N. D., & Sandman, P. M. (1992). A model of the precaution adoption process: Evidence from home radon testing. *Health Psychology, 11,* 170–180.

Wurtele, S. K., & Maddux, J. E. (1987). Relative contributions of protection motivation theory components in predicting exercise intentions and behavior. *Health Psychology, 6,* 453–466.

Zola, I. K. (1973). Pathways to the doctor—From person to patient. *Social Science and Medicine, 7,* 677–689.

3

Cognitive Representations of Health and Illness

Richard R. Lau

INTRODUCTION

A simplistic view of illness, not uncommon in the Western industrialized world, holds that people are healthy until some external, tangible stimulus (e.g., a germ, a carcinogen, a severe blow) somehow "invades" the body to disrupt normal functioning. In some cases, the body's own defenses or regenerative processes or both are sufficient to "fight off" the invader; in other cases, a professionally trained medical expert must intervene to repair the damage, either with medicine or, in extreme cases, with surgery. "Patients" are assumed to be universally motivated to *want* to return to good health and thus to be highly motivated to follow "doctor's orders" to do so (Idler, 1979; Parsons, 1951; Parsons & Fox, 1952). If the damage is successfully repaired, the person is once again healthy; if the damage cannot be fully repaired, the person may die, and at best must

spend the remainder of life somehow physically handicapped.

With such a view of illness, one would have little reason to examine psychological, social, or cultural factors. By this view, within a reasonably narrow range of parameters, a given external stimulus (e.g., a germ or injury) should cause the same symptoms or bodily damage in people everywhere and should be ameliorated by the same treatment. Consequently, if this treatment is not successful, there is a physical or organic explanation (e.g., malnutrition caused by poverty; culturally determined dietary practices that somehow interact with prescribed treatment) for the failure of the illness to follow its "normal" course and of the treatment to have its "normal" effectiveness.

Such a simplistic view, however, is no longer shared by many people (including many physicians) who have spent much time thinking about the topic (e.g., Epstein et al., 1987; Ware, Brook, Davies, & Lohr, 1981). There is far too much cultural variation in the prevalence and "experience" of disease, far too many social factors related to morbidity and mortality, indeed far too much individual-level variation (even within a given culture and social context) in the course of

Richard R. Lau • Institute for Health, Health Care Policy, and Aging Research, Rutgers University, New Brunswick, New Jersey 08903.

Handbook of Health Behavior Research I: Personal and Social Determinants, edited by David S. Gochman. Plenum Press, New York, 1997.

disease and the efficacy of prescribed treatments for this simplistic view to hold much sway.

This chapter will review the literature on cognitive representations of (or, in more common parlance, the perception of) health and illness. Although the focus will be on the individual, and thus on cognitive/psychological factors, social factors that influence the perception of health and illness cannot be ignored. Further, though most of the empirical evidence is drawn from samples in Eurocentric industrialized societies, it should be borne in mind that cross-cultural differences could increase the complexity of any conclusions.

The chapter begins with a review of the literature on the meaning of "health"—for how can one understand the meaning of "illness" without first understanding the meaning of health? It then turns to the more extensive literature on cognitive representations of illness. Leventhal's self-regulatory model is presented in some detail. It also briefly examines cross-cultural evidence that is consistent with this general model. These two major sections of the chapter both discuss theoretical and practical implications of the models presented. The chapter concludes by discussing future directions for research, in particular suggesting how commonsense representations of both health and illness can help illuminate reported links between self-assessed health and mortality.

To begin, however, some important terms must be carefully defined and distinguished. The term *disease* will be reserved for some biological/organic abnormality in a human organism. The term *illness*, on the other hand, refers to the subjective perception of abnormality, to the subjective perception that "something is wrong" or that "I am sick." The two are not the same: A "disease" can exist (in a pre- or asymptomatic state) in the absence of any perceived illness, while an "illness" can exist in the absence of any determinable disease, e.g., a "psychosomatic" illness (Williams, 1983). Indeed, it is the discrepancy between the two that is the focus of the second part of this chapter.

Stating that disease and illness are not the same certainly does not argue that they are unrelated. There is a large amount of interpersonal consistency in the illness associated with many diseases. It is this consistency that gives physicians much of their ability to diagnose. It is also true, however, that illness can vary tremendously among people with the same disease. In fact, perceptions of illness and their consequences can actually influence the course of the disease.

Before the chapter can examine how illnesses are perceived and cognitively represented, however, it must first try to describe what it means to be "healthy."

COGNITIVE REPRESENTATIONS OF "GOOD HEALTH"

What does it mean to be "healthy"? At its founding, the World Health Organization (1947) defined health as "a state of complete physical, mental and social well-being" (p. 29). This classic multidimensional definition has guided most of the subsequent research on assessing health status; additionally, by including "mental" and "social" well-being as part of the definition, it opened the process of assessing health to social scientists. While physicians can best assess physical health, psychologists, sociologists, and social workers are better attuned to assessing mental and social well-being.

Indeed, a case could be made that individuals are best able to assess their own health, particularly when health is so broadly defined. Scores of studies in the health field have asked participants a simple question such as, "In general, would you say your health is excellent, good, fair, poor, or bad?" Responses to this single question correlate quite strongly with more "objective" indicators of health status such as use of health services and clinical judgments by physicians (e.g., Hulka & Wheat, 1985; Mechanic, 1979; Wolinsky & Arnold, 1988). The discussion at the end of the chapter will return to this simple self-assessment of health status.

Empirical Validation of the World Health Organization Definition

A few studies have tried to determine whether people, in assessing their own health, have a multidimensional view similar to that of the World Health Organization. Bauman (1961) took the straightforward approach of asking a sample of 462 clinic patients and medical students what they thought "most people" mean when they say they are in good health or good physical condition. Responses fell into three large categories: [absence of] symptoms, [positive] feeling states, and performance [of normal physical activities]. These three categories map fairly well onto physical, mental, and social well-being. Over half of Bauman's subjects gave responses falling into more than one category, suggesting a multidimensional conception of health. Natapoff (1978), studying 1st-, 4th-, and 7th-grade children, basically replicated these same three general categories.

Laffrey (1986) developed a 28-item Likert scale designed to measure four different conceptions of health: (1) *clinical*, defined as the absence of disease or symptoms or both; (2) *functional/role performance*, defined as the ability to carry out various role functions satisfactorily; (3) *adaptive*, defined as the ability to adapt to flexible circumstances and environmental stress; and (4) *eudaimonistic*, defined in terms of exuberant well-being or self-actualization (see also Smith, 1981). These four subscales, which were administered to a sample of 141 master's students in a school of nursing, were all found to have high internal consistency and test–retest reliability. Most interestingly, the maximum (absolute) correlation between these four subscales was 0.15, suggesting four fairly distinct conceptions of health.

Hall, Epstein, and McNeil (1989) asked 590 elderly (70 and older) members of a health maintenance organization (HMO) a variety of questions aimed at measuring their cognitive functioning, emotional experience (three scales: anxiety, depression, overall well-being), functional status (four scales: ambulation, body care and movement, home management, mobility), social activity (two scales: family and nonfamily contact), and self-perceived health. In addition, these patients' primary physicians rated them on their "current physical and mental health" and their "likelihood of deterioration." An audit of the patients' medical records also noted the prevalence of 24 medical conditions common in geriatric populations.

These 13 summary scales were subjected to a second-order exploratory principal-components analysis. For current purposes, the three-factor solution (with orthogonal rotation) is most revealing. The four functional status scales had high loadings on the first factor (but on no other), the three emotional experience scales had high loadings on the second factor (but on no other), and the cognitive-functioning and family social activity scales both loaded highly on the third factor (but on no other; nonfamily social activity did not have a high loading on any of the first three factors). What is most interesting is that self-perceived health had a heavy loading on *both* of the first two factors. Thus, in this population at least, "health" would seem to be comprised of both physical functioning and emotional experience (mental health), but not so much social functioning. Ware et al. (1981) and Guralnik (1988) reported similar findings, in that social health seems to be distinct from and largely unrelated to mental and physical health. Thus, like Laffrey (1986), Hall et al. (1989) found *distinct* conceptions of health.

A second interesting finding from this study is that the two "objective" indicators of health (the physician rating and the chart audit) both loaded highly on the first factor, but on no other. Physicians, it would seem, focus on physical functioning, giving little thought to mental and social factors in assessing their patients' health, and presumably equally little thought to mental and social factors in diagnosing and treating illnesses. Indeed, it is likely that physicians know little or nothing about their patients' mental and social well-being because they do not often ask about such matters (Lau, Williams, Williams, Ware, & Brook, 1982). This divergence between the perceptions of laypersons, on one hand, and physicians and other medically trained personnel, on the other, is one theme that runs throughout this literature.

As part of a much larger medical outcomes study, Hays and Stewart (1990) studied the physical and mental health perceptions of 1980 adults with a chronic illness (e.g., advanced coronary artery disease, depression, diabetes, or hypertension). These adults were all patients of small fee-for-service practices, large multispecialty groups, or HMOs in Boston, Chicago, or Los Angeles. Physical health was defined by scales measuring physical functioning, mobility, satisfaction with physical abilities, and role limitations due to physical health. Mental health was measured by scales tapping anxiety, depression, feelings of belonging, and positive affect. All of these measures were collected via a self-administered questionnaire. Because of previous research indicating that social health is unrelated to physical and mental health, no attempt was made to measure it in this study. A second-order confirmatory factor analysis indicated, as expected, that the first four scales loaded significantly on a "Physical Health" factor and the next four on a "Mental Health" factor. Of more interest is the correlation between these two factors, $r = 0.46$, indicating a shared variance of about 21%. Hays and Stewart reject on statistical grounds two alternative models, the first specifying a single factor, the second specifying two orthogonal factors.

At first glance, the findings of Hays and Stewart (1990) are inconsistent with those reported by Laffrey (1986) and by Hall et al. (1989) to the extent that Hays and Stewart found distinct but correlated physical and mental health factors, while Laffrey and Hall et al. found that physical, mental, and social health were all uncorrelated with each other. While orthogonal factors are good for expository purposes, the world is rarely structured so neatly. While Laffrey (1986) examined intercorrelations between factors and found

them to be quite low, Hall et al. (1989) never looked at intercorrelations. Fortunately, Hall et al. provided sufficient information in their article to allow a reanalysis of their data with a series of confirmatory factor analyses similar to those performed by Hays and Stewart.

Following their results, I tested a confirmatory factor analysis model that had four subscales loading on a functional (or physical) health factor and three subscales loading on an emotional experience (psychological health) factor. In addition, a distinct physician rating subscale was created with two indicators (rather than allowing these two variables to load on the physical health factor), and single subscales defining non-family social well-being, family social well-being, cognitive well-being, and self-assessed health were included. Following the analytical strategy of Hays and Stewart, two alternative factor structures were examined, one in which correlations among the four health factors were fixed at 0 (but each was allowed to correlate freely with the other factors in the model) and a second in which the physical, mental, and two social health factors were allowed to correlate with each other (and with the other factors in the model). If there is little or no correlation between the four health factors, the data should fit these two models equally well.

As suspected, however, the results of a reanalysis of the Hall et al. (1989) data basically replicated the findings reported by Hays and Stewart in two primary respects. First, a model in which factors representing different dimensions of health were allowed to correlate was statistically superior to one in which those factors were forced to be orthogonal: $\chi^2 (6) = 131.85$, $p < 0.001$. Second, physical, mental, and non-family social health all had modest positive correlations with each other in the 0.41–0.45 range. These correlations are reported in Table 1. Moreover, all three scales correlated highly (0.46–0.57) with self-assessed health, suggesting that people *do* think about and consider all three dimensions when assessing their own health status.

Table 1. Intercorrelations of Measures of Health Status[a]

Physical health	1.0						
Psychological health	0.41[b]	1.0					
Nonfamily social well-being	0.44[b]	0.45[b]	1.0				
Family social well-being	0.20[b]	0.26[b]	0.17	1.0			
Physician ratings	0.74[b]	0.42[b]	0.42[b]	0.12	1.0		
Cognitive well-being	0.18[b]	0.09	0.06	0.06	0.20[b]	1.0	
Self-assessed health	0.56[b]	0.57[b]	0.46[b]	0.27[b]	0.77[b]	0.08	1.0

[a]Table entries are Pearson correlations between latent factors.
[b]$p < 0.01$.

What Does It Mean to Be "Healthy"?

These two major studies examined populations in which "health" would be expected to be quite salient because it could not be taken for granted: All of Hall et al.'s (1989) respondents were above 70 years of age, while all of Hays and Stewart's (1990) respondents had a chronic illness that could have become life-threatening had it not been properly managed. In such samples, at least, physical, mental, and social health are distinct but modestly interrelated dimensions of what it means to people to be healthy. Half of Bauman's (1961) respondents and all of Laffrey's (1986) were medical professionals—or at least students becoming professionals. But what about the rest of the population, who are not elderly, who do not currently have a serious chronic illness, and who have not chosen to become part of the medical establishment? It is quite possible that relatively healthy lay people do not make these distinctions (or make different distinctions) in thinking about their own health.

This question can be addressed with data gathered from a relatively small subsample of healthy young adults who were participating in a much larger longitudinal study of the development of preventive health beliefs and health behaviors (Lau, Bernard, & Hartman, 1989; Lau, Quadrel, & Hartman, 1990). In a very real sense, this sample is the extreme opposite of the samples of Hall et al. (1989) and Hays and Stewart

(1990), in that if there is ever a set of people who take their health for granted, for whom "good health" is barely salient, it is healthy young adults.

A random subsample of participants in the larger study had been asked to provide brief weekly "health diaries," and the 156 subjects whose responses are reported here not only agreed to participate (56% of those who were asked), but also returned at least 10 of the 13 weekly diaries (92% of those who initially agreed to participate).

The relevant data come from week 7 of the diary study. That week, subjects were instructed to write in their own words "what being healthy means to you." As summarized in Table 2, when these healthy young adults were asked to define spontaneously what they mean by "being healthy," their responses fell primarily into five major categories. The largest category is physiological/physical—fully 75% of all subjects reported some physiological or physical meaning. Almost as large a category is the 56% who gave some clearly psychological meaning. And over half (52%) of all subjects explicitly mentioned both physiological and psychological definitions, giving strong support to the World Health Organization's comprehensive definition of "health."

Another set of responses clearly reflect behavioral manifestations of being healthy (e.g., "I can do the things I normally do") that were mentioned by a quarter of the subjects. A fourth category of responses reflect the future conse-

Table 2. Open-Ended Definitions of Being "Healthy"

Question asked: *In general, what do you mean when you say you are "healthy"?*

Responses	Mentioned by
I feel good (nonspecific: can't code as clearly physiological or psychological)	9%
Physiological/physical	
Feel good physiologically	40%
Good condition, physically capable	40%
Have energy	21%
Don't tire easily	15%
Total mentioning *any* physiological/physical	*75%*
Psychological	
Feel good psychologically, emotionally, mentally	23%
Don't think/worry about my health	2%
Positive self-image	16%
Happy, energetic	22%
Social: Enjoy family, friends	1%
Can cope with problems	15%
Total mentioning *any* psychological	*56%*
Total mentioning *both* physiological/physical *and* psychological	*52%*
Behavioral	
Can do (fun) things I normally do	10%
Can do work, obligations	1%
Eat, sleep properly	14%
Don't smoke, drink	2%
Total mentioning *any* behavioral	*24%*
Future consequences	
My body resists illness; live longer	8%
"Health" is the absence of:	
Not sick; nothing wrong; no disease; no symptoms	58%
No injury, physical constraints	7%
No psychological ailment	11%
Total mentioning *any* absence of	*65%*
Total mentioning *only* absence of	*9%*
Residual	
Other; uncodeable above	2%

quences of being healthy (e.g., "My body resists illness").

A final and quite large category of responses define health *negatively*—as the *absence of* illness (see also Millstein & Irwin, 1987; Williams, 1983). If most of the 65% of subjects who gave any response in this final category had given *only* responses in this category, then one might conclude that a large proportion of these subjects

had a conception of health that was not distinct from illness. This was not the case, however: Fewer than 10% of all subjects gave responses that fell exclusively in this general category, suggesting that most people do have a positive definition of "being healthy."

These studies together largely confirm empirically the very broad definition of health offered by the World Health Organization. They suggest that people—at least people in industrialized countries—define or think of health in terms that clearly encompass more than physical/physiological factors. At the very least, people also very frequently include a psychological component (that may or may not include a social component, the evidence being less clear on this point).

Implications

The literature on the cognitive representation of health is rather small, probably because until recently the subject seemed largely of only academic interest. What people mean by "being healthy," however, is of both practical and theoretical importance. This discussion has gone to some length to document that most people have a fairly broad definition of health similar to that offered by the World Health Organization (1947) because the implications of such a broad definition of health are different from those associated with a narrower definition that focuses exclusively on physiological factors.

At the practical or policy-oriented level, any attempt to assess the efficacy of different treatments for a particular disease, or the value of entire comprehensive health plans, should consider and attempt to assess both physiological and psychological criteria of success. Such an assessment approach is influencing health-policy making in three ways. First, the various health insurance proposals considered by the 103rd and 104th Congresses differed not only in how they would be financed but also in the comprehensiveness of the benefits offered. The more "generous" proposals (e.g., the plan passed by the Senate Labor and Human Resources committee) expanded upon the mental health benefits proposed by President Clinton; the less generous proposals (e.g., those developed by the Senate Finance Committee) did not. There is certainly a trade-off between cost and comprehensiveness of coverage; one could argue, however, that any health insurance plan that covers only the treatment of physiological diseases should be called "health" insurance only in a very narrow sense.

Second, if "managed" competition in the health insurance industry is to help keep costs down, then consumers wanting to make informed choices (or government regulators trying to make sure the public is getting the biggest bang for its buck) have the right to know not only the cost of the services being provided by HMOs or other health service providers, but also their quality. Assessments of quality of care should be as comprehensive as definitions of what it means to be healthy: They should measure the impact of care on psychological and social functioning, as well as on physiological or physical functioning. This is the assessment strategy taken most prominently by Ware and his colleagues in their "medical outcomes study approach" (Stewart & Ware, 1992; Ware, 1987; Ware et al., 1981; Ware & Sherbourne, 1992), and it is an approach to be emulated as the movement to assess the quality of care delivered by different health care providers picks up steam.

Third, as policy makers struggle increasingly with ways to keep health care costs down, explicit proposals for "rationing" health services are beginning to be heard. Indeed, the state of Oregon has adopted one such proposal, whereby various illnesses are ranked in terms of the cost and effectiveness of treatment and the social consequences of leaving the illness untreated. Again, any judgments about the effectiveness of available treatment should be based on a comprehensive assessment of that treatment. Society might conclude, for example, that the quality of life of patients on renal dialysis is so low that it does not warrant the cost of treatment, given other patients on whom and other illnesses on which those same health care dollars could be spent.

At the theoretical level, it is important to know how people cognitively represent health because that representation is a baseline against which people determine whether or not they are "sick." Most people spend most of their lives in a relatively "healthy" state, and it makes intuitive sense that people will begin to realize they are "sick" when they perceive changes in their normal healthy state. Thus, knowing what people mean by and consider when they think of "being healthy" is theoretically important because it is deviations from that state—however narrowly or comprehensively defined—that they notice and use to define themselves as "ill." Knowing what people mean by "health" is the basis of Leventhal's self-regulatory model of illness representation to be discussed below (Leventhal, Nerenz, & Strauss, 1982). To begin, however, what do people mean when they say they are "sick"?

COGNITIVE REPRESENTATIONS OF ILLNESS

What Does It Mean to Be "Sick"?

The same healthy young adults who had described what they meant by "being healthy" had earlier (week 2) described, in the same open-ended manner, what they meant by "being sick." A categorization of their responses is shown in Table 3. About half of the respondents said being sick meant not being "normal," not feeling "right," reinforcing their aforementioned notion that "being healthy" is the normal state of affairs. Over three quarters of the sample mentioned, as an example, some specific symptoms they experienced when they felt sick, and almost half mentioned a specific disease. About 4% of the sample mentioned a time line associated with the illness, e.g., "I am sick when symptoms last more than one day." About a third of the sample also mentioned some consequence associated with the illness, such as not being able to exercise or go to class. Finally, more than a quarter of the sample defined being sick negatively—as what they did *not* mean, rather than what they did mean. Only 1

Table 3. Open-Ended Definitions of Being "Sick"

Question asked: *In general, what do you mean when you say you are "sick"?*

Responses	Mentioned by
I'm not "normal," I don't feel right	51%
Symptoms	
Physiological	75%
Psychological, emotional	17%
Total symptoms (either of the two)	78%
Labels	
Some specific serious disease (e.g., cancer)	15%
Some specific virus (e.g., a cold)	36%
Psychological illness (e.g., depression)	12%
Other specific (minor) disease	2%
Injury	6%
Total labels (any of the five)	47%
Total mentioning *both* physiological and psychological	*15%*
Time line: Symptoms last more than 1 day	4%
Consequence: Normal activity impossible	32%
I do *not* mean:	
Minor physiological symptoms	16%
Emotional/psychological symptoms	4%
An injury	12%
Total defining negatively	*28%*
Total mentioning *only* negative definitions	*1%*
Other, uncodeable	2%

person defined being sick exclusively in a negative manner, however, suggesting (as with the case for being "healthy") that virtually everyone has a good idea of what it means to be "sick."

Several differences between the types of definitions these subjects gave for being "healthy" and being "sick" are worth noting. First, more than twice as many people defined what it means to be "healthy" negatively than was the case for what it means to be "sick." As noted above, few people gave exclusively negative responses; consequently, these "negative" codes can be interpreted as attempts to elaborate or refine one's initial definition, and thus as indications of a perception that one's initial definition was not sufficiently clear. That so many more people felt it necessary to resort to such clarifications in defining "healthy" compared to defining "sick" suggests that in general, people believed that their definition of "healthy" *needed* clarification much more than their definition of being sick—and thus a general sense on the part of these subjects that they shared (with the investigators) a culturally universal conception of what it means to be sick, but less confidence that they shared a similarly universal conception of what it means to be healthy. This interpretation is consistent with the fact that people felt it necessary to give longer definitions of what it means to be healthy than of what it means to be sick [3.5 codeable responses compared to 2.9 codeable responses, $t(168) = 4.07$, $p < 0.001$]. Again, this interpretation is consistent with the idea that a healthy state is a general norm or perceptual background that is taken for granted with little cognitive awareness. People consequently must struggle more when asked to define a state to which they give little thought. Just as fish do not realize they are wet, so many healthy people take no cognizance of being healthy until a wave of illness hurls them onto shore and they notice a change from their normal environment.

A second difference worth mentioning is that while over half of the sample included both physiological and psychological components in their definition of being healthy, only 15% included both physiological and psychological components in their definition of being sick. This difference can probably be explained by the social stigma associated with mental illness: While there is nothing wrong with admitting one is psychologically healthy, in American culture there is still a strong stigma associated with having some psychological or mental illness.

Commonsense Representations of Illness

The data in Table 3 came from relatively healthy people defining what they mean by being sick *in general*, in the abstract. Much more research has been conducted on people describing specific illnesses (Lau et al., 1989; Lau & Hartman, 1983; Leventhal, Meyer, & Nerenz, 1980; Meyer, Leventhal, & Gutmann, 1985). For example, my colleagues and I have generally asked healthy respondents to "think back to the last time you were sick" and to "tell us everything you remember about this illness." "Sick" is intentionally left undefined. By the nature of illness in our society, the "most recent illness" most people describe is a relatively minor, contagious disease (e.g., a cold or the flu). On the other hand, Leventhal and his colleagues have more typically interviewed clinic populations of patients who have a fairly serious chronic disease such as hypertension or diabetes.

Despite the different methodologies and subject populations employed, this research all suggests that lay or "commonsense" representations of illness have the following five attributes:

1. An *identity*—a label, and symptoms that are associated with the illness.
2. A set of *consequences* (beyond the immediate somatic symptoms). For example: "How will my life be affected by this illness [e.g., socially, economically]? Will I die from this illness?"
3. A *time line*: "How long will this illness [and thus any symptoms, and larger consequences] last? Is this illness acute [and therefore relatively short-lived] or chronic [and therefore much more long-term]?"
4. A *cause*: "Why did I get sick? Was the illness

preventable? Was it my own [or someone else's] fault?"

5. Finally, most illness representations also have some notion of *cure or control*: "What can I do to avoid or minimize the consequences associated with this illness?"

These five attributes describe a cognitive "architecture" or "superstructure" that not only aids people in the orderly processing and recalling of information about illnesses, but also tells them what to "expect" or "look for" when they believe they are getting sick.

Supporting Evidence

Open-ended survey questions, much less structured but more free-flowing interviews, have a serious drawback when it comes to reporting their results: Actual responses tend to be idiosyncratic and far too numerous to be reported in "raw" form. They must be categorized or structured in some way *by the researcher* before they can be reported in summary form. A legitimate concern in such instances is the extent to which any resulting structure is more a research artifact than one built by the respondents.

Fortunately, there are several lines of evidence suggesting that this is not the case in this investigation. First, Lau et al. (1989) gave a naive sample of 20 subjects 65 representative statements taken from the descriptions of "your most recent illness." These 20 subjects were shown the question that had generated these statements and instructed to sort them into piles that "made sense to them." Analyses showed that the groupings made by these naive subjects agreed substantially (but less formally in the case of 17 of the 20) with the categorization of those same 65 items by the authors into the five components described above. The greatest difference was the tendency of many subjects to distinguish between labels and symptoms, rather than put them in a single "identity" pile.

A second line of evidence comes from research by Bishop and his colleagues (for a review,

see Bishop, 1991). Bishop argued that if there is a shared understanding of illness and disease within a culture, certain hypotheses (based on the social cognition literature [see Fiske & Taylor, 1991; Rosch, 1978]) about how people process information about illness and disease ought to be true. For example, if a set of symptoms are prototypically assumed to be associated with an illness, then that symptom set ought to more readily yield a specific diagnosis (a label), and those specific symptoms ought to be recalled more easily and accurately (Bishop & Converse, 1986).

Testing this hypothesis experimentally, Bishop and Converse presented subjects with brief descriptions of people who were each experiencing six different symptoms. Subjects were instructed to form impressions of the symptoms experienced by each of the different people. In a high-prototype scenario, all six symptoms had been rated by pretest subjects as commonly associated with a specific disease (e.g., chicken pox, hay fever, heart attack, ulcer); in a low-prototype scenario, only two of the six symptoms were commonly associated with a disease. As predicted, when given an unexpected memory test, subjects could more accurately recall the symptoms from the high-prototype scenario than those from the low. Furthermore, subjects were much more likely to believe that the symptom set was indicative of a particular disease, and to name it accurately, in the high-prototype scenario than in the low.

More to the point here, Bishop, Briede, Cavazos, Grotzinger, and McMahon (1987) further hypothesized that if a set of symptoms are prototypic of a disease, then more than just symptoms and a label ought to be associated with that prototype: If the five-component model of disease representations presented above is correct, then people should also make many schema-based associations that fall into the consequences, time line, cause, and cure categories. To test this hypothesis, Bishop et al. presented subjects with symptom sets that varied in how prototypically they were associated with a particular disease and asked them to think about and write down "what else might be associated with the person's situation" (i.e., the person who was experiencing these symptoms). Subjects offered a little more than four additional associations, of which 91% were categorized as falling into one of the five components outlined above. Subjects were very likely to give associations that fell into the identity, cause, and cure categories, moderately likely to make associations falling into the consequences category, and not very likely to give associations falling into the time line category (Bishop et al., 1987).

In summary, the same five components of identity, consequences, time line, cause, and cure have emerged from samples of healthy and sick adults, in patients who have coped for years with a chronic diseases, and in patients recently diagnosed with a life-threatening disease (e.g., cancer [Leventhal, Easterling, Coons, Luchterhand, & Love, 1986]). Widely different methodologies have been employed by different research teams to gather the evidence (e.g., face-to-face structured interviews, self-administered open-ended questions, experiments), with essentially similar results. Thus, there is a great deal of convergent evidence for this model of how people commonly understand illnesses.

A Self-Regulatory Model of Illness Behavior

Leventhal and his colleagues (Leventhal et al., 1980, 1982) enveloped this commonsense cognitive representation of illness in a more fully elaborated self-regulatory model of behavior (see also Dubos, 1965; Schlenger, 1976). Self-regulatory models (which are certainly applicable to many domains other than health [e.g., see Carver, 1979]) begin with the reasonable assumption that most people, when faced with a problem, will actively try to solve or cope with it. There are three general stages in the problem-solving process: (1) *interpretation*, triggered by some change in a normal, equilibrated environment, in which a representation or understanding of the problem

is reached; (2) *coping*, when an ameliorative course of action is planned and executed, with the aim of returning to the equilibrium state; and (3) *appraisal*, when the success of the coping strategy is assessed and, if that strategy has been unsuccessful, a new interpretation and coping strategy are developed. This process continues until a successful coping strategy is reached.

In the domain of health, the interpretation stage might be triggered by changes in somatic sensations. For example, a person might begin experiencing itchy eyes and a runny nose, or suffer aching joints, or discover a lump in a breast. Such symptoms would be noticed and trigger the self-regulatory process only if they are deviations from a normal state: A person who chronically suffers from arthritis, say, would hardly notice aching joints or think they augur some new health threat. As another example, a cue to a health danger might come from a physician's finding an abnormal result on a diagnostic test conducted during an annual checkup, without the patient's having had any prior somatic sensation. The self-regulatory model holds that somatic and social messages such as these will motivate the performance of various procedures that allow a person to define the meaning of these somatic problems, to act to remove any risk, and to return to a normal, "healthy" equilibrium. The person relies on stored knowledge (from personal experience with these same or similar symptoms or by learning about them from friends or the media) to *construct* an initial interpretation of or label for the problem; e.g., the itchy eyes and runny nose mean an allergy attack; the lump means cancer. Confirmatory evidence for this initial assessment is often sought; e.g., a cold front has blown in from Canada, and such fronts usually bring new allergens with them.

Once an initial interpretation of the problem has been made, ameliorative actions can be taken to correct or at least cope with the problem. These actions may include a decision to take an antihistamine to clear up the problem or to call a doctor for a mammogram. Many times, the decision may be to "wait and see" if the problem clears up (as have most prior symptoms) or if any further symptoms develop.

After a coping procedure has been adopted, one can appraise its outcome. Have the symptoms been reduced or eliminated? If the answer is yes, the person can accept a diagnosis that the condition is benign and return to other concerns. If the coping procedure proves ineffective, the person might try another (e.g., take a different antihistamine) or consider an alternative interpretation of the problem (maybe I'm getting a cold and I should take a cold remedy). In other words, the success of the coping strategy adopted in stage 2 determines whether the self-regulatory process starts over again. The initial diagnosis (label) may be questioned; at the very least, a new coping strategy will be tried, and it will subsequently be appraised for efficacy, perhaps leading to the seeking of expert help. The feedback loop continues until a successful coping strategy is achieved.

What makes this self-regulatory mechanism different from the illness schemata or common-sense representations of common illnesses already discussed is the assumption that almost always, a cognitive representation *and* an emotional reaction are simultaneously triggered when a deviation from equilibrium is noticed. The emotions can be the *direct* result of the same somatic symptoms that triggered the initial cognitive interpretation stage (e.g., pain can lead directly to fear or to depression), or they can be a *consequence of* the initial interpretation (e.g., a diagnosis of cancer would cause most people to be fearful). Moreover, an emotional reaction can influence the initial interpretation of the problem. For instance, a strong emotional reaction could cloud clear thinking or could lead to an initial interpretation (e.g., a strained chest muscle) that is less fear provoking than another (a heart attack).

Moreover, any coping mechanism must deal with both the cognitive *and* the emotional consequences of the initial representation of the health threat. A person fearful of cancer might delay seeking confirmation of this diagnosis from a physician—even though *cognitively* the person knows that delaying treatment can only allow the cancer (if that is what the lump is) to become worse—because the person cannot cope with the *emotions*, the fear, of having cancer.

This process is illustrated in Figure 1. The most important points include:

1. When a person notices potential threat to health, the person *constructs* an interpretation of the threat (both cognitive and emotional) based on prior personal experience with illness and disease, i.e., the person's own phenomenological knowledge base.
2. The cognitive and emotional interpretation of the health threat guides the selection and performance of some plan designed to cope with the threat. This plan is directed toward two successive purposes:
   • Defining the health threat more precisely (if the incoming cues were somewhat ambiguous, as they often are, and the initial "diagnosis" was consequently uncertain).
   • Eliminating the health threat (or at least minimizing its consequences).
3. The initial interpretation not only guides the action/coping plan, but also establishes criteria for assessing its success. If the assessment is negative—i.e., if the initial coping strategy was unsuccessful—the process starts over again.

Cross-Cultural Variations

All the research considered so far has been conducted in Eurocentric, industrialized societies in which the "germ" model of disease is widely accepted. No studies seeking to determine whether the same five dimensions of illness representations exist in non-Eurocentric societies have been conducted. On one hand, the lack of cross-cultural validation is somewhat surprising, because illness is a universal phenomenon. People everywhere might be expected to have a basic need to label or identify an illness, to

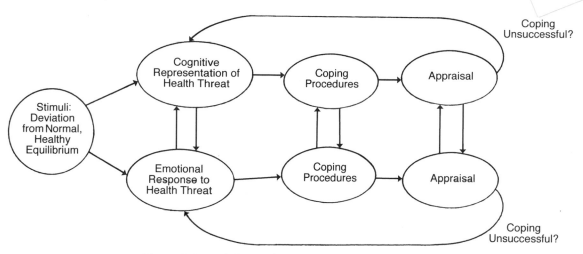

Figure 1. Leventhal's self-regulatory model of illness appraisal.

be curious about its cause and the potential for curing or at least ameliorating it, and to want to know what consequences an illness has and how long it will last. While culturally specific *answers* to these questions would be expected, it is surprising that these questions have not been asked (Kleinman, 1981; Kleinman, Eisenberg, & Good, 1978).

On the other hand, cultural anthropology, the social science that has most closely studied this topic, has very different research traditions than those generally employed in the studies cited above, and it may be too much to expect to find precise comparability. A thorough review of the anthropological literature is well beyond the scope of this chapter, but there is some cross-cultural research that has found results broadly similar to those presented above. For example, Weller (1984) conducted a multidimensional scaling study of cultural conceptions of different illnesses among English-speaking Americans and Spanish-speaking Guatemalans and came up with two broad dimensions of contagion (which is certainly a cause) and severity (the magnitude of consequences and the duration of the time line) that were shared by both cultures (see also Bishop, 1991; D'Andrade, 1973; Young, 1978).

Chrisman (1977), focusing on subculture variations in health-seeking behaviors within a broader culture, includes symptom definition, shifts in role behavior (consequences), and treatment actions (cure) among the five components derived from the medical anthropology literature. Thus, there is some converging cross-cultural evidence for how people think about or cognitively represent illnesses.

The degree of cross-cultural similarity should not be over-emphasized, however, because culturally specific findings are almost always reported in the anthropological literature. For example, D'Andrade, Quinn, Nerlove, and Romney (1972) found a "hot–cold" dimension to best characterize how Spanish-speaking Mexicans categorized disease, and Weller (1984) was very careful to warn of the necessity to examine the *variability* within each culture on the common dimensions that are found across cultures, with the idea that a certain dimension is more salient within a culture when it has less variability.

Implications

The practical implications of cognitive representations of illness representations are many.

One warning emerging from the anthropological literature is to be aware of possible professional-lay differences in understanding disease and illness even within a given culture. Any professional subculture develops its own special language, its own particular categories and ways of thinking about the problems it studies that are certainly a product of the larger culture of which it is a part, but also partially distinct from those of the larger culture (Brown, 1985). Indeed, a number of studies have found broad variation in what lay people, and professionals, think a "disease" is. For example, Hayes-Bautista (1978) asked a group of medical practitioners and their Hispanic patients to conceptualize what they meant by an illness. Professional conceptualizations were very formal, acquired in structured settings from a narrow set of sources, and were designed to achieve clarity by eliminating contradictions and ruling out alternative causes. Lay conceptualizations, on the other hand, were quite informal, acquired somewhat randomly from a wide variety of sources, and displayed a tendency toward increasing comprehensiveness that resulted in frequent (although not always perceived) contradictions and only partial clarity (see also Eisenberg, 1977; Hadlow & Pitts, 1991).

Any lay-professional differences in understandings of disease can have important implications for doctor-patient communication and ultimately for acceptance of medically prescribed treatment regimens (see Chapter 1 in Volume II of this *Handbook*). There are many different reasons for nonadherence to treatment regimens. The point here is to emphasize one of them: nonadherence due to a lack of shared understanding of the illness and thus perhaps a lack of understanding of the treatment regimen itself. For example, Marteau, Johnston, Baum, and Bloch (1987) found not only that parents and physicians had significantly different understandings of childhood diabetes, but also that adherence to treatment for the disease was strongly affected by the parents' understanding of their child's disease and their own goals for treatment, i.e., their own criteria for determining whether treatment is "effective." Similarly, Leventhal et al. (1980) found that hypertension patients who adopted a "chronic" time line for their disease were more likely to stay in treatment than patients who believed that hypertension was an "acute" illness that was cured when symptoms "disappeared."

Another set of implications comes from a basic human motivation: the need to "make sense of" or "come to grips with," cognitively and emotionally, any illness or deviation from a normal health equilibrium. Given a set of symptoms, a person will seek a label for those symptoms (as well as information about consequences, causes, cures, and time lines). Conversely, *given a label, a person will seek symptoms that seem to be consistent with that label* (Bauman, Cameron, Zimmerman, & Leventhal, 1989; Croyle & Sande, 1988; Lau, Leventhal, & Leventhal, 1992; Leventhal, Diefenbach, & Leventhal, 1992; Meyer et al., 1985). One level of consistency is semantic: A cold should be accompanied by "chills," hypertension by a tension in the shoulder muscles. Another level of consistency is physiological: "Heart problems" should be accompanied by chest pains, but less plausibly by pain in the extremities. This point puts a cognitive interpretation on at least some of what are referred to as "psychosomatic" illnesses—illnesses that apparently have no biological or physiological causes.

This same need to make sense of an illness could influence the type of causes that are most likely to be associated with it and the cures that are most likely to be adopted. It is easier to understand that hypertension is caused by too much stress in one's life than by too much salt in one's diet, and therefore it is easy to predict from this perspective which recommendation (all else being equal) is more likely to be followed.

The very decision to seek professional help in the first place is a function of first deciding that such help is needed. The labeling of a set of symptoms as a "serious illness" is not directly a function of those symptoms themselves, but rather the *interpretation* that is given to those symptoms—and that interpretation is based on past experience with disease. For example, Cameron, Leventhal, and Leventhal (1993) found that symptom experience was necessary but not sufficient to explain care seeking in a community-dwelling clinic population. Care seekers (compared to matched controls who were also experiencing new symptoms but did not elect to seek help) were more likely to rate their symptoms as serious and more likely to identify possible consequences. Matthews, Siegel, Kuller, Thompson, and Varat (1983) even found significant variation in how quickly professional help was sought among patients suffering from a heart attack (who presumably were all experiencing fairly severe symptoms) as a function of how those symptoms were labeled.

FUTURE RESEARCH DIRECTIONS

New research should prove particularly productive in several areas. To begin with, an instrument that would make the *measurement* of health and illness representations both easier and more comparable across studies would be immensely helpful. Such an instrument should be general enough to apply to (or at least be easily adapted to) many different types of illnesses. An instrument for measuring illness representations is currently being developed and tested by Petrie and Weinman (1994) and their colleagues in England and New Zealand. Their 40-item Illness Perception Questionnaire has good internal and test–retest reliability and has been found to explain more variance in adjustment to chronic fatigue syndrome than standard measures of coping strategies (Moss-Morris, Petrie, & Weinman, in press) and to mediate the effectiveness of a therapeutic treatment for relieving arthritis pain (Pimm, Byron, Curson, & Weinman, 1994). This instrument, once it is in the literature and widely available, should greatly facilitate research on illness representations.

A second issue concerns the *development* of cognitive representations of health and illness.

If these representation have the proposed theoretical and practical implications, it is important to learn how they develop. Commonsense representations of illnesses are suggested to be based on past experience with illness not because of evidence that is specifically relevant to this point, but rather because the suggestion seems commonsensical and seems to be true for cognitive representations of many other physical and social objects (i.e., cognitive "schemata"). But what *types* of experience are important? Personal experience with an illness? "Vicarious experience" with an illness via a close family member or friend? Is a vivid media depiction of an illness episode sufficient? Are all of these experiences more or less equally important, or do some experiences (e.g., personal experience) have stronger effects than others?

A third topic for future research concerns *links* between cognitive representations of illness and cognitive representations of health. At first glance, one might think the two obviously must be related, but in fact they may not be if they are based on two very different types of experience. Yet if deviations from what it means to an individual to be healthy are cues for the occurrence of an illness (as in Leventhal's self-regulatory model), then the two must at the very least have an impact upon each other, although exactly how and why is not immediately clear.

Tying It All Together? Subjective Perceptions of Health Status

A fourth example of future research directions would be how *cognitive* representations of health and illness affect *subjective* perceptions of health status. A case has been made earlier in this chapter that individuals are best able to assess their own health, particularly when "health" is broadly defined, citing as evidence correlations between a single self-assessment of health question and more "objective" measures of health such as clinical ratings by physicians or health services use. In fact, there is compelling (and continually growing) evidence that this single

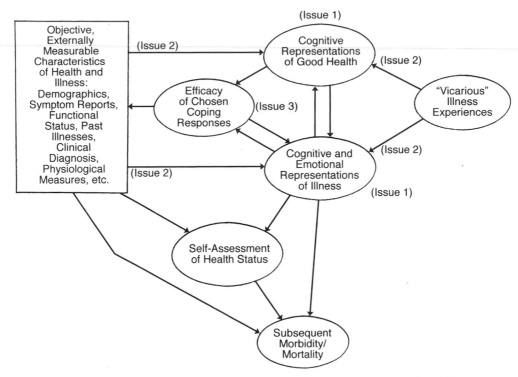

Figure 2. Directions for future research on cognitive representations of health and illness.

self-assessment question taps some *unique* aspect of an individual's health that is independent of any evidence that can be obtained by an outside observer—by a physician. As reviewed by Idler (1992, 1993), there are at least 13 longitudinal studies reporting that self-assessment of health has a significant effect on *mortality, controlling for a variety of more objective measures,* such as demographic factors known to be associated with mortality, self-reports of symptoms, functional disabilities, physician ratings, medication use, pain reports, and so on. The *meaning* of this relationship, however, is still unclear. Why is there some aspect of self-assessed health that cannot be explained by the most sophisticated measurement tools available to the medical and social sciences but that laypersons are aware of when assessing their own health?

More important, how is this unique, unexplained variance associated with mortality?

Figure 2 suggests one possible answer to these questions. This figure is meant to represent the dynamic interrelationships among seven conceptual variables: objective, externally observable measures of a person's health status; other "vicarious experiences" that person has had with illness; cognitive representations of health; cognitive and emotional representations of illness; mechanisms designed to cope with illness; self-assessment of health status; and subsequent morbidity/mortality. A partial answer to the lack of explanation of all of the real variance in self-assessed health status is that none of the studies in this literature has attempted to measure what it means to the individuals in the study to be healthy and what it means to them to be sick. Yet these meanings, these cognitive representations, are certainly available to the individuals when they are assessing their health and quite plausibly influence those assessments. Cognitive representations of health and illness are going to be influenced by the same sort of objective, externally measurable characteristics of prior and current health status that affect self-assessments of health status, as depicted in Figure 2. But any unique variance in self-assessed health status that can be explained by illness representations must come from some source *other than* those external factors that have typically been used in studies of self-assessed health status and mortality—such as what I have called "vicarious experience" with illness, or the emotional reactions that go hand in hand with cognitive representations of illness, or both.

How can this unique variance in self-assessed health status be related to mortality independent of all of the factors that have been measured and controlled for in this literature? Figure 2 suggests one possible reason: that the *actual* efficacy of the coping mechanisms adopted by the self-regulating individual is only partially measured by standard physiological responses. Such coping responses are often dictated by a physician; even when they are, however, it would be extremely rare if *all* coping responses adopted by an individual were suggested by a physician. Only the *patient* can assess the success of his or her own unique coping responses, which in turn feeds back into a cognitive and emotional representation of the illness, which could independently influence self-assessments of health status and might certainly be reflected in higher mortality and morbidity.

Figure 2 alone represents a huge research agenda. It also parenthetically illustrates the first three topics for future research mentioned above: the need for better measurement of health and illness representations (Issue 1), the need for a better understanding of how such representations develop (Issue 2), and the need for better theory and evidence explaining how (or whether) cognitive representations of health and illness

interact and mutually affect each other (Issue 3). Figure 2 suggests many more relationships than could possibly be examined in any one study, of course, and there are undoubtedly many important factors that have been omitted from the figure. As reviewed in this chapter, there is ample evidence that cognitive representations of health and illness are important factors in helping appreciate how people understand and try to maintain their own health and how they understand and try to cope with illness episodes. But there is far more that is not known, far more still to learn, than has been discovered already.

REFERENCES

Bauman, B. (1961). Diversities in conceptions of health and physical fitness. *Journal of Health and Human Behavior*, 2, 39–46.

Bauman, L. J., Cameron, L. D., Zimmerman, R. S., & Leventhal, H. (1989). Illness representations and matching labels with symptoms. *Health Psychology*, 8, 449–469.

Bishop, G. D. (1991). Understanding the understanding of illness: Lay disease representations. In J. A. Skelton & R. T. Croyle (Eds.), *The mental representation of health and illness*. New York: Springer-Verlag.

Bishop, G. D., Briede, C., Cavazos, L., Grotzinger, R., & McMahon, S. (1987). Processing illness information: The role of disease prototypes. *Basic and Applied Social Psychology*, 8, 21–43.

Bishop, G. D., & Converse, S. A. (1986). Illness representations: A prototype approach. *Health Psychology*, 5, 21–43.

Brown, W. M. (1985). On defining "disease." *Journal of Medicine and Philosophy*, 10, 311–328.

Cameron, L., Leventhal, E. A., & Leventhal, H. (1993). Symptom representations and affect as determinants of care seeking in a community-dwelling adult sample population. *Health Psychology*, 12, 171–179.

Carver, C. S. (1979). A cybernetic model of self-attention processes. *Journal of Personality and Social Psychology*, 37, 1251–1281.

Chrisman, N. J. (1977). The health seeking process: An approach to the natural history of illness. *Culture, Medicine and Psychiatry*, 1, 351–377.

Croyle, R. T., & Sande, G. N. (1988). Denial and confirmatory search: Paradoxical consequences of medical diagnosis. *Journal of Applied Social Psychology*, 18, 473–490.

D'Andrade, R. G. (1973). Cultural constructions of reality. In L. Nader & T. W. Maretzk (Eds.), *Culture, illness, and health*. (pp. 115–127). Washington, D.C.: American Anthropological Association.

D'Andrade, R. G., Quinn, N., Nerlove, S. B., & Romney, A. K. (1972). Categories of disease in American-English and Mexican-Spanish. In A. K. Romney, R. N. Shepard, & S. B. Nerlove (Eds.), *Multidimensional scaling: Theory and applications in the behavioral sciences: Vol. 2.* (pp. 9–54). New York: Seminar Press.

Dubos, R. (1965). *Man adapting.* New Haven, CT: Yale University Press.

Eisenberg, L. (1977). Disease and illness: Distinctions between professional and popular ideas of sickness. *Culture, Medicine, and Psychiatry, 1,* 9–23.

Epstein, A. M., Hall, J. A., Besdine, R., Cumella, E., Jr., Feldstein, M., McNeil, B. J., & Rowe, J. W. (1987). The emergence of geriatric assessment units: The "new technology of geriatrics." *Annals of Internal Medicine, 106,* 299.

Fiske, S. T., & Taylor, S. E. (1991). *Social cognition* (2nd ed.). New York: McGraw-Hill.

Guralnik, J. M. (1988). Assessment of health status in older persons. *Quality of Life and Cardiovascular Care, 4,* 151–155.

Hadlow, J., & Pitts, M. (1991). The understanding of common health terms by doctors, nurses and patients. *Social Science and Medicine, 32,* 193–196.

Hall, J. A., Epstein, A. M., & McNeil, B. J. (1989). Multidimensionality of health status in an elderly population: Construct validity of a measurement battery. *Medical Care, 27,* S168–S177.

Hayes-Bautista, D. E. (1978). Chicano patients and medical practitioners: A sociology of knowledge paradigm of lay-professional interaction. *Social Science and Medicine, 12,* 83–90.

Hays, R. D., & Stewart, A. L. (1990). The structure of self-reported health in chronic disease patients. *Psychological Assessment, 2,* 22–30.

Hulka, B. S., & Wheat, J. R. (1985). Patterns of utilization: The patient perspective. *Medical Care, 23,* 438–460.

Idler, E. L. (1979). Definitions of health and illness and medical sociology. *Social Science and Medicine, 13A,* 723–731.

Idler, E. L. (1992). Self-assessed health and mortality: A review of studies. In S. Maes, H. Leventhal, & M. Johnston (Eds.), *International review of health psychology* (pp. 33–54). New York: Wiley.

Idler, E. L. (1993). *Self-ratings of health: Mortality, morbidity, and meaning.* Paper presented at the Conference on Cognitive Aspects of Self-Reported Health Status, National Center for Health Statistics, Hyattsville, MD.

Kleinman, A. (1981). On illness meaning and clinical interpretations: Not "rational man," but a rational approach to man the sufferer/man the healer. *Culture, Medicine, and Psychiatry, 5,* 373–377.

Kleinman, A., Eisenberg, L., & Good, B. (1978). Clinical lessons from anthropologic and cross-cultural research. *Annals of Internal Medicine, 88,* 251–258.

Laffrey, S. C. (1986). Development of a health conception scale. *Research in Nursing and Health, 9,* 107–113.

Lau, R. R., Bernard, T. M., & Hartman, K. A. (1989). Further explorations of common-sense representations of common illnesses. *Health Psychology, 8,* 195–219.

Lau, R. R., & Hartman, K. A. (1983). Common sense representations of common illnesses. *Health Psychology, 2,* 167–185.

Lau, R. R., Leventhal, E. A., & Leventhal, H. (1992). *Policy implications of a self-regulatory model of response to health threats.* Paper presented at the 3rd SPSSI-sponsored conference, Social Science and Health Policy: Building Bridges between Research and Action. Bethesda, MD, March 4–6, 1992.

Lau, R. R., Quadrel, M. J., & Hartman, K. A. (1990). Development and change of young adults' preventive health beliefs and behavior: Influence from parents and peers. *Journal of Health and Social Behavior, 31,* 240–259.

Lau, R. R., Williams, H. S., Williams, L. C., Ware, J. E., Jr., & Brook, R. H. (1982). Psychosocial problems in chronically ill children. *Journal of Community Health, 7,* 250–261.

Leventhal, H., Diefenbach, M., & Leventhal, E. A. (1992). Illness cognition: Using common sense to understand treatment adherence and affect cognition interactions. *Cognitive Therapy and Research, 16,* 143–163.

Leventhal, H., Easterling, D. V., Coons, H., Luchterhand, C., & Love, R. R. (1986). Adaptation of chemotherapy treatments. In B. Andersen (Ed.), *Women with cancer.* (pp. 172–203). New York: Springer-Verlag.

Leventhal, H., Meyer., D., & Nerenz, D. (1980). The common sense representation of illness danger. In S. Rachman (Ed.), *Medical psychology: Vol. II* (pp. 7–30). New York: Pergamon Press.

Leventhal, H., Nerenz, D., & Strauss, A. (1982). Self-regulation and the mechanisms for symptom appraisal. In D. Mechanic (Ed.), *Monograph series in psychosocial epidemiology 3: Symptoms, illness behavior, and help-seeking* (pp. 55–86). New York: Neale Watson.

Marteau, T. M., Johnston, M., Baum, J. D., & Bloch, S. (1987). Goals of treatment in diabetes: A comparison of doctors and parents of children with diabetes. *Journal of Behavioral Medicine, 10,* 33–49.

Matthews, K. A., Siegel, J. M., Kuller, L. H., Thompson, M., & Varat, M. (1983). Determinants of decisions to seek medical treatment by patients with acute myocardial infarction symptoms. *Journal of Personality and Social Psychology, 44,* 1144–1156.

Mechanic, D. (1979). Correlates of physician utilization: Why do major multivariate studies of physician utilization find trivial psychosocial and organizational effects? *Journal of Health and Social Behavior, 20,* 387–396.

Meyer, D., Leventhal, H., & Gutmann, M. (1985). Common-sense models of illness: The example of hypertension. *Health Psychology, 4,* 115–135.

Millstein, S. G., & Irwin, C. E. (1987). Concepts of health and illness: Different constructs or variations of a theme? *Health Psychology, 6,* 515–524.

Moss-Morris, R., Petrie, K., & Weinman, J. (in press). Functioning in chronic fatigue syndrome: Do illness perceptions and coping play a regulatory role? *British Journal of Clinical Psychology*.

Natapoff, J. N. (1978). Children's views of health: A developmental study. *American Journal of Public Health*, *68*, 995-999.

Parsons, T. (1951). Illness and the role of the physician: A sociological perspective. *American Journal of Orthopsychiatry*, *21*, 452-460.

Parsons, T., & Fox, R. (1952). Illness, therapy, and the modern urban American family. *Journal of Social Issues*, *8*, 31-44.

Petrie, K., & Weinman, J. (1994). *The IPQ: A new method for assessing illness representations*. Paper presented at the Annual Meeting of the American Psychological Association, Los Angeles.

Pimm, T. J., Byron, M. A., Curson, D. M., & Weinman, J. (1994). *Personal illness models and the self management of arthritis*. Paper presented at the American College of Rheumatologists/Association of Rheumatology Health Professionals Annual Conference, Minneapolis, October.

Rosch, E. (1978). Principles of categorization. In E. Rosch & B. B. Lloyd (Eds.), *Cognition and categorization*. Hillsdale, NJ: Erlbaum.

Schlenger, W. E. (1976). A new framework for health. *Inquiry*, *13*, 207-214.

Smith, J. A. 1981. The idea of health: A philosophical inquiry.

Advances in Nursing Science, *3*(3), 43-50.

Stewart, A. L., & Ware, J. E., Jr. (Eds.). (1992). *Measuring functioning and well-being: The medical outcomes study approach*. Durham, NC: Duke University Press.

Ware, J. E., Jr. (1987). Standards for validating health measures: Definition and content. *Journal of Chronic Disease*, *40*, 473-480.

Ware, J. E., Jr., Brook, R. H., Davies, A. R., & Lohr, K. N. (1981). Choosing measures of health status for individuals in general populations. *American Journal of Public Health*, *71*, 620-625.

Ware, J. E., Jr., & Sherbourne, C. D. (1992). The MOS 36-Item Short-Form Health Survey SF-36. *Medical Care*, *30*, 473-483.

Weller, S. S. (1984). Cross cultural concepts of illness: Variables and validation. *American Anthropologist*, *86*, 341-351.

Williams, R. (1983). Concepts of health: An analysis of lay logic. *Sociology*, *17*, 185-205.

Wolinsky, F. D., & Arnold, C. L. (1988). A different perspective on health and health services utilization. *Annual Review of Gerontology and Geriatrics*, *8*, 71-101.

World Health Organization. (1947). *Constitution of the World Health Organization*. Geneva, Switzerland: Author Basic Documents.

Young, J. (1978). Illness categories and action strategies in a Tarascan town. *American Ethnologist*, *5*, 81-97.

4

The Health Belief Model and Health Behavior

Victor J. Strecher, Victoria L. Champion, and Irwin M. Rosenstock

INTRODUCTION

Since the 1950s, the health belief model (HBM) has been one of the most widely used conceptual frameworks in the health behavior field. The HBM has been used to explain change and maintenance of health-related behaviors, as a guiding framework for health behavior interventions, and as a guide in evaluating intervention programs. The HBM has been expanded, broken down into components, compared to other frameworks, and analyzed using a wide array of multivariate analytical techniques. It is likely that the HBM has been *misused* in the health behavior area more than most other conceptual frameworks have been used. This overuse is due in part

to the lack of specification of the relationships among the content, importance, and measurement of health beliefs (Ronis, 1992; Weinstein, 1993). The HBM has become to some extent a projective test that users interpret in ways that best match their concept of health behavior change. With broad concepts set into only roughly specified relationships, it is not suprising to see so many interpretations of the HBM.

Since the 1970s, however, more research has been conducted to specify measures of health beliefs and relationships among those beliefs. In addition, other models of health-related behaviors have received increasing attention; there are now new perspectives for explaining, predicting, and intervening in health-related behaviors. These new models have provided new insight into more dynamic relationships among health beliefs.

This chapter reviews the ideas embodied in the HBM that remain vital. It also examines other psychosocial constructs that further explain relationships within the HBM. It is not another review of HBM research findings, such as those that have been done in the two previous decades (Becker, 1974a; Janz & Becker, 1984). Even mid-1990s research continues to look at individual

Victor J. Strecher • University of Michigan Comprehensive Cancer Center, University of Michigan, Ann Arbor, Michigan 48109. **Victoria L. Champion** • School of Nursing, Indiana University, Indianapolis, Indiana 46202-5117. **Irwin M. Rosenstock** • College of Health and Human Services, California State University (Emeritus), Long Beach, California 90801.

Handbook of Health Behavior Research I: Personal and Social Determinants, edited by David S. Gochman. Plenum Press, New York, 1997.

health beliefs, placing them in multivariate analyses and looking at their predictive qualities. This type of analysis adds little to the specificity of measurement or the relationships among health beliefs. Instead, this chapter focuses on three aspects of the HBM: measurement of HBM constructs, the relationships among HBM constructs, and how to use the HBM for real problems in field situations.

The chapter begins by describing the origins of the HBM and its place in psychosocial theory. It then discusses in some detail issues related to the measurement of and relationships among HBM constructs, areas that have received only minimal attention. The chapter then discusses how the HBM can be used to explain and intervene in AIDS-related behavior and in addictive behaviors. These examples are used because they represent two very different, behaviorally based public health problems in our society. Finally, the chapter offers recommendations for researchers and journal reviewers.

ORIGINS OF THE HEALTH BELIEF MODEL

The health belief model was initially developed in the 1950s by a group of social psychologists in the U.S. Public Health Service in an effort to explain the widespread failure of people to participate in programs to prevent or to detect disease (Hochbaum, 1958; Rosenstock, 1966). Later, the model was extended to apply to people's responses to symptoms (Kirscht, 1974) and to their behavior in response to diagnosed illness, particularly compliance with medical regimens (Becker, 1974b). Although the model evolved gradually in response to very practical programmatic concerns to be described below, its basis in psychological theory is provided as an aid to understanding its rationale as well as its strengths and weaknesses.

During the early 1950s, academic social psychology was engaged in developing an approach to understanding behavior that grew out of a confluence of learning theories derived from two major sources: stimulus–response (S–R) theory (Hull, 1943; Thorndike, 1898; Watson, 1925) and cognitive theory (Kohler, 1925; Lewin, 1935, 1936, 1951; Lewin, Dembo, Festinger, & Sears, 1944; Tolman, 1932). S–R theory itself represents a marriage of classic conditioning theory (Pavlov, 1927) and instrumental conditioning theory (Thorndike, 1898).

In simple terms, S–R theorists believe that learning results from events (termed *reinforcements*) that reduce physiological drives that activate behavior. In the case of punishment, behavior that avoids punishment is learned because it reduces the tension set up by the punishment. The concept of drive reduction, however, is not necessary to S–R theory. Skinner (1938) formulated the widely accepted hypothesis that the frequency of a behavior is determined by its consequences (or reinforcements). For Skinner, the mere temporal association between a behavior and an immediately following reward is sufficient to increase the probability that the behavior will be repeated. Such behaviors are termed *operants*; they operate on the environment to bring about changes that result in reward or reinforcement. In this view, no mentalistic concepts such as "reasoning" or "thinking" are required to explain behavior.

Cognitive theorists emphasize the role of subjective hypotheses or expectations held by the subject (e.g., Lewin et al., 1944). In this perspective, behavior is a function of the subjective *value* of an outcome and of the subjective probability, or *expectation*, that a particular action will achieve that outcome. Such formulations are generally termed *value–expectancy* theories. Mental processes such as thinking, reasoning, hypothesizing, and expecting are critical components of all cognitive theories. Cognitive theorists, along with behaviorists, believe that reinforcements, or consequences of behavior, are important. For cognitive theorists, however, reinforcements operate by influencing expectations (or hypotheses) regarding the situation, rather than by influencing behavior directly (Bandura, 1977).

The HBM is a value–expectancy theory. When value–expectancy concepts were gradually reformulated in the context of health-related behavior, the translations were as follows: (1) the desire to avoid illness or to get well (value) and (2) the belief that a specific health action available to a person would prevent (or ameliorate) illness (expectation). The expectancy was further delineated in terms of the individual's estimate of personal susceptibility to and severity of an illness and of the likelihood of being able to reduce that threat through personal action.

The development of the HBM grew out of real concerns with the limited success of various programs of the Public Health Service in the 1950s. One such early example was the failure of large numbers of eligible adults to participate in tuberculosis screening programs provided at no charge and in mobile X-ray units conveniently located in various neighborhoods. The program operators were concerned with identifying those factors that were facilitating or inhibiting participation.

Beginning in 1952, Hochbaum (1958) studied probability samples of more than 1200 adults in three cities that had conducted recent TB screening programs in mobile X-ray units. He assessed their "readiness" to obtain X rays, which included their beliefs that they were susceptible to TB and their beliefs in the personal benefits of early detection. Perceived susceptibility to TB itself comprised two elements: (1) the respondents' beliefs about whether contracting TB was a realistic (not merely a mathematical) possibility for them personally and (2) the extent to which they accepted the fact that one might have TB in the absence of any symptoms.

The measure of perceived personal benefits of early detection also included two elements: whether respondents believed that X rays could detect tuberculosis prior to the appearance of symptoms and whether they believed that early detection and treatment would improve the prognosis. For the group of persons that exhibited both beliefs, i.e., belief in their own susceptibility to TB and the belief that overall benefits

would accrue from early detection, 82% had had at least one voluntary chest X ray during a specified period preceding the interview. Of the group exhibiting neither of these beliefs, only 21% had obtained a voluntary X ray during the criterion period. In short, 4 of 5 people who exhibited both beliefs (susceptibility and benefits) took the predicted action, while 4 of 5 people who accepted neither of the beliefs had not taken the action. Hochbaum thus demonstrated with considerable precision that a particular action to screen for a disease was strongly associated with the two interacting variables—perceived susceptibility and perceived benefits.

Hochbaum also thought that the readiness to take action (perceived susceptibility and perceived benefits) could be potentiated only by other factors, particularly by "cues" to instigate action, such as bodily events, or by environmental events, such as media publicity. He did not, however, study the role of cues empirically. Indeed, while the concept of cues as a trigger mechanism is appealing, it has been most difficult to study in explanatory surveys; a cue can be as fleeting as a sneeze or the barely conscious perception of a poster.

COMPONENTS OF THE HEALTH BELIEF MODEL

Over the years since Hochbaum's survey, many investigations have helped to expand and clarify the health belief model and to extend it beyond screening behaviors to include all preventive actions to illness behaviors and to sick role behavior (see the summaries in Becker, 1974b; Janz & Becker, 1984; Kirscht, 1974). In general, it is now believed that individuals will take action to ward off, to screen for, or to control ill-health conditions if they regard themselves as susceptible to the condition, if they believe it to have potentially serious consequences, if they believe that a course of action available to them would be beneficial in reducing either their susceptibility to or the severity of the condition, and if they believe that the anticipated barriers to (or costs of) taking the action are outweighed by its benefits. The definitions and commentary that follow specify the key variables in greater detail.

Perceived Susceptibility. This dimension refers to one's subjective perception of the risk of contracting an illness. In the case of medically established illness, the dimension has been reformulated to include acceptance of the diagnosis, personal estimates of resusceptibility, and susceptibility to illness in general.

Perceived Severity. Feelings concerning the seriousness of contracting an illness or of leaving it untreated include evaluations of both medical and clinical consequences (e.g., death, disability, and pain) and possible social consequences (such as effects of the conditions on work, family life, and social relations). The combination of perceived susceptibility and severity has come to be labeled *perceived threat.*

Perceived Benefits. While acceptance of personal susceptibility to a condition that is also believed to be serious (perceived threat) produces a force leading to behavior, the particular course of action taken depends upon beliefs regarding the effectiveness of the various available actions in reducing the disease threat, termed the *perceived benefits* of taking health action. Other factors include non-health-related benefits (e.g., quitting smoking to save money, getting a mammogram to please a family member). Thus, an individual who exhibits an optimal (high) level of beliefs in susceptibility and severity would not be expected to accept any recommended health action unless that action was perceived as potentially efficacious.

Perceived Barriers. The potential negative aspects of a particular health action, or the perceived barriers, may act as impediments to undertaking the recommended behavior. A nonconscious cost-benefit analysis occurs wherein the individual weighs the expected effectiveness of the action against perceptions that it may be expensive, dangerous (having negative side effects or iatrogenic outcomes), unpleasant (painful, difficult, upsetting), inconvenient, time-consuming, and so forth. Thus, in the words of Rosenstock (1974, p. 332), "The combined levels of susceptibility and severity provided the energy or force to act and the perception of benefits (less barriers) provided a preferred path of action."

Cues to Action. In various early formulations of the HBM, the concept of cues that trigger action were discussed. These cues may ultimately prove to be important, but they have not been systematically studied.

Other Variables. Diverse demographic, sociopsychological, and structural variables may affect the individual's perceptions and thus indirectly influence health-related behavior. Specifically, sociodemographic factors, particularly educational attainment, are believed to have an indirect effect on behavior by influencing the perception of susceptibility, severity, benefits, and barriers.

Self-Efficacy. In 1977, Bandura introduced the concept of self-efficacy, or efficacy expectation, as distinct from outcome expectation (Bandura, 1977, 1986), which must be added to the HBM in order to increase its explanatory power (Rosenstock, Strecher, & Becker, 1988). Outcome expectation, defined as a person's estimate that a given behavior will lead to certain outcomes, is quite similar to the HBM concept of perceived benefits. Self-efficacy is defined as "the conviction that one can successfully execute the behavior required to produce the outcomes" (Bandura, 1977, p. 79). Lack of efficacy is viewed as a perceived barrier to taking a recommended health action.

It is not difficult to see why self-efficacy was never explicitly incorporated into early formulations of the HBM. The original focus of the early model was on circumscribed preventive actions, usually of a one-shot nature, such as accepting a screening test or an immunization—actions that generally were simple behaviors for most people to perform. Since it is likely that most prospective members of target groups for those programs had adequate self-efficacy for performing those simple behaviors, that dimension was not even recognized.

The situation is vastly different, however, in working with lifestyle behaviors requiring long-term changes. The problems involved in modifying lifelong habits concerning eating, drinking, exercising, smoking, and sexual practices are obviously far more difficult to surmount than are those for accepting a one-time immunization or a screening test. One must have a good deal of confidence that one can alter such behaviors before one can successfully change them. Thus, for behavior change to succeed, people must (as the original HBM theorizes) feel threatened by their current behavioral patterns (perceived susceptibility and severity) and believe that change of a specific kind will be beneficial by resulting in a valued outcome at acceptable cost, but they must also feel themselves competent (self-efficacious) to overcome perceived barriers to taking action. A growing body of literature supports the importance of self-efficacy in helping to account for initiation and maintenance of behavioral change (Bandura, 1986; Strecher, DeVellis, Becker, & Rosenstock, 1986).

The original HBM focused on cognitive variables. Efforts to change cognitions about health matters, however, have often involved attempts to arouse fear through threatening messages (Leventhal, 1970). According to protection motivation theory (Rogers, 1975), the most persuasive communications are those that arouse fear while enhancing perceptions, central to the HBM, of the severity of an event, the likelihood of exposure to that event, *and* the efficacy of responses to that threat. More recently, Rogers (1983) incorporated self-efficacy into his theory. This view of the joint role of fear and reassurance

in persuasive communications is generally accepted.

Summary. As a convenient way of summarizing the HBM components, the key variables are subsumed under three categories, which are summarized in Figure 1.

EVIDENCE FOR AND AGAINST THE HEALTH BELIEF MODEL

In 1974, *Health Education Monographs* devoted an entire issue to "The Health Belief Model and Personal Health Behavior" (Becker, 1974a). That monograph summarized findings from research on the HBM to understand why individuals did or did not engage in a wide variety of health-related actions. The monograph provided considerable support for the model in explaining behavior pertinent to prevention and behavior in response to symptoms or to diagnosed disease. During the decade following publication of the monograph, the HBM continued to be a major organizing framework for explaining and predicting acceptance of health and medical care recommendations. Accordingly, an updated critical review was made of HBM studies conducted between 1974 and 1984, which also combined the new results with earlier findings to permit an overall assessment of the model's performance (Janz & Becker, 1984). Space limitations do not permit more than a brief summary of the findings of the detailed reviews of 1974 and 1984; the interested reader should consult those sources for details.

Included in the 1984 review were such preventive health and screening behaviors as influenza inoculations, practice of breast self-examination, and attendance at screening programs for Tay-Sachs carrier status, high blood pressure, seat belt use, exercise, nutrition, smoking, visits to physicians for checkups, and fear of being apprehended while under the influence of alcohol. Sick role behaviors included compliance with

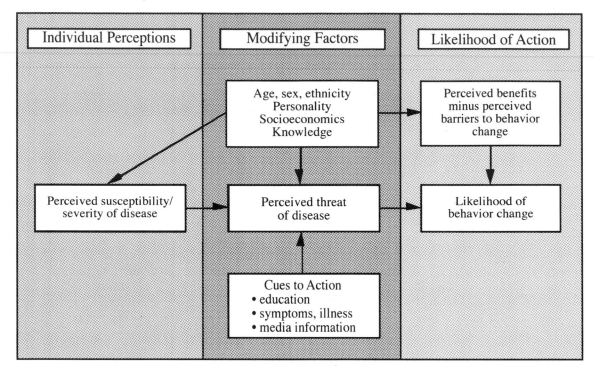

Figure 1. Summary of the key variables in the health belief model.

antihypertensive regimens, diabetic regimens, end-stage renal disease regimens, medication regimens for parents to give their children with otitis media, weight loss regimens, and medication regimens for parents to give to asthmatic children.

Summary results provided substantial empirical support for the HBM, with findings from prospective studies at least as favorable as those obtained from retrospective research. Perceived barriers was the most powerful single predictor of the HBM dimensions across all studies and behaviors. While both perceived susceptibility and perceived benefits were important overall, perceived susceptibility was a stronger predictor of preventive health behavior than sick role behavior, while the reverse was true for perceived benefits. Overall, perceived severity was the least powerful predictor; however, this dimension was strongly related to sick role behavior.

Researchers have frequently attempted to operationalize concepts related to the HBM. Although measures have been developed for specific studies, researchers have not always adequately addressed validity and reliability issues. In addition, many researchers have worked in isolation with few attempts to build on previous work. Given the futility of exploring a theory without simultaneously addressing measurement issues, the following section discusses some of the major attempts to conceptualize and operationalize HBM concepts. Issues related to measurement of the HBM are addressed, as well as suggestions for future studies.

FACTOR ANALYSES AND DEFINITIONS

The development of measures for health belief model concepts has spanned several decades. One of the early attempts was published by

Maiman, Becker, Kirscht, Haefner, and Drachman (1977), who specified constructs such as general health motivation, perceived susceptibility, perceived severity, perceived benefits, and perceived barriers. In this report, the general health concern index included a mother's concerns about her child's general health, her health behavior practices related to the health of the child, and her concern about her own health. Perceived susceptibility was defined as the mother's sense of the probability of a child's developing acute or chronic conditions. Perceived seriousness ratings referred to the same acute or chronic conditions. Perceived benefits included faith in the ability of the medical care system to cure conditions and the perceived benefits of weight loss (a dependent variable). Barriers consisted of likelihood of diet-related problems and perceived safety of diet. Reliability findings using consistency coefficients were reported for separate scales and for overall health concern, threat, and diet benefits. Regression analyses yielded results supporting the significance of general health concern, susceptibility, seriousness, and benefits in predicting weight loss. The authors of this study are to be applauded for their attempt to develop indices to measure HBM concepts; however, their measures require greater specificity and direction. For instance, perceived susceptibility and severity do not relate to a specific disease. Benefits are not behavior-specific and barriers refer only to diet-related problems.

A more comprehensive attempt at HBM construct validation was conducted by Cummings, Jette, and Rosenstock (1978). In this study, a multitrait, multimethod design was used to measure concepts of health interest, control, susceptibility, severity, benefits, and barriers. Although health interest and health locus of control related to general health matters, susceptibility, severity, benefits, and barriers were specific to influenza vaccination. Each construct was measured by fixed alternative multiple-choice scale, vignette, and Likert scale. The multimatrix, multimethod correlation matrix supported multiple choice and Likert formats, whereas measurement by vignette resulted in significantly lower correlations. In addition, discriminant validity was indicated by perceptions of benefits and barriers that differed substantially from those that pertained to susceptibility or severity. Because a convenience sample of 85 graduate students was used, however, generalization is limited. Nonetheless, these initial attempts at construct validation were important forerunners of later studies.

An important contribution to concept measurement of scales was added by Jette, Cummings, Brock, Phelps, and Naessens (1981), who questioned the lack of attention given to validity and reliability of measures. Three important questions were addressed by these investigators: distinctions among concepts, reliability of indices of concepts, and stability across samples. In this study, questionnaires were developed with items measuring susceptibility, seriousness, general health motivation, general health concerns, barriers to taking prescribed medication, health locus of control, trust in physicians, and health status. Questions were borrowed from previous studies in an appropriate attempt to build on previous work. Two independent probability samples were used, and factor analysis supported the structural similarity of some health belief measures across two independent samples. Reliability coefficients ranged from 0.31 to 0.72. Interpretable factors that emerged from both samples included general health threat, perceived barriers to taking medication, perceived severity, perceived susceptibility, health locus of control, trust in physician, and concern about general health. Caution was recommended in interpreting findings, since general and specific questionnaire items were mixed in the same index.

Another factor analysis was used to test the validity of HBM variables in 1987 (Cockburn, Fahey, & Sanson-Fisher, 1987). In this study, the HBM was used as the conceptual base for data collection, and the initial pool of items was drawn from literature, previous scales, and structured interview. Principal components analysis with varimax rotation was used to analyze the data. Results compared the a priori theoretical grouping of items with factor results. The first identified factor related to perceived severity of a condition and perceived susceptibility to illness in general, while the second factor included items related to perceived barriers of taking medication. Other factors included medical motivation (concern or trust in physician) and perceived control. Cronbach's alpha for the illness threat scale was an acceptable 0.82. Alpha coefficients for barriers, medical motivation, and control were low. Susceptibility and severity items were not differentiated by this factor analysis, nor were items related to benefits and barriers.

Eisen and Zellman (1986) developed a multi-item attitude scale that tested the concepts of susceptibility, seriousness, benefits, and barriers pertaining to contraceptive measures with 203 teenagers. Items were developed using the original conceptual definitions from the HBM and the adolescent sexuality literature. Items were grouped according to specific content area, and factor analysis was used to construct summed rating scales using principal components analysis with varimax rotation. Items were specific to sexual and contraceptive behaviors and scored on a 5-point Likert scale ranging from "strongly agree" to "strongly disagree." Internal consistency reliabilities ranged from 0.56 to 0.70. Results of factor analysis indicated five stable factors relating to HBM concepts: (1) susceptibility to pregnancy, (2) seriousness of pregnancy, (3) interpersonal benefits of contraceptive usage, (4) ideological/structural barriers to contraceptive usage, and (5) psychosocial/physical barriers to contraceptive usage. Four of the five HBM-based attitude scales (all but psychosocial barriers) were significant predictors of level of sexual and contraceptive knowledge.

HBM concepts also were measured in a Michigan blood pressure survey in which 32 questionnaire items measured general health-related beliefs (Weissfeld, Brock, Kirscht, & Hawthorne, 1987; Weissfeld, Kirscht, & Brock, 1990). Except for barriers, all health belief constructs were measured using several items. Exploratory and confirmatory factor analyses were used in

addition to reliability analysis. The primary purpose of the study was to examine consistency in results across demographic subgroups. Scales resulting from factor analysis included general health motivation, general health threat, susceptibility, severity, benefit of medical care, and self-help benefit. The inclusion of only one barrier item prevented scale analysis.

In an effort to correct generality problems in measuring concepts, Given, Given, Gallin, and Condon (1983) developed scales to measure beliefs representing basic HBM concepts, but with behaviors specific to diabetic patients. Given et al. (1983) voiced concern about the infrequent use of similar measures and the failure to report scale reliability. Items were developed using previous instruments related to HBM, review of diabetic patient education material, and in-depth interviews with a convenience sample of 25 patients. In all, 76 statements were identified to measure 12 concepts related to beliefs. All items except one were scored on a 5-point Likert scale ranging from "strongly agree" to "strongly disagree." One item, "How serious do you believe your diabetes to be?" was measured with ordinal-level seriousness responses. A total of 156 diabetic patients completed the scales. A confirmatory factor analysis was used to test the data fit to the proposed model. The fit was cross-validated by a second sample of 92 diabetic patients. Six scales were confirmed after scale refinement and were considered reproducible across the two samples of diabetic patients. The refined scales included control of effects of diabetes, barriers to following diet, social support for diet, barriers to taking medication, impact of job on therapy, and commitment to benefits of therapy. Alpha coefficients ranged from 0.68 to 0.87.

Hyman and Baker (1992) also found that few population-specific scales have been developed with adequate attention to measurement issues, thus necessitating the development of an instrument to measure HBM constructs as applied to mammography. A 39-item questionnaire with reverse-scored items using a 6-point Likert format measured the components of susceptibility, barriers, and benefits in their patients. Perceived seriousness was not incorporated because prior studies had found limited variance in this construct when subjects considered breast cancer. In one of the few attempts at content validity, Hyman and Baker had items checked by a researcher experienced with the HBM. This questionnaire was administered to two samples, one of 104 employees and another of 89 patients. Using a principal-components factor analysis, a three-factor structure was retained: benefits, barriers, and susceptibility. Items with low factor loading were discarded, leaving 7 for the benefit scale, 10 for the barrier scale, and 5 for the susceptibility scale. Intercorrelations among the total scores were low. Using known group comparisons for validity, t-tests comparing constructs were significant between those seeking mammography and those with other health conditions. Little information was given, however, on the advisability of comparing these two groups. In correlating the scales with recent mammography use, susceptibility items correlated at 0.25 and 0.22, benefits at 0.14 and 0.17, and barriers at 0.08 and 0.15. Alpha coefficients ranged from 0.60 to 0.83, while test–retest reliabilities ranged from 0.49 to 0.69.

Using LISREL analysis to test HBM concepts, Ronis and Harel (1989) reported on a survey of 619 Detroit-area women. The four concepts of susceptibility, seriousness, benefits, and barriers were measured, with the focus being breast self-examination (BSE) and clinical breast examination (CBE). Separate sets of questions addressed barriers to breast cancer screening when breast cancer is treated late as opposed to early. Ronis and Harel identified an additional dimension of severity, noting that differences in perception of severity depend upon whether the condition is treated early or late. For instance, a condition like breast cancer has less serious consequences if treated early; therefore, perceptions of benefits to breast cancer screening might be different depending upon whether the cancer is at an early or a late stage. Conceptually, Ronis and Harel (1989) believed that perceived benefit is dependent upon perceived susceptibility and two components of perceived severity: severity given inaction and severity given action. The dependent behavioral variables for this study were frequency of BSE and frequency of obtaining CBE. Five independent constructs were identified: health beliefs related to benefits of BSE, cost of BSE, severity of outcome given delay of treatment, severity of outcome given prompt treatment, and beliefs about personal susceptibility.

As a first step in this study, confirmatory factor analysis with LISREL was used to test a refined measurement model for BSE and CBE. The second-stage analyses involved testing causal relationships among the constructs by fitting path models to the data. As an outcome, severity was further broken into: (1) clinical problems with discovering breast cancer late, (2) clinical problems with discovering breast cancer early, (3) social problems with discovering breast cancer late, and (4) social problems with discovering breast cancer early. Clinical problems with discovering breast cancer late were positively related to benefit, as anticipated. High severity when detected early was inversely related to benefits and had effects on BSE only through benefits. Benefits did not mediate the effects of susceptibility on behavior; rather, susceptibility had direct effects. Susceptibility also did not interact with severity, contrary to suggestions by Becker (1974a,b). Perceived cost (barriers) was a better predictor of behavior than other constructs. Since severity functioned through benefits, the only direct effects on behavior were susceptibility, benefits, and barriers. This approach to looking at HBM variables may explain the lack of significance in previous studies of perceived severity.

In a similar attempt to use the HBM with more complicated measurement strategies, Stein, Fox, Murata, and Morisky (1992) examined the role of health beliefs and screening mammography among a community-based sample of 1057 women over the age of 35. Perceived susceptibility, barriers, benefits, cues to action, prior mammography, and future intentions were measured. Items were developed for each of these constructs and were subjected to confirmatory factor analysis. A path model between predictor and outcome variables was then assessed. Perceived susceptibility and barriers were significant, with physician communication (viewed as a cue to action) being the most important as a predictor of both prior mammography and future intentions. Indirect paths were found among some of the HBM variables, as well as among cues to action, socioeconomic status, and HBM variables.

Bond, Aiken, and Somerville (1992) reported on developing scales to measure HBM concepts in adolescents with insulin-dependent diabetes. Although the sample size was small ($N = 56$), factor analysis confirmed the concepts and a more thorough measurement of HBM variables resulted. Initially, health motivation, perceived susceptibility, perceived severity, perceived benefits, perceived barriers, and cues to action were developed. Between 4 and 9 items were identified for each scale. Any subscale with an alpha coefficient of less than 0.6 was deleted from the measurement model. The general health motivation scale was deleted because of an alpha coefficient of 0.35. A single threat measure was constructed from severity and susceptibility items, and a second construct was composed of benefits minus costs. In addition, a single indicator measured perceived cues. The measured threat and benefits minus cost scales exhibited adequate internal consistency coefficients, and testing the model with summed scales resulted in the best fit being obtained by using threat as one construct and benefits minus cost as a separate construct. HBM components were associated with questionnaire measures of compliance and with diabetic management assessment score. Cues were also associated with adherence. When threat was low, a positive effect for benefits minus cost was observed, suggesting that high threat with chronic disease may diminish the impact of perceived benefits of the medical regimen. The interaction of threat with benefits suggested, as did the work of Ronis and Harel (1989),

a need to modify the HBM for application to chronic long-term diseases.

Tiedje, Kingry, and Stommel (1992) developed an instrument to measure HBM constructs related to health behaviors during pregnancy. Focus groups, literature review, and consultation with an HBM expert were used to generate items to measure perceived susceptibility, perceived seriousness, perceived benefits, and perceived barriers. A total of 127 women were tested, and data were analyzed using confirmatory factor analysis. As an outcome of the factor analysis loading, a scale measuring susceptibility and seriousness was developed. A separate benefits and barriers scale for prenatal care was developed, as well as a susceptibility–seriousness scale and a benefits–barriers scale related to drinking. Similar scales were developed for nutrition and smoking, each of which included behavior–specific items. Reliability analyses for each of the subscales were conducted. Results suggested a three-factor solution with susceptibility and seriousness combining on one scale, benefits on a second, and barriers on a third. Only two subscales could be distinguished with respect to smoking. For smoking, a scale combining susceptibility, seriousness, and benefits was developed. Results from this study also demonstrated the utility of combining susceptibility and seriousness into one construct and even suggested that differences between susceptibility and seriousness are artificial. Barriers stood consistently as a singular construct across all behaviors.

Hurley (1990) described a process used to evaluate the HBM scale in relation to diabetes. An original diabetes scale from Given et al. (1983) was used to modify and validate an HBM scale for individuals with diabetes. Hurley (1990) described the necessity of assessing content validity prior to actual testing. A sample of 269 middle-aged adults was used for three phases of data collection: (1) an outpatient pilot, (2) an inpatient pilot, and (3) a prospective study. Reliability estimates were completed with pilot and prospective data. Construct validity was tested by factor analyses. Criterion validity was assessed by comparing relationships between scale scores and external variables. Three significant factors emerged: barriers, benefits, and seriousness.

Champion (1984) developed an instrument to measure the HBM concepts of susceptibility, seriousness, benefits, barriers, and health motivation. She included 20–24 items for each concept, all of which were based on past literature. Content validity was established by submitting items to judges who were familiar with HBM constructs. Construct validity as well as internal consistency and test–retest reliability were computed, with resulting consistency reliabilities of 0.61–0.78 and test–retest reliabilities of 0.47–0.46. A revision of this scale reported in 1993 again used a process of assessing content validity, construct validity, and test–retest reliability (Champion, 1993). An additional scale for self-efficacy or confidence related to BSE was added. Exploratory factor analysis showed five factors with eigen values ranging from 2.11 to 7.69. Except for one item on each of the confidence, seriousness, health motivation, and barrier scales, all items loaded at 0.45 or above. Predictive validity was established through the bivariate correlation between subscales and BSE. Multiple regression of BSE behavior on subscales accounted for 24% of the variance. The Cronbach alpha for scales ranged from 0.80 to 0.93, with test–retest reliability ranging from 0.45 to 0.70.

Others have revised Champion's scale for use with different health behaviors. Kim, Horan, Gendler, and Patel (1991) developed an osteoporosis health belief scale using the Champion (1984) scale. Items were reflective of susceptibility, seriousness, and health motivation, with separate items for benefits of calcium or exercise and barriers of calcium and exercise scales. Consistent with the theoretical expectation, Kim et al. (1991) developed behavior-specific measures resulting in two scales for benefits and barriers. Data collection took place over a 3-month period and used a sample of 150 elderly individuals. Items were subjected to factor analysis with varimax rotation, resulting in a six-factor solution consisting of susceptibility, seriousness, health

motivation, benefits and barriers related to calcium, and benefits and barriers related to exercise; for the barriers concept, items for exercise and calcium loaded on the same factor. Because the instrument was intended for use in determining relationships for calcium intake and exercise as distinct behaviors, 35 items were separated into two scales. Each scale shared three common subscales composed of 15 items that measured susceptibility, seriousness, and health motivation, and several unique items related separately to calcium or exercise. Internal consistencies ranged from 0.61 to 0.80, with factor results supporting scale independence. Discriminant analysis was used to test the relationship between HBM variables with calcium and exercise, resulting in barriers and health motivation being significant predictors.

Russell (1991) used the original Champion (1984) HBM scales to assess benefits and barriers to maternal behavior for childhood injury prevention. Content validation as well as internal consistency and validity testing were completed, yielding scales with Cronbach alphas ranging from 0.83 to 0.98 and significant test–retest correlations. Concurrent validity assessment demonstrated that scales were significantly correlated with maternal injury prevention behavior.

Hahn (1993) used a convenience sample of 200 parents or primary caregivers of preschool children to develop scales related to the HBM constructs initially developed by Champion (1984). Scales included susceptibility, seriousness, barriers, benefits, control, and health motivation, with the number of items per construct ranging from 4 to 9. Cronbach alphas for scales ranged from 0.79 to 0.87. To test validity, the relationship between scales and parental health behaviors was assessed. Susceptibility, seriousness, and health motivation differed significantly according to whether they related to tobacco or illicit drug use. In addition, there were significant differences between smokers and nonsmokers for susceptibility and health motivation scales.

Summarizing these studies, it is clear that one of the most important deficits in the research on the HBM has been inconsistent measurement of HBM concepts. Although some of the more thorough attempts at measuring HBM concepts have been briefly reviewed in this chapter, it is readily apparent that almost every study used different ways to operationalize constructs. In addition, the vast majority of the reports in the literature have failed to establish validity or reliability prior to model testing. Another concern related to HBM variables is the confusion about the relationships among these variables. Some researchers have attempted to establish each of the four major concepts — susceptibility, seriousness, benefits, and barriers — as independent; others have tried multiplicative approaches. Most recently, investigators have been most successful when looking at models that measure direct as well as indirect effects of variables on behavior.

Critics of the HBM have stressed the small amounts of variance explained in reported studies. As indicated by Rosenstock (1991), the HBM is a psychosocial model and as such is limited in predicting individual behaviors. This limitation may be especially important when addressing entrenched behaviors with physiological components such as smoking, drug addiction, or alcohol use.

Another problem related to measurement of constructs has been the inconsistency in specific versus general item development. Ajzen and Timko (1986) state that predictability of health behaviors is contingent upon measurement correspondence. Researchers have attempted at times to use items such as perceived susceptibility to illness in general and have tried to predict behaviors in response to a specific condition. These attempts led to inconsistent results. Researchers also have attempted to mix general and specific measures on the same scales.

The nature of the condition is also an issue that should receive further attention in HBM research. Ronis and Harel (1989) attempted to look at susceptibility and severity separated for early- and late-stage breast cancer. Indeed, beliefs about HBM variables might be contingent upon whether the women believed a behavior had already occurred. For instance, a person might rate severity of breast cancer lower if she was a consistent user of mammography and believed that any breast cancer, if it did occur, would be at a curable stage. Most attempts to measure HBM variables have not considered this issue. Explicit instructions might increase measurement specificity for the HBM.

Another issue pertains to the relationships among variables. In some studies, correlations between outcome variables and HBM predictor variables may be hidden by the indirect relationships among variables. For example, the Ronis and Harel (1989) study highlighted complex relationships among HBM constructs. More attention needs to be paid to complex, indirect relationships among HBM constructs. In other words, the HBM should be examined like a model — not like a simple collection of variables.

One final issue related to measurement of the HBM constructs is that of temporality. Most studies have used cross-sectional data with no attempt to determine whether attitudes did in fact precede behavior. If attitudes were measured currently and behavior was retrospectively recalled, any belief–behavior relationships might well be spurious. Janz and Becker (1984) addressed this issue, recommending that cross-sectional studies be eschewed in favor of predictive studies.

Given the current state of measurement of the HBM constructs, one question that surfaces is whether it is possible to develop general stem items for each of the relevant concepts that, with a few changes, can be made behavior-specific. Initial attempts at such development were reported by Champion (1993) and by subsequent researchers who modified initial scales for different behaviors. This approach seemed more feasible when measuring the constructs for severity, susceptibility, and general health motivation, as opposed to benefits or barriers. Benefits and barriers constructs may need to be more behavior-specific and may not as readily share item stems.

In addition, the relationship between theory and measurement cannot be underestimated. Measuring abstract concepts presents a clear challenge to social researchers, however. Consequently, it is imperative that researchers using the HBM be mindful of issues related to developing valid and reliable scales. Operationalizing constructs requires the researcher to be familiar with the theory as well as with the processes needed for operationalizing concepts relevant to measurement issues. One mistake often made in using theory to guide instrument development is the failure to recognize that the construct measuring the theory may be inconsistent with the theory. Any flaw in measurement procedures results in flaws in the conclusions about the theory. Adequate measures are necessary conditions for research.

Scale development takes a great deal of knowledge, planning, and work and is an ongoing, iterative process. Even when valid and reliable measures are used, these measures must be revalidated with each data collection. Validity and reliability are sample-specific and may change depending on sample characteristics. When testing theory, researchers need to seriously investigate measurement issues. Measurement is an integral part of theory development and a prerequisite to valid conclusions.

APPLICATIONS OF THE HEALTH BELIEF MODEL

Two examples of how the health belief model can be employed to better understand a health-related behavior are presented in the following section. These examples are included because (1) each represents an area of public health concern and (2) the factors that predict the two sets of quite different behaviors are complex and multifactorial. In both cases, the HBM provides a framework for better understanding the complexity of these behaviors.

AIDS-Protective Behaviors

Ideally, with AIDS-related behaviors as well as other health-related behaviors, one should ex-

amine the predictive utility of the total HBM, i.e., the likelihood that individuals with various *combinations* of health beliefs will engage in higher- or lower-risk AIDS preventive behaviors. For example, one would predict perceptions of susceptibility and severity to be associated largely with an *intention* to take action, similar to the predicted functions of attitudes in the theory of reasoned action (Ajzen & Fishbein, 1980). As Catania, Kegeles, and Cortes's (1990b) theoretical analysis notes, for individuals who objectively exhibit high-risk behaviors, perceived susceptibility is a factor required before commitment to changing these risky behaviors can occur. The HBM goes on to hypothesize that those committed to taking action would then assess the benefits of taking a recommended health action and the barriers to taking the action. If the benefits outweighed the barriers, the individual would be more likely to take the recommended health action.

Unfortunately, *none* of the research on the utility of the HBM in predicting AIDS-preventive behavior examined for this chapter analyzed the constructs in this manner. In fact, every study treated the constructs separately. Analyses that threw all health belief constructs into a multiple regression model did not test the HBM in the suggested manner. For example, among those with high perceived threat, perceptions of benefits and barriers would be more predictive of behavior change. Appropriate tests of this hypothesis would require analyses of subgroups (e.g., testing the effects of benefits and barriers only for those with high perceived threat) or multivariate analyses involving a carefully constructed series of interaction terms.

Perceived Threat

Reviewing research that examined associations between perceived susceptibility and AIDS-protective behavior yielded very mixed results. In a longitudinal study of gay men's AIDS-protective behavior, Aspinwall, Kemeny, Taylor, Schneider, and Dudley (1991) found decreases in numbers of sexual partners (anonymous and known) chiefly among seronegative men, who had earlier perceived themselves to be at increased risk of contracting HIV. Cross-sectional studies (e.g., Allard, 1989; Basen-Engquist, 1992; Hays, Kegeles, & Coates, 1990; Hingson, Strunin, Berlin, & Heeren, 1990) also have found significant susceptibility–behavior associations. Countering these findings are a number of longitudinal studies (e.g., McKusick, Coates, Morin, Pollack, & Hoff, 1990; Montgomery et al., 1989) and cross-sectional studies (e.g., Catania et al., 1990a; Walter et al., 1992).

Of particular interest is whether trends in a susceptibility–behavior association differed among higher-risk versus lower-risk groups, in cross-sectional versus longitudinal study designs, and in various methods of measuring susceptibility. This analysis found little to suggest a higher or lower susceptibility–behavior association among gay men, among the general adult population, or among adolescents. It also found no trend among longitudinal versus cross-sectional studies. It did find, however, variation in results by the methods used to measure susceptibility. A number of articles used a behavioral anchor in their susceptibility measures, e.g., asking the question "*If you do not practice safer sex*, how likely are you to become infected with the AIDS virus?" as opposed to simply "How likely are you to become infected with the AIDS virus?" Research by Ronis (1992) strongly supported the importance of asking susceptibility questions that are clearly conditional on action or inaction. Unconditional susceptibility measures can lead to a pattern of personalized interpretation—respondents who indicate that their risk of infection is great largely *because* they are not practicing safer sex.

Perceptions of AIDS severity must address the perceived costs of being HIV-positive and of having AIDS. As mentioned previously, perceived seriousness refers to personal evaluations of the probable biomedical, financial, and social consequences of contracting HIV and having AIDS. Ostensibly, one would think that items reflecting this construct would focus on the life changes involved in an increasingly debilitative disease

such as AIDS, the interpersonal effects, the agony of the dying process, and the perceived impact of one's death. Then, as previously stated, this measure should interact with the perception of susceptibility to form a perception of AIDS threat.

Some might argue that asking about AIDS severity would be a waste of respondent time—everyone would report that AIDS is an extremely severe disease. Unfortunately, most measures in the research literature did not focus directly on these elements of AIDS severity. Items thought to be most closely related to perceived severity included a general measure of AIDS seriousness, "How serious a health problem is AIDS?" (Aspinwall et al., 1991), and a measure of the likelihood of dying from AIDS (Hingson et al., 1990). These measures, however, still did not directly address personal evaluations of the probable biomedical, financial, and social consequences of contracting HIV and having AIDS. Would most respondents report that contracting HIV and AIDS, and dying from AIDS, would be severe? This would seem the most likely response; however, fear of death or the perception of death as being severe may not always obtain for high-risk individuals. It is not unreasonable to view drug abuse or even cigarette smoking in some individuals as a self-perceived form of slow suicide. In a study of HIV-risk taking among young men, Hays et al. (1990) cited a poignant statement of an HIV-positive respondent: "It seems like nobody cares if I die anyway" (p. 905). Consideration must also be given to the possibility that the severity of the fear of rejection and not being loved may exceed the perceived severity of the infection and thus lead to unsafe sexual practices. These comments speak to the need for sophisticated measurement of perceived severity of all aspects of AIDS, including dying from the disease.

Most measures of AIDS severity focused on the anxiety that AIDS produced. For example, the personal severity measure used by Montgomery et al. (1989) in a study of gay men in Chicago concerned the "stress of AIDS." Anxiety and worry could certainly be found in those who perceive AIDS as a serious disease. Anxiety from

AIDS is likely to be low, however, unless an individual also feels *susceptible* to the risk of acquiring AIDS. In other words, anxiety is not just a function of perceived severity.

Studies using AIDS anxiety measures have found mixed associations with AIDS-related behaviors. For example, Montgomery and colleagues found perceived severity to be the most consistent longitudinal predictor of AIDS-protective behavior changes out of all HBM constructs. Allard (1989) found cross-sectional associations between severity measures (many of which were related to AIDS anxiety) and AIDS-protective behaviors. Walter et al. (1992) and Catania et al. (1990a), however, also in cross-sectional studies, did not find such associations. Catania et al. (1990a) found that individuals getting tested for HIV who had greater AIDS anxiety were *less* likely to return for their test results.

Perceived Benefits and Barriers

For any level of perceived threat of AIDS beyond a threshold, the HBM would hypothesize that AIDS-protective behavior decisions become largely a function of perceptions of benefits minus perceived barriers to behavior change. If the perception of AIDS threat is not high, strong perceived benefits of AIDS-protective behavior may still influence behavior change. For example, a person who uses condoms because his partner prefers them may adopt and maintain condom-use behavior regardless of his perception of AIDS threat. Although there are perceived benefits in this example, they are not directly related to AIDS-protective behavior, but rather to the benefits of pleasing one's partner. If the perceptions of AIDS threat and benefits are not high, it is not likely that low perceived barriers would necessarily influence AIDS-preventive behavior.

Of the possible benefits, "response efficacy," or the perception that adopting and maintaining AIDS-preventive behaviors will reduce AIDS risk, is one of the most commonly researched. Measures of response efficacy (e.g., Allard, 1989; Aspinwall et al., 1991; Hingson et al., 1990) have

been associated with AIDS-preventive behaviors in cross-sectional and longitudinal studies. The HBM would hypothesize that these associations would be even stronger among those reporting strong perceptions of AIDS threat. This hypothesis is consistent with Catania et al.'s (1990b) theoretical analysis suggesting that response efficacy will be most relevant once a decision to commit to changing sexual behaviors has been made.

Other benefits of AIDS-preventive behaviors have been examined by Catania et al. (1991). Positive personal feelings resulting from condom use and positive regard from the respondent's sex partner for condom use distinguished men who always used condoms from those who did not. A nearly significant trend ($p < 0.06$) was found for the effects of condom use on sexual pleasure. The perception that condoms enhanced sexual pleasure distinguished men who always used condoms from those who did not use condoms.

In Catania et al. (1991), as well as others, condom use is generally perceived as a barrier to sexual pleasure. Relationships between perceived barriers and AIDS-preventive behaviors have been mixed across both longitudinal and cross-sectional studies. Unfortunately, a number of the studies reviewed included questionable measures of barriers. Montgomery et al. (1989), for example, used "barriers" measures that included knowledge of the virus and modes of transmission, whether the respondent was ever paid for sex, and belief in a vaccine or a potential cure; the study did not include lack of sexual enjoyment as a barrier. These measures were unrelated to subsequent AIDS-protective behavior changes. Another study with negative results (Allard, 1989) used only two "barriers to [AIDS] treatment" items—not at all relevant to preventive practices.

Studies using more relevant barriers measures tended to find results in the expected direction. Basen-Engquist (1992) found strong associations in the expected direction between perceived barriers and both intention to use condoms and actual condom use. Seven barriers were aggregated to form a single scale; examples of barriers included "embarrassment caused by practicing safer sex, moral implications of condom use, and satisfaction involved in practicing safer sex." Aspinwall et al. (1991) used barrier measures that included temptation to engage in sex with numerous partners and importance and difficulty of refraining from doing so. This study found that gay men without primary partners who reported strong barriers reported higher numbers of anonymous sexual partners at follow-up. Baseline reports of strong barriers to changing unprotected receptive anal intercourse also predicted subsequent unprotected receptive anal intercourse with partners whose HIV status was unknown.

As these studies suggest, the concepts of benefits and barriers are rather open-ended and can include wide domains of factors, including emotional, physical, and social. One of the most important barriers to engaging in AIDS-preventive behaviors may be lack of self-efficacy, which, as noted earlier, has been suggested for inclusion in the HBM.

Researchers must continue efforts to determine just which benefits and barriers exist and which benefits and barriers have the greatest influence on AIDS-preventive behaviors. As with the perceived susceptibility construct, this review found that the adequacy of the benefits and barriers measures used, judged by their face validity, often were the most important predictors of whether a positive or negative association with AIDS-protective behavior was found. Unfortunately, most studies reviewed failed to specify the actual measures used.

Cues to Action

According to the HBM, if perceived AIDS threat is high and perceived benefits outweigh perceived barriers, a cue to action can prompt or trigger an individual to adopt and maintain AIDS-preventive behavior, in effect stimulating the belief–action link. Again, it is suggested that the cue to action construct be analyzed in concert with perceived threat. Cues to action are hypothesized to be more strongly associated with AIDS-preventive behavior among individuals who have a high perceived AIDS threat. None of the studies reviewed analyzed the cue to action construct for the strength of this association.

As indicated earlier, the cue to action construct is, in general and in the area of AIDS prevention, the least-studied construct in the HBM. This neglect is unfortunate, since a good deal of anecdotal evidence supports the importance of brief though salient cues that stimulate a decision to act. Similar to the case of perceived barriers and benefits, it is important to determine what cues to action exist as well as their relative efficacy in influencing AIDS-preventive behaviors.

Cues to action were examined in the Hingson et al. (1990) and the Aspinwall et al. (1991) studies. Among a general population of adolescents, Hingson et al. asked the respondents whether they had read or heard about AIDS from media sources; whether they ever discussed AIDS with a family member, teacher, or physician; and whether they knew someone with AIDS. Having discussed AIDS with friends or with a physician was positively associated with condom use. Knowing someone with AIDS, however, was *negatively* associated with condom use. Aspinwall et al. (1991) asked how many close friends had AIDS-related complex (ARC), how many had AIDS, and how many had died of AIDS or ARC in the past year. A summed index of these potential cues to action did not predict AIDS-protective behavior changes. Of course, it is not known how many of these adolescents felt threatened by AIDS, and perceived threat is a necessary condition for events to serve as true cues to action.

Addictive Behaviors

Perceived Threat

Viewing perceived threat as the primary construct of the HBM may have attenuated its popularity in the addictive behavior fields. This decline in favor is a result of consistent findings that the vast majority of cigarette smokers and other addictive substance users already perceive a threat from their habit(s). The common thinking in this regard is that "smokers already perceive a health threat—you don't need to scare them any more." Field research (Strecher, Kreuter, & Kobrin, 1994) conducted in the University of North Carolina Health Communications Research Laboratory has found that patients who smoke are indeed more likely to perceive a heightened personal risk of heart attack, cancer, and stroke when compared with patients who do not smoke; however, a much larger proportion of smokers compared to nonsmokers tended to *underestimate* their actual risk of heart attack, cancer, and stroke (measured by Health Risk Appraisal). In other words, smokers do tend to perceive a health risk, but they underestimate the *magnitude* of their health risk.

These findings suggest that in clinical situations, perceived threat *relative to the patient's actual health threat* should be assessed. Smokers or other addictive substance abusers who perceive their threat as being moderately above average still may not have a realistic estimate of their risk. A realistic estimate of threat is necessary before the patient is likely to make a cognitive evaluation of the benefits of taking a recommended health action (i.e., quitting smoking) or of the barriers to taking the health action.

Perceived Benefits and Barriers

While acceptance of personal susceptibility to a condition that also poses a serious perceived threat produces a force that leads to behavior, the particular course of action that will be taken depends upon beliefs regarding the effectiveness of the various available actions in reducing the disease threat, termed the *perceived benefits* of taking health action. Thus, an individual exhibiting an optimal level of belief in susceptibility and severity would not be expected to accept any recommended health action unless that action was perceived as potentially efficacious.

Research in the Health Communications Research Laboratory among family practice patients (Strecher et al., 1994) included the measurement of perceived benefits and barriers among patients who smoke and among patients who may have alcohol problems (measured by the CAGE questionnaire). Perceived benefits of quitting smoking included health maintenance, encouragement from family and friends, and cost savings from not buying cigarettes. These benefits were seen in a number of United States studies (e.g., Ewing, 1984) and appear to encompass the vast majority of reasons for quitting. The perceived benefits of reducing alcohol consumption were very similar to those found among smokers. They included health improvement, taking greater control over their life, and setting a better example for their family.

In the Strecher et al. (1994) study and in the research of others, barriers to quitting smoking consistently included a fear of stress or anxiety when refraining from cigarettes, fear of significant weight gain (often "significant" can mean only a few pounds to a patient!), pressure from other smokers to relapse, and a general fear of relapse. Perceived barriers among patients with alcohol problems included fear of stress or anxiety when cutting back on alcohol and peer pressure from friends who drink. Another important barrier to many substance abusers is lack of self-efficacy.

Cues to Action

If perceived threat is high and perceived benefits outweigh perceived barriers, a cue to action can prompt or trigger an individual to take a particular health action, in effect stimulating the belief–action link. Cues to action may be internal (e.g., symptoms) or external (e.g., media information). As an example, for individuals already highly motivated to quit smoking, receiving strong advice from a physician to set an actual date to quit smoking may well serve as an external cue to take action.

RECOMMENDATIONS TO RESEARCHERS AND JOURNAL REVIEWERS

The following recommendations are offered for researchers and reviewers of manuscripts submitted for publication that examine health belief model variables:

1. Test the health belief model as a model or, at a minimum, as a combination of constructs—not as a collection of equally weighted variables operating simultaneously. It makes little sense to throw health belief variables into a multivariate analysis, select the "strongest swimmers," and claim that these are the factors on which to intervene. The following hypotheses could serve as a starting point for testing the health belief model as a model:

a. Perceived threat is a sequential function of perceived severity and perceived susceptibility. A state of high perceived severity is required before perceived susceptibility becomes a powerful predictor. Given this state of high perceived severity, perceived susceptibility will be a stronger predictor of intention to engage in health-related behaviors than of actual engagement in health-related behaviors.

b. Perceived benefits and barriers will be stronger predictors of behavior change when perceived threat is high than when it is low. Under conditions of low perceived threat, benefits of and barriers to engaging in health-related behavior will not be salient. The only exception to this condition may be that when certain benefits of the recommended behavior are perceived to be high (e.g., a partner's encouragement for safe sex), perceived threat may not need to be high.

c. Self-efficacy, a factor now included in the health belief model, will be a strong predictor of many health-related behaviors. Self-efficacy will be a particularly strong predictor of behaviors that require significant skills to perform.

d. Cues to action will have a greater influence on behavior in situations in which perceived threat is great. The cue to action construct is a little-studied phenomenon: Little is known about what cues to action exist or about their relative impact.

2. Specify the measures used to study belief constructs in publications. An important reason for variance in results between studies is due to large variations in the specific measures used. When the actual questions were included in the article or could be readily determined, a disconcertingly large proportion did not appear to be good indicators of HBM constructs.

3. Researchers should delay aggregating items that measure benefits, barriers, and cue to action into general constructs; such items are often unrelated to one another and have low interitem correlations. To the practitioner charged with creating programs that will contain health messages, analysis of single items can often offer more relevant information than a general grouped construct.

4. Include a behavioral anchor when measuring perceived susceptibility. For example, a behaviorally anchored question for AIDS-preventive behavior would ask "*If you do not practice safer sex*, how likely are you to become infected with the AIDS virus?" as opposed to "How likely are you to become infected with the AIDS virus?" Ronis (1992) found strong evidence for the importance of asking susceptibility questions that are conditional on action or inaction.

SUMMARY

This chapter has described both strengths and limitations of the health belief model as formulated to date. It is hoped that future theory-building or theory-testing research will direct efforts more toward strengthening the HBM where it is weak than toward repeating what has already been established. More work is needed on experimental interventions to modify health beliefs and health behavior than on surveys to reconfirm already established correlations. More work is also needed to specify and measure factors that need to be added to the HBM to increase its predictive power. The addition of self-efficacy to the traditional HBM should improve explanation and prediction, particularly in the area of lifestyle practices.

It is timely for professionals who are attempting to influence health-related behaviors to make use of the health belief variables, including self-efficacy, in their program planning, both in needs assessment and in program strategies. Programs to deal with a health problem should be based, in part, on knowledge of how many and which members of a target population feel susceptible to a particular health-related outcome, believe the health-related outcome to constitute a serious health problem, and believe that the threat of having the health-related outcome could be reduced by changing their behavior at an acceptable psychological cost. Moreover, health professionals should also assess the extent to which clients possess adequate self-efficacy to carry out the prescribed action(s), over a long period of time if necessary.

The collection of data on health beliefs, along with other data pertinent to the group or community setting, permits the planning of more effective programs than would otherwise be possible. Interventions can then be targeted to the specific needs identified by such an assessment, whether the problems to be dealt with are those of individual patients, of groups of clients, or of entire communities. In planning programs to influence the behavior of large groups of people for long periods of time, the role of the HBM (including self-efficacy) must be considered in context. Permanent changes in behavior can rarely be wrought solely by direct attacks on belief systems. Even more, when the behavior of large groups is the target, interventions at societal levels (e.g., social networks, work organizations, the physical environment, the legislature) along with interventions at the individual level will likely prove more effective than single-level interventions. It should never be forgotten, however, that a crucial way station on the road to improved health is in the beliefs and behavior of each of a number of individuals.

REFERENCES

Ajzen, I., & Fishbein, M. (1980). *Understanding attitudes and predicting behavior*. Englewood Cliffs, NJ: Prentice-Hall.

Ajzen, I., & Timko, C. (1986). Correspondence between health attitudes and behavior. *Basic and Applied Social Psychology*, 7(4), 259–276.

Allard, R. (1989). Beliefs about AIDS as determinants of preventive practices and of support for coercive measures. *American Journal of Public Health*, 79, 448–452.

Aspinwall, L., Kemeny, M., Taylor, S., Schneider, S., & Dudley, J. (1991). Psychosocial predictors of gay men's AIDS risk-reduction behavior. *Health Psychology*, 10(6), 432–444.

Bandura, A. (1977). Self-efficacy: Toward a unifying theory of behavior change. *Psychological Review*, 84, 191–215.

Bandura, A. (1986). *Social foundations of thought and action*. Englewood Cliffs, NJ: Prentice-Hall.

Basen-Engquist, K. (1992). Psychosocial predictors of "safer sex" behaviors in young adults. *AIDS Education & Preventions*, 4, 120–134.

Becker, M. H. (Ed.). (1974a). The health belief model and personal health behavior. *Health Education Monographs*, 2, 324–473.

Becker, M. H. (1974b). *The health belief model and personal health behavior*. Thorofare, NJ: Charles B. Slack.

Becker, M. H., & Maiman, L. A. (1980). Strategies for enhancing patient compliance. *Journal of Community Health*, 6, 113–135.

Bond, G. G., Aiken, L. S., & Somerville, S. C. (1992). The health belief model and adolescents with insulin-dependent diabetes mellitus. *Health Psychology*, 11(3), 190–198.

Catania, J., Coates, T., Kegeles, S., Fullilove, M., Peterson, J., Marin, B., Siegel, D., & Hulley, S. (1991). Condom use in multi-ethnic neighborhoods of San Francisco: The population-based AMEN (AIDS in Multi-Ethnic Neighborhoods) study. *American Journal of Public Health*, 182(2), 284–287.

Catania, J., Coates, T., Stall, R., Bye, L., Kegeles, S., Capell, F., Henne, J., McKusick, L., Morin, S., Turner, H., & Pollack, L. (1991). Changes in condom use among homosexual men in San Francisco. *Health Psychology*, 10(3), 190–199.

Catania, T., Kegeles, J., & Coates, T. (1990a). Psychosocial predictors of people who fail to return for their HIV test results. *AIDS*, 4(3), 261–262.

Catania, T., Kegeles, J., & Coates, T. (1990b). Towards an understanding of risk behavior: An AIDS risk reduction model (AARM). *Health Education Quarterly*, 17(1), 53–72.

Champion, V. L. (1984). Instrument development of health belief model constructs. *Advances in Nursing Science*, 6(3), 73–85.

Champion, V. L. (1993). Instrument refinement for breast cancer screening behaviors. *Nursing Research*, *42*(3), 139–143.

Cockburn, J., Fahey, P., & Sanson-Fisher, R. W. (1987). Construction and validation of a questionnaire to measure the health beliefs of general practice patients. *Family Practice*, *4*(2), 108–116.

Cummings, K. M., Jette, A. M., & Rosenstock, I. M. (1978). Construct validation of the health belief model. *Health Education Monographs*, *6*(4), 394–405.

Eisen, M., & Zellman, G. L. (1986). The role of health belief attitudes, sex education, and demographics in predicting adolescents' sexuality knowledge. *Health Education Quarterly*, *13*(1), 9–22.

Ewing, J. (1984). Detecting alcoholism: The CAGE questionnaire. *Journal of the American Medical Association*, *252*, 1905–1907.

Given, C. W., Given, B. A., Gallin, R. S., & Condon, J. W. (1983). Development of scales to measure beliefs of diabetic patients. *Research in Nursing and Health*, *6*, 127–141.

Gochman, D. S., (Ed.). (1988). *Health behavior: Emerging research perspectives*. New York: Plenum Press.

Hahn, E. J. (1993). Parental alcohol and other drug (AOD) use and health beliefs about parent involvement in AOD prevention. *Issues in Mental Health Nursing*, *14*, 237–247.

Hays, R., Kegeles, S., & Coates, T. (1990). High HIV risk-taking among young gay men. *AIDS*, *4*(9), 901–907.

Hingson, R., Strunin, L., Berlin, B., & Heeren, T. (1990). Beliefs about AIDS, use of alcohol and drugs, and unprotected sex among Massachusetts adolescents. *American Journal of Public Health*, *80*(3), 295–299.

Hochbaum, G. M. (1958). *Public participation in medical screening programs: A sociopsychological study*. PHS Publication No. 572. Washington, DC: U.S. Government Printing Office.

Hull, C. L. (1943). *Principles of behavior*. New York: Appleton-Century-Crofts.

Hurley, A. C. (1990). The health belief model: Evaluation of a diabetes scale. *Diabetes Educator*, *16*(1), 44–48.

Hyman, R. B., & Baker, S. (1992). Construction of the Hyman–Baker mammography questionnaire, a measure of health belief model variables. *Psychological Reports*, *71*, 1203–1215.

Janz, N. K., & Becker, M. H. (1984). The health belief model: A decade later. *Health Education Quarterly*, *11*, 1–47.

Jette, A. M., Cummings, M., Brock, B. M., Phelps, M. C., & Naessens, J. (1981). The structure and reliability of health belief indices. *Health Services Research*, *16*(1), 81–98.

Kaplan, R., Sallis, J., & Patterson, T. (1993). *Health and human behavior*. New York: McGraw-Hill.

Kim, K. K., Horan, M. L., Gendler, P., & Patel, M. K. (1991). Development and evaluation of the Osteoporosis Health Belief Scale. *Research in Nursing and Health*, *14*, 155–163.

Kirscht, J. P. (1974). The health belief model and illness behavior. *Health Education Monographs*, *2*, 387–408.

Kohler, W. (1925). *The mentality of apes*. New York: Harcourt Brace.

Leventhal, H. (1970). Findings and theory in the study of fear communications. In L. Berkowitz (Ed.), *Advances in experimental social psychology: Vol. 5*. New York: Academic Press.

Lewin, K. (1935). *A dynamic theory of personality*. New York: McGraw-Hill.

Lewin, K. (1936). *Principles of topological psychology*. New York: McGraw-Hill.

Lewin, K. (1951). The nature of field theory. In M. H. Marx (Ed.), *Psychological theory*. New York: Macmillan.

Lewin, K., Dembo, T., Festinger, L., & Sears, P. S. (1944). Level of aspiration. In J. Hunt (Ed.), *Personality and the behavior disorders*. New York: Ronald Press.

Maiman, L. A., Becker, M. H., Kirscht, J. P., Haefner, D. P. & Drachman, R. H. (1977). Scales for measuring health belief model dimensions: A test of predictive value, internal consistency, and relationships among beliefs. *Health Education Monographs*, 215–230.

McKusick, L., Coates, T., Morin, S., Pollack, L., & Hoff, C. (1990). Longitudinal predictors of reductions in unprotected anal intercourse among gay men in San Francisco: The AIDS behavioral research project. *American Journal of Public Health*, *80*(8), 978–983.

Montgomery, S., Joseph, J., Becker, M., Ostrow, D., Kessler, R., & Kirscht, J. (1989). The health belief model in understanding compliance with preventive recommendations for AIDS: How useful? *AIDS Education and Prevention*, *1*(4), 303–323.

Pavlov, I. (1927). *Conditioned reflexes*. Oxford, England: Oxford University Press.

Petosa, R., & Jackson, K. (1991). Using the health belief model to predict safer sex intentions among adolescents. *Health Education Quarterly*, *18*(4), 463–476.

Rogers, R. W. (1975). A protection motivation theory of fear appeals and attitude change. *Journal of Psychology*, *91*, 93–114.

Rogers, R. W. (1983). Cognitive and psychological in fear appeals and attitude change: A revised theory of protection motivation. In J. Cacioppo & R. Petty (Eds.), *Social psychophysiology*. New York: Guilford Press.

Ronis, D. (1992). Conditional health threats: Health beliefs, decisions, and behaviors among adults. *Health Psychology*, *11*(2), 127–134.

Ronis, D., & Harel, Y. (1989). Health beliefs and breast examination behaviors: Analysis of linear structural relations. *Psychology and Health*, *3*, 259–285.

Rosenstock, I. M. (1960). What research in motivation suggests for public health. *American Journal of Public Health*, *50*, 295–301.

Rosenstock, I. M. (1966). Why people use health services. *Milbank Memorial Fund Quarterly*, *44*, 94–124.

Rosenstock, I. M. (1974). Historical origins of the health belief model. *Health Education Monographs*, *2*, 328–335.

Rosenstock, I. M. (1991). The health belief model: Explaining health behaviors through expectancies. In K. Glanz, F. M. Lewis, & B. Rimer (Eds.), *Health behavior and health education* (pp. 39–62). San Francisco: Jossey-Bass Health Series.

Rosenstock, I. M., Strecher, V. J., & Becker, M. H. (1988). Social learning theory and the health belief model. *Health Education Quarterly, 15*(2), 175–183.

Russell, K. (1991). Development of an instrument to assess maternal childhood injury health beliefs and social influence. *Issues in Comprehensive Pediatric Nursing, 14*, 163–177.

Skinner, B. F. (1938). *The behavior of organisms.* New York: Appleton-Century-Crofts.

Stein, J. A., Fox, S. A., Murata, P. J., & Morisky, D. E. (1992). Mammography usage and the health belief model. *Health Education Quarterly, 19*(4), 447–462.

Strecher, V. J., DeVellis, B. M., Becker, M. H., & Rosenstock, I. M. (1986). The role of self-efficacy in achieving health behavior change. *Health Education Quarterly, 13*, 73–92.

Strecher, V. J., Kreuter, M. W., & Kobrin, S. C. (1995). Do cigarette smokers have unrealistic perceptions of their heart attack, cancer and stroke risks? *Journal of Behavioral Medicine, 18*(1).

Tiedje, L. B., Kingry, M. J., & Stommel, M. (1992). Patient attitudes concerning health behaviors during pregnancy: Initial development of a questionnaire. *Health Education Quarterly, 19*(4), 481–493.

Thorndike, E. L. (1898). Animal intelligence: An experimental study of the associative processes in animals. *Psychological Monographs, 2*(8) (entire issue).

Tolman, E. C. (1932). *Purposive behavior in animals and men.* New York: Appleton-Century-Crofts.

Walter, H., Vaughan, R., Gladis, M., Ragin, D., Kasen, S., & Cohall, A. (1992). Factors associated with AIDS risk behaviors among high school students in an AIDS epicenter. *American Journal of Public Health, 82*(4), 528–532.

Watson, J. B. (1925). *Behaviorism.* New York: Norton.

Weinstein, N. D. (1993). Testing four competing theories of health-protective behaviors. *Health Psychology, 12*(4), 324–333.

Weissfeld, J. L., Brock, B. M., Kirscht, J. P., & Hawthorne, V. M. (1987). Reliability of health belief indexes: Confirmatory factor analysis in sex, race, and age subgroups. *HSR: Health Services Research, 21*(6), 777–793.

Weissfeld, J. L., Kirscht, J. P., & Brock, B. M. (1990). Health beliefs in a population: The Michigan blood pressure survey. *Health Education Quarterly, 17*(2), 141–155.

5

Beliefs about Control and Health Behaviors

John W. Reich, Kristi J. Erdal, and Alex J. Zautra

LOCUS OF CONTROL: AN ENDURING CONSTRUCT

A Brief History of the Construct

Few other characterizations of stable personality or trait dispositions have received as much research attention as that of locus of control (LOC). Deriving from Phares's (1957) and Rotter's (1966) social learning theory approach to personality, the construct refers to the individual's expectancy that personal behaviors will result in desired outcomes: The higher one's degree of such belief, the greater the confidence that one's own internal states can lead to achievement of desired goals (an "internal" belief system); the lower one's belief, the more one feels that other people, chance, or other powers beyond one's control are responsible for one's outcomes (an "external" orientation). In the earlier social learning

John W. Reich, Kristi J. Erdal, and Alex J. Zautra • Department of Psychology, Arizona State University, Tempe, Arizona 85287-1104.

Handbook of Health Behavior Research I: Personal and Social Determinants, edited by David S. Gochman. Plenum Press, New York, 1997.

theory formulations of internal/external (IE) theory, these tendencies were conceptualized as stable beliefs and perceptions concerning expectancies of receiving reinforcement and the value of that reinforcement (Lefcourt, 1976; Phares, 1976; Rotter, 1966). The popularity of the concept, however, has extended its use far beyond the original formulations, and it is now employed quite generally without specific reference to reinforcement/learning processes. The continuing high rate of publication of papers employing control instruments (Lefcourt, 1992) attests to the concept's continuing expansion throughout the body of psychological science. It has had a particularly strong impact on research involving human health behaviors, which are the topic of this chapter.

The chapter reviews the basic properties of the construct, proposes that it be placed within a "person–environment fit" conceptualization, and reviews research and theory demonstrating the strong role that social influence processes play in LOC processing. The chapter then reviews specific LOC–health behavior relationships. Following Gochman (1988), health behavior is considered here to be action and activities that "people do or refrain from doing" that relate to maintaining, restoring, or improving their health.

The concept of health itself is complex and multifaceted, and there is a developing body of literature that attempts to determine the latent measurement structure of a physical health construct. We present an original study on the structure of health and then employ that structure to determine the relationships between LOC and social influence processes in health behavior. This original research is presented as an attempt to develop a more comprehensive model of person–environment relationships related to health behavior.

Some Properties of the Internality Construct

Over the years, there has been considerable refinement of LOC theory and methodology, with a resultant increase in detail and specification. Especially significant has been the trend toward increasing measurement precision because it was recognized, even in early formulations, that the construct was not uniform or homogeneous. Collins (1974) and, more recently, Marshall (1991) found in factor analytical studies that the Rotter IE scale was not unidimensional. Levenson (1973, 1981) created a new instrument to assess control by the self, by others, and by chance factors. In a major shift, B. S. Wallston, K. A. Wallston, Kaplan, and Maides (1976) developed a scale specifically to assess LOC for health issues, a scale now widely employed. That scale has subscales of internality, powerful others, and chance, but the content of the items was focused strictly on health matters. Following the general meaning of the construct, internals are those people who believe that their health is under their own control, while externals are those who believe that external factors such as luck or chance determine their health. A whole host of topic-specific scales are now available (e.g., Lefcourt, 1991), with most investigators now following Rotter's (1975) suggestion that more specific measures will be better able to detect significant

relationships among variables. In fact, K. A. Wallston and Smith (1993) explicitly argued against summing or averaging the subscales into a total score, since the scales often assess quite distinct, unrelated processes. Similarly, Gregory (1978) found it useful to distinguish between LOC for positive events and that for negative events, finding quite distinctly different results when they were assessed separately.

Although research on LOC has continued in the personality/psychometric tradition, other research areas on control have arisen and are continuing in their own lines more or less independently of the LOC tradition. Two separate traditions have emerged and will be mentioned briefly to provide a broader framework for reviewing LOC–health behavior research.

Event-Based Control. The first tradition to appear is what might be called the "event-based tradition." In this tradition, perceptions of how much individuals believe that they have caused an event to occur, or not to occur, are assessed. This assessment, of course, involves attributions of causation and of responsibility. This area of application is expanding rapidly in the health area. Researchers are exploring the extent to which people think that, for instance, they themselves or other people are responsible for their medical conditions or the cure of those conditions. Affleck, Tennen, Pfeiffer, and Fifield (1987), Helgeson (1993), and Taylor, Helgeson, Reed, and Skokan (1991), and Thompson, Sobolew-Shubin, Galbraith, Schwankovsky, and Cruzen (1993) have all found that attributions of personal control over an illness have very different consequences than attributions that others have control, and these differing attributions in turn have different consequences when attributions about curing the illness are made. Zautra, Reich, and Newsom (1994) melded both internal and external control in a study of older adults. They found an interaction between the onset of an illness that reduced behavioral autonomy and beliefs in personal control over life events. Loss of autonomy led to changes for the worse in mental health except in those subjects who held strong beliefs in personal control; these beliefs acted as a buffer against the deleterious consequences of loss of autonomy. Although quite promising for illuminating health behavior processes, these studies typically do not involve trait measures of LOC. Integrating the event-based approach with the trait approach would appear to provide a valuable linkage of two productive research traditions (Reich & Zautra, 1990a).

Also in this general "event-based" area, we include the experimental/manipulational approach, in which subjects are provided control over stimulus conditions, as, for example, Weiss (1970), Glass and Singer (1972), Langer and Rodin (1976), and Schulz and Hanusa (1978). These studies made clear to the subjects that they do have or can have control over the events of either the experimental arrangements or their lives in general. Almost without exception, this research finds that people who are provided control handle stress better and report higher mental health and well-being.

Self-Efficacy Control. The second tradition is what might be called the "self-efficacy tradition." Beginning most formally with Bandura's (1977) pioneering work, this research focuses on two areas: persons' beliefs that they will be able to carry out a given task and the degree of confidence that they will be able to carry out the task successfully. Thus, the concept refers, not to the ability to achieve desired end states or outcomes (which are often not under one's control), but to which tasks can be accomplished by the individual's exercise of skill, talent, and competence. For instance, one may be able to manifest a wide range of health behaviors, but that ability, per se, does not guarantee that a health problem will not arise. If one is self-efficacious, one can retain a sense of competence and capability by claiming "I did all I could do" to avoid it. This approach narrows the concept of control to situation- or task-specific control and thus can assess the complexity of the various types of self-efficacy in many different domains of life.

All of these constructs are insightful and heuristic approaches to personal variables in a wide range of applications. Again, however, these studies tend not to include the traditional dispositional LOC construct. Each in its own way involves control beliefs and perceptions as its core constructs, so future research could be moved forward if all these types of measures could be interrelated in studying health variables.

A Person–Environment Fit Approach to Control Beliefs

The LOC research tradition has been focused largely on detecting the nature of the relationship of the IE variable with other variables. Within the conceptual framework presented in this chapter, we would call such research "main effect" research: showing differences between "internals" (Is) and "externals" (Es) in some relationship with a manipulated or assessed variable. There is enough evidence about internality, however, that a more complex, integrative, interactional approach is possible, and certainly advisable. The framework for such an approach is already available.

The important relationships can be conceptualized in what is traditionally called the "person–environment fit" approach. Stemming most directly from Lewin's (1951) early formulation, $B = f(P,E)$ (in which B is behavior, P is person, and E is environment), more recent formulations have elaborated the basic framework into a more interactional approach: $B = f(P,E,P \times E)$ (Carp & Carp, 1984; Lawton, 1982; Lawton & Nahemow, 1973). The key concept is that the interaction term that incorporates both person and environment variables simultaneously can be assessed. Statistically, this formulation implies that the interaction term, $P \times E$, has to be shown to be significant over and above the variance accounted for by the main effect P and E terms. Review of the person–environment literature (e.g., Bowers, 1973; Endler, 1976) in fact shows that interaction terms commonly account for more variance than either the P or the E term alone.

The fundamental issue is to determine the "fit" between the individual's perception of control and the amount of encouragement or restriction of control by the environment. Most studies generally support the notion that fit relates to improved outcomes (Compass, Banez, Malcarne, & Worsham, 1991; Taylor et al., 1991; Thompson & Spacapan, 1991). Summarizing this extensive literature briefly, high internals tend to respond most favorably when their environment offers them a high degree of choice or freedom of action, while externals respond more adaptively when the environment is not objectively controllable.

In the health literature, this type of approach has involved perceptions of controllability over, for instance, disease treatment and cure (e.g., Affleck et al., 1987; Burish et al., 1984). K. A. Wallston and Smith (1993) showed that "the action is in the interaction" and that analyses of people with health problems should focus not only on their dispositional control beliefs about their health, but also on the amount of controllability in the health situation itself.

As this review of the LOC–health behavior literature will show, there are extensive differences between Is and Es in their health behaviors; almost invariably, Is show greater levels than Es of behaviors to maintain, restore, and enhance their health. That "main effect" approach provides a firm foundation for moving on to a more integrative level of analysis in which variables that mediate or moderate this basic effect can be discovered. The $P \times E$ fit concept offers a promising approach for analyzing these more complex relationships, but to date there is little systematic conceptualization or empirical research specifically focused on health behaviors. Since the internality–externality dimension relates directly to how much persons believe that they have control over life's events and outcomes, it is especially relevant to personal health and well-being. This review of the IE literature points to an important class of moderator variables that have

been discovered but not yet fully integrated into health behavior research. The next section describes that class of variables and a later section presents some research data employing that class of variables, operating within a basic $P \times E$ fit framework.

Control Beliefs and Social Relationships

One general trend has arisen in the IE literature with enough consistency that it suggests a heuristic addition to a $P \times E$ fit approach: There is differential responsiveness to social processes and social relations by internals and externals. Internals tend to outperform externals in cognitive and problem-solving tasks, but externals tend to respond more to the social component involved in task and problem-solving situations. Externals respond more to social cues from the experimenter, conform more, and are more cooperative (Biondo & MacDonald, 1971; Davis & Davis, 1967; Doctor, 1971; Pines & Julian, 1972); in nonlaboratory research, externals tend to report having larger social networks (Sandler & Lakey, 1982) and, while internals respond favorably to control-enhancing social interactions, externals respond more favorably to friendly social contacts while demonstrating little or no reactivity to control-enhancement manipulations (Reich & Zautra, 1990b).

There is, of course, an extensive literature on social factors in health processes, assessing the role of caregivers and support networks in coping, and adjustment processes in samples of ill patients (e.g., Cohen & Syme, 1985; Cutrona, 1986; Minkler, 1985). While these results have been detected in a wide range of settings, health behaviors per se have not yet been investigated in this framework. The following review of the literature summarizes what has been found concerning IE and health behaviors. The results, however, are mostly "main effect" results: Interactional $P \times E$ findings are rare, largely because the issue has not yet received the full attention of the research community. Following the literature survey, we will present our own results, which were explicitly analyzed within a $P \times E$ framework.

CONTROL BELIEFS AND HEALTH BEHAVIORS

The Literature up to 1978

Strickland (1978, 1979) provided a comprehensive survey and interpretation of the research literature on locus of control and health behavior. Its more salient findings are summarized here, highlighting the central issues and, especially, issues on which new research should be focused.

If any one result stands out clearly from the Strickland review, it is the consistent evidence that high internals manifest more health-related activity than externals. Strickland (1978) points out that the putative cognitive and motivational constructs underlying LOC research lead one to expect that "… internals, in contrast to externals, would be more sensitive to health messages, would have increased knowledge about health conditions, would attempt to improve physical functioning and might even, through their own efforts, be less susceptible to physical and psychological dysfunction" (p. 1193).

The research literature supports those expectations. Research has shown with reasonable consistency that internals, relative to externals, seek out more health-related information, assume more responsibility for their health, and take greater health-protection precautions. They engage more in physical exercise, are more likely to quit smoking or never to have taken it up, and, for females, are more likely to practice birth control.

Strickland (1978) and others (e.g., Kirscht, 1983; Rodin, 1986; Rodin & Timko, 1992) have been clear to point out that not all studies consistently show internals to be superior in health behaviors. Furthermore, Strickland assumes that some studies resulted in nonsignificant effects and thus were not published, resulting in an artificially high proportion of published data showing superiority for internals. Although the clearest trend in the literature up to 1978 was a tendency to show that those high in internality are those most concerned with and most active in relation to their health, there are enough inconsistencies to render this view more of a guideline for hypotheses than an established fact.

Research and Methodological Issues: The Literature since 1978

More recent developments in LOC research have continued the main theme of searching for differences between internals and externals. As yet, there have been few conceptual or theoretical alterations in the fundamental approach. Several distinct new areas have appeared, however, and they will be reviewed next.

Increased Assessment Specificity

There has been a good deal of activity surrounding assessment and methodological concerns. Most significant has been the increasing specificity of assessment. Whereas the original LOC measures were generalized, more recent developments have resulted in highly domain-specific measures of LOC. Perhaps most central to health issues, B.S. Wallston et al. (1976) stimulated an extensive line of research with their Health Locus of Control (HLOC) measure. This multidimensional instrument assesses three components of subjects' beliefs in control over their health: their own control (Internal), control by Powerful Others, and by Chance factors (External). All three scales were modeled after the three-component model of Levenson (1973, 1981).

Lau and Ware (1981) developed scales for a closely related four-factor structure. Others have developed scales that focus on assessing control over specific types of health behaviors: Carnahan (1979) in dental health, Saltzer (1981) in weight control behaviors, and Donovan and O'Leary (1983) in control of drinking behavior. Generally, main effects were found, with internals demonstrating more healthy behaviors, but Saltzer found that LOC had significant effects on weight reduction behaviors only when it interacted with components of health beliefs.

More recent reviews of the literature by K. A. Wallston and B. S. Wallston (1981) and Rodin and Timko (1992) continued to support the earlier results of Strickland's (1978) review: In general, internals tended to demonstrate higher levels of health activity than externals; they tended to gather more information about illness, were less likely to drop out of exercise programs, were more likely to quit smoking, and complied more consistently with dietary and medication recommendations by physicians. Again, however, K. A. Wallston and B. S. Wallston (1981) cautioned against too much enthusiasm for the patterns of relationships showing internals to be superior to externals in health activity: They reported on a number of studies in which no significant differences between internals and externals were found, among which were studies on female college students' exercise, dental care, and alcohol drinking behaviors and blue-collar workers' health care behaviors (Weitzel, 1989) and Murray and Corney's (1989) study of visits to the doctor in a sample of middle-aged British women.

Inconsistency in the findings of these studies is difficult to explain, but more recent developments in the LOC methodology may prove to be helpful. K. A. Wallston's view that an interactional approach should be employed (K. A. Wallston, 1989; K. A. Wallston & Smith, 1993) suggests that an interaction with other variables may be involved. A small subset of studies have begun investigations in this area, and significant interaction effects have begun to appear.

Interactional Approach

K. A. Wallston's approach to interactional analysis incorporates one or more of the three subscales of the HLOC scale and tests the interaction of that variable with subjects' ratings of the degree to which they value health. The latter variable, valuing, is very much in line with Rotter's original conceptualization, since it deals directly with the reinforcement value of a given

behavior, in this case health beliefs. Kaplan and Cowles (1978) found that such an interaction term significantly predicted smoking cessation behavior; those subjects who were higher in internality, and had stronger beliefs in the value of health were more successful at cessation of smoking.

In related research, K. A. Wallston (1989) tested the interaction of HLOC beliefs and perceived competence, a measure based on Bandura's self-efficacy model. In a study of chronic obstructive pulmonary disease patients, a significant interaction of the two variables on exercise behaviors was found: Internals who scored higher on self-efficacy engaged in higher amounts of exercise. On the other hand, Lau (1988) reported on one of his projects in which women received breast self-examination (BSE) brochures, half emphasizing self-control variables in health and the other half emphasizing that getting cancer was a matter of luck. It was shown that the greatest increases in BSE occurred among those who were internal for health care and received the control message and among those who were external for health care and received the chance message.

As in tests of simple LOC main effects, however, other tests of interaction effects have not been successful. Bundek, Marks, and Richardson (1993) entered Hispanic women's scores on beliefs in Internality and in Powerful Others (subscales of the Wallston instrument) to predict BSE behaviors. Both were significantly positively correlated with higher degrees of self-examination behaviors, but their interaction was not significant.

Overall, there has been a decline in the number of studies employing LOC as a correlate of health activity. While the causes of this decline are not immediately obvious, it may well be that most investigators regard the matter as essentially resolved: The reviews of Strickland, the Wallstons, and others leave the distinct impression that while there are inconsistencies and failures to find significance, in general it appears that internals are more active in their health behaviors than externals. With that "fact" established, it appears that most investigators have little motivation to pursue the matter further.

The more complex, integrative models that pursue tests of interactions offer the promise of a rejuvenation of interest in the issue. At this point, however, there are relatively few studies of interaction tests of LOC with other independent variables, and the results of these studies are somewhat inconsistent. Certainly the interactional model seems to be the most promising avenue of approach, since in principle it should be able to account for more variance than single-variable models.

Locus of Control Interactions with Social Support Processes

Researchers (e.g., Lefcourt, Martin, & Saleh, 1984; Sandler & Lakey, 1982) have shown an interaction between dispositional control and social support processes. People who reported low levels of internal control beliefs ("externals") reported having a more extensive social network than internals, but the latter demonstrated greater positive benefits from their social network: Internality acted as a stress buffer against negative events, while externals did not have comparable benefits.

One area of agreement is that externals appear to be responsive to social network relationships. Early research on the control variable showed that whereas internals are task-oriented, externals are more responsive to the social processes involved in experimental arrangements (Coppell & Smith, 1980; Davis & Phares, 1967), conform more (Biondo & MacDonald, 1971; Doctor, 1971), and are more responsive to social evaluation (Pines & Julian, 1972). These relationships would be expected to be especially pronounced in social situations relating to dependency.

It seems likely that physical health variables would similarly be related to beliefs about control and to social support processes. Seeman, Seeman, and Sayles (1985) found evidence that externals with high levels of reliance on their social relations reported poorer health. Such results should be interpreted within the framework established earlier by Johnson and Sarason (1978), who showed that for externals, there were significant positive correlations between life stresses and depression and anxiety. People who perceive that they have relatively little control over life events would be expected to show more adverse effects when their social networks are unsupportive.

Although it may seem common sense to assume that all persons would want to be in control of their lives, it has been shown that the issue is in fact far more complicated. In some domains of life, particularly physical health, people may desire to cede control to others such as physicians (K. A. Wallston & B. S. Wallston, 1987). This phenomenon suggests the value, if not the necessity, of developing a more complex and integrated model of control, one in which control is studied in relation to the context of life in which one finds oneself. These types of relationships should be conceptualized within the general framework of a large body of research showing that social relationships play an influential role in the etiology and course of physical illness (Cohen, 1988; Cohen & Wills, 1985; Kiecolt-Glaser et al., 1984; B. S. Wallston, Alagna, DeVellis, & DeVellis, 1983; Wortman & Conway, 1985; Wortman & Dunkel-Schetter, 1987).

MODELS OF MEASUREMENT STRUCTURE OF PHYSICAL HEALTH

The relationships between physical health and mental health, personality, and social relationships are complex. A major problem in understanding them is that of conceptualizing the multidimensional nature of a term as complex as health. Liang (Liang, 1986; Liang, Lawrence, Bennett, & Whitelaw, 1987) has determined a latent causal structure of five components of health: chronic illness, number of sick days, physical self-maintenance, instrumental activities of daily living, and subjective ratings of one's own health. Wolinsky, Coe, Miller, and Prendergast (1984) found similar components, but also found significant clusters of items relating to sensory functions. Ware (1984) found a five-factor model (physical health, mental health, social health, general health perceptions, and role). Rothman et al. (1990) were able to replicate the Ware model, but only by splitting the social health factor into two components. In general, then, the data of various independent studies show that multidimensional models of health tend to fit empirical results better than unidimensional models (Ware, 1986).

PHYSICAL HEALTH–MENTAL HEALTH RELATIONSHIPS

A number of investigations have assessed the relationships between physical health and mental health indicators (for useful summaries, see Cohen & Syme, 1988; Sarafino, 1990). As might be expected, the research literature provides evidence for a positive relationship (e.g., Okun, Stock, Haring, & Witter, 1984). The relationship, however, is not always a strong one (Ware, 1986). For instance, Mechanic and Angel (1987) reported that patients of equal levels of physical symptomatology reported significantly different levels of psychological distress. Liang (1986) highlighted the current status of this area of research by noting (p. 258): "Given the often suggested connection between physical health and psychological well-being ... it would be interesting to examine such linkages by incorporating multidimensional structural formulations of both constructs."

A STUDY: CONTROL BELIEFS, SOCIAL RELATIONS, AND HEALTH BELIEFS AND BEHAVIORS

Purpose of the Study

A generalized Person × Environment model provides a framework for conceptualizing an empirical approach to the analysis of how control beliefs influence health behavior. Although com-

plex, such an approach suggests the value of testing for main and interaction effects involving all the central components discussed to this point. One of our projects has in fact employed these variables in an extensive longitudinal examination of a sample of older adults. Details of this project are available in other publications (e.g., Zautra, Guarnaccia, & Reich, 1988; Zautra, Reich, & Guarnaccia, 1990). Reported here are a set of analyses that illustrates how a $P \times E$ model might be employed in attempting to disentangle the complex relationships among personal, social, and physical and mental health variables. Of course, this is only one approach to a particular class of subjects, older adults; there is a need for other models of analyses with other classes of respondents, to provide a fuller picture of these types of relationships.

This section presents data on the measurement and determination of the latent structure of a battery of instruments that assess physical health variables and relates that structure to LOC, illness occurrences, social relationships, and mental health outcomes.

Hypotheses

The research literature led to a set of interrelated hypotheses. The first was that it would be possible to confirm a multiconstruct model of the self-reported health of older adults. Evidence in the literature indicated the likelihood of a four-factor structure, and such a structure was hypothesized.

Second, it was expected that poor physical health would show a direct relationship with the psychological distress aspect of mental health, and vice versa. Poor physical health was assessed both as health status and as health downturns: Illness-worsening events occurring over the 8 months between the first and second assessments were included to assess the role of changing health and how it might relate to the other physical, psychological, and social components of the model.

Third, on the basis of our prior research

(Finch, Okun, Barrera, Zautra, & Reich, 1989), it was expected that positive social relations would relate to better mental health (lowered psychological distress) and negative social relations to poorer mental health (higher psychological distress). Given that externals show greater sensitivity to social relations than internals, we predicted that externals would show a significant relationship between their positive and negative social network interactions and their physical and mental health; internal subjects were predicted to show no such relationships.

Project Design

This study involved a prospective design; subjects were assessed repeatedly on a monthly schedule for 10 months. The study employed a wide range of measures of personality, minor daily and major life events, social network variables, and detailed measures of physical and mental health. The analyses presented here relate to the LOC–social relationship variables and how they are related to physical health, illness events, and health behavior variables as well as their subsequent relationships with mental health outcomes.

Subjects

The project involved 269 adults between the ages of 60 and 80 years. These respondents came from two at-risk samples of male and female subjects who had recently experienced a major physical health stressor ($N = 61$) or death of a spouse ($N = 62$) (Zautra, 1988). Control samples matched on age, sex, and income, but who had not experienced the stressors, served as comparison groups.

Interview Instruments

A total of nine subscales composed of 105 items were organized into an interview instrument. The items that assessed the various health variables were selected from standard instruments (Dohrenwend, Shrout, Egri, & Mendelson,

1980; Duke University Center, 1978; Gurland et al., 1983; Mossey & Shapiro, 1982; Murrell, 1982; Reich, Zautra, & Guarnaccia, 1989). Internality was assessed with the Internal Control subscale of the Levenson I-E scale (Levenson, 1973, 1981). The dependent variable, psychological distress, taken from two mental health scales, was assessed by items that measured depression, anxiety, helplessness–hopelessness, suicidal ideation, and confused thinking (see Zautra et al., 1988). Social support was assessed with an abridged version of the scale developed by Fischer (1982). Confirmatory factor analyses (Finch et al., 1989) determined the presence of two independent factors of social support: positive support, e.g., instrumental and emotional support, and negative social ties, i.e., the presence of people who cause problems for the individual. In turn, these dimensions were shown to relate to mental health: Positive social relationships related positively to psychological well-being; negative relationships related positively to psychological distress and negatively to psychological well-being. In accord with results of Finch et al. (1989), it was expected that negative social support would relate directly to psychological distress, while positive socially supportive experiences would be unrelated to such distress.

Procedure

The interviews were conducted in the respondents' homes by a member of a staff of trained older adult female interviewers. The initial interviews took 2–3 hours on average to complete. A telephone interview instrument composed of a subset of scales that assessed health and other variables was then readministered every month for the next 8 months, and the final, 10th interview was again conducted in-home with the full set of scales. In addition, respondents were given a pencil-and-paper questionnaire with questions about psychological symptoms to complete and return by mail. Subjects were paid a total of $30 for their participation.

Results[1]

Table 1 presents the basic intercorrelations, means, and standard deviations for all of the study's variables.

Structure of Physical Health. The measurement structure underlying the various health measures at the first assessment was determined by employing the EQS structural equations program of Bentler (1989).

Initial tests of the latent construct loadings suggested by the Liang five-factor model resulted in a significant χ^2/df ratio: 20.05(10), $p < 0.02$. A better fit was sought by exploratory testing of other models to determine what patterns of loadings might improve the fit. These explorations led to the development and testing of a three-construct model that resulted in a nonsignificant χ^2/df ratio of 14.741/11 or 1.34, indicating a good fit to the data.

The resultant model's three latent constructs, their dependent variables, and their loadings are presented in Table 2. In addition to the individual items' loadings on the latent constructs, the intercorrelations of the constructs also were determined by the EQS analysis. All were significant. The correlation between the perceived health problems construct and the medications construct was 0.42; between the medications construct and the medical services utilization construct, 0.50; and between the perceived health problems and the medical services utilization constructs, 0.67. The p values for the t-tests of these relationships were all significant at < 0.01.

Testing of the Latent Construct Relationships over Time. After estimation of the physical health measurement model, the next step in the analyses employed the LISREL VI program of Jöreskög and Sörbom (1985) to determine the interrelationships among the physical health, mental health, LOC, and social support constructs over time, using the full longitudinal data

[1]A more detailed report of the analyses involved in this chapter may be obtained from any of the authors.

set of 10 monthly interviews. First, we tested the hypothesized model of the relationships between the three health constructs at Time 1 and at Time 10, illness-worsening events recorded from Time 2 to Time 9, and psychological distress measured at Time 1 and Time 10. The model for this test is presented in Figure 1.

The fit of this model was very good [$\chi^2(20) = 31.12$, $p = 0.054$, Tucker & Lewis (1973) Index (TLI) = 0.98]. The path from distress at Time 1 to health problems at Time 10 reached only marginal significance ($p = 0.10$). When we attempted to trim the model by dropping this path, however, the fit decreased slightly, so this path was retained in the model. In Figure 1, all paths have positive signs.

As Figure 1 shows, the three health constructs showed considerable stability over time, as did psychological distress with itself over time. Individual differences in physical and mental health were trait-like to a large extent; clearly, the best predictor of level of health, distress, and medical services utilization was the older adults' prior status on those variables. The model also showed that health problems (Time 1) were associated with an increase in subsequent illness-worsening events. Illness-worsening events (Time 2 to Time 9) in turn affected all three health constructs, in that illness-worsening events increased health problems, medications taken, and medical services utilization at Time 10. Health problems also were associated with greater psychological distress at both Time 1 and Time 10.

Internality, Social Relations, and Physical Health Interactions. Next, we sought to determine how this model of the relationship between health and distress was affected by internality, social support variables, and the possible interaction of the two. The positive social support and negative social support variables were added to the model as exogenous concepts. The eight paths from positive support and negative support to Time 1 variables (health problems, medications, medical services utilization, and psychological distress) were set free to be estimated.

Table 1. Intercorrelations, Means, and Standard Deviations of the Basic Variables of the Study

Variable	1	2	3	4	5	6	7	8	9	10
1. Instrumental activities of daily living	—	0.51	0.29	0.32	0.68	0.42	0.51	−0.18	0.14	−0.26
2. Medication usage		—	0.26	0.28	0.51	0.35	0.41	−0.14	0.11	−0.20
3. Medical services utilization			—	0.18	0.29	0.16	0.27	−0.01	0.02	−0.07
4. Psychophysiological symptomatology				—	0.40	0.32	0.55	−0.03	0.28	−0.17
5. Self-report of health status					—	0.45	0.59	−0.21	0.09	−0.22
6. Illness-worsening events						—	0.45	−0.12	0.25	−0.20
7. Everyday health symptoms							—	−0.08	0.25	−0.22
8. Positive social support								—	0.14	0.19
9. Negative social support									—	0.25
10. Internal control										—
Mean:	4.3	2.4	8.8	0.81	1.94	1.05	0.46	19.6	1.6	36.3
Standard deviation:	6.11	2.3	10.8	0.80	0.50	1.01	0.38	13.0	2.6	7.4

The sample was then divided at the median of LOC to create two mutually exclusive groups (externals and internals) and the models run conjointly to compare the model's fit were constrained to be equal versus allowed to vary between groups.

It was hypothesized that the paths from both positive support and negative support to health and mental health would be different for externals compared with internals. Also, we expected that the three paths from illness-worsening events to the three health constructs at Time 10 would differ as a function of internality. It was hypothesized that these named paths would be stronger for the external group due to their being more affected by external situations and to their sensitivity to social variables being greater than internals. The results are presented in Figure 2.

The only significant difference between the groups in the relations between the support variables and the physical health and mental health variables was in the path from negative support to psychological distress at Time 1 [$\chi^2(93) = 121.50$]. There was a significant χ^2 change [$\chi^2(1) = 5.13, p < 0.05$] when this path was allowed to vary between groups in comparison to a model in which the paths were constrained to be equal. This path was significant and positive for the externals, but close to 0.0 and nonsignificant for the internals, a finding in line with theoretical predictions. Also as predicted, the externals with more negative social ties showed more distress; internals did not show the same relationship.

There was a significant difference between the groups in the relation between illness-worsening events and health problems as well, as revealed by a significant χ^2 difference when this

Table 2. Latent Constructs and Their Dependent Variables

Construct	Constituent subscales	Factor loadings
1. Perceived health	Instrumental activities of daily living	0.51
	Health symptoms	0.73
	Psychophysiological symptomatology	0.29
	Self-report of health status	0.82
2. Medications	Medication usage	1.0
3. Medical services utilization	Number of times seeing a doctor in past 6 months	0.76
	Small daily event, "seeing a doctor"	0.59

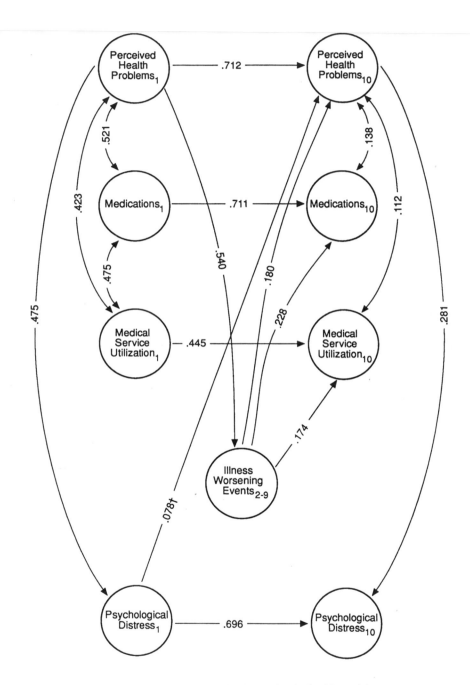

Figure 1. Standardized solution for the health model.

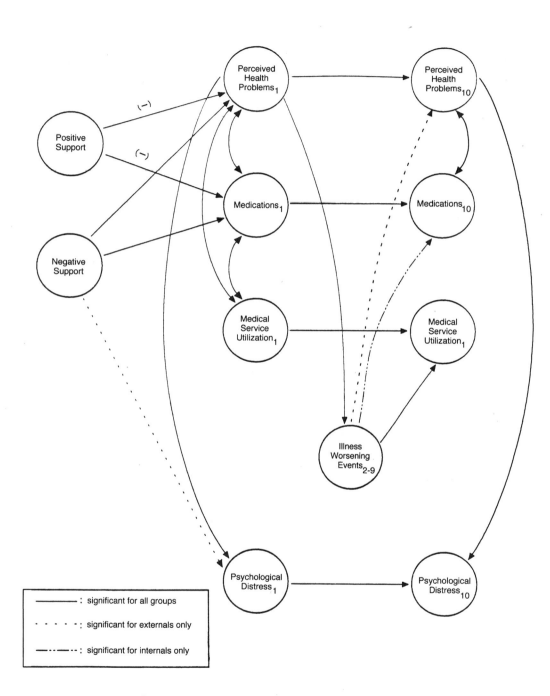

Figure 2. Standardized solution for the complete causal model.

path was freed between the groups [$\chi^2(94)$ = 126.63, χ^2 change, $\chi^2(1) = 4.32, p < 0.05$]. This path was significant for externals only, again as predicted.

There was a significant difference between the groups in the relation between illness-worsening events and medications, as revealed by a significant χ^2 change value [$\chi^2(95) = 130.95; \chi^2$ change, $\chi^2(1) = 15.45, p < 0.001$]. This path was significant only for internals and was counter to the original hypothesis. Internals were more likely to show greater medication use after illness events than were externals.

Discussion

To fully examine $P \times E$ transactions, the relationships among many classes of variables need to be investigated. We were concerned with four major classes: physical health, mental health, personality, and social support. Our interpretation of the research literature on those variables was clear enough to allow the formulation of a set of interrelated hypotheses. We expected that physical health would be characterized by four latent constructs, that physical and mental health variables would be related to each other, and that these processes would be influenced differentially by individual differences in locus of control in interaction with social support variables. The first hypothesis was not fully supported: A three-construct measurement model provided a better fit of the data than the four-construct model we hypothesized. The other hypotheses received support, and additional relationships were found that, while not predicted, provided useful information elaborating on $P \times E$ interactions.

Structure of Physical Health. Although the data of this study did not match the hypothesized four-component model reported by Liang (1986) and Liang et al. (1987), other studies also have obtained different models with different numbers and types of constructs. All studies are more alike than it would appear, however, differ-

ing in details but agreeing in overall content. We summarize our picture of the structure of physical health by noting that it was shown to have a construct comprising both perceptions of actual health conditions (factor 1) and more objective health behavior/behavioral constructs (factors 2 and 3) and that these components operated in different ways in their relationships with the personality and social support components of our causal model. Thus, these data argue for researchers to employ more differentiated models of health activity. Taking medications and going to the physician were shown to be related but nevertheless distinct constructs. Both were distinct from perceptions that one has a health problem, although of course all three constructs were correlated with each other. These relationships were significantly influenced by the subject's sense of control and the social network in which the subject was embedded.

Physical Health–Mental Health Relationships. The data showed several interrelated sets of effects of physical health and health activities on mental health. First, poorer health at Time 1 was related to an exacerbation of illness-worsening events in the next 8 months, which in turn led to an increase in subsequent health problems and, ultimately, increased psychological distress. Having health problems acts as a risk factor for enhancing the probability that one will later experience increases in ill health and psychological distress. Distress did not, in itself, influence later medication or medical services usage. The subjects who felt that they had health problems also became more psychologically distressed. Most of these effects were accounted for in the perceived health problems constructs. Thus, it was at the psychological level of perceptions of health that much of the mediating relationships between physical and mental health occurred, a finding reported by other researchers as well (e.g., Burckhardt, 1985; Young, 1992).

Perceived Control and Social Support Processes. The third set of hypothesized relationships concerned perceived control (internality) and social support relationships and their interaction relating to each other and to the physical and mental health measures. Positive support was related to decreased reports of health problems and medications, but not to medical services utilization or to psychological distress. Negative support did relate to greater psychological distress along with increased perceptions of health problems and medication usage, but not to medical services utilization. Thus, medical services utilization was not influenced by either positive social support or negative social ties, indicating that this type of activity is not generally under the control of social support, at least as assessed here. Presumably, utilization of health services is a major activity under the influence of other classes of variables, such as a serious illness or a medical emergency, adequate financial resources, or insurance coverage, that may have overshadowed the influence of the variables assessed in this study.

This differentiated pattern is in line with a general two-factor model of mental health, in which negative social ties have their effect largely on negative outcomes such as distress, while positive states do not (e.g., Zautra & Reich, 1983; Zautra et al., 1990). Other researchers have noted the similar patterns in the relations of positive and negative states with different outcome variables (e.g., Erdal & Zautra, 1993; Fontana, Marcus, Dowds, & Hughes, 1980).

Some support was found for the prediction that social support would interact with dispositional internal control. Prior research has shown that externals are especially sensitive to social relations (Reich & Zautra, 1991; Seeman et al., 1985), and that was shown to be the case here. The effects occurred only with the negative social support construct: Externals showed greater distress as they reported higher levels of negative social support, while, as expected, no effect was found for internals.

As predicted, internality also had significant effects on health. The externals demonstrated an increase in Time 10 perceived health problems

the more they experienced illness-worsening events in the preceding 9 months. Only one interaction effect on these causal paths was found for internals: They were more likely to report increased medication usage as illness-worsening events increased over the interim between the two assessment periods, while externals did not show any such relationship. In retrospect, it does not seem surprising that those who profess high levels of belief in their ability to control their lives would report higher levels of taking medications when ill if this behavior is interpreted as being a means of actively coping with and attempting to control disease effects.

Perhaps the clearest implication of our results is the *transactional* nature of the findings. All subjects experienced increased medical services utilization as illness-worsening events increased. That relationship was not differentially affected by internality or social support. Experiences of negative social support, however, differentially affected external and internal subjects in their mental health. At Time 1, externals with greater negative social supports suffered increased psychological distress. At Time 1, increased health problems were related to increased negative social support. An increased degree of vulnerability to illness-worsening events resulted. This was moderated by LOC, however, when the externals reported an increase in subsequent health problems.

Internals, on the other hand, did not experience the same degree of vulnerability and did not show particularly favorable or unfavorable patterns of changes among the social and physical components of their lives as the externals did. These differences might be expected from control theory: Causation is internally structured in their lives, and their mental and physical health are less sensitive to negative social relationships.

Critique and Implications

Several methodological issues must be highlighted to put the data of this study into context. First, many of the analyses involved cross-sectional data (e.g., the mental health–physical health relationships and the social support relationships were both studied at Time 1). It is possible that the direction of causality specified in the structural model could have operated the other way: People with increased health problems might have suffered a loss of positive social relations and an increase of negative ones (Cohen & Syme, 1985; Dooley, 1985). The structural model fit well and did not call for modification in the order of causal paths we specified. Nevertheless, other measures or tests more focused on reverse relationships might have obtained a different pattern of data. We regard the findings from this test of ordered paths as tentative because of the possibility of some reversals in causal ordering. On the other hand, these relationships were tested longitudinally, controlling for Time 1 status, in analyses of the Time 10 relationships. This design has the effect of controlling for spurious relationships related to measurement error and increasing the sensitivity of the measures.

The expected path from Time 1 distress to Time 10 perceived health problems was only a trend. The lengthy time gap of 9 months between the assessment of the two constructs might understandably have made detection of the relationship difficult. A shorter time period might have provided a more powerful test of the path, but it was not possible to make the time shorter within the framework of the design. This path is an important one to show mutual influence between mental health and physical health variables, so a more focused study of temporal factors in these relationships would be useful.

The results of this study appear to be encouraging for the use of Person × Environment models of dispositional, social, and health variables in understanding the adjustment process. These data suggest the types of considerations that might be involved in tailoring therapeutic interventions. Interventions aimed at enhancing adjustment can be focused with somewhat greater precision, recognizing that certain people respond differently from others when, for instance, their social network relationships are negative or when they express low rather than high levels of dispositional internality. Such interactions have direct consequences on their physical health and, subsequently, their mental health. Larger-scale assessments incorporating transactional paths and focusing therapeutic interventions on the types of relationships found in this study are a promising next step for theory, research, and practice.

ACKNOWLEDGMENTS. This project was supported in part by a National Institute of Health Grant to Arizona State University (Institutional Biomedical Grant No. BRSG 2 SO7 RR07112) and in part by a National Institute on Aging Grant (RO1-AG04924-01-05). Support by both agencies is gratefully acknowledged. Also, the authors would like to acknowledge the many valuable contributions of Dr. John Finch to this project.

Portions of this report were presented at the Third Biennial Conference on Community Research and Action, Division 27 of the American Psychological Association, June 1991.

Correspondence concerning this chapter should be addressed to John W. Reich, Department of Psychology, Arizona State University, Tempe, AZ 85287-1104.

REFERENCES

Affleck, G., Tennen, H., Pfeiffer, C., & Fifield, C. (1987). Appraisals of control and predictability in adapting to a chronic disease. *Journal of Personality and Social Psychology, 53,* 273-279.

Bandura, A. (1977). Self-efficacy: Toward a unifying theory of behavioral change. *Psychological Review, 84,* 191-215.

Bentler, P. M. (1989). *EQS: Structural equations program manual.* Los Angeles: BMDP Statistical Software.

Biondo, J., & MacDonald, A. P., Jr. (1971). Internal–external locus of control and response to influence attempts. *Journal of Personality, 39,* 407-419.

Bowers, K. S. (1973). Situationism in psychology: An analysis and a critique. *Psychological Review, 80,* 309-336.

Bundek, N. I., Marks, G., & Richardson, J. L. (1993). Role of health locus of control beliefs in cancer screening of elderly Hispanic women. *Health Psychology, 12,* 193-199.

Burckhardt, C. S. (1985). The impact of arthritis on quality of life. *Nursing Research, 34,* 11-16.

Burish, T. G., Carey, M. P., Wallston, K. A., Stein, M. J., Jamison, R. N., & Lyles, J. N. (1984). Health locus of control and chronic disease: An external orientation may be advantageous. *Journal of Social and Clinical Psychology, 2,* 326–332.

Carnahan, T. M. (1979). *The development and validation of the multidimensional dental locus of control scales.* Unpublished doctoral dissertation. State University of New York at Buffalo.

Carp, F. M., & Carp., A. (1984). A complementary/congruence model of well-being or mental health for the community elderly. In I. Altman, M. P. Lawton, & J. F. Wohlwill (Eds.), *Elderly people and the environment* (pp. 279–336). New York: Plenum Press.

Cohen, S. (1988). Psychosocial models of the role of social support in the etiology of physical disease. *Health Psychology, 7,* 269–297.

Cohen, S., & Syme, S. L. (1985). *Social support and health.* New York: Academic Press.

Cohen, S., & Wills, T. A. (1985). Stress, social support, and the buffering hypothesis. *Psychological Bulletin, 98,* 310–357.

Collins, B. E. (1974). Four components of the Rotter Internal–External Scale: Belief in a difficult world, a just world, a predictable world, and a politically responsive world. *Journal of Personality and Social Psychology, 29,* 381–391.

Compass, B. E., Banez, G. A., Malcarne, V., & Worsham, N. (1991). Perceived control and coping with stress: A developmental perspective. *Journal of Social Issues, 47,* 23–34.

Coppell, D., & Smith, R. E. (1980). Acquisition of stimulus-outcome and response-outcome expectancies as a function of locus of control. *Cognitive Therapy and Research, 4,* 179–188.

Cutrona, C. E. (1986). Behavioral manifestations of social support: A microanalytic investigation. *Journal of Personality and Social Psychology, 51,* 201–208.

Davis, W. L., & Davis, E. D. (1972). Internal–external control and attribution of responsibility for success and failure. *Journal of Personality, 60,* 123–126.

Davis, W. L., & Phares, E. J. (1967). Internal–external control as a determinant of information-seeking in a social influence situation. *Journal of Personality, 35,* 547–561.

Doctor, R. M. (1971). Locus of control of reinforcement and responsiveness to social influence. *Journal of Personality, 39,* 542–551.

Dohrenwend, B. P., Shrout, P. E., Egri, G., & Mendelson, F. S. (1980). Nonspecific psychological distress and other dimensions of psychopathology. *Archives of General Psychiatry, 37,* 1229–1236.

Donovan, D. M., & O'Leary, J. R. (1983). Control orientation, drinking behavior, and alcoholism. In H. Lefcourt (Ed.), *Research with the locus of control construct: Vol. 2* (pp. 107–153). New York: Academic Press.

Dooley, D. (1985). Causal inference in the study of social support. In S. Cohen & S. L. Syme (Eds.), *Social support and health.* New York: Academic Press.

Duke University Center for the Study of Aging and Human Development. (1978). *Multidimensional functional assessment: The OARS methodology.* Durham, NC: Duke University.

Endler, N. S. (1976). The case for person–situation interaction. In N. S. Endler & D. Magnusson (Eds.), *Interactional psychology and personality* (pp. 58–70). New York: Hemisphere.

Erdal, K. J., & Zautra, A. J. (1993). *The psychological impact of illness downturns: A comparison of new versus chronic conditions.* Paper presented at the 14th annual Scientific Session of the Society of Behavioral Medicine, San Francisco, March.

Finch, J. F., Okun, M. A., Barrera, M., Jr., Zautra, A. J., & Reich, J. W. (1989). Positive and negative social ties among older adults: Measurement models and the prediction of psychological distress and well-being. *American Journal of Community Psychology, 17,* 585–605.

Fischer, C. S. (1982). *To dwell among friends.* Chicago: University of Chicago Press.

Fontana, A. F., Marcus, J. L., Dowds, B. N., & Hughes, L. A. (1980). *Psychosomatic Medicine, 42,* 279–288.

Glass, D. C., & Singer, J. E. (1972). *Urban stress.* New York: Academic Press.

Gochman, D. S. (1988). Health behavior: Plural perspectives. In D. S. Gochman (Ed.), *Health behavior: Emerging research perspectives* (pp. 3–17). New York: Plenum Press.

Gregory, W. L. (1978). Locus of control for positive and negative outcomes. *Journal of Personality and Social Psychology, 36,* 840–849.

Gurland, B. J., Copeland, J. R., Kuriansky, J., Kelleher, M. J., Sharpe, L., & Dean, L. L. (1983). *The mind and mood of aging.* New York: Haworth.

Helgeson, V. S. (1993). The onset of chronic illness: Its effect on the patient–spouse relationship. *Journal of Social and Clinical Psychology, 12,* 406–428.

Johnson, J. H., & Sarason, I. G. (1978). Life stress, depression and anxiety: Internal–external control as a moderator variable. *Journal of Psychosomatic Research, 22,* 205–208.

Jöreskög, K. G., & Sörbom, D. (1985). *LISREL VI: Analysis of linear structural relationships by the method of maximum likelihood.* Mooreville, IN: Scientific Software.

Kaplan, G. D., & Cowles, A. (1978). Health locus of control and health value in the prediction of smoking reduction. *Health Education Monographs, 6,* 129–137.

Kiecolt-Glaser, J. K., Ricker, D., George, J., Messick, G., Speicher, C. E., Warner, W., & Glaser, R. (1984). Urinary cortisol levels, cellular immunocompetency, and loneliness in psychiatric inpatients. *Psychosomatic Medicine, 46,* 15–23.

Kirscht, J. P. (1983). Preventive health behavior: A review of research and issues. *Health Psychology, 2,* 277–301.

Langer, E. J., & Rodin, J. (1976). The effects of choice and enhanced personal responsibility for the aged: A field experiment in an institutional setting. *Journal of Personality and Social Psychology, 34,* 191–198.

Lau, R. (1988). Beliefs about control and health behavior. In D. S. Gochman (Ed.), *Health behavior: Emerging research perspectives* (pp. 43-62). New York: Plenum Press.

Lau, R. R., & Ware, J. F. (1981). Refinements in the measurement of health-specific locus-of-control beliefs. *Medical Care, 19,* 1147-1158.

Lawton, M. P. (1982). Competence, environmental press, and the adaptation of older people. In M. P. Lawton, P. G. Windley, & T. O. Byerts (Eds.), *Aging and the environment: Theoretical approaches* (pp. 35-39). New York: Springer.

Lawton, M. P., & Nahemow, L. (1973). Ecology and the aging process. In C. Eisdorfer & M. P. Lawton (Eds.), *Psychology of adult development and aging* (pp. 619-674). Washington, DC: American Psychological Association.

Lefcourt, H. M. (1976). *Locus of control: Current trends in theory and research.* Hillsdale, NJ: Erlbaum.

Lefcourt, H. M. (1991). Locus of control. In J. P. Robinson, P. R. Shaver, & L. S. Wrightsman (Eds.), *Measures of personality and social psychological attitudes* (pp. 413-499). San Diego: Academic Press.

Lefcourt, H. M. (1992). Durability and impact of the locus of control construct. *Psychological Bulletin, 112,* 411-414.

Lefcourt, H. M., Martin, R. A., & Saleh, W. E. (1984). Locus of control and social support: Interactive moderators of stress. *Journal of Personality and Social Psychology, 47,* 378-389.

Levenson, H. (1973). Multidimensional locus of control in psychiatric patients. *Journal of Consulting and Clinical Psychology, 41,* 397-404.

Levenson, H. (1981). Differentiating among internality, powerful others and chance. In H. M. Lefcourt (Ed.), *Research with the locus of control construct: Vol. 1. Assessment methods* (pp. 15-31). New York: Academic Press.

Lewin, K. (1951). In D. Cartwright (Ed.), *Field theory in social science: Selected theoretical papers.* New York: Harper.

Liang, J. (1986). Self-reported physical health among aged adults. *Journal of Gerontology, 41,* 248-260.

Liang, J., Lawrence, R. H., Bennett, J. M., & Whitelaw, N. (1987). *Appropriateness of composites when utilizing a multiple indicators model of self-reported physical health.* Paper presented at the annual meeting of the Gerontological Society of America, Washington, DC, November.

Marshall, G. N. (1991). A multidimensional analysis of internal health locus of control beliefs: Separating the wheat from the chaff? *Journal of Personality and Social Psychology, 61,* 483-491.

Mechanic, D., & Angel, R. J. (1987). Some factors associated with the report and evaluation of back pain. *Journal of Health and Social Behavior, 28,* 131-139.

Minkler, M. (1985). Social support and health of the elderly. In S. Cohen & S. L. Syme (Eds.), *Social support and health* (pp. 199-216). New York: Academic Press.

Mossey, J. M. & Shapiro, E. (1982). Self-rated health: A predic-

tor of mortality in the aged. *American Journal of Public Health, 72,* 800-808.

Murray, J., & Corney, R. (1989). Locus of control in health: The effects of psychological well-being and contact with the doctor. *International Journal of Social Psychiatry, 35,* 361-369.

Murrell, S. (1982). *Resources, stress, and older persons.* Fieldwork No. 4. Louisville, KY: Urban Studies Center, University of Louisville.

Okun, M. A., Stock, W. A., Haring, M., & Witter, R. A. (1984). Health and subjective well-being. *International Journal of Aging and Human Development 18-19,* 111-132.

Phares, E. J. (1957). Expectancy changes in skill and chance situations. *Journal of Abnormal and Social Psychology, 54,* 339-342.

Phares, E. J. (1976). *Locus of control in personality.* Morristown, NJ: General Learning Press.

Pines, H. A., & Julian, J. W. (1972). Effects of task and social demands on locus of control differences in information processing. *Journal of Personality, 40,* 407-416.

Reich, J. W., & Zautra, A. J. (1990a). Dispositional control beliefs and the consequences of a control-enhancing intervention. *Journal of Gerontology, 45,* P46-51.

Reich, J. W., & Zautra, A. J. (1990b, August). *Analysis of the social components of internality in control-enhancing interventions.* Paper delivered at the Symposium, "Understanding the Factors Responsible for Support Intervention Success and Failure" (K. Heller, Chair), presented at the 98th Annual Convention of the American Psychological Association, Boston.

Reich, J. W., & Zautra, A. J. (1991). Experimental and measurement approaches to internal control in at-risk older adults. *Journal of Social Issues, 47,* 143-158.

Reich, J. W., Zautra, A. J., & Guarnaccia, C. A. (1989). The effects of disability and bereavement on the mental health and recovery of older adults *Psychology and Aging, 4,* 57-65.

Rodin, J. (1986). Health, control, and aging. In M. M. Baltes & P. B. Baltes (Eds.), *The psychology of control and aging* (pp. 139-163). Hillsdale, NJ: Erlbaum.

Rodin, J., & Timko, C. (1992). Sense of control, aging, and health. In M. G. Ory, R. P. Abeles, & P. D. Lipman (Eds.), *Aging, health, and behavior* (pp. 174-206). Newbury Park, CA: Sage.

Rotter, J. B. (1966). Generalized expectancies of internal versus external control of reinforcement. *Psychological Monographs, 80,* 1-28.

Rotter, J. B. (1975). Some problems and misconceptions related to the construct of internal versus external control of reinforcement. *Journal of Consulting and Clinical Psychology, 43,* 56-67.

Saltzer, E. B. (1981). Cognitive moderators of the relationship between behavioral intentions and behavior. *Journal of Personality and Social Psychology, 41,* 260-271.

Sandler, I. S., & Lakey, B. (1982). Locus of control as a stress moderator: The role of control perceptions and social support. *American Journal of Community Psychology, 10,* 65–80.

Sarafino, E. P. (1990). *Health psychology.* New York: Wiley.

Schulz, R., & Hanusa, B. H. (1978). Long-term effects of control and predictability-enhancing interventions: Findings and ethical issues. *Journal of Personality and Social Psychology, 36,* 1194–1201.

Seeman, M., Seeman, T., & Sayles, M. (1985). Social networks and health status: A longitudinal analysis. *Social Psychology Quarterly, 48,* 237–248.

Strickland, B. R. (1978). Internal–external expectancies and health-related behaviors. *Journal of Consulting and Clinical Psychology, 46,* 1192–1211.

Strickland, B. R. (1979). Internal–external expectancies and cardiovascular functioning. In L. C. Perlmuter & R. A. Monty (Eds.), *Choice and perceived control* (pp. 221–231). Hillsdale, NJ: Erlbaum.

Suls, J., & Ritterhouse, J. D. (1987). Personality and physical health [Special Issue]. *Journal of Personality, 55*(2).

Taylor, S. E., Helgeson, V. S., Reed, G. M., & Skokan, L. A. (1991). Self-generated feelings of control and adjustment to physical illness. *Journal of Social Issues, 47,* 91–109.

Tesser, R., & Mechanic, D. (1978). Psychological distress and perceived health status. *Journal of Health and Social Behavior, 19,* 254–262.

Thompson, S. C., Sobolew-Shubin, A., Galbraith, M. E., Schwankovsky, L., & Cruzen, D. (1993). Maintaining perceptions of control: Finding perceived control in low-control circumstances. *Journal of Personality and Social Psychology, 64,* 293–304.

Thompson, S. C., & Spacapan, S. (1991). Perception of control in vulnerable populations. *Journal of Social Issues, 47,* 1–21.

Tucker, L. R., & Lewis, C. (1973). A reliability coefficient for maximum likelihood factor analysis. *Psychometrika, 48,* 1–10.

Wallston, B. S., Alagna, S. W., DeVellis, B. M., & DeVellis, R. F. (1983). Social support and physical illness. *Health Psychology, 2,* 367–391.

Wallston, B. S., Wallston, K. A., Kaplan, G. D., & Maides, S. A. (1976). The development and validation of the health related locus of control (HLC) construct. *Journal of Consulting and Clinical Psychology, 44,* 580–585.

Wallston, K. A. (1989). Assessment of control in health-care settings. In A. Steptoe & A. Appels (Eds.), *Stress, personal control, and health* (pp. 85–105). New York: Wiley.

Wallston, K. A., & Smith, M. S. (1993). Issues of control and health: The action is in the interaction. In G. Penny, P.

Bennett, & M. Herbert (Eds.), *Health psychology: A lifespan perspective* (pp. 153–168).

Wallston, K. A., & Wallston, B. S. (1981). Health locus of control scales. In H. Lefcourt (Ed.), *Research with locus of control scales: Vol. 1* (pp. 189–243). New York: Academic Press.

Wallston, K. A., & Wallston, B. S. (1987). Age and health care beliefs: Self-efficacy as a mediator of low desire for control. *Psychology and Aging, 2,* 3–8.

Ware, J. E. (1984). Conceptualizing disease impact and treatment outcomes. *Cancer, 53,* 2316–2326.

Ware, J. E. (1986). The assessment of health status. In L. H. Aiken & D. Mechanic (Eds.), *Applications of social science to clinical medicine and health policy.* New Brunswick, NJ: Rutgers University Press.

Weiss, J. M. (1970). Somatic effects of predictable and unpredictable shock. *Psychosomatic Medicine, 32,* 397–409.

Weitzel, A. H. (1989). A test of the health promotion model with blue collar workers. *Nursing Research, 38,* 99–104.

Wolinsky, F. D., Coe, R. M., Miller, D. K., & Prendergast, J. M. (1984). Measurement of the global and functional dimensions of health status in the elderly. *Journal of Gerontology, 39,* 88–92.

Wortman, C. B., & Conway, T. L. (1985). The role of social support in adaptation and recovery from physical illness. In S. Cohen & S. L. Syme (Eds.), *Social support and health* (pp. 281–302). New York: Academic Press.

Wortman, C. B., & Dunkel-Schetter, C. (1987). Interpersonal relationships and cancer: A theoretical analysis. *Journal of Social issues, 35,* 120–155.

Young, L. (1992). Psychological factors in rheumatoid arthritis. *Journal of Consulting and Clinical Psychology, 60,* 619–627.

Zautra, A. J., Guarnaccia, C. A., & Reich, J. W. (1988). Factor structure of mental health measures for older adults. *Journal of Consulting and Clinical Psychology, 56,* 514–519.

Zautra, A. J., & Reich, J. W. (1983). Life events and perceptions of life quality: Developments in a two-factor approach. *Journal of Community Psychology, 11,* 121–132.

Zautra, A. J., Reich, J. W., & Guarnaccia, C. A. (1990). Some everyday life consequences of disability and bereavement for older adults. *Journal of Personality and Social Psychology, 59,* 550–561.

Zautra, A. J., Reich, J. W., & Newsom, J. T. (1994). Autonomy and a sense of control among older adults: An examination of their effects on health. In L. Bond, S. Cutler, & A. Grams (Eds.), *Promoting successful and productive aging* (pp. 153–170). Newbury Park, CA: Sage.

6

Protection Motivation Theory

Ronald W. Rogers and Steven Prentice-Dunn

INTRODUCTION

Unhealthful behavior continues to sicken and kill us. As the 21st century approaches, the majority of deaths in Western societies are due to "lifestyle illnesses" caused by improper diet, lack of exercise, alcohol and tobacco use, and risk-taking behaviors (Kaplan, Sallis, & Patterson, 1994). Lifestyle is responsible for many cancers in humans (Hermo, 1987). Individual actions may affect the health of others as well. Those affected by secondhand smoke are often spouses and children. Injuries, largely preventable, kill more children than the next six causes combined (Peterson & Roberts, 1992). Clearly, maladaptive habits take their toll in poorer life quality and premature death.

Motivating people to act to protect themselves presents an excellent reason for focusing on the role played by the threat to their health. A major source of motivation to take preventive actions is to avoid the unpleasant consequences of not taking those actions. Prevention programs frequently provide people with information about unpleasant, but avoidable, health consequences. Even if the threatening information is not mentioned explicitly or is deliberately omitted, the perception of danger motivates people to take healthful, protective action. As Schwarzer (1992, p. 235) stated, "A minimum level of threat or concern must exist before people start contemplating the benefits of possible actions and ruminate their competence to actually perform them." Would people refrain from smoking cigarettes if there were no threat of lung and heart problems? Would men, if their female partners were on some form of contraception, use condoms if there were no threat of AIDS and other sexually transmitted diseases? Thus, because the threat of pain and suffering motivates people to take protective action, the motivational role of threats is important.

Protection motivation theory is one formulation of the effects of threatening health information on attitude and behavior change. Rogers (1975, 1983) provided a complete description of the theory, and Prentice-Dunn and Rogers (1986) and Schwarzer (1992) compared protection motivation theory to the health belief model. Olson and Zanna (1993, p. 139) stated: "Fear appeals have probably received more research attention than any other message characteristic. The dominant theoretical framework in this literature is

Ronald W. Rogers and Steven Prentice-Dunn • Department of Psychology, University of Alabama, Tuscaloosa, Alabama 35487-0348.

Handbook of Health Behavior Research I: Personal and Social Determinants, edited by David S. Gochman. Plenum Press, New York, 1997.

Rogers's (1983) protection motivation theory....
Recent research within this framework has supported its utility for understanding the influence of messages on a variety of issues." This chapter provides an updated description of protection motivation theory, reviews the research of the past 15 years, and poses questions for future research.

STRUCTURE AND PROCESSES OF PROTECTION MOTIVATION THEORY

Protection motivation theory (PMT) originated to explain the effects of fear appeals on persuasion. The revised version (Rogers, 1983) of the initial formulation (Rogers, 1975) has received the most attention and will be the focus of this chapter.

Although PMT may be used to study static, existing beliefs, it emphasizes the changes produced by persuasive communications. Such research has used persuasive messages to stimulate central, systematic processing of the content of the messages. Such experimentally induced cognitions might not be salient in a survey study that did not activate the theoretically relevant beliefs in an attempt to change selected health attitudes and behaviors. A diagram of PMT is shown in Figures 1 and 2.

Sources of Information

As may be seen in Figure 1, many sources of information may initiate the cognitive mediating processes that are the focus of PMT. These sources may be categorized as either environmental or intrapersonal. Examples of the former are verbal persuasion (especially fear appeals) and observational learning (seeing what happens to others) (Rogers, 1983). Intrapersonal sources include the individual's personality or dispositional characteristics and prior experience with similar threats, the latter being perhaps the most underappreciated component in these sources. Such "feedback from coping activity" (Rogers, 1983, p. 167) may influence subsequent reactions to health threats; however, such feedback remains largely unexplored in PMT studies.

Cognitive Mediating Processes

Information about a health threat initiates cognitive mediating processes. These processes appraise maladaptive response(s) or adaptive response(s). For many health problems, there may be only one maladaptive and one adaptive response (e.g., smoking and smoking cessation); for others (e.g., improper diet, lack of exercise), there may be more than one response of each kind.

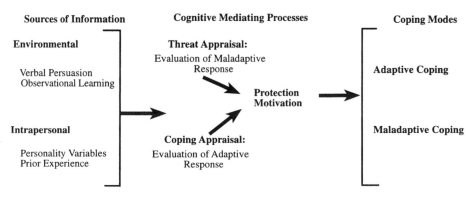

Figure 1. Overall model of protection motivation theory.

Cognitive Mediating Processes

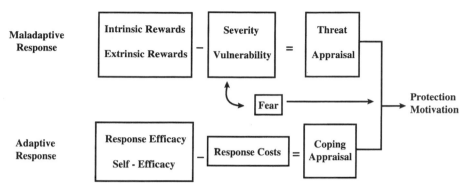

Figure 2. Cognitive mediating processes of protection motivation theory.

The mediating processes are illustrated in detail in Figure 2. Threat appraisal evaluates the maladaptive response, which may be a current behavior (e.g., unprotected sex) or one that could be started (e.g., abusing alcohol). The threat appraisal factors that increase the probability of the maladaptive response include intrinsic rewards (e.g., physical and psychological pleasure) and extrinsic rewards (e.g., peer approval, social norms as described in the theory of reasoned action). The threat appraisal factors that decrease the likelihood of the maladaptive response are the severity of the threat and the expectancy of being exposed to the threat. The latter was defined in the original PMT as "the conditional probability that the event will occur provided that no adaptive behavior is performed or there is no modification of an existing behavioral disposition" (Rogers, 1975, p. 97); it is now labeled vulnerability. Severity refers to the degree of physical harm, psychological harm (e.g., self-esteem), social threats (e.g., family and work relationships), economic harm (e.g., higher energy prices), dangers to others rather than oneself, and even threats to other species. It is assumed that the appraisal of these factors sums algebraically to produce the final appraisal of threat.

Fear plays only an indirect role in threat appraisal. Research reviewed by Rogers (1983) found that fear influences attitude and behavior change, not directly, but indirectly by affecting the appraisal of the severity of the danger. Rippetoe and Rogers (1987) discovered that fear can have an indirect and detrimental effect on attitude change by inducing maladaptive coping, specifically defensive avoidance.

The coping appraisal process evaluates one's ability to cope with and avert the threatened danger. As shown in Figure 2, the coping appraisal factors that increase the probability of the adaptive response(s) are the belief that the recommended coping response is effective—response efficacy (e.g., stopping smoking is an effective way to avoid the dangers associated with smoking)—and that one can successfully perform the coping response—self-efficacy (e.g., one can overcome the difficulty of smoking cessation). Coping appraisal is the summation of these appraisals of response efficacy and self-efficacy, minus any physical and psychological "costs" of adopting the recommended preventive response.

Although response costs and self-efficacy are related, it is useful to differentiate them conceptually. Self-efficacy refers to beliefs about one's ability and effort (e.g., "I doubt my willpower"), which can be independent of the response costs in any particular situation. Thus, people with weak beliefs in their self-efficacy may persist against those same response costs.

With respect to the temporal sequence of the cognitive mediating processes, Rogers (1975) stated in the original formulation of PMT (p. 93): "In the research paradigm designed to investigate the effects of fear appeals upon attitude change, an individual typically is exposed to persuasive communications that depict the noxious consequences accruing to a specified course of action. Recommendations are presented that can avert the danger if the individual adopts the appropriate attitudes and acts upon them." PMT experiments always present information in the same order, i.e., threatening information followed by coping information. Furthermore, the original studies of fear appeals and attitude change (see Hovland, Janis, & Kelley, 1953) adopted the instrumental-avoidance-learning paradigm in general and the fear-as-acquired-drive model in particular. Thus, PMT assumes that motivation must be supplied first to initiate the coping process.

The amount of protection motivation elicited is a function of the threat and coping appraisal processes. Like any intervening variable or logical construct, protection motivation can be measured several ways, but it is assumed that the best measure is behavioral intentions. Studies in PMT have sought to motivate people to make the decision to accept the communicator's health recommendation. Thus, behavioral intentions are an index of the effects of persuasion.

Two final points should be made about the mediational processes in PMT. First, the factors involved in threat appraisal and coping appraisal have rich meanings that may be conceptualized in a variety of ways. For example, Paterson and Neufeld (1987) inferred from the literature on stress that severity is composed "of the number of goals threatened, the importance of each goal, and the extent to which the goals will be unavailable should the event occur" (p. 413). Other dimensions of severity may be found in instrumental conditioning procedures for avoidance and punishment (e.g., intensity, duration, frequency, and rate of onset). To consider one more

example, self-efficacy can refer to ability, effort, initiation of action, and persistence. Thus, one of the major frontiers for future research will be to find different facets of PMT components that have theoretical and practical importance.

Second, PMT does not assume that the decision maker is rational. People can exhibit self-defeating behavioral tendencies, and there are differences in how individuals process information. Well-established findings in research on formal reasoning show that people often inadvertently change the meaning of information, fail to consider all possible interpretations, and fail to consider more than one way of combining information (see Galotti, 1989). There are numerous other biases in human thinking (e.g., confirmation bias, availability heuristic, belief perseveration, premature closure) and entire theories that explore them (e.g., prospect theory, image theory, cognitive–experiential self-theory, fuzzy logic models). With respect to just one component of PMT, vulnerability, Abelson and Levi (1985) reviewed numerous difficulties that humans have in estimating outcome probabilities: (1) overweighting of positive instances, (2) the availability heuristic, (3) instances that conform to preconceived ideas, and (4) the shift from statistical evidence to global intuition. Each of the appraisal processes will be affected by these cognitive and motivational biases. Although these relatively nonrational processes will prevent a veridical mapping of the objective information, it is important to note that the final threat and coping appraisals will reflect them and thus correspond closely with the amount of protection motivation elicited.

Coping Modes

Protection motivation eventuates in maladaptive coping or adaptive coping (especially acceptance of the communicator's recommendation) or both. In their dichotomy, maladaptive and adaptive coping are similar, respectively, to intrapsychic and direct action, internal and external adjustments, fear control and danger control, and emotion-focused and problem-focused coping. Although fear control and defense mechanisms are adaptive in that they can reduce emotional distress, coping modes are labeled maladaptive if they do not directly manage the threat to physical well-being by dealing with the reality of the external situation.

Any changes in coping will feed back as a source of information in the model of protection motivation as "prior experience" (see Figure 1). Although PMT does not have the "action" and "maintenance" stages of some theories (e.g., Prochaska, DiClemente, & Norcross, 1992; Schwarzer, 1992; Weinstein & Sandman, 1992), it is important to note that feedback from adaptive and maladaptive coping will force reappraisals of the threat and coping resources.

Of course, changes in attitudes and behavior produced by health information are bombarded by inimical forces. For example, sustaining the acceptance of a communicator's recommendation (e.g., to negotiate the four stages of the smoking career: initiation, maintenance, cessation, and relapse) may require additional interventions such as relapse prevention training, booster treatments, and attempts to deal with any abstinence violation effect. Nevertheless, successfully motivating or persuading people to protect themselves is an important step in disease prevention and health promotion.

The Combinatorial Rule and Interaction Effects

PMT initially assumed that the components of the model would combine multiplicatively because this is the rule in the family of expectancy–value theories from which PMT was derived. This combinatorial rule had to be rejected because PMT research has never found the higher-order interaction effects predicted by the multiplicative rule (see Rogers, 1983). The rule has also been disconfirmed by other investigators of health persuasion, including Mulilis and Lippa (1990), Ronis (1992), Sutton and Eiser (1984, 1990), and Witte (1992c).

Jonas (1993) also concluded that studies in health behavior have rejected the multiplicative rule. He presented evidence that the reason for the lack of support for the rule is its overly demanding assumption that individuals assign other than ordinal values to the different factors on subjective scales, convert them to a common scale, and perform trade-offs between valences and expectancies. A conjoint measurement analysis showed that the violation of the multiplicative rule was due to the cognitive difficulty of performing the trade-offs. Although a minority of the subjects did use the rule, it was under highly facilitative conditions (e.g., within-subjects designs) and would be of little importance in realistically demanding conditions.

Furthermore, according to economic utility theories, the relationship between the amount of something and its utility is nonlinear. Thus, the concept of diminishing marginal returns (the greater the value, the less the added utility of additional amounts) would work against the multiplicative rule. Diminishing marginal utility can also yield subadditivity effects, which is the type of interaction effect typically found. For example, Birnbaum and Sotoodeh (1991) scaled the stresses induced by life changes and found that in a series of three stressors of equal value, the third stressful event contributed less than half as much as the first.

Although an additive model holds within each appraisal process, when components of the threat and coping appraisal processes are combined, subadditive interaction effects occur (see Figure 3). If people believe they can cope with a threat, the greater the danger, the greater the intentions to perform those coping responses. On the other hand, if people do not believe they will be able to cope with the danger, as that danger becomes greater, intentions to perform the coping response actually diminish (e.g., people actually plan to drink or smoke more!). This "boomerang" interaction effect, with coping operationalized as either response efficacy or response efficacy plus self-efficacy, has been confirmed in several of our experiments and by other

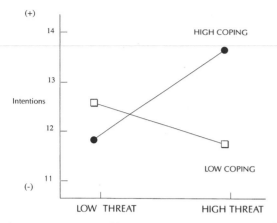

Figure 3. Interaction of threat and coping. From Sturges and Rogers (1996).

investigators as well (see the later section on review of the interaction).

REVIEW OF RESEARCH ON PROTECTION MOTIVATION THEORY

Since its inception, protection motivation theory has generated a large number of tests of its four central variables: severity, vulnerability, response efficacy, and self-efficacy. Fewer studies have assessed rewards for the maladaptive response and response costs of the adaptive action. This section will focus on those studies that explicitly manipulated or measured components of PMT variables, but will not review research covered in other chapters in this volume (e.g., the health belief model).

The published research that has investigated components of PMT is shown in Tables 1 and 2. Several points may be made from an examination of the main effects found in PMT research. First, studies have been conducted on a diverse array of topics: disease prevention, health promotion, injury prevention, protecting others, political issues, and environmental concerns. PMT has been applied to over 30 different topics. Second, although most dependent measures have been be-

havioral intentions, several have been overt behaviors. Similar results have been found for the two categories of measures. Third, comparatively few investigators have failed to find predicted effects. Fourth, hypothesized effects of PMT variables have been found with both experimental and correlational research. Finally, research on PMT appears to be increasing, especially since the mid-1980s.

Threat Appraisal

Among the most consistent findings in PMT research has been that increases in severity or vulnerability or both lead to greater intentions to behave in a healthful way. Although our meta-analysis of the research on PMT has not been completed, a simple frequency count of studies that reported significant or nonsignificant effect is promising. The number of studies that reported a significant effect and the total number of studies are, respectively, 21 of 23 for severity, 17 of 18 for vulnerability, and 7 of 8 for the combination of severity plus vulnerability.

Strong manipulations of threat (especially vulnerability) may be needed to overcome the optimistic bias held by most individuals (cf. Weinstein, 1993). It should be noted, however, that subjective assessments of vulnerability are not always overly optimistic. Two studies have found that those whose sexual practices place them at increased risk for HIV infection do have realistic perceptions of vulnerability (Van der Velde, van der Plight, & Hooykas, 1994; Van der Velde, Hooykas, & van der Plight, 1992).

Clearly, the rewards associated with the maladaptive response have been the least investigated of the PMT variables. In a survey of adolescents about skin cancer, rewards associated with tanning were associated with weaker intentions to take precautions (Mermelstein & Riesenberg, 1992). Results of an experiment on the same topic (Prentice-Dunn, Jones, & Floyd, in press) also indicate that rewards decrease intentions in predicted ways.

Coping Appraisal

Sutton (1982) performed a meta-analysis on 38 studies of fear-arousing communications published between 1953 and 1980. One of his major conclusions was that "increasing the efficacy of the recommended action strengthens intentions to adopt that action" (p. 323). As can be seen in Table 2, more recent research corroborates Sutton's conclusion. The number of studies that reported a significant effect and the total number of studies are, respectively, 28 of 31 for response efficacy, 24 of 26 for self-efficacy, and 3 of 3 for the combination of response plus self-efficacy.

In general, findings from the frequent studies of self-efficacy suggest that beliefs that one can carry out the health recommendation are very important to one's decision to act. Self-efficacy may play an even greater role in children's health. Sturges and Rogers (1996) found that these beliefs were much more malleable in children than in adolescents or adults.

Fewer tests have been conducted on the response costs associated with the adaptive response. The consistent conclusion, however, is that intentions to act adaptively are damaged by response costs.

Interaction of Threat Appraisal and Coping Appraisal

Threat and coping appraisal variables have been found to interact in about one half of the studies in which both classes of variables have been tested (Brouwers & Sorrentino, 1993; Kleinot & Rogers, 1982; Maddux & Rogers, 1983; Mulilis & Lippa, 1990; Rogers & Mewborn, 1976; Self & Rogers, 1990; Sturges & Rogers, 1996; Witte, 1992c; Wurtele & Maddux, 1987). The interactions tend to appear when the threat manipulation is especially strong. Almost all are boomerang interactions. For example, Self and Rogers (1990) found that increasing the level of threat strengthened intentions to moderate alcohol consumption only if people believed they could cope with the threat. If people did not believe they could cope effectively with the threat, increases in threat produced intentions to drink more alcohol.

The boomerang interaction effect has been found when coping has been operationalized either as response efficacy or as response efficacy plus self-efficacy. Only one study has differentiated self-efficacy from response efficacy and manipulated them orthogonally (Maddux & Rogers, 1983). In this study, the form of the interaction depended on the level of self-efficacy. The boomerang interaction occurred under conditions of low self-efficacy, but the interaction under conditions of high self-efficacy was interpreted in terms of precaution and hyperdefensive decision-making strategies.

Several interpretations of the boomerang interaction effect may be advanced. First, the effect may be understood if individuals are assumed to act with some restraint in their health behaviors. Should people come to believe that a danger cannot be avoided, they may find no reason to continue to restrain themselves. Second, Rogers (1985) acknowledged that when people are confronted with a real danger, many cognitive and motivational processes may prevent an optimal (i.e., multiplicative) integration of information, whereas an experiment may demonstrate that people respond in an eminently rational fashion when confronted with a hypothetical threat. Confronting an actual danger (e.g., the threat of breast cancer) may evoke defensive, maladaptive coping that could short-circuit the multiplicative integration of information (Janis & Feshbach, 1953; Rippetoe & Rogers, 1987).

A third possible interpretation of the boomerang effect concerns uncontrollability. Because controllability is related to interest in taking beneficial action (Weinstein, 1982), it is likely that the individuals who feel less able to determine their fate act with less regard for the consequences. Fourth, it may be that individuals respond to the uncontrollability by attempting to restore perceived control of their fate. An individ-

Table 1. Threat Appraisal Variables Tested in Prior Research

Study	Topic[a]
Severity	
Rogers & Thistlethwaite (1970)	Smoking (I)
Hass, Bagley, & Rogers (1975)	Smoking (I)
Rogers & Deckner (1975)	Smoking (B)
Griffeth & Rogers (1976)	Safe driving (I), driving errors (B)
Rogers & Mewborn (1976)	Smoking (I)
Rogers, Deckner, & Mewborn (1978)	Smoking (B)
Mewborn & Rogers (1979)	Avoidance of sexually transmitted diseases (I)[b]
Shelton & Rogers (1981)	Helping endangered species (I)
Rogers (1985)	Inoculation against a virus (I)
Wolf, Gregory, & Stephan (1986)[c]	Action against nuclear war (I)
Wurtele & Maddux (1987)	Regular exercise (B)
Robberson & Rogers (1988)	Regular exercise (I)
Allard (1989)[c]	AIDS-preventive actions (B)
Rhodes & Wolitski (1990)	Perceived effectiveness of AIDS poster (B)
Seydel, Taal, & Wiegman (1990)[c]	Breast self-examination (I)
Sutton, Marsh, & Matheson (1990)[c]	Smoking (I)
Ahia (1990)[c]	Safe-sex behaviors (I)
Axelrod & Newton (1991)[c]	Action against nuclear war (I)
Hine & Gifford (1991)	Commitment to stop pollution (I), financial donations (B), time commitment (I)[b]
Smith Klohn & Rogers (1991)	Osteoporosis prevention (I)
Weinstein, Sandman, & Roberts (1991)	Radon testing kit (B), use of kit (I)
Allen (1993)	Action against nuclear war (I)
Lynch et al. (1992)[a]	Exercise program for high cholesterol (B)
Vulnerability	
Hass, Bagley, & Rogers (1975)	Energy conservation (I)[b]
Mewborn & Rogers (1979)	Avoidance of sexually transmitted diseases (I)
Maddux & Rogers (1983)	Smoking (I)
Rogers (1985)	Inoculation against a virus (I)
Wolf, Gregory, & Stephan (1986)[c]	Action against nuclear war (I)
Wurtele & Maddux (1987)	Regular exercise (B)
Wurtele (1988)	Calcium intake (B), calcium intake (I)
Allard (1989)[c]	AIDs-preventive actions (B)
Tanner, Day, & Crask (1989) ·	Condom use (I)
Steffan (1990)[c]	Testicular self-examination (I)
Ahia (1990)[c]	Safe-sex behaviors (B)
Aspinwall, Kemeny, Taylor, Schneider, & Dudley (1991)[c]	Number of anonymous sex partners of homosexual men (B)
Axelrod & Newton (1991)[c]	Action against nuclear war (I)
Weinstein, Sandman, & Roberts (1991)	Radon testing kit orders (B)
Liberman & Chaiken (1992)	Caffeine consumption (I)
Mermelstein & Riesenberg (1992)[c]	Precautions against skin cancer (I), sunscreen use (B)
Vaughan (1993)[c]	Protection against pesticide misuse (B)
Sutton, Bickler, Sancho-Aldridge, & Saidi (1994)[c]	Mammography (B)
Combination of severity and vulnerability	
Stainback & Rogers (1983)	Alcohol abstention (I)
Calantone & Warshaw (1985)	Political election (I)
Rippetoe & Rogers (1987)	Breast self-examination (I)
Knapp (1991)	Reduction in tooth plaque (B)

Table 1. (*Continued*)

Study	Topic[a]
Combination of severity and vulnerability (*cont.*)	
Gleicher & Petty (1992)	Crime prevention (I)
McElreath, Prentice-Dunn, & Rogers (1997)	Children's use of bicycle helmets (I)
Pointer & Rogers (1994)	Moderation of drinking alcohol (I)
Sturges & Rogers (1996)	Smoking (I)[b]
Rewards	
Mermelstein & Riesenberg (1992)[c]	Precautions against skin cancer (I), sunscreen use (B)[b]
Prentice-Dunn, Jones, & Floyd (in press)	Precautions against skin cancer (I)

[a]The letter in parentheses indicates whether the topic was assessed with measures of intention (I) or with behavioral measures (B).
[b]No main effect or interaction was found with the independent variable.
[c]The independent variable was not manipulated.

ual might think, "If a bad thing is going to happen, it will happen because I choose to make it happen."

Another possible explanation may stem from the fact that the interaction effect seems to occur primarily with health behaviors that occur in a social context and produce immediately pleasurable and rewarding effects (e.g., drinking, smoking, actions associated with sexually transmitted diseases).

Witte (1992b) attempted to explain the boomerang effect by extending Leventhal's (1970) danger control process and fear control process. Danger control deals with how people realistically try to prevent a danger from occurring; fear control concerns how people handle their affective emotional states. Witte argued that when perceived efficacy is low, attempts to control the fear (e.g., defensive avoidance, denial) dominate attempts to control the danger. Although Self and Rogers (1990) found a tendency for people in their low-coping/high-threat condition to resort to wishful thinking, religious faith, defensive avoidance, and feelings of hopelessness and fatalism, the effect was not significant. Clearly, there is a need for research that directly addresses the mediator(s) of the boomerang effect.

Overall Tests of the Theory

Community interventions using PMT are rare, but are beginning to appear in the literature. For example, Rhodes, Wolitski, and Thornton-Johnson (1992) used videos, role plays, and discussions based on three PMT variables to influence females whose sex partners were intravenous drug users. The authors reported several adaptive changes, including an increase in condom use. Stanton, Black, Kaljee, and Ricardo (1993) used ethnographic methods to summarize the perceptions of urban children and adolescents on each of the PMT variables applied to sexual behavior.

Attempts to test PMT as a whole have typically failed to include rewards and response costs (Flynn, Lyman, & Prentice-Dunn, 1995; Van der Velde & van der Plight, 1991) or have included additional variables (Wallerstein & Sanchez-Merki, 1994). Nonetheless, all three studies supported the general framework of the model. Future tests of the entire theory using structural equation modeling are needed.

Modes of Coping

There is now a comprehensive literature illustrating that people respond to threats in a variety of ways. This chapter explicitly acknowledges that persuasive health messages may lead, under some circumstances, to maladaptive ways of coping with a health threat. There also may be coping modes (e.g., rational problem solving, seeking social support) that serve as adaptive precursors to behavioral intentions.

Table 2. Coping Appraisal Variables Tested in Prior Research

Study	Topic[a]
Response efficacy	
Rogers & Thistlethwaite (1970)	Smoking (I)
Rogers & Deckner (1975)	Smoking (B)
Rogers & Mewborn (1976)	Smoking (I), safe driving (I), avoidance of sexually transmitted diseases (I)
Shelton & Rogers (1981)	Helping endangered species (I)
Maddux & Rogers (1983)	Smoking (I)
Rogers (1985)	Inoculation against a virus (I)
Stanley & Maddux (1986)	Regular exercise (I)
Wolf, Gregory, & Stephan (1986)[c]	Action against nuclear war (I)
Rippetoe & Rogers (1987)	Breast self-examination (I)
Calnan & Rutter (1988)[c]	Breast self-examination (B)
Sutton & Hallett (1988)[c]	Smoking (I)
Wurtele (1988)	Calcium intake (I)
Campis, Prentice-Dunn, & Lyman (1989)	Parental education of children about child sexual abuse (I)
Sutton & Hallett (1989a)[c]	Smoking (I)
Sutton & Hallett (1989b)[c]	Seat belt use (I)
Peterson, Farmer, & Kashani (1990)[c]	Parental action to prevent children's injuries (B)
Rhodes & Wolitski (1990)	Perceived effectiveness of AIDS poster (B)[b]
Seydel, Taal, & Wiegman (1990)[c]	Cancer prevention (I), cancer prevention (B)[b]
Steffen (1990)[c]	Testicular self-examination (I)
Sutton, Marsh, & Matheson (1990)[c]	Smoking (I)
Aspinwall, Kemeny, Taylor, Schneider, & Dudley (1991)[c]	Number of anonymous sex partners of homosexual men (B)
Ahia (1990)[c]	Safe sex behaviors (B)
Axelrod & Newton (1991)[c]	Action against nuclear war (I)
Kelly, Zyzanski, & Alemagno (1991)[c]	Smoking (I), stress reduction (I), proper nutrition (I), seat belt use (I), regular exercise (I)
Lynch et al. (1992)[c]	Exercise program for high cholesterol (B)
Marcus & Owen (1992)[c]	Regular exercise (B)
Vaughan (1993)[c]	Protection against pesticide misuse (B)
Wulfert & Wan (1993)[c]	Condom use (I)
McElreath, Prentice-Dunn, & Rogers (1997)	Children's use of bicycle helmets (I)[b]
Plotnikoff (1994)[c]	Cardiovascular disease prevention (I)
Sutton, Bickler, Sancho-Aldridge, & Saidi (1994)[c]	Mammography (B)
Self-efficacy	
Maddux & Rogers (1983)	Smoking (I)
Sutton & Eiser (1984)[c]	Smoking (I)
Stanley & Maddux (1986)	Regular exercise (I)
Wolf, Gregory, & Stephen (1986)[c]	Action against nuclear war (I)
Rippetoe & Rogers (1987)	Breast self-examination (I)
Sutton, Marsh, & Matheson (1987)[c]	Smoking (I)
Wurtele & Maddux (1987)	Regular exercise (B)
Campis, Prentice-Dunn, & Lyman (1989)	Parental education of children about child sexual abuse (I)
Sutton & Hallett (1989a)[c]	Smoking (I)
Tanner, Day, & Crask (1989)	Condom use (I)
Seydel, Taal, & Wiegman (1990)[c]	Cancer prevention (I), cancer prevention (B)[b]
Ahia (1990)[c]	Safe-sex behaviors (B)
Aspinwall, Kemeny, Taylor, Schneider, & Dudley (1991)[c]	Numbers of anonymous sex partners of homosexual men (B)

Table 2. (*Continued*)

Study	Topic[a]
Self-efficacy (*cont.*)	
Axelrod & Newton (1991)[c]	Action against nuclear war (I)
Fruin, Pratt, & Owen (1992)[c]	Regular exercise (I)
Kelly, Zyzanski, & Alemagno (1991)[c]	Smoking (I), stress reduction (I), proper nutrition (I), seat belt use (I), regular exercise (I)
Tedesco, Keffer, & Fleck-Kandath (1991)[c]	Tooth brushing (B), flossing (B)
Ho (1992)[c]	Smoking (I)
McCauley (1992)[c]	Regular exercise (I)
Marcus & Owen (1992)[c]	Regular exercise (B)
Winett et al. (1992)	HIV preventive skills (B)
Taal, Rasker, Seydel, & Wiegman (1993)[c]	Regimen for rheumatoid arthritis (B)
Vaughan (1993)[c]	Protection against pesticide misuse (B)
Wulfert & Van (1993)[c]	Condom use (B)
McElreath, Prentice-Dunn, & Rogers (1997)	Children's use of bicycle helmets (I)[b]
Plotnikoff (1994)[c]	Cardiovascular disease prevention (I)
Combination of response efficacy and self-efficacy	
Campis, Prentice-Dunn, & Lyman (1989)	Parental education of children about child sexual abuse (I)
Self & Rogers (1990)	Safe-sex behaviors (I)
Sturges & Rogers (1996)	Smoking (I), smokeless tobacco (I)
Response costs	
Campis, Prentice-Dunn, & Lyman (1989)	Parental education of children about child sexual abuse (I)
Ronis & Kaiser (1989)[c]	Breast self-examination (B)
Peterson, Farmer, & Kashani (1990)[c]	Parental action to prevent children's injuries (B)
Sutton, Marsh, & Matheson (1990)[c]	Smoking (I)
Fruin, Pratt, & Owen (1992)[c]	Regular exercise (I)
Marcus & Owen (1992)[c]	Regular exercise (B)
Vanweesenbeeck, de Graaf, van Zessen, Straver, & Visser (1993)[c]	Protective behaviors among male clients of female prostitutes (I)

[a]The letter in parentheses indicates whether the topic was assessed with measures of intention (I) or with behavioral measures (B).
[b]No main effect or interaction was found with the independent variable.
[c]The independent variable was not manipulated.

Rippetoe and Rogers (1987) found that high response efficacy produced stronger intentions to perform breast self-examinations and greater use of rational problem solving, relative to low response efficacy. The low-response-efficacy message produced higher levels of fatalism and use of religious faith. High self-efficacy (compared to low self-efficacy) resulted in greater intentions, more rational problem solving, and less hopelessness.

Rippetoe and Rogers found that high threat led to use of both adaptive and maladaptive modes of coping. Other investigators have found that the nature of the threat is likely to produce more of one class of coping than the other. For example, Hansell, Thorn, Prentice-Dunn, and Floyd (1997) found that women who viewed their gynecological problem (breast reexamination or return for a Pap smear) as a threat tended to use less rational action, more wishful thinking, and more fatalism than did women who saw their problem as a challenge. On the other hand, Schaefer, Schaefer, Bultena, and Hoiberg (1993) found that subjects who viewed unsafe food as a serious and probable health threat used more adaptive coping modes than did subjects who did not see food in a similar manner.

Self and Rogers (1990) found that depressed people, compared to normal individuals, engaged in more maladaptive thinking about the health topics of drinking, exercise, and sexually transmitted diseases. Tendencies toward reality distortion and mildly disordered thinking are posited by cognitive theories of depression. Interestingly, antisocial personalities engaged in less maladaptive thinking than the normals. Beliefs that one could not cope produced some maladaptive coping among normal individuals, but had no effect on the depressed or antisocial personalities.

Individual Differences

A range of individual difference and personality variables have been assessed in conjunction with PMT components, including health locus of control, ethnicity, gender, political orientation, and environmental concern. With few exceptions, individual difference variables have not had an influence on the outcomes of PMT investigations.

Brouwers and Sorrentino (1993) reasoned that some inconsistencies in PMT research could be due to the neglect of uncertainty orientation. Uncertainty-oriented people, compared to certainty-oriented ones who tend to avoid potentially threatening information, are motivated to process information when there is uncertainty and would behave according to PMT. Brouwers and Sorrentino found that these people requested more information under high-efficacy conditions than under low-efficacy conditions, and the difference was greater under high-threat conditions than under low-threat conditions.

Depressed and antisocial personalities were compared to normal individuals by Self and Rogers (1990). The coping variable (high versus low levels of response efficacy and self-efficacy) had the predicted effect on intentions to practice safe sex among normals, but did not affect depressed individuals because they are characterized by feelings of inadequacy and ineffectiveness. The antisocial personalities, too, were not affected by the coping information, but for a different reason. They have an egoistic incapacity to realize the effects of their behavior on others and have minimal concern for their sexual partners.

Another variable that may affect PMT re-

search outcomes is concern for one's appearance. For some, appearance motivation is as large a factor in behavior as concern for health (Hayes & Ross, 1987; Jones & Leary, 1994). Indeed, Prentice-Dunn et al. (in press) found that appearance motivation adversely affected intentions to reduce skin cancer risk.

One variable that does appear to matter is age (or cognitive developmental level). Results of two studies (McElreath, Prentice-Dunn, & Rogers, 1997; Sturges & Rogers, 1996) suggested that children may process health information differently than do adolescents and adults. Verbal persuasion has been studied extensively with adults, but much less is known about changing the attitudes of children. Indeed, can a cognitive model devised to explain adults' health-decision making be applied to children? PMT's interaction between threat and coping was found in a study on the prevention of cigarette smoking among adults and 15-year-old adolescents (see Figure 3), but not among 10-year-old children. The children did not show the hypothesized cognitive deficits in processing information about health threats and how to cope with them. The major difference between the children and the adults and adolescents was that the children's self-efficacy beliefs could be either built up or devastated rather easily. These 10-year-old children were in Erikson's stage of Industry versus Inferiority, and beliefs in self-efficacy may have been easily manipulated because the children had not completed this developmental stage. These studies indicate the importance of adding a developmental perspective to theories of preventive health psychology.

MULTIPLE ROUTES TO PERSUASION: IMPLICATIONS OF THE ELABORATION LIKELIHOOD MODEL AND THE HEURISTIC–SYSTEMATIC MODEL FOR PROTECTION MOTIVATION THEORY

There is a great deal of criticism in cognitive psychology of traditional rational choice theories that assume that people maximize utility functions (e.g., Frisch & Clemen, 1994). It is usually argued that rational choice theories are normative but not descriptive (e.g., Herrnstein, 1990). Many theories in cognitive psychology and in social psychology offer alternatives to logical–rational models. For example, to explain automatic decision making, Mitchell and Beach (1990) proposed image theory, which is based on the fit between choice alternatives and images or between principles and plans. Epstein (1994) discussed several multiple processing theories that involve parallel, interacting modes of information processing, each following its own set of rules. Epstein's cognitive–experiential self-theory has two information-processing systems (cf. Kirkpatrick & Epstein, 1992). The rational system functions according to rational rules of logic and evidence. The experiential system represents events concretely, is heavily influenced by emotional events, and operates automatically. There are also microlevel models that, like the experiential system, attempt to account for the transformation of objective probabilities into subjective probabilities that appear irrational: (1) Hendrickx, Vlek, and Calje (1992) differentiated relative frequency information, which refers to past outcomes, from cognitive scenario information, which refers to information that aids the construction of images of the processes that lead to danger; and (2) Slovic (1987) distinguished "risk perception" (qualitative dreaded and unknown characteristics of the risk) from "risk assessment" (morbidity and mortality statistics) information.

Within the field of social psychology, two process theories of attitude change have become extremely influential: Petty and Cacioppo's (1986) elaboration likelihood model (ELM) and Chaiken's heuristic–systematic model (HSM) (see Chaiken, Liberman, & Eagly, 1989). Petty and Cacioppo's ELM postulates a continuum of the likelihood that elaboration will occur in response to a persuasive message. The elaboration likelihood continuum is anchored at one end by central processing and at the other end by peripheral processing, the two routes to persuasion. In central processing, persuasion results from close scrutiny and consideration of issue-relevant arguments in a persuasive message. In peripheral processing, persuasion occurs without any close scrutiny of issue-relevant arguments, but rather is based on simple, issue-irrelevant cues. Persuasion resulting from central processing tends to be enduring, while persuasion from peripheral processing tends to be temporary. Central processing is highly similar to Chaiken and her colleagues' (cf. Chaiken et al., 1989; Jepson & Chaiken, 1990) systematic processing, but the conceptualization of heuristic processing is narrower than that of peripheral processing.

According to both theories, the motivation to process a message is the factor that determines whether processing will be predominantly central or peripheral, and the most important motivational variable is involvement or the personal relevance of the topic. According to ELM's and HSM's analysis of fear appeals and attitude change, whether central or peripheral processing is invoked depends on an individual's motives, or goals. Gleicher and Petty (1992) interpreted their data to mean that if people are motivated to protect themselves, they will engage in a thoughtful analysis of the message; if they believe new information might challenge their sense of reassurance, they will engage in biased processing or be affected via the peripheral route. Liberman and Chaiken (1992) argued similarly that if people are realistically motivated to protect themselves, personal relevance increases systematic processing, but if they are not motivated to be objective and instead seek a particular conclusion, then personal relevance will increase defensive, biased, systematic processing.

PMT assumes that fear appeals initiate cognitive mediating processes (Rogers, 1983). Increasing the amount of threat in a fear appeal is postulated to increase involvement and central processing. There is evidence that health-threat communications involve central, systematic processing. Rippetoe and Rogers's (1987) path analysis demonstrated that the variables manipulated in their experiment (threat, response efficacy, and self-efficacy) did not have a direct effect on attitude change, as might be expected if they operate as peripheral or heuristic cues, but that the effects of the manipulated variables were mediated by thoughts about adaptive and maladaptive ways of coping. To indicate the breadth and comprehensiveness of this elaboration, the threat manipulation affected cognitions about two adaptive coping mechanisms and five defensive processes (which were all that were measured).

Pointer and Rogers (1994) reasoned that a threat to one's health qualifies as "involving" and "personally relevant" because these terms imply significant, personal consequences. They conducted a direct test of these ideas and included measures of message processing typically used in ELM and HSM research. A factorial experiment manipulated threat, argument quality, and source expertise to illuminate the central, systematic versus the peripheral, heuristic processing of a fear appeal. Greater agreement with the recommendation to drink moderately was produced by high than by low threat, by strong than by weak arguments, and by an expert than by a nonexpert. The assumption of PMT that threat increases central, systematic processing was confirmed.

The manipulation of threat had positive main effects on the measures of (1) perceived threat, (2) self-reports of involvement, and (3) cognitive responses or thought listing. Jepson and Chaiken (1990, p. 62) had asked, "Does fear increase or decrease systematic processing?" These findings showed that threat can increase systematic processing. Jepson and Chaiken also wondered whether people accept a communicator's recommendation under high-threat conditions because they have closely scrutinized the message or accepted it blindly without much elaboration. The data supported the PMT assumption that recommendations are accepted after individuals carefully appraise the threat and how they can cope with it.

In Pointer and Rogers's (1994) study, however, threat did not have the predicted interaction effects with argument quality and expertise on the measures of attitude and behavioral intention, revealing that the persuasive effect of threat is not identical to that of involvement.

There are at least two plausible interpretations of why the predicted interaction effects, derived from ELM and HSM, were not confirmed. A major difference between the Pointer and Rogers study and most investigations of ELM is the issue of personal control or the necessity for people to do something to avoid the threatening outcomes described in the messages. Typical studies of ELM assess attitudes toward issues that would affect people, but over which they have no personal control; furthermore, there is no attempt to persuade them to do anything. In contrast, the raison d'être of studies of fear appeals is to persuade people to adopt the communicator's recommendations (e.g., to moderate their drinking).

The remaining interpretation follows from both ELM and HSM. Petty and Cacioppo (1986) acknowledged that some variables can have multiple effects, such as enhancing and reducing message processing or shifting elaboration from relatively objective to relatively biased processing. The heuristic–systematic model postulates that in addition to being motivated to hold correct attitudes, processing can also serve the defensive motive of defending a particular position (Liberman & Chaiken, 1992). Rippetoe and Rogers (1987) found that threat affected intentions (as did Pointer and Rogers) and also activated three specific types of defenses: avoidance (trying not to think about the danger), hopelessness (believing there is no solution without being able to accept this state of affairs), and wishful thinking (dreaming about unrealistic solutions). Thus, Rippetoe and Rogers demonstrated that threat can initiate processing that serves two goals or motives: (1) the goal to have a realistic appraisal of the threat and how best to cope with it, which would be concerned about the information in the messages; and (2) the goal to defend one's unhealthy habits, which would be less concerned about the quality of arguments. These goals eventuate in adaptive coping and maladaptive coping, respectively. Although the research reviewed in this chapter clearly demonstrates that the components of PMT produce adaptive coping, these same components simultaneously elicit specific maladaptive forms of coping (see Rippetoe & Rogers, 1987).

EXTENSIONS OF PROTECTION MOTIVATION THEORY

PMT has been extended in numerous directions. First, it has been confirmed that the same variables that induce self-protection induce other-protection (Shelton & Rogers, 1981). Three studies (Campis, Prentice-Dunn, & Lyman, 1989; Flynn et al., 1995; Peterson, Farmer, & Kashani, 1990) illustrate that PMT may be extended to actions on the behalf of another person's health. Each study concerned parents' behavior on behalf of their children (education about sexual abuse, adherence to a medical regimen for muscular dystrophy, and prevention of childhood injuries). In every instance, coping appraisal variables were central to affecting parental intentions and behavior. The evidence suggested that these variables may play a greater role in the protection of children than in the protection of adults. Wallerstein and Sanchez-Merki's (1994) work expanded PMT to include "other-protective efficacy" or socially responsible behavior. These authors emphasized the social and political embeddedness of intervention programs that have individual and community aspects.

Response efficacy works, not just to help oneself, but to help others when the help must be mediated by a social organization (Shelton & Rogers, 1981). Wolf, Gregory, and Stephan (1986) extended PMT to a political domain by showing that response efficacy was instrumental in producing a willingness to engage in active antinuclear behaviors. Axelrod and Newton's (1991) survey of efforts to prevent nuclear war found a similar effect and concluded that such research can "discover effective avenues toward public education and the strengthening of societal supports for sustained participation in democratic action to influence public policies toward major reduction in the threat of nuclear war" (pp. 38–39).

PMT is not limited to physical, health concerns, but has been extended to social and psychological threats as well (Robberson & Rogers, 1988). Fear appeals have been compared to, and found to be superior to, positive appeals (Robberson & Rogers, 1988). Other research reviewed in this chapter has extended the theory to children (McElreath et al., 1997; Sturges & Rogers, 1996) and to clinically relevant personality types (Self & Rogers, 1990).

Several theorists have elaborated PMT. Maddux (1993) offered an integrated social–cognitive model that weaves PMT and the HBM into the theory of planned behavior. Witte (1992a,b) proposed an extended parallel process model (EPPM). It incorporates PMT's explanation of the danger control process and expands the study of the fear control process to focus on why fear appeals are rejected. The model predicts that when perceived threat exceeds perceived efficacy, fear control processes will dominate. In fact, the fourth proposition of the EPPM is that "as perceived threat increases when perceived efficacy is low, people will do the opposite of what is advocated (boomerang)" (Witte, 1992b, p. 341). There is a critical point at which fear control processes dominate danger control ones. The EPPM also assumes that fear is a direct cause of maladaptive responding.

In a revision of PMT referred to as ordered protection motivation theory, Tanner, Hunt, and Eppright (1991) emphasized the role of fear, ordered the appraisal processes, addressed the issue of maladaptive coping, and examined normative components. More recently, Eppright, Tanner, and Hunt (1994) emphasized the role of two types of knowledge: generalized and experiential.

Among many stage models of health behavior (e.g., Prochaska et al., 1992; Weinstein & Sandman, 1992), Schwarzer (1992) proposed the health action process approach, which distinguishes between a motivational and an action stage. The former phase incorporates familiar concepts from cognitive models, including PMT, but the new focus of the theory is the action stage, which is composed of action plans, action control, and situational barriers and support.

IMPORTANT RESEARCH QUESTIONS

This chapter concludes by highlighting a few issues that may be among the more important ones for future research. First, dimensions of the message components (e.g., different aspects of severity, different ways to present information about vulnerability) should be differentiated and manipulated orthogonally.

Second, research is needed to address the similarities and differences between response costs and (1) self-efficacy and (2) intrinsic and extrinsic rewards.

Third, assumptions of temporal order have not been tested. The threat is presented, followed by information on how to cope. What if the order were reversed? That more adaptive coping would be elicited by presenting information about the threat before information about coping remains an untested assumption.

Fourth, although several studies have conducted behavioral follow-ups, there is a woeful lack of knowledge of how people's long-term coping behavior feeds back into and affects the cognitive mediating processes.

Fifth, under what conditions will central, systematic processing occur, and under what conditions will peripheral, heuristic processing occur?

Sixth, a fruitful area of research involves longitudinally tracking individuals with a demonstrated health threat (e.g., hypertensive patients) on protection motivation theory variables. There is some initial evidence that PMT variables operate differently in medical compliance situations than in situations in which the health threat may not yet be manifest (Flynn et al., 1995).

The most important issues have been saved for last. Many differing interpretations of the Threat × Coping interaction effect have been offered. Most studies to date have not attempted to explain why it is so prevalent. Although a few studies (e.g., Self & Rogers, 1990; Witte, 1992c) have tested one explanation, there has been no strong support for any single mechanism, nor have two or more mediators been tested simultaneously.

Finally, because most people do not respond to health information with the adaptive coping recommended by the communicator, more work is needed on all facets of the maladaptive coping modes. How many independent types are there? How do they rank on a continuum of maladaptivity? How are they affected by different aspects of persuasive health appeals? How are they affected by PMT's cognitive mediating processes? How does maladaptive coping ebb and flow over time?

CONCLUSION

This chapter presented a revision of protection motivation theory, one theory of how health-threat information can persuade people to adopt a health communicator's recommendations. A review of published research investigating PMT revealed that the predicted main effects were confirmed in over 90% of these studies. The chapter then presented some implications of two cognitive processing theories, the elaboration likelihood model and the heuristic–systematic model, for PMT and the processing of health-threat messages. Finally, extensions of the 1983 version of PMT were described, and some of the more interesting theoretical and empirical issues were identified.

The morbidity and mortality associated with unhealthful lifestyles are largely preventable conditions (e.g., improper diet, lack of exercise, alcohol abuse, smoking, risk-taking behaviors). The prevention of disease and promotion of health can be achieved, in large part, by persuading people to adopt more healthful lifestyles. It is hoped that conceptual and empirical work on PMT can contribute modestly to helping people live longer and healthier lives.

ACKNOWLEDGMENTS. We express our appreciation to Jody L. Jones for her assistance on the project and to Lani Greening, Lisa McElreath, and Donna Floyd for their helpful comments on the manuscript.

REFERENCES

Abelson, R., & Levi, A. (1985). Decision making and decision theory. In G. Lindzey & E. Aronson (Eds.), *Handbook of social psychology: Vol. I. Theory and method* (3rd ed.) (pp. 231–310). New York: Random House.

Ahia, R. N. (1990). Compliance with safer-sex guidelines among adolescent males: Application of the health belief model and protection motivation theory. *Journal of Health Education, 22,* 49–52.

Allard, R. (1989). Beliefs about AIDS as determinants of preventive practices and of support for coercive measures. *American Journal of Public Health, 79,* 448–452.

Allen, B. (1993). Frightening information and extraneous arousal: Changing cognitions and behavior regarding nuclear war. *Journal of Social Psychology, 133,* 459–467.

Aspinwall, L. G., Kemeny, M. E., Taylor, S. E., Schneider, S., & Dudley, J. (1991). Psychosocial predictors of gay men's AIDS risk-reduction behavior. *Health Psychology, 10,* 432–444.

Axelrod, L. J., & Newton, J. W. (1991). Preventing nuclear war: Beliefs and attitudes as predictors of disarmist and deterrentist behavior. *Journal of Applied Social Psychology, 21,* 29–40.

Birnbaum, M., & Sotoodeh, Y. (1991). Measurement of stress: Scaling the magnitudes of life changes. *Psychological Science, 2,* 236–243.

Brouwers, M. C., & Sorrentino, R. M. (1993). Uncertainty orientation and protection motivation theory: The role of individual differences in health compliance. *Journal of Personality and Social Psychology, 65,* 102–112.

Calantone, R. J., & Warshaw, P. R. (1985). Negating the effects of fear appeals in election campaigns. *Journal of Applied Psychology, 70,* 627–633.

Calnan, M., & Rutter, D. R. (1988). Do health beliefs predict health behaviour? A follow-up analysis of breast self-examination. *Social Science and Medicine, 26,* 463–466.

Campis, L. K., Prentice-Dunn, S., & Lyman, R. D. (1989). Coping appraisal and parents' intentions to inform their children about sexual abuse: A protection motivation theory analysis. *Journal of Social and Clinical Psychology, 8,* 304–316.

Chaiken, S., Liberman, A., & Eagly, A. H. (1989). Heuristic and systematic information processing within and beyond the persuasion context. In J. S. Uleman & J. A. Bargh (Eds.), *Unintended thought* (pp. 212–252). New York: Guilford Press.

Eppright, D., Tanner, J., & Hunt, J. (1994). Knowledge and the ordered protection motivation model: Tools for presenting AIDS. *Journal of Business Research, 30,* 13–24.

Epstein, S. (1994). Integration of the cognitive and the psychodynamic unconscious. *American Psychologist, 49,* 709–724.

Flynn, M. F., Lyman, R. D., & Prentice-Dunn, S. (1995). Protec-

tion motivation theory and adherence to medical regimens for muscular dystrophy. *Journal of Social and Clinical Psychology, 14,* 61–75.

Frisch, D., & Clemen, R. (1994). Beyond expected utility: Rethinking behavioral decision research. *Psychological Bulletin, 43,* 46–54.

Fruin, D. J., Pratt, C., & Owen, N. (1992). Protection motivation theory and adolescents' perceptions of exercise. *Journal of Applied Social Psychology, 22,* 55–69.

Galotti, K. (1989). Approaches to studying formal and everyday reasoning. *Psychological Bulletin, 105,* 331–351.

Gleicher, F., & Petty, R. (1992). Expectations of reassurance influence the nature of fear-stimulated attitude change. *Journal of Experimental Social Psychology, 28,* 86–100.

Griffeth, R., & Rogers, R. (1976). Effects of fear arousing components of driver education on trainee's attitudes and simulator performance. *Journal of Educational Psychology, 69,* 501–506.

Hansell, P. L., Thorn, B. E., Prentice-Dunn, S., & Floyd, D. L. (1997). *The effects of primary appraisals of infertility and other gynecological stressors on coping.* Manuscript submitted for publication.

Hass, J., Bagley, G., & Rogers, R. W. (1975). Coping with the energy crisis: Effects of fear appeals upon attitudes toward energy consumption. *Journal of Applied Psychology, 60,* 754–756.

Hayes, D., & Ross, C. E. (1987). Concern with appearance, health beliefs, and eating habits. *Journal of Health and Social Behavior, 28,* 120–130.

Hendrickx, L., Vlek, C., & Calje, H. (1992). Effects of frequency and scenario information on the evaluation of large-scale risks. *Organizational Behavior and Human Decision Processes, 52,* 256–275.

Hermo, H. (1987). Chemical carcinogenesis: Tumor initiation and promotion. *Occupational Medicine, Occupational Cancer, and Carcinogenesis, 2,* 1–25.

Herrnstein, R. (1990). Rational choice theory: Necessary but not sufficient. *American Psychologist, 45,* 356–367.

Hine, D. W., & Gifford, R. (1991). Fear appeals, individual differences, and environmental concern. *Journal of Environmental Education, 23,* 36–41.

Ho, R. (1992). Cigarette health warnings: The effects of perceived severity, expectancy of occurrence, and self-efficacy on intentions to give up smoking. *Australian Psychologist, 27,* 109–113.

Hovland, C., Janis, I. L., & Kelly, H. (1953). *Communication and persuasion.* New Haven, CT: Yale University Press.

Janis, I. L., & Feshbach, S. (1953). Effects of fear-arousing communication. *Journal of Abnormal and Social Psychology, 48,* 78–92.

Jepson, C., & Chaiken, S. (1990). Chronic issue-specific fear inhibits systematic processing of persuasive communications. Communication, cognition, and anxiety [Special Issue]. *Journal of Social Behavior and Personality, 5,* 61–84.

Jonas, K. (1993). Expectancy–value models of health behavior: An analysis by conjoint measurement. *European Journal of Social Psychology*, *23*, 167–183.

Jones, J. L., & Leary, M. R. (1994). Effects of appearance-based admonitions against sun exposure on tanning intentions in young adults. *Health Psychology*, *13*, 86–90.

Kaplan, R. M., Sallis, J. F., Jr., & Patterson, T. L. (1994). *Health and human behavior*. New York: McGraw-Hill.

Kelly, R. B., Zyzanski, S. J., & Alemagno, S. A. (1991). Prediction of motivation and behavior change following health promotion: Role of health beliefs, social support, and self-efficacy. *Social Science and Medicine*, *32*, 311–320.

Kirkpatrick, L., & Epstein, S. (1992). Cognitive–experiential self-theory and subjective probability: Further evidence for two conceptual systems. *Journal of Personality and Social Psychology*, *63*, 534–544.

Kleinot, M. C., & Rogers, R. (1982). Identifying effective components of alcohol misuse prevention programs. *Journal of Studies on Alcohol*, *43*, 802–811.

Knapp, L. G. (1991). The effects of type of value appealed to and valence of appeal on children's intentions and dental health behavior. *Journal of Pediatric Psychology*, *16*, 675–686.

Leventhal, H. (1970). Findings and theory in the study of fear communications. In L. Berkowitz (Ed.), *Advances in experimental social psychology: Vol. 5* (pp. 119–186). New York: Academic Press.

Liberman, A., & Chaiken, S. (1992). Defensive processing of personally relevant health messages. *Personality and Social Psychology Bulletin*, *18*, 669–679.

Lynch, D. J., Birk, T. J., Weaver, M. T., Cohara, A. F., Leighton, R. F., Repka, F. J., & Walsh, M. E. (1992). Adherence to exercise interventions in the treatment of hypercholesterolemia. *Journal of Behavioral Medicine*, *15*, 365–377.

Maddux, J. (1993). Social cognitive models of health and exercise behavior: An introduction and review of conceptual issues. *Journal of Applied Sport Psychology*, *5*, 116–140.

Maddux, J., & Rogers, R. (1983). Protection motivation and self-efficacy: A revised theory of fear appeals and attitude change. *Journal of Experimental Social Psychology*, *19*, 469–479.

Marcus, B. H., & Owen, N. (1992). Motivational readiness, self-efficacy and decision-making for exercise. *Journal of Applied Social Psychology*, *22*, 3–16.

McCauley, E. (1992). The role of efficacy cognitions in the prediction of exercise behavior in middle-aged adults. *Journal of Behavioral Medicine*, *15*, 65–68.

McElreath, L. H., Prentice-Dunn, S., & Rogers, R. W. (1997). *Protection motivation theory and children's modes of coping with a health threat*. Manuscript submitted for publication.

Mermelstein, R. J., & Riesenberg, L. A. (1992). Changing knowledge and attitudes about skin cancer risk factors among adolescents. *Health Psychology*, *11*, 371–376.

Mewborn, C., & Rogers, R. (1979). Effects of threatening and reassuring components of fear appeals on physiological and verbal measures of emotion and attitudes. *Journal of Experimental Social Psychology*, *15*, 242–253.

Mitchell, T., & Beach, L. (1990). "... Do I love thee? Let me count ..." Toward an understanding of intuitive and automatic decision making. *Organizational Behavior and Human Decision Processes*, *47*, 1–20.

Mulilis, J. P., & Lippa, R. (1990). Behavioral change in earthquake preparedness due to negative threat appeals: A test of protection motivation theory. *Journal of Applied Social Psychology*, *20*, 619–638.

Olson, J., & Zanna, M. (1993). Attitudes and attitude change. In L. Porter & M. Rosenzweig (Eds.), *Annual review of psychology: Vol. 4* (pp. 117–154). Palo Alto, CA: Annual Reviews.

Paterson, R., & Neufeld, R. (1987). Clear danger: Situational determinants of the appraisal of threat. *Psychological Bulletin*, *101*, 404–416.

Peterson, L., Farmer, J., & Kashani, J. H. (1990). Parental injury prevention endeavors: A function of health beliefs? *Health Psychology*, *9*, 177–191.

Peterson, L., & Roberts, M. C. (1992). Complacency, misdirection, and effective prevention of children's injuries. *American Psychologist*, *47*, 1040–1044.

Petty, R. E., & Cacioppo, J. T. (1986). *Communication and persuasion: Central and peripheral routes to attitude change*. New York: Springer-Verlag.

Plotnikoff, R. C. (1994). *An application of protection motivation theory to coronary heart disease risk factor behaviour in three Australian samples: Community adults, cardiac patients, and school children*. Unpublished doctoral dissertation. University of Newcastle, Australia.

Pointer, J., & Rogers, R. (1994). *Cognitive processing and persuasive effects of threat, argument quality, and source expertise*. Manuscript submitted for publication.

Prentice-Dunn, S., Jones, J. L., & Floyd, D. L. (in press). Persuasive appeals and the reduction of cancer risk: A protection motivation theory analysis. *Journal of Applied Social Psychology*.

Prentice-Dunn, S., & Rogers, R. (1986). Protection motivation theory and preventive health: Beyond the health belief model. *Health Education Research*, *1*, 153–161.

Prochaska, J., DiClemente, C., & Norcross, J. (1992). In search of how people change: Applications of addictive behaviors. *American Psychologist*, *47*, 1102–1114.

Rhodes, F., & Wolitski, R. J. (1990). Perceived effectiveness of fear appeals in AIDS education: Relationship to ethnicity, gender, age, and group membership. *AIDS Education and Prevention*, *2*, 1–11.

Rhodes, F., Wolitski, R. J., & Thornton-Johnson, S. (1992). An experiential program to reduce AIDS risk among female sex partners of injection-drug users. *Health and Social Work*, *17*, 261–272.

Rippetoe, P., & Rogers, R. (1987). Effects of components of

protection motivation theory on adaptive and maladaptive coping with a health threat. *Journal of Personality and Social Psychology, 52,* 596–604.

Robberson, M., & Rogers, R. (1988). Beyond fear appeals: Negative and positive persuasive appeals to health and self-esteem. *Journal of Applied Social Psychology, 18,* 277–287.

Rogers, R. (1975). A protection motivation theory of fear appeals and attitude change. *Journal of Psychology, 91,* 93–114.

Rogers, R. (1983). Cognitive and physiological processes in fear-based attitude change: A revised theory of protection motivation. In J. Cacioppo & R. Petty (Eds.), *Social psychophysiology: A sourcebook* (pp. 153–176). New York: Guilford Press.

Rogers, R. (1985). Attitude change and information processing in fear appeals. *Psychological Reports, 56,* 179–182.

Rogers, R., & Deckner, C. (1975). Effects of fear appeals and physiological arousal upon emotion, attitudes, and cigarette smoking. *Journal of Personality and Social Psychology, 32,* 222–230.

Rogers, R., Deckner, W., & Mewborn, C. (1978). An expectancy-value theory approach to the long-term modification of smoking behavior. *Journal of Clinical Psychology, 34,* 562–566.

Rogers, R., & Mewborn, C. (1976). Fear appeals and attitude change: Effects of a threat's noxiousness, probability of occurrence, and the efficacy of coping responses. *Journal of Personality and Social Psychology, 34,* 54–61.

Rogers, R., & Thistlethewaite, D. (1970). Effects of fear arousal and reassurance on attitude change. *Journal of Personality and Social Psychology, 15,* 227–233.

Ronis, D. (1992). Conditional health threats: Health beliefs, decisions, and behaviors among adults. *Health Psychology, 11,* 127–134.

Ronis, D., & Kaiser, M. (1989). Correlates of breast self-examination in a sample of college women: Analyses of linear structural relations. *Journal of Applied Social Psychology, 19,* 1068–1084.

Schaefer, R. B., Schaefer, E., Bultena, G., & Hoiberg, E. (1993). Coping with a health threat: A study of food safety. *Journal of Applied Social Psychology, 23,* 386–394.

Schwarzer, R. (1992). Self-efficacy in the adoption and maintenance of health behaviors: Theoretical approaches and a new model. In R. Schwarzer (Ed.), *Self-efficacy: Thought control of action* (pp. 217–243). Washington, DC: Hemisphere.

Self, C. A., & Rogers, R. W. (1990). Coping with threats to health: Effects of persuasive appeals on depressed, normal, and antisocial personalities. *Journal of Behavioral Medicine, 13,* 343–357.

Seydel, E., Taal, E., & Wiegman, O. (1990). Risk appraisal, outcome and self-efficacy expectancies: Cognitive factors in preventive behaviour related to cancer. *Psychology and Health, 4,* 99–109.

Shelton, M., & Rogers, R. (1981). Fear-arousing and empathy-arousing appeals to help: The pathos of persuasion. *Journal of Applied Social Psychology, 11,* 366–378.

Slovic, P. (1987). Perceptions of risk. *Science, 236,* 280–285.

Smith Klohn, L., & Rogers, R. W. (1991). Dimensions of the severity of a health threat: The persuasive effects of visibility, time-of-onset, and rate-of-onset on intentions to prevent osteoporosis. *Health Psychology, 10,* 323–329.

Stainback, R. D., & Rogers, R. (1983). Identifying effective components of alcohol abuse prevention programs: Effects of fear appeals, message style, and source expertise. *International Journal of the Addictions, 18,* 393–405.

Stanley, M. A., & Maddux, J. E. (1986). Cognitive processes in health enhancement: Investigation of a combined protection motivation and self-efficacy model. *Basic and Applied Social Psychology, 7,* 101–113.

Stanton, B. F., Black, M., Kaljee, L., & Ricardo, I. (1993). Perceptions of sexual behavior among urban adolescents: Translating theory through focus groups. *Journal of Early Adolescence, 13,* 44–66.

Steffen, V. J. (1990). Men's motivation to perform the testicular self-exam: Effects of prior knowledge and an educational brochure. *Journal of Applied Social Psychology, 20,* 681–702.

Sturges, J., & Rogers, R. (1996). Preventive health psychology from a developmental perspective: An extension of protection motivation theory. *Health Psychology, 15,* 158–166.

Sutton, S. (1982). Fear-arousing communications: A critical examination of theory and research. In J. Eiser (Ed.), *Social psychology and behavioral medicine* (pp. 303–337). London: Wiley.

Sutton, S. (1989). Relapse following smoking cessation: A critical review of current theory and research. In M. Gossop (Ed.), *Relapse and addictive behavior* (pp. 41–72). London: Routledge.

Sutton, S., Bickler, G., Sancho-Aldridge, J., & Saidi, G. (1994). Prospective study of predictors of attendance for breast screening in inner London. *Journal of Epidemiology and Community Health, 48,* 65–73.

Sutton, S., & Eiser, J. (1984). The effect of fear-arousing communications on cigarette smoking: An expectancy-value approach. *Journal of Behavioral Medicine, 7,* 13–33.

Sutton, S., & Eiser, J. (1990). The decision to wear a seat belt: The role of cognitive factors, fear and prior behavior. *Psychology and Health, 4,* 111–123.

Sutton, S., & Hallett, R. (1988). Understanding the effects of fear-arousing communications: The role of cognitive factors and amount of fear aroused. *Journal of Behavioral Medicine, 11,* 353–360.

Sutton, S., & Hallett, R. (1989a). The contribution of fear and cognitive factors in mediating the effects of fear-arousing communications. *Social Behavior, 4,* 83–98.

Sutton, S., & Hallett, R. (1989b). Understanding seat belt intentions and behavior: A decision-making approach. *Journal of Applied Social Psychology, 19,* 1310–1325.

Sutton, S., Marsh, A., & Matheson, J. (1987). Explaining

smokers' decisions to stop: Test of an expectancy–value approach. *Social Behavior, 2*, 35–49.

Sutton, S., Marsh, A., & Matheson, J. (1990). Microanalysis of smokers' beliefs about the consequences of quitting: Results from a large population sample. *Journal of Applied Social Psychology, 20*, 1847–1862.

Taal, E., Rasker, J. J., Seydel, E. R., & Wiegman, O. (1993). Health status, adherence with health recommendations, self-efficacy and social support in patients with rheumatoid arthritis. *Patient Education and Counseling, 20*, 63–76.

Tanner, J. F., Day, E., & Crask, M. (1989). Protection motivation theory: An extension of fear appeals theory in communication. *Journal of Business Research, 19*, 267–276.

Tanner, J. F., Hunt, J. B., & Eppright, D. R. (1991). The protection motivation model: A normative model of fear appeals. *Journal of Marketing, 55*, 36–45.

Tedesco, L. A., Keffer, M. A., & Fleck-Kandath, C. (1991). Self-efficacy, reasoned action, and oral health behavior reports: A social cognitive approach to compliance. *Journal of Behavioral Medicine, 14*, 341–355.

Van der Velde, F. W., & van Der Plight, J. (1991). Coping, protection motivation and previous behavior. *Journal of Behavioral Medicine, 14*, 429–451.

Van der Velde, F. W., van Der Plight, J., & Hooykaas, C. (1994). Perceiving AIDS-related risk: Accuracy as a function of differences in actual risk. *Health Psychology, 13*, 25–33.

Van der Velde, F. W., Hooykaas, C., & van Der Plight, J. (1992). Risk perception and behavior: Pessimism, realism, and optimism about AIDS-related health behavior. *Psychology and Health, 6*, 23–38.

Vanweesenbeeck, I., de Graaf, R., van Zessen, G., Straver, C. J., & Visser, J. H. (1993). Protection styles of prostitutes' clients: Intentions, behavior, and considerations in relation to AIDS. *Journal of Sex Education and Therapy, 19*, 79–92.

Vaughan, E. (1993). Chronic exposure to environmental hazard: Risk perceptions and self-protective behavior. *Health Psychology, 12*, 74–85.

Wallerstein, N., & Sanchez-Merki, V. (1994). Freirian praxis in health education: Research results from an adolescent prevention program. *Health Education Research, 9*, 105–118.

Weinstein, N. D. (1982). Unrealistic optimism about suscep-tibility to health problems. *Journal of Behavioral Medicine, 5*, 441–460.

Weinstein, N. D. (1993). Testing four competing theories of health-protective behavior. *Health Psychology, 12*, 324–333.

Weinstein, N. D., & Sandman, P. M. (1992). A model of the precaution adoption process: Evidence from home radon testing. *Health Psychology, 11*, 170–180.

Weinstein, N. D., Sandman, P. M., & Roberts, N. E. (1991). Perceived susceptibility and self-protective behavior: A field experiment to encourage home radon testing. *Health Psychology, 10*, 25–33.

Winett, R. A., Anderson, E. S., Moore, J. F., Sikkema, K. J., Hook, R. J., Webster, D. A., Taylor, C. D., Dalton, J. E., Ollendick, T. H., & Eisler, R. M. (1992). Family/media approach to HIV prevention: Results of a home-based, parent-teen video program. *Health Psychology, 11*, 203–206.

Witte, K. (1992a). Preventing AIDS through persuasive communications: A framework for constructing effective culturally-specific health messages. In F. Korzenny & S. Ting-Toomey (Eds.), *International and Intercultural Communication Annual, 16*, 67–86.

Witte, K. (1992b). Putting the fear back into fear appeals: The extended parallel process model. *Communication Monographs, 59*, 329–349.

Witte, K. (1992c). The role of threat and efficacy in AIDS prevention. *International Quarterly of Community Health Education, 12*, 225–249.

Wolf, S., Gregory, L., & Stephan, W. G. (1986). Protection motivation theory: Prediction of intentions to engage in anti-nuclear war behaviors. *Journal of Applied Social Psychology, 16*, 310–321.

Wulfert, E., & Wan, C. K. (1993). Condom use: A self-efficacy model. *Health Psychology, 12*, 346–353.

Wurtele, S. K. (1988). Increasing women's calcium intake: The role of health beliefs, intentions, and health value. *Journal of Applied Social Psychology, 18*, 627–639.

Wurtele, S. K., & Maddux, J. E. (1987). Relative contributions of protection motivation theory components in predicting exercise intentions and behavior. *Health Psychology, 6*, 453–466.

7

Behavioral Intentions in Theories of Health Behavior

James E. Maddux and Kimberley A. DuCharme

INTRODUCTION

Most people try to predict what others will do by asking them what they *intend* or *plan* to do. Likewise, the major theories of health behavior also assume that intentions are good predictors of health-related behavior. Behavioral intentions play an important role in several important social–cognitive models of health behavior: the theory of reasoned action (Fishbein & Ajzen, 1975), the theory of planned behavior (Ajzen, 1988), protection motivation theory (see Chapter 6), and self-efficacy theory (Bandura, 1977, 1986). This chapter discusses the role of behavioral intentions in theory and research on health behavior. It begins with a description of the models in which behavioral intentions play the most crucial role—the theory of reasoned action and the theory of planned behavior. It then presents re-

James E. Maddux • Department of Psychology, George Mason University, Fairfax, Virginia 22030-4444.   **Kimberley A. DuCharme** • Department of Physical Education, Wilfrid-Laurier University, Waterloo, Ontario N2L 3C5, Canada.

Handbook of Health Behavior Research I: Personal and Social Determinants, edited by David S. Gochman. Plenum Press, New York, 1997.

search from studies of exercise behavior and discusses briefly the role of behavioral intentions in several other prominent models of health behavior. Finally, it presents a revised theory of planned behavior that attempts to integrate the major components of the models described and includes work on stages of change and habits.

THEORY OF REASONED ACTION AND THEORY OF PLANNED BEHAVIOR

Theory of Reasoned Action

The theory of reasoned action (Fishbein & Ajzen, 1975) and its recent extension, the theory of planned behavior (Ajzen, 1988), assume that people make rational decisions about their behavior based on information or beliefs about the target behavior. The theories propose that the most important determinants and predictors of behavior are *intentions* and that intentions are a function of a person's *attitude toward the behavior* and the person's perceptions of *social norms* regarding the behavior. Attitude toward the behavior and perceived social norms consist of sets of beliefs about expected consequences and the importance of those consequences. The theories also assume that the behaviors to be predicted are under the person's *volitional control*—that the person can decide at will to perform or not perform the behaviors.

Fishbein and Ajzen (1975) defined an *intention* as "the person's subjective probability that he will peform the behavior in question" (p. 12) and said it should be measured by "a procedure which places the subject along a subjective-probability dimension involving a relation between himself and some action" (pp. 12–13). This definition of intention, although seemingly straightforward, has been the subject of considerable debate. For example, this definition can be viewed as one's *estimate* or *prediction* that one will (or will not) perform the behavior in question, rather than as one's *intent* or *plan* to perform the behavior. Measures of intention based on this definition are therefore inconsistent with the everyday definition of intention.

To be good predictors of behavior, intentions need to be measured with a high degree of *specificity* with regard to the *action* to be performed, the *target* at which the action is directed, the *context* in which the action is performed, and the *time* at which it is performed. For example, to predict attendance at an aerobics class, it is necessary to assess a person's attitude toward aerobics (the action) in a particular scheduled aerobics class (the target) at a particular time of day (the context) and for a specified period of time (the class duration). The greater the specificity of intentions and behavior on these four features, the better intentions will predict behavior.

Attitude toward the behavior refers to the person's favorable/unfavorable evaluation of the behavior based on the *expected consequences* (outcomes) of the behavior and the *value* or *importance* of those consequences (both benefits and costs). *Perceived social norms* are beliefs about the probability that other people will or will not support or approve of the behavior in question. Perceived social norms consist of *normative beliefs*—beliefs that salient others think

the person should or should not engage in the behavior—and *motivation to comply* with those others' preferences. Thus, perceptions of social norms include *expectations* about the reactions of other people and the *value or importance* of those people and their reactions. Both attitude toward the behavior and perceived social norms can be defined and measured in the common currency of *outcome expectancy* (or means–end expectancies) and *outcome value* as defined in traditional expectancy–value theories of choice and behavior.

The *theory of reasoned action* (TRA) is concerned with intentional behavior, but not all human behavior is the direct result of deliberate deciding and intending at the moment it is performed. The notion of a *habit*, in both everyday language and health psychology, assumes that much behavior is the product of automatic rather than deliberate cognitive processes (Ronis, Yates, & Kirscht, 1989). Consistent with this notion, the TRA does *not* assume that people always deliberately assess their attitudes before forming their intentions or that they consciously form intentions each time they act. Thus, not all action is reasoned in the sense of being the result of an on-the-spot analysis. Instead, the theory assumes that attitudes toward a behavior and beliefs about social norms develop over time as people develop expectations about the consequences of the behaviors and beliefs about the importance of these consequences.

Likewise, intentions are reasoned products of those attitudes and perceived social norms. People do not analyze these expectations, values, and norms, however, in each situation that offers the possibility for performing the behavior. For example, people do not consider the consequences of buckling or not buckling their seat belts each time they get into an automobile; the practice of buckling up or not buckling up develops as a result of considering the practical and social consequences of doing so or not doing so. In this sense, attitudes, perceived social norms, and intentions may become automatically activated in the presence of certain situational cues, although the behavior remains under volitional control in that the person decides to perform it or not. The consideration of situational cues and the automaticity of attitudes, norms, and intentions lead to consideration of the processes by which a behavior moves out of volitional control over time and becomes a habit. The issue of volitional control will be discussed in a later section of the chapter.

All behavioral decisions involve choices among behaviors, even if the decision is simply to perform or not to perform a behavior. For this reason, the TRA can be viewed as a theory of *choice* between two or more behavioral alternatives, rather than simply a theory about the performance of a single behavior in isolation. In fact, Fishbein and Ajzen advocate assessing differences in the intentions associated with alternative behaviors and indicate that doing so enhances the prediction of behavior (Ajzen & Fishbein, 1980; Jaccard & Becker, 1985).

Reviews of the research on the theory demonstrate that, together, attitude toward the behavior and perceived social norms are good predictors of behavior. Ajzen and Fishbein's (1973) review of 10 studies reported a mean multiple R of 0.81 using attitude and social norms to predict behavior. Van der Putte's (1991) meta-analysis of 113 studies found a mean multiple R of 0.68 for predicting intention from attitude toward the behavior and perceived social norm, and a mean r of 0.62 between intention and behavior. Shephard, Hartwick, and Warshaw's (1988) meta-analysis of 87 estimates found similar results. Both of these meta-analyses, however, found considerable variability across studies in predicting behavior from intentions.

Theory of Planned Behavior

An important assumption of the theory of reasoned action as originally proposed is that the behavior to be predicted must be under *volitional* control. Because few behaviors are under complete volitional control, however, this assumption places serious limitations on the range of behaviors encompassed by the theory. To remedy this problem, Ajzen (1988) added a component concerned with belief in volitional control over the behavior in question, which he termed *perceived behavioral control* and defined as "the person's belief as to how easy or difficult performance of the behavior is likely to be" (Ajzen & Madden, 1986, p. 457). He named the revised theory the *theory of planned behavior* (TPB). According to this revised theory, perceived behavioral control influences behavior both directly and through its influence on behavioral intentions.

The relative importance of intention and perceived behavioral control in the prediction of behavior is assumed to vary across situations and across behaviors. When the behavior or situation allows a person complete control over the behavior, intention alone should predict behavior. The less the person's volitional control over a behavior, however, the greater will be the importance of perceived behavioral control in determining behavior. Perceived behavioral control is similar to *perceived self-efficacy* (Bandura, 1986) because it involves beliefs that one has both the resources and the opportunities to execute a behavior or attain a goal.

Despite its relatively straightforward definition, the measurement of perceived behavioral control presents some ambiguities. Early studies assessed perceived control in terms of perceived barriers to performing a behavior (e.g., Ajzen & Madden, 1986), but assessing beliefs about barriers is at best an indirect way to measure beliefs about personal control. Also unclear is whether perceived behavioral control should be measured as control over the *behavior* or control over *goal attainment* (e.g., Madden, Ellen, & Ajzen, 1992). For example, "getting an A" in a course is not a behavior but an outcome or goal that can be attained by performing a number of behaviors effectively (Ajzen & Madden, 1986). Thus, one might assess perceived control over "getting an A" or perceived control over any number of the behaviors that affect grades, such as attending class, studying, and taking tests.

In some TPB studies, the assessment of perceived control is concerned with the expectation of attaining a specific *goal* rather than performing specific behaviors or executing a specific plan of action that is expected to lead to the goal. For example, in Schifter and Ajzen's (1985) study of weight loss, perceived control was measured by items concerning "the likelihood that if you try you will manage to reduce weight over the next six weeks" and "your best estimate that an attempt on your part to reduce weight will be successful." These measures do not address the person's beliefs about his or her ability to perform a behavior effectively or execute a plan of action that may lead to weight loss, such as "reducing your caloric intake by 25%" or "engaging in moderate exercise three times a week." Instead, these items entail a somewhat vague assessment of the effectiveness of "trying" and "attempting" and the likelihood that one will reach the goal of losing weight. Other studies have remedied this problem, however, by assessing subjects' beliefs that they will be able to perform relatively specific behaviors or plans of action (e.g., DeVellis, Blalock, & Sandler, 1990).

Research has strongly supported the predictive utility of perceived behavioral control. Much of this support is provided indirectly by the scores of studies that have shown that *self-efficacy beliefs* are powerful determinants of behavior (Bandura, 1986; Maddux, 1995a). Support also has come from studies that specifically examined perceived behavioral control in the context of the TPB. For example, in the prediction of weight loss (Schifter & Ajzen, 1985), attending college classes (Ajzen & Madden, 1986), and course grades (Ajzen & Madden, 1986), perceived control added to the prediction of intention beyond that predicted by attitude and social norm. Intention predicted weight loss only in an *interaction* with perceived control (Schifter & Ajzen, 1985), predicting weight loss only for people who indicated high perceived control. Perceived control did not add to the prediction of class attendance beyond that predicted by attitude and social norms, possibly because of the

high degree of actual control people have over *behaviors* (such as attending class) versus *goals* (such as losing weight) that are the result of many behaviors. Because losing weight is not a behavior but an outcome of the performance of a variety of behaviors, it should be much more difficult to predict from intentions. The TPB assumes that prediction of behavior from intentions will be improved as the measurement of intention and the opportunity for performance of the behavior are closer in time. Consistent with this assumption, Ajzen and Madden (1986) found that perceived control assessed near the *end* of the semester instead of the beginning did improve the prediction of course grades.

In a review of 12 studies employing a variety of behaviors (e.g., playing video games, voting, shoplifting), Ajzen (1991) reported that perceived control usually improved the prediction of intentions beyond attitude and social norms (mean R for predicting intentions was 0.71). Ajzen (1991) reported multiple correlations ranging from 0.20 to 0.78 (mean = 0.51) for the prediction of behavior from intentions and perceived control. Perceived control improved the prediction of behavior in most of these studies and in others (e.g., Netemeyer & Burton, 1990); in most of these studies, however, intentions remained the stronger predictor of behavior.

SIMILARITIES AMONG
HEALTH BEHAVIORS

Numerous studies have indicated that the theories of reasoned action and planned behavior are useful in predicting a wide range of health-related behaviors (e.g., Ajzen, 1988; Ajzen & Fishbein, 1980; Fisher, Fisher, & Rye, 1995; Godin, 1993; McAuley & Courneya, 1993). It is unnecessary to review all these numerous and diverse applications, however, to achieve a basic understanding of a theory's major strengths and problems. From the standpoint of theory, the health behaviors that have received the most attention from researchers—smoking, exercise, diet, compliance with medical regimens, safer sex practices—are more similar than different. For example, if one could strip away the rhetoric, politics, and emotions that so often accompany discussions about HIV and AIDS, and could view the disease strictly through the lens of social–cognitive theory, one would discover that the behaviors that lead to HIV infection are more similar to than different from the behaviors that cause or contribute to the development of most serious health problems with a behavioral genesis, such as smoking, excessive alcohol use, unhealthful dietary practices, and chronic sedentariness (Maddux, 1994). In each of these examples, the behaviors involved are easy and simple. Putting on a condom or putting down a cigarette is less complicated and requires less effort, for example, than skiing down a steep, icy slope. At the same time, however, these behaviors are associated with powerful human urges and powerful pleasures that are not easily resisted, especially when a person is in a situation in which these urges and pleasures are salient. Sexual drives are powerful forces indeed, but so are hunger, thirst, cravings for alcohol and nicotine, and the desire to avoid physical pain and discomfort.

These behaviors also share obstacles to change. The major obstacle to changing from an unhealthful behavior to a healthful behavior is the conflict between proximal (immediate) and distal (future) consequences and the power that proximal consequences exert over behavior. Most unhealthful behaviors are unhealthful only in the long run, yet immediately pleasurable and gratifying. Likewise, changing from unhealthful to healthful behavior (e.g., starting an exercise program, giving up high-fat foods) almost always results in initial pain or discomfort. This conflict makes it difficult for people to adopt safer sexual practices, quit smoking, reduce the amount of fat in their diets, and engage in regular exercise. Sex, smoking, high-fat foods, and sedentariness are immediately pleasurable and gratifying, while the costs of these behaviors exist only in an imagined and indefinite future. Likewise, giving up these activities involves immediate loss of pleasure and an increase in discomfort. Changing health-related behavior also has social repercussions, as the theories of reasoned action and planned behavior and supporting research indicate. Major changes in a person's behavior can greatly affect the important people in the person's life; thus, effectively changing and maintaining changes in sexual behavior, addictive behaviors, diet, and exercise depends largely on the person's ability to manage personal relationships and the emotions inherent in these relationships.

Certainly each health problem and health behavior presents a unique challenge. For example, efforts to convince people to exercise regularly will differ in important ways from efforts to convince sexually active people to use condoms. Despite these differences, however, the processes or mechanisms of change that are the focus of theory are the same. The fears, expectations, goals, and obstacles related to condom use differ from those associated with exercise, but these behaviors are not governed by different mechanisms. Thus, there is no need for different theories and models for these different behaviors. The theories of reasoned action and planned behavior do stress *specificity* in the assessment and prediction of health-related beliefs and behaviors. The kind of specificity they stress, however, is not specificity of *process*, but specificity of the details that must be included in the assessment of problems and situations and in the measure of the constructs employed (i.e., specific goals, plans, expectancies, and situations). This specification is not always an easy job, but it is a technical problem, not a theoretical one (see also Maddux, 1994; Maddux, Brawley, & Boykin, 1995).

The difference between specificity of process and specificity of content or detail is underscored by two recent studies of health-related behavior change. First, in a study of inner city women's AIDS-risk behavior, Hobfoll, Jackson, Lavin, Britton, and Shepherd (1994) compared the effectiveness of training in generic health-promotion skills with training in AIDS-related risk behavior that taught identical general competencies yet targeted AIDS-risk behavior specifically. Both training programs were more effective in promoting behavior change (condom acquisition) than no training, but the AIDS-specific training was more effective than the generic training. Additional support is provided by a recent study by Prochaska et al. (1994) examining the transtheoretical stages of change model and 12 problem behaviors, most of which are health-related. Prochaska et al. (1994, p. 39) found that "clear commonalities were observed across the 12 areas, including both the internal structures of the measures and the pattern of changes in decisional balance across stages." Both studies indicated that the same generic social–cognitive variables and the same generic skills can be applied effectively in understanding and changing a wide range of health-related behaviors.

RESEARCH ON EXERCISE BEHAVIOR

A review of research on numerous health behaviors is not necessary to achieve an understanding of the basic processes in the relationship between intentions and health-related behavior; a single, well-researched health behavior will suffice. *Exercise* has been the topic of considerable research and provides a good vehicle for understanding TRA/TPB because it has multiple and diverse behavioral manifestations (e.g., aerobics, running, walking, lifting weights) that each have multiple yet specific behavioral components. In addition, regular exercise is a cornerstone of healthful living. Not only is exercise an important strategy for preventing disease and promoting health (e.g., decreasing risk of heart disease), but also it can lead to additional healthful behavior changes (e.g., weight loss). People who exercise regularly then find it easier to make other healthful changes such as reducing or giving up smoking and eating more healthful food (e.g., changing to a low-fat diet). Finally, exercise shares problems and barriers with most other important health-related behaviors. As with sexual behavior, smoking, and diet, changing from a sedentary pattern of behavior to an active one that involves regular, vigorous exercise involves

giving up some immediate pleasures and comforts and enduring some displeasure, discomfort, boredom, and pain (sometimes more imagined than actual) for the sake of benefits that, although fairly certain and valuable, are not seen for months or even years. For these reasons, what has been learned from the study of exercise can enhance understanding of other health-related behaviors.

From a review of 21 studies, Godin (1993) concluded that the theory of reasoned action has been useful in understanding the decision-making process that underlies exercise behavior. He found that approximately 30% of the variance in exercise intentions was explained by the attitudinal and social norm measures. Consistent with research on other health behaviors, the attitude component seems to be a more stable and significant predictor of intentions to exercise than perceived social norms. Godin (1993) also reported that all of the 12 studies that investigated the association between intentions and behaviors found the relationship to be statistically significant.

Godin (1993) concluded that the results of six published studies provided only partial support for the utility of the theory of planned behavior in predicting exercise behavior. Only two studies reported that perceived behavioral control predicted a significant additional amount of variance in exercise behavior beyond that predicted by attitudes and perceived social norms. Godin, Valois, and LePage (1993) suggested that perceived behavioral control does not contribute to the prediction of exercise behavior beyond the components of the theory of reasoned action because exercise behavior is fully volitional.

METHODOLOGICAL AND RESEARCH ISSUES

Problems in Definition and Conceptualization

Questions concerning the correct application of the theories of reasoned action and planned behavior to exercise behavior have been raised by several authors (Courneya & McAuley, 1993; Godin, 1993; Poag-DuCharme, Brawley, Rodgers, & Robinson, 1992, October). Some of the confusion in the current exercise research is due to two methodological problems in the published research (Godin, 1993). The first problem is a failure to implement the theory in its most complete form. For example, Godin (1993) indiciates that some studies have failed to measure intentions in terms of time, context, and action, as Fishbein and Ajzen stipulate.

The second methodological problem concerns the operational definition of constructs, in which two basic problems occur (Godin, 1993). First, measures of the same construct are sometimes given different labels by different researchers. For example, Dzewaltowski, Noble, and Shaw (1990) found a correlation of 0.81 between self-efficacy and intention. Correlations this high create suspicion that the measures may be assessing the same construct. Second, a given measure may not be measuring what a researcher claims it is measuring. For example, Sallis et al.'s (1989) assessment of lack of interest in and enjoyment of exercise as a measure of perceived barriers may correspond better to the intention and attitudinal components than to perceived barriers.

Of central importance in the theories of reasoned action and planned behavior is the relationship between intention and behavior. Two key issues in this relationship are the *conceptualization* and *measurement* of intentions (Poag-DuCharme et al., 1992, October). Definition and measurement of intentions have been the subject of some disagreement among researchers. Some have measured intentions consistent with Fishbein and Ajzen's original definition of one's subjective probability or prediction of performing a specified behavior. Others have defined and measured intentions as what one intends or plans to do. Of course, what one plans to do can be very different from what one predicts one will do, possibly because when formulating a prediction, people consider a wider range of possible influences than when formulating an intention (Sheppard et al., 1988). For example, research found

that *estimates* (predictions) of future performance were better predictors of behavior ($r = 0.57$) than were stated *intentions* to perform the behavior ($r = 0.49$) (Sheppard et al., 1988).

Concerning the conceptualization of intentions, Warshaw and Davis (1985) suggested that many researchers are measuring expectation or estimation of behavior but reporting that they are measuring intention (see the previous discussion). Warshaw and Davis (1985) defined behavioral intention as "the degree to which a person has formulated conscious plans to perform or not perform some specified future behavior" (p. 214). They differentiated this notion of intention from behavioral expectation, which they defined as "the individual's estimation of the likelihood that he or she actually will perform some specified future behavior" (p. 215). Courneya and McAuley (1993) suggested that understanding the conceptual difference between intention and expectation might help explain the modest and highly variable relationship between intention and exercise behavior.

Likewise, Fishbein and Stasson's (1990) discussion of intention differentiates behavioral *self-prediction* (i.e., "I will perform the action") from behavioral *intention* (e.g., "I will try to …", "I am aiming to …"; "I intend to …"). This distinction is concerned with whether perceived behavioral control (sometimes measured as self-efficacy) correlates more strongly with self-prediction than with intention. If it does, then the theory of planned behavior should be a better predictor of self-prediction than of intention, whereas the theory of reasoned action, which does not include perceived behavioral control, should predict these constructs equally well.

This issue was examined by Poag-DuCharme et al. (1992, October), using data from four different prospective studies of exercise. Robinson (1992) found that behavioral intention and behavioral self-prediction were differentially predicted by attitudes, social norms, and self-efficacy in active and inactive elderly persons. For the active subjects, attitude and social norms significantly predicted 58% of the variance in behavioral intention. Adding self-efficacy as a predictor did not provide an additional contribution to the prediction of intention. Attitude and social norms, however, predicted only 13% of the variance in self-prediction. Adding self-efficacy as a predictor increased the amount of variance in behavioral self-prediction to 56%. The same pattern of results was found with the group of nonactive elderly subjects. Consistent with Fishbein and Stasson's (1990) suggestion, attitude and social norms were significantly better predictors of intention than was self-prediction. Also consistent with their argument was the finding that self-efficacy, attitude, and social norms (as in the theory of planned behavior) best predicted behavioral self-prediction.

Likewise, Poag-DuCharme and Brawley (1993) examined the participation of 207 adult community-based fitness participants and found that self-efficacy for in-class exercise was a stronger predictor of self-prediction than intention in week 1 of the program. Exercise self-efficacy at week 7 also predicted self-prediction better than it predicted intention. These studies indicated strongly that the distinction between intention and self-prediction of behavior is sufficiently important to require additional investigation.

Measurement Issues

A common problem with the measurement of intention is the use of single-item measures that do not allow respondents to report variability in intention strength and to commit to more challenging behavior. Several exercise investigators have used multiple-item assessments of intention for both conceptual and psychometric reasons (i.e., Poag-DuCharme & Brawley, 1993). For example, Rodgers and Brawley (1991a) had 60 campus fitness participants indicate strength of their intention to exercise 1, 2, and 3 times per week, using Likert scales of 1–9 points. Although classes were scheduled 3 times per week, presenting multiple intentions allowed for variable commitment levels to be assessed. Results indicated that strength of intentions declined as attendance increased for each intention assessed (1

time/week, mean = 8.2; 2 times/week, mean = 7.9; 3 times/week, mean = 5.6). Similar trends were found by Poag-DuCharme and Brawley (1993) for 62 exercise initiates who recently had joined a women's health club for unstructured exercise. Rodgers and Brawley (1991b, June) also found that this pattern was reliable across several weeks of a structured exercise program. For the adherers, the strength of the relationship between self-efficacy to attend and perform exercise and intentions differed for the different intentions. Specifically, for intention to exercise once a week, self-efficacy predicted intention only later in the program (week 7; R^2 adj. = 0.23, $p < 0.02$). However, self-efficacy predicted intention to exercise 2 and 3 times per week throughout the program (R^2 adj. from 0.19 to 0.52, all p's < 0.01).

With respect to intentions and actual exercise class attendance, Poag-DuCharme and Brawley (1993) found that when the strength (scale: 1–9) of multiple intentions to attend the health club (1–4 times per week) was adjusted to represent the individual's strongest level of intention, intention significantly predicted weekly club attendance at weeks 9–16 (R^2 adj. = 0.16, $p < 0.01$).

These findings indicate that the strength of behavioral intention varies with the frequency of exercise and with the time individuals have been involved in the exercise program. The prediction of actual behavior may therefore improve when adjusting for "true" intention. The challenge facing exercise behavior researchers is to reconsider the conceptualization and measurement of intention to increase the prediction of actual behavior.

RELATED MODELS

Several additional models incorporate a number of elements found in the theories of reasoned action and planned behavior. Understanding of the role of intention in health-related behaviors will be better achieved by understanding these other models.

Protection Motivation Theory

Protection motivation theory (PMT) was developed originally to explain inconsistencies in the research on fear appeals and attitude change but has since been employed primarily as a model for health decision making and action (see Chapter 6). PMT is concerned with decisions to protect oneself from harmful or stressful life events, although it can also be viewed as a theory of coping with such events. In PMT, decisions to engage (or not engage) in health-related behaviors are influenced by two primary cognitive processes: *threat appraisal*, an evaluation of the factors that influence the likelihood of engaging in a potentially unhealthy behavior (e.g., smoking, sex without a condom), and *coping appraisal*, an evaluation of the factors that influence the likelihood of engaging in a recommended preventive response (e.g., exercise, using a condom). The most common index of protection motivation is a measure of *intention* to perform the recommended preventive behavior.

Threat appraisal and coping appraisal are both concerned with the expected consequences of engaging or not engaging in a specific health behavior *and* the importance of those consequences; thus, they are conceptually identical to attitude toward the behavior in TRA/TPB. In addition, perceptions of social norms—expectations about the reactions of other people—can be considered aspects of threat appraisal and coping appraisal. Strong support has been found for utility of the PMT in predicting health-related intentions and behavior (Maddux & Rogers, 1983; Stanley & Maddux, 1986; Wurtele & Maddux, 1987) (see also Chapter 6).

Health Belief Model

The health belief model (HBM) (Rosenstock, 1974) consists of four major cognitive components: (1) perceived susceptibility to a particular health threat, (2) perceived severity of the health threat, (3) perceived benefits of the behavior recommended to reduce the threat, and (4) perceived barriers to action (perceptions of the possible undesirable consequences of the preventive behavior). In addition, the likelihood of taking action will be influenced by a *cue to action*—an external event (e.g., mass media message) or internal event (e.g., symptom of possible illness) that prompts the individual to act on the aforementioned perceptions—and by demographic and sociocultural variables. The HBM has received considerable support in numerous investigations of preventive health behaviors and compliance with medical regimens (Janz & Becker, 1984; Rosenstock, 1974). Although the HBM does not include a specific component comparable to behavioral intention, its other components are similar or identical to the TRA/TPB's attitudes toward the behavior and perceived social norms. Research also has shown that *social support* is an important addition to the original components (e.g., Uzark, Becher, Dielman, & Rocchini, 1987), consistent with research supporting the role of perceived social norms in the theories of reasoned action and planned behavior.

Self-Efficacy Theory

Self-efficacy theory proposes that the initiation of and persistence in behaviors and courses of action are determined primarily by judgments and expectations concerning behavioral skills and capabilities and the likelihood of being able to successfully cope with environmental demands and challenges (Bandura, 1977, 1986). These expectations determine choice of goals and goal-directed actions, expenditure of effort in the pursuit of goals, persistence in the face of adversity, and emotional or affective reactions (Bandura, 1986). Beliefs about self-efficacy influence health in two ways. First, self-efficacy influences the adoption of healthful behaviors, the cessation of unhealthful behaviors, and the maintenance of these behavioral changes in the face of challenge and difficulty (Maddux et al., 1995). Second, self-efficacy affects the body's physiological response to stress, including endogenous opioid activity and the immune system (O'Leary, 1995).

Hundreds of studies have shown that self-efficacy beliefs are good predictors of behavior (Bandura, 1986; Maddux, 1995b). Research has shown that self-efficacy beliefs directly influence behavioral intentions, behavior, and affect (Bandura, 1986; Maddux, 1995a). A few studies suggest that some of the influence of self-efficacy on behavior is mediated by behavioral intentions (e.g., McAuley & Rowney, 1990).

Self-efficacy beliefs are distinguished from *outcome expectancies*, which are beliefs about the probability that a specified course of action will lead to certain outcomes or consequences (Bandura, 1977). The relationship between self-efficacy and outcome expectancy has been a source of confusion and controversy, and well-designed studies of their relationship and relative predictive utility are few (see Maddux, 1991, 1995a). When defined and measured carefully and in a manner consistent with the conceptual distinction, self-efficacy expectancy and outcome expectancy can each be important in the prediction of intentions and behavior (Maddux, 1995a; Maddux, Norton, & Stoltenberg, 1986).

Stages of Change Models

Several theories of behavior change are based on the premise that behavior change occurs in stages or phases and the factors that influence behavior may change from one stage to another. The *transtheoretical model* (TM) (Prochaska, DiClemente, & Norcross, 1992) and the *precaution adoption process model* (Weinstein, 1988) are the best-developed stage models. Although the number and names of the stages differ among the models, these models agree on the importance of distinguishing among awareness of a health issue, engagement in or contemplation of the issue (e.g., thinking about the pros and cons of changing behavior), committing and planning to change behavior, actively changing behavior, and maintaining the behavior change. These models also assume that progression from phase to phase is not linear and constantly forward and that people move back and forth and in

and out of these phases as they encounter new information, attempt new behaviors, and encounter success and failure.

The TM stages of change model and the theory of planned behavior (TPB) share several important elements (Courneya, 1995). The "pros" and "cons" in TM are with respect to the expected consequences and values that comprise attitude toward the behavior in the TPB. Also, as noted earlier, perceived behavioral control in the TPB is similar to self-efficacy. Intentions are also important in the early stages of readiness in the TM. Research has found that self-efficacy, pros and cons, and intentions are related to stage of readiness (Courneya, 1995). In a study of exercise behavior using a sample of 288 older adults (60 and older), Courneya (1995) found linear relationships between each TPB construct and the stage of physical activity (based on self-reports of exercise behavior) and found that intention, attitude, and perceived behavioral control distinguished among the stages of change of the TM.

In addition, a path analysis found that intention, perceived behavioral control, and attitude were related directly to stages of readiness and that other variables were related to stages through these variables. The variables from the TPB shared 63% of the variance with the TM's stages of readiness. This finding is consistent with other studies of exercise (e.g., Marcus, Selby, Niaura, & Rossi, 1992). Also in Courneya (1995), people in the precontemplation stage had more negative attitudes and lower control beliefs than people in the more advanced contemplation stage. Precontemplators also reported weaker intentions, more negative attitudes toward the behaviors, weaker expectations of social support, and less perceived behavioral control than persons in the other more advanced stages of change. Courneya suggested that the TPB provides a useful framework for understanding the cognitions related to stages of change in the TM.

Implicit in stage models is the assumption that, initially, behavior change is largely under the control of deliberate cognitive processes, such as those described in the TRA/TPB. As the new behavior is repeated over time, however, situational cues to decisions begin to elicit the cognitive processes that result in decisions and intentions. As these cues become more numerous and powerful, the person may enter a maintenance stage in which situational cues easily elicit the decision-making process but elicit few behaviors. As decisions and intentions lead to action, and as actions are maintained and repeated over time, actions may come to be performed automatically in response to situational cues such that they are no longer under volitional control. In some cases, a *habit stage* may evolve in which behavior is primarily controlled by cues to action. For example, frequent repetition of buckling a seat belt when getting into the driver's side of one's own car probably will lead to automatic performance of buckling under those specific conditions, although buckling the seat belt when getting into the passenger side of someone else's car may still require engagement of controlled cognitive processes.

TOWARD AN INTEGRATED MODEL

The similarities among the theories of reasoned action and planned behavior and the other major health behavior models strongly suggest that they are not different models but simply different arrangements of the same basic conceptual buiding blocks. For this reason, no consensus concerning which model is the most useful has yet been achieved. Empirical comparisons that have pitted one model against another have been few (Weinstein, 1993). Indeed, studies that place one model in competition against another are unlikely to be informative because there are so few differences on which to base competing hypotheses. A better approach is to attempt to incorporate the major features of the relevant models into a single model and then attempt to determine the relative importance of the features of the new inclusive model.

Because it includes most of the major components of the other models, the theory of planned behavior provides a good vehicle for integration. It offers several advantages. First, perceived behavioral control includes (although it is not identical to) the notion of self-efficacy. Second, the TPB includes a perceived social norms component that is not featured prominently in the other models. Third, the requirement for definition and measurement of attitudes toward the behavior incorporates outcome expectancy and outcome value in its assessment of beliefs about expected consequences and the importance of those consequences. Fourth, the theory includes intention as a variable that links attitudes and beliefs to behavior.

Basic Building Blocks

An integrative model can be built from five basic building blocks. If it is assumed that a person has the necessary skills for engaging in a behavior and that the environment provides an opportunity for its performance (i.e., no insurmountable barriers), then the major *psychological* factors that influence behavior change are (1) outcome expectancy, (2) outcome value, (3) self-efficacy expectancy, (4) intention, and (5) habitual cue-based responses.

Outcome Expectancy

An outcome expectancy is the belief that certain behaviors probably will or will not result in certain outcomes or goals. Outcome expectancies can be categorized into *stimulus expectancies*, beliefs about external events that might result from an action, and *response expectancies*, beliefs about nonvolitional responses such as emotions or pain (Kirsch, 1995). For many health-related behaviors, response expectancies may be more important than stimulus expectancies. For example, most people want to avoid injury and illness because these conditions are uncomfortable and painful. In addition, the major desired outcomes that lead people to engage in health-promoting behaviors are feelings of physical and psychological well-being, not material goods or financial rewards, and the major costs associated with most health-related behaviors are nonvolitional responses (e.g., anxiety, pain, discomfort, inconvenience, loss of pleasure).

Outcome expectancies appear in the health belief model and protection motivation theory as perceived vulnerability or susceptibility and the expected benefits and costs of the recommended health behavior. The theories of reasoned action and planned behavior include outcome expectancies in the assessment of attitudes toward the behavior (i.e., expected outcomes) and social norms (i.e., probable reactions of other people). The TRA and TPB do not specify a perceived vulnerability component, but their assessments of attitude toward the behavior may presuppose that people engage in protection and detection behavior because they perceive some personal vulnerability.

Outcome Value

Outcome value is the value or importance attached to specific outcomes in specific contexts or situations, sometimes referred to as *reinforcement value* or *incentive value*. An outcome can be important because a person wishes to attain it (money, better health) or because the person wishes to avoid it (e.g., cancer, obesity). In protection motivation theory and the health belief model, the perceived severity of the health threat component is an outcome value. In the TRA and TPB, outcome value is evident in the assessment of attitudes toward the behavior (evaluation of expected outcomes) and social norms (importance placed on reactions of significant others).

Self-Efficacy

Self-efficacy expectancy or belief is a judgment concerning one's ability to execute a behavior or course of action. Self-efficacy beliefs influence choice of goals and goal-directed actions, expenditure of effort in the pursuit of goals, persistence in the face of adversity, and

emotional or affective reactions (Bandura, 1986). Self-efficacy has been incorporated into the health belief model, protection motivation theory, and the TRA and TPB. As noted previously, however, the lack of clarity in the definition and measurement of perceived behavior control in studies of the TRA and TPB leaves some questions about their similarity to self-efficacy. In addition, research on self-efficacy is also plagued by the inconsistent definition and measurement of self-efficacy (Maddux, 1995a).

Intention

An intention is what one says one plans to do. Research on the theory of reasoned action has shown that intentions are good predictors of behavior. Although intention seems a simple notion, problems in its measurement have occured, as noted previously. In addition, in a number of common situations relevant to health behavior, the distinctions between intentions, self-efficacy expectancy, and outcome expectancy become fuzzy, especially in situations in which people may expect a behavior to lead to fear, pain, or discomfort (Kirsch, 1995). Fear and pain expectancies are response expectancies, which are a type of outcome expectancy (Kirsch, 1995). When people anticipate aversive outcomes such as fear or pain and are not willing to engage in behavior that may produce those aversive outcomes (e.g., engaging in vigorous exercise, approaching a snake), their linguistic habit is to say they *cannot* perform the behavior (a report of low self-efficacy), rather than that they *will not* perform it. Measures of willingness may simply be measures of intention. In situations in which fear or pain is anticipated, therefore, people's reports of perceived ability to perform the behavior (self-efficacy) may be reports of intention to perform the behavior, which is determined primarily by pain or fear expectancies. The mislabeling of intention and perceived ability may occur in other important health domains in which people are asked to engage in behaviors that may lead to immediate discomfort, such as dieting and exercising.

Habitual Cue-Based Responses

A *habit* is a behavior that has been performed repeatedly so that it is performed automatically without the necessity for a conscious decision that involves the consideration of at least one other alternative course of action (Ronis et al., 1989). Health-related behaviors are likely to be most effective if performed habitually, but many important health-related behaviors become habitual only with great difficulty, if at all. The TRA and TPB consider habit to be an external influence on behavior in that habits can influence behavior without being mediated by attitudes and intentions. Most habits, however, begin as intentional behaviors and become habitual over time with repeated performance. Understanding how behaviors become habits is therefore important for understanding the role of behavioral intentions in health behavior.

Several attitude theorists have explored the notion of habit. For example, Bentler and Speckart's (1979) model of the attitude–behavior relationship included *past behavior* as an influence on behavior. They proposed that past behavior influences behavior both directly and indirectly through its influence on intentions. Triandis's (1980) model of the attitude–behavior relationship defined habit as behavior that has become automatic and is performed without self-instruction.

The most complete theory of habit, however, was offered by Ronis (e.g., Ronis et al., 1989). It is based on the distinction between *controlled cognitive processes*—those that are intentional and require conscious effort—and *automatic cognitive processes*—those that are so well-learned through repetition that they do not require conscious effort but are set in motion by *situational cues* (Schneider & Shiffrin, 1977). A health behavior that is performed frequently (e.g., tooth brushing, using a seat belt) may eventually come under the control of these situational cues. Behaviors performed less frequently (e.g., vaccinations, medical checkups, HIV testing) remain under the control of conscious cognitive processes and deliberate decisions and intentions. These behaviors therefore remain under

volitional control and thus are the types of behaviors encompassed by the TRA and TPB.

Situational cues influence behavior in two ways—as *cues to decisions* and as *cues to action*. For frequently repeated behaviors that come under the control of situational cues, the situation contains cues to action (e.g., automatically locking the doors when getting into the driver's side of an automobile). For health behaviors that never become habitual and that continue to be influenced primarily by controlled cognitive processes and intentions, situational cues will retain indirect influence over these behaviors because the situation will contain cues to decision that elicit controlled cognitive processes and decision making. For example, clear weather or the sight of one's running shoes or bicycle may initiate a process of deciding whether or not to go for a run or a ride. Seeing a television commercial for athletic gear or a health club may be a cue for deciding whether or not to exercise. These cues do not elicit the behavior itself, but they do elicit the social cognitive factors involved in the formation of intentions and plans.

The distinction between cues to decision and cues to action suggests that beliefs, attitudes, and intentions will be most influential at the *initiation* of a new health behavior and in the early stages of its performance, but will become less important if the behavior is repeated frequently under consistent conditions. For example, if a behavior becomes habitual, measures of intentions will remain highly *correlated* with behavior, but will not influence behavior because habitual behaviors are automatic and not the result of decisions, intentions, and plans.

A final conceptual issue concerns the putative causal role of past behavior and habit in influencing current behavior. A habit is a behavior that is automatically triggered by certain situational cues. It is not a *cause* of behavior; it is a certain kind of *behavior*, one that is triggered automatically by situational cues and occurs without deliberation. Thus, to say that a habit is a cause of current automatic behavior (habit) is to say that a behavior causes itself. Not only can a behavior not cause itself, but also a past behavior cannot influence a current behavior. Past behavior is important in the development of habits because frequency of performance of an intentional behavior in the presence of certain situational cues influences the strength of the acquired association between situational cues and the behavior. Yet, current behavior is influenced by situational cues and by cognitive associations strengthened over time, not by past behavior. Thus, if anything can be said to cause automatic or habitual behavior, it is the *cues*, not past behavior or "habit."

A Revised Theory of Planned Behavior: From Reasoned Action to Habit

These five basic building blocks can be used to construct an integrated model of health behavior that incorporates the best of each individual model. The theory of planned behavior provides a useful vehicle for integration because it already includes most of the major elements from the other models. Some modification of the theory will be helpful, however, in an attempt at integration. Modifications of the theory of planned behavior derived from the other models would include the following:

1.   Perceived vulnerability or susceptibility (as found in the health belief model and protection motivation theory) should be incorporated specifically into the attitude component as an outcome expectancy for the negative health consequences that might result from maintaining one's present health behavior (e.g., "If I continue my sedentary lifestyle, I will increase my chances of developing heart disease").

2.   A perceived severity component (as found in the health belief model and protection motivation theory) should be incorporated into the attitude component in the form of the importance of the negative health consequences of maintaining one's current health behavior.

3.   Incorporating the concept of situational cues and the distinction between cues to decision and cues to action provides a foundation for expanding the theory of planned behavior into a stage or phase theory. This revision would include the concept of *habit* and would assume (as do other stage models) that people move in and out of stages or phases as they attempt to make difficult behavioral changes.

Figure 1 offers an integrated model of health behavior based on the theory of planned behavior. It incorporates what research on the other models suggests about the important influences on health and exercise behavior. In this model, behavior is the result of three influences: self-efficacy for the new behavior, situational cues to action, and intentions. Intentions are the most immediate and powerful determinant of behavior. Self-efficacy influences behavior both directly and indirectly through its influence on intentions. Situational cues influence behavior directly when a behavior has been performed repeatedly in the presence of the same cues and is prompted automatically by these cues. When situational cues automatically prompt behavior, these cues are referred to as cues to action and the behavior is referred to as a habit.

Intentions are determined by four factors: self-efficacy for the new behavior, attitude toward the new behavior, attitude toward the current behavior, and perceived social norms. Independent assessment of attitudes toward the current (unhealthful) and new (more healthful) behavior is important because people who are considering changing their behavior will engage in a comparative analysis of the benefits and costs of the current and new behaviors. Attitude toward the new and current behaviors consists of outcome expectancies (expected benefits and costs) and outcome values (importance of these benefits and costs). Assessment of attitude toward the new behavior must also include an assessment of perceived vulnerability to the relevant negative health outcomes and perceived severity of these expected negative health outcomes (as noted in protection motivation theory and the health belief model).

Self-efficacy expectancy for the new behavior replaces perceived behavioral control. Although perceived behavioral control, as em-

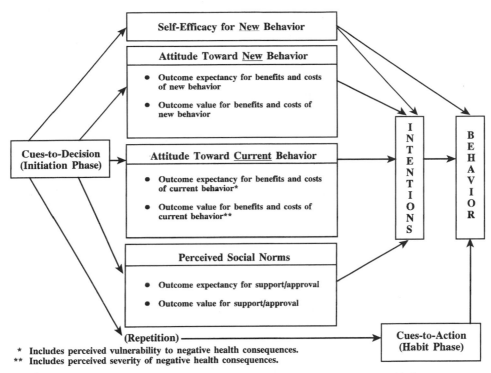

Figure 1. A revised theory of planned behavior incorporating cues and habits.

ployed in research on the theory of planned behavior, incorporates both self-efficacy expectancy and outcome expectancy, theory and research suggest that these two expectancy components should be given separate consideration. Another reason for limiting the definition and measurement of perceived control to self-efficacy is that this model incorporates outcome expectancies in the assessment of attitude toward the behavior (e.g., expected outcomes and their value or importance). Thus, to include outcome expectancies in a measure of perceived control would be redundant. For this reason, perceived behavioral control should be defined and measured as a self-efficacy expectancy rather than a hybrid of self-efficacy expectancy and outcome expectancy. The extensive theory and research on the development of self-efficacy and its influence on behavior would then be directly applicable to this new definition of perceived behavioral control.

Because perceived social norms also are concerned with expected consequences and the importance of these consequences (i.e., the expected reactions of others and the importance of those reactions), perceived social norms are also assessed by a combination of outcome expectancy measures (e.g., "If I attend my aerobics class, my spouse will approve of/support me") and outcome value measures (e.g., "My spouse's approval/support is very important to me"). Thus, perceived social norms could be included in the assessment of attitude toward the behavior. The research on the TRA and TPB suggests, however, that the strong influence of social norms warrants giving expected social outcomes consideration separately from other types of expected nonsocial outcomes.

These cognitive influences are automatically triggered by situational cues that may be either external (e.g., a television commercial for sneakers that triggers cognitions about the pros and cons of exercise) or internal (e.g., a cough that triggers cognitions about trying to quit smoking). Situational cues that trigger the cognitive process that leads to behavioral intentions to behave but do not automatically prompt the behavior itself are called cues to decision. For complex sequences of behaviors that require some deliberation and planning for their execution, cues to decision will remain important over time. If the decision-making process and the behavior are repeated sufficiently over time in the presence of the same cues, however, these initial cues to decision may become cues to action, a process that may take considerable time for some behaviors.

As cues to decision become cues to action and behavior becomes less deliberate and more automatic, the individual gradually moves into habit phase and acts without the information processing (i.e., considering beliefs, expectancies, and social norms) that influenced the initial intentions to act. This movement into a habit phase is roughly equivalent to the movement from the preparation stage to the action stage and then to the maintenance stage as described in the transtheoretical stages of change model. As a result of this movement from intentional behavior to automatic behavior, the social–cognitive factors important for the initiation of a behavior and the early period of maintenance will become, for some behaviors, less important over time. What begins as a reasoned action and a planned behavior becomes, with repeated performance over time, a habit.

PROBLEMS WITH INTENTIONAL AND COGNITIVE EXPLANATIONS OF BEHAVIOR: A PEEK INTO PANDORA'S BOX

The study of the role of behavioral intentions in health behavior raises not only empirical issues and problems but also philosophical ones. The most vexing issue is the role of volition in human behavior, an issue related to the issue of

the role of cognition in human behavior because the cognitive models of behavior change assume that people are capable of controlling or regulating their own behavior. The theories of reasoned action and planned behavior, as well as the other major theories of health behavior, begin with the assumption that people can exercise some degree of *volition* or *free will*. To say that behavior is intentional and volitional is to say that it is purposeful, goal-directed, and to some degree freely chosen. These assumptions are inherent in the phrases *reasoned action* and *planned behavior*. Indeed, the general social–cognitive psychology to which these theories belong assumes that people are to a great extent free agents who are capable of making relatively rational decisions and choices about their behavior and about the situations in which they place themselves. The assumption that human behavior can be intentional and that volition can be a cause of behavior has not gone unquestioned. Some have gone so far as to claim that intentional explanations of behavior have no place in a scientific psychology (Baum & Heath, 1992).

The question of the extent to which human behavior is under the control of volition rather than determined exclusively by external forces cannot be discussed in detail here. Of course, to assume that humans exercise volition is not to say that they are always, or even usually, rational and deliberate in choosing and behaving, only that they are capable of rationality and volition and can learn to exercise these abilities more often and more efficiently.

In addition to being a volitional construct, intention is a cognitive construct, as are attitudes, expectancies, and social norms. According to Lee (1989), theories of behavior based on these constructs share a number of problems: They confuse description of behavior change with explanation of behavior change, they rely on poorly defined and unobservable interactions among poorly defined variables, and they cannot make precise predictions about behavior. Lee (1989) concluded that social–cognitive models are not testable and are therefore not useful. The pros and cons of employing cognitive constructs in explanations of human behavior have been discussed repeatedly since the days of Watson and Pavlov and cannot be given full treatment here.

It is true that constructs such as attitudes, expectancies, self-efficacy, and intentions present definitional and measurement problems. Refinement and consistency in definition and measurement are likely to develop, however, as theorists and researchers become aware of these difficulties and address them. Furthermore, the wholesale dismissal of the importance of human thought in human behavior is at odds with hundreds of studies that demonstrate the centrality of cognition in human social behavior (e.g., Bandura, 1986). Decades of research on such social-cognitive constructs as attributions, expectancies, goals, and intentions amply demonstrate the measurability of covert variables and their utility in at least *predicting* behavior. Whether theories based on these constructs truly *explain* behavior remains a question on which psychology's philosophers of science have not yet agreed.

CONCLUSION

The theory of reasoned action and its more recent variant, the theory of planned behavior, are concerned with the role of expected consequences, both material and social, in people's decisions and intentions to engage in health-related behavior. Considerable research on both theories has provided evidence for the utility of attitude toward the behavior and perceived social norms in predicting behavioral intentions and the utility of intentions in predicting behavior. In addition, research on the theory of planned behavior has provided evidence for the additional utility of perceived behavioral control in predicting intentions beyond what is predicted by attitudes and social norms. This research also indicates that perceived behavioral control is an important direct predictor of behavior. Support for the importance of perceived behavioral control is also provided by the con-

siderable research on self-efficacy, a construct similar but not identical to perceived behavioral control.

Research on exercise behavior illustrates the utility of the theories of reasoned action and planned behavior in the prediction of health-related behavior. The research also illustrates some of the conceptual and methodological problems and controversies concerning these theories. This chapter offers a revised theory of planned behavior that explicitly incorporates the notion of cognitive and behavioral habits based on the distinction between situational cues to decision and situational cues to action. The revision offers a rudimentary explanation of the process by which initially deliberate and intentional behaviors become more automatic and less under the control of deliberate decision process as they are performed repeatedly over time. Since so many of the major benefits of health behaviors require prolonged maintenance of the behavior over time, understanding the transition of intentional behavior to habitual behavior is crucial for developing strategies for healthful living.

ACKNOWLEDGMENT. The authors thank Ted Gessner for his helpful comments on an earlier version of this chapter.

REFERENCES

Ajzen, I. (1988). *Attitudes, personality, and behavior*. Chicago: Dorsey Press.

Ajzen, I. (1991). The theory of planned behavior. *Organizational Behavior and Human Decision Processes, 50,* 179-211.

Ajzen, I., & Fishbein, M. (1973). Attitudinal and normative variables as predictors of specific behaviors. *Journal of Personality and Social Psychology, 27,* 41-57.

Ajzen, I., & Fishbein, M. (1980). *Understanding attitudes and predicting social behavior*. Englewood Cliffs, NJ: Prentice-Hall.

Ajzen, I., & Madden, T. J. (1986). Prediction of goal-directed behavior: Attitudes, intentions, and perceived behavioral control. *Journal of Experimental Social Psychology, 22,* 453-474.

Bandura, A. (1977). Self-efficacy: Toward a unifying theory of behavioral change. *Psychological Review, 84,* 191-215.

Bandura, A. (1986). *Social foundations of thought and action*. New York: Prentice-Hall.

Baum, W. M., & Heath, J. L. (1992). Behavioral explanations and intentional explanations in psychology. *American Psychologist, 47*, 1312–1317.

Bentler, P. M., & Speckart, G. (1979). Models of attitude–behavior relations. *Psychological Review, 86*, 452–464.

Courneya, K. S. (1995). Understanding readiness for regular physical activity in older individuals: An application of the theory of planned behavior. *Health Psychology, 14*, 80–87.

Courneya, K. S., & McAuley, E. (1993). Predicting physical activity from intention: Conceptual and methodological issues. *Journal of Sport and Exercise Psychology, 15*, 50–62.

DeVellis, B. M., Blalock, S. J., & Sandler, R. S. (1990). Predicting participation in cancer screening: The role of perceived behavioral control. *Journal of Applied Social Psychology, 20*, 639–660.

Dzewaltowski, D. A., Noble, J. M., & Shaw, J. M. (1990). Physical activity participation: Social cognitive theory versus the theories of reasoned action and planned behavior. *Journal of Sport and Exercise Psychology, 12*, 388–405.

Fishbein, M., & Ajzen, I. (1975). *Belief, attitude, intention, and behavior: An introduction to theory and research*. Reading, MA: Addison-Wesley.

Fishbein, M., & Stasson, M. (1990). The role of desires, self-predictions, and perceived control in the prediction of training session adherence. *Journal of Applied Social Psychology, 20*, 173–198.

Fisher, W. A., Fisher, J. D., & Rye, B. J. (1995). Understanding and promoting AIDS-preventive behavior: Insights from the theory of reasoned action. *Health Psychology, 14*, 255–264.

Godin, G. (1993). The theories of reasoned action and planned behavior: Overview of findings, emerging research problems, and usefulness for exercise promotion. *Journal of Applied Sport Psychology, 5*, 141–157.

Godin, G., Valois, P., & LePage, L. (1993). The pattern of influence of perceived behavioral control upon exercising behavior: An application of Ajzen's theory of planned behavior. *Journal of Behavioral Medicine, 16*, 81–102.

Hobfoll, S. E., Jackson, A. P., Lavin J., Britton, P. J., & Shepherd, J. B. (1994). Reducing inner-city women's AIDS risk activities: A study of single, pregnant women. *Health Psychology, 13*, 397–403.

Jaccard, J. J., & Becker, M. A. (1985). Attitudes and behavior: An information integration perspective. *Journal of Experimental Social Psychology, 21*, 440–465.

Janz, N. K., & Becker, M. H. (1984). The health belief model: A decade later. *Health Education Quarterly, 11*, 1–47.

Kirsch, I. (1995). Self-efficacy and outcome expectancies: A concluding commentary. In J. E. Maddux (Ed.), *Self-efficacy, adaptation, and adjustment: Theory, research, and application* (pp. 331–345). New York: Plenum Press.

Lee, C. (1989). Theoretical weaknesses lead to practical problems: The example of self-efficacy theory. *Journal of Behavior Therapy and Experimental Psychiatry, 20*, 115–123.

Madden, T. J., Ellen, P. S., & Ajzen, I. (1992). A comparison of the theory of planned behavior and the theory of reasoned action. *Personality and Social Psychology Bulletin, 1*, 3–9.

Maddux, J. E. (1991). Self-efficacy. In C. R. Snyder & D. R. Forsyth (Eds.), *Handbook of social and clinical psychology* (pp. 57–78). New York: Pergamon Press.

Maddux, J. E. (1994). Social cognitive theories of behavior change: Basic principles and issues in the prevention of AIDS. *General Psychologist, 30*(3), 90–95.

Maddux, J. E. (1995a). Self-efficacy theory: An introduction. In J. E. Maddux (Ed.), *Self-efficacy, adaptation, and adjustment: Theory, research, and application* (pp. 3–36). New York: Plenum Press.

Maddux, J. E. (Ed.). (1995b). *Self-efficacy, adaptation, and adjustment: Theory, research, and application*. New York: Plenum Press.

Maddux, J. E., Brawley, L., & Boykin, A. (1995). Self-efficacy and healthy decision-making: Protection, promotion, and detection. In J. E. Maddux (Ed.), *Self-efficacy, adaptation, and adjustment: Theory, research, and application* (pp. 173–202). New York: Plenum Press.

Maddux, J. E., Norton, L. W., & Stoltenberg, C. D. (1986). Self-efficacy expectancy, outcome expectancy, and outcome value: Relative effects on behavioral intentions. *Journal of Personality and Social Psychology, 51*, 783–789.

Maddux, J. E., & Rogers, R. W. (1983). Protection motivation and self-efficacy: A revised theory of fear appeals and attitude change. *Journal of Experimental Social Psychology, 19*, 469–479.

Marcus, B. H., Selby, V. C., Niaura, R. S., & Rossi, J. S. (1992). Self-efficacy and the stages of exercise behavior change. *Research Quarterly for Exercise and Sport, 63*, 60–66.

McAuley, E., & Courneya, K. S. (1993). Adherence to exercise and physical activity as health-promoting behaviors: Attitudinal and self-efficacy influences. *Applied and Preventative Psychology, 2*, 65–77.

McAuley, E., & Rowney, T. (1990). Exercise behavior and intentions. The mediating role of self-efficacy cognitions. In L. VanderVelden & J. H. Humphrey (Eds.), *Psychology and sociology of sport: Vol. 2* (pp. 3–15). New York: AMS Press.

Netemeyer, R. G., & Burton, S. (1990). Examining the relationships between voting behavior, intention, perceived behavioral control, and expectation. *Journal of Applied Social Psychology, 20*, 661–680.

O'Leary, A. (1995). Self-efficacy and the physiological stress response. In J. E. Maddux (Ed.), *Self-efficacy, adaptation, and adjustment: Theory, research, and application* (227–248). New York: Plenum Press.

Poag-DuCharme, K. A., & Brawley, L. R. (1993). Self-efficacy theory: Use in the prediction of exercise behavior in the community setting. *Journal of Applied Sport Psychology, 5*, 178–194.

Poag-DuCharme, K. A., Brawley, L. R., Rodgers, W., & Robinson, K. (1992, October). *Behavioral intention to exercise: Conceptualization and measurement*. Paper presented at the annual meeting of the Association for the Advancement of Applied Sport Psychology, Colorado Springs, CO.

Prochaska, J. O., DiClemente, C. C., & Norcross, J. C. (1992). In search of how people change: Applications to addictive behaviors. *American Psychologist, 47*, 1102–1114.

Prochaska, J. O., Velicer, W. F., Rossi, J. S., Goldstein, M. G., Marcus, B. H., Rakowski, W., Fiore, C., Harlow, L. L., Redding, C. A., Rosenbloom, D., & Rossi, S. R. (1994). Stages of change and decisional balance for 12 problem behaviors. *Health Psychology, 13*, 39–46.

Robinson, K. (1992). *Predicting the physical activity of the elderly: Use of the theory of planned behavior*. Unpublished masters dissertation. University of Waterloo, Waterloo, Ontario, Canada.

Rodgers, W. M., & Brawley, L. R. (1991a). The role of outcome expectancies in participation motivation. *Journal of Sport and Exercise Psychology, 13*, 411–427.

Rodgers, W. M., & Brawley, L. R. (1991b, June). *Evaluating fitness messages promoting involvement: Effects on attitudes and behavioural intentions*. Paper presented at the annual meeting of the North American Society for the Psychology of Sport and Physical Activity, Kent, OH.

Ronis, D. L., Yates, J. F., & Kirscht, J. P. (1989). Attitudes, decisions, and habits as determinants of behavior. In A. R. Pratkanis, S. J. Breckler, & A. G. Greenwald (Eds.), *Attitude structure and function* (pp. 213–239). New York: Erlbaum.

Rosenstock, I. M. (1974). The health belief model and preventive health behavior. *Health Education Monographs, 2*, 354–386.

Sallis, J. F., Hovell, M. F., Hofstetter, C. R., Faucher, P., Elder, J. P., Blanchard, J., Casperson, C. J., Powell, K. E., & Christenson, G. H. (1989). A multivariate study of determinants of vigorous exercise in a community sample. *Preventive Medicine, 18*, 20–34.

Schifter, D. B., & Ajzen, I. (1985). Intention, perceived control, and weight loss: An application of the theory of planned behavior. *Journal of Personality and Social Psychology, 49*, 843–851.

Schneider, W., & Shiffrin, R. M. (1977). Controlled and automatic human information processing. I. Detection, search, and attention. *Psychological Review, 84*, 1–66.

Sheppard, B. H., Hartwick, J., & Warshaw, P. R. (1988). The theory of reasoned action: A meta-analysis of past research with recommendations for modifications and future research. *Journal of Consumer Research, 15*, 325–345.

Stanley, M. A., & Maddux, J. E. (1986). Cognitive processes in health enhancement: Investigation of a combined protection motivation and self-efficacy model. *Basic and Applied Social Psychology, 7*, 101–113.

Triandis, H. C. (1980). Values, attitudes, and interpersonal behavior. In H. E. Howe, J. Page, & M. M. Page (Eds.), *Nebraska Symposium on Motivation, 1979: Vol. 27* (pp. 195–259). Lincoln: University of Nebraska Press.

Uzark, K. C., Becher, M. H., Dielman, T. E., & Rocchini, A. P. (1987). Psychosocial predictors of compliance with a weight control intervention for obese children and adolescents. *Journal of Compliance in Health Care, 2*, 167–178.

van den Putte, B. (1991). *20 years in the theory of reasoned action of Fishbein & Ajzen: A meta-analysis*. Unpublished manuscript. University of Amsterdam, The Netherlands.

Warshaw, P. R., & Davis, F. D. (1985). Disentangling behavioral intention and behavioral expectations. *Journal of Experimental Social Psychology, 21*, 213–228.

Weinstein, N. D. (1988). The precaution adoption process. *Health Psychology, 7*, 355–386.

Weinstein, N. D. (1993). Testing four competing theories of health-protective behavior. *Health Psychology, 12*, 324–333.

Wurtele, S. K., & Maddux, J. E. (1987). Relative contributions of protection motivation theory components in predicting exercise intentions and behavior. *Health Psychology, 6*, 453–466.

8

Health Services Utilization Models

Lu Ann Aday and William C. Awe

INTRODUCTION

Andersen's behavioral model of health services utilization (often referred to as the "health services utilization model") has provided a defining research agenda for the study of health care utilization since it was introduced in the late 1960s. Andersen initially developed and empirically tested his model in a nationwide personal interview survey of 2367 families conducted in 1964 (Andersen, 1968). The model organized and integrated an array of correlates of health and health care behavior from the disparate literatures in sociology, psychology, economics, and medicine into predisposing, enabling, and need predictors of families' use of physician, hospital, and dentist services.

The 1964 survey, for which Andersen was Study Director, was the third in a series conducted at 5-year intervals by the Health Information Foundation and the National Opinion Research Center at the University of Chicago to obtain information about the types and amounts of health services used during the 1-year period prior to the interview, the costs of these services, and how families paid for them.

In his 1968 monograph, *A Behavioral Model of Families' Use of Health Services*, based on analyses of the 1964 data guided by his new and innovative framework, Andersen argued for an explicit consideration of the role of social contexts in influencing individuals' and families' health care decision making and behavior (Andersen, 1968). This perspective is manifest in his delineation of the role that family composition (e.g., family size, gender of family head) and social structure (employment, social class, and occupation of main wage earner) play in predisposing families' use of services, as well as the importance of the availability of both family resources (income, savings, insurance) and community resources (physicians and hospital beds) in enabling them to do so. The focus on families' aggregate use of services also acknowledged the essential and intimate family context in which health and health care decisions are made and the direct influence of different stages of the family life cycle (premarriage through marriage and the birth and growth of children, children's transition to adulthood, divorce, retirement, and widowhood) on the profile and magnitude of both families' and individual members' utilization of health care services.

Lu Ann Aday and William C. Awe • School of Public Health, University of Texas at Houston, Houston, Texas 77225.

Handbook of Health Behavior Research I: Personal and Social Determinants, edited by David S. Gochman. Plenum Press, New York, 1997.

Andersen's model has subsequently been modified, expanded, and applied to examining the predictors of an array of health care behaviors. The discussion that follows describes Andersen's model, as well as revised approaches based on the original model developed by Andersen and his colleagues.

ORIGINAL MODEL: ANDERSEN'S BEHAVIORAL MODEL

Andersen's behavioral model is displayed in Figure 1 (Andersen, 1968). The terms *model* and *framework* are used interchangeably in discussing Andersen's contributions. A model is an actual example or replica of a phenomenon of interest. A framework is more the plan or scheme for organizing the components of that phenomenon. Andersen's "model" has in fact been used for both purposes: (1) to display and test complex causal models of health care–seeking behavior and (2) to simply order and array relevant predictors and indicators of utilization. The defining contributions of Andersen's model to subsequent research on health care services utilization

behavior will serve as a point of reference in describing the original and revised and expanded models, highlighting the body of empirical research over the last three decades based on his model, and presenting the criticisms and suggested adaptations of the model. These contributions are, in general, as follows:

1. Systematically characterizing the array of predictors of health services utilization (*independent variables*) as predisposing, enabling, and need factors.
2. Delineating the indicators of health services utilization (*dependent variables*) according to the type of service (hospital, physician, dentist) and reason for use (discretionary or nondiscretionary).
3. Specifying the hypothesized relationships (*causal pathways*) between the predictors and indicators of utilization.
4. Providing an integrated theoretical and empirical approach that has widespread applicability (*generalizability*) to diverse populations (international, national, and local) and important health policy problems (access, equity).

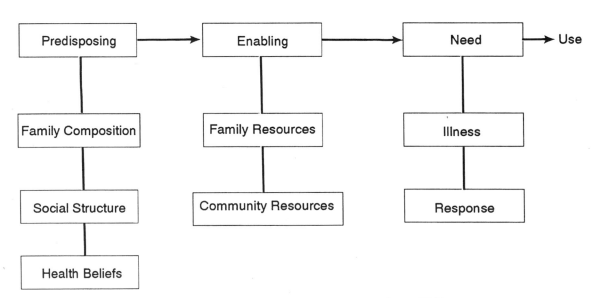

Figure 1. Andersen's behavioral model. From Andersen (1968).

Independent Variables

Predisposing variables include those that describe the propensity of family members to use services—including family composition (family size; gender marital status, and age of family head; ages of oldest and youngest family members), social structure (employment, social class, and occupation of main wage earner; education of family head; ethnicity; race), and health beliefs (value of health services, physicians, good health, health insurance; attitude toward health services and physician use; knowledge of disease).

For example, age is highly correlated with the need for care. Variables such as ethnicity, education, and occupation suggest the importance of lifestyle and environmental influences on individuals' decisions to seek care. People who believe strongly in the value of health care or physicians might be more likely to seek care than those who do not have these beliefs.

The *enabling* component describes the means individuals have available to them for the use of services. Both resources specific to families (income, savings, health insurance, regular source of care, and welfare care) and attributes of the community in which they live (physician and hospital bed ratios, residence, region) are included. Place of residence—e.g., whether one lives in a rural or urban area—may indicate geographic proximity to a source of care as well as prevailing community attitudes toward medical care.

Need refers to health status or illness, which is the most immediate and important cause of health service use. The need for care may be reflected in evidence of the presence of illness (symptoms, disability days, health level, free care for major illness), responses to it (seeing doctor for symptoms), or steps to prevent it (regular physical examinations).

Dependent Variables

Andersen drew an important distinction between *discretionary* and *nondiscretionary* utilization. Behavior that is highly discretionary means either that the seriousness of an individual's ill health does not compel seeing a provider, or that the family or individual would be the primary decision maker with respect to whether care is actually sought, or both. Nondiscretionary behavior would be either behavior dictated by a person's experiencing serious health problems or behavior attributable to decisions that are usually made by the providers of services. Andersen hypothesized that when little discretion can be exercised by the patient or family (e.g., in the decision to be hospitalized), need is likely to be the principal predictor of use. When there is considerable opportunity for discretion, the predisposing and enabling components would be more important.

Andersen also devised a mechanism for combining and aggregating various types of use (e.g., hospital, physician, dentist, drugs) across individuals for the purposes of measuring families' total utilization of services. This approach involved weighting the various types of services by standard or relative prices for each. Actual units or quantities of services (e.g., visits, admissions, ancillary services) were weighted by these standardized "prices." The resulting "dollar equivalents" or "units of use" were then added to derive aggregate measures of hospital, physician, dentist, or total services utilization for each family.

Causal Pathways

Andersen (1968, pp. 19–20) formulated and tested three major hypotheses regarding the relationship of the predisposing, enabling, and need components to health services utilization:

1. The amount of health services used by a family will be a function of the predisposing and enabling characteristics of the family and its need for medical care. Each of these three components will make an independent contribution to the understanding of differences in use of health services.
2. The explanatory components of the model will vary in their contribution to the explanation of total use. Need will be more im-

portant than the predisposing and enabling components because it represents factors most directly related to use.

3. The contribution of each component will vary according to the type of health service: (a) The contribution of need will be greatest for hospital services; (b) the contribution of the predisposing and enabling components will be greatest for dental services; and (c) all of the components will contribute to understanding physician services.

The first and second hypotheses were supported by his analysis. The third hypothesis was supported, in general, for physician and dentist use, but not for hospital use. Need was the primary determinant of a family's hospital utilization, but a predisposing factor (age of youngest family member) was also important, suggesting that families at the reproductive stage of the family life cycle were likely to have admissions associated with obstetrical care.

Generalizability

Andersen (1968) points out in the conclusions to his 1968 monograph that although the family is a relevant and important context for health care decision making, there may also be considerable heterogeneity within families, which should be taken into account in determining the relevant unit of analysis (individual or family) for addressing a given research question.

With considerable insight into a central and continuing policy issue, Andersen sought to illuminate the policy implications of his framework and analysis for the empirical and normative assessment of equity in the distribution of health care services. He argued that in an equitable system, the need for care and associated family life cycle factors (or compositional factors) would be the principal determinants of health services utilization, while other predisposing factors (social structure, health beliefs) and enabling factors should be much less influential determinants of who *did* and *did not* get care.

Andersen's formulation, analysis, and interpretation of the findings emanating from his research presaged many of the important theoretical and policy-relevant questions to be addressed with respect to the delivery and distribution of health care in the United States and other countries in the ensuing decades. Correspondingly, his creative and careful approach to measuring key study concepts and hypothesizing their probable relationships provided a theoretical and empirical compass to guide succeeding utilization researchers.

EXPANDED BEHAVIORAL MODEL: ANDERSEN AND NEWMAN UTILIZATION FRAMEWORK

Approximately ten years after the study on which Andersen's original model was based, Andersen and Newman formulated an expanded model (Figure 2), adding or elaborating compo-

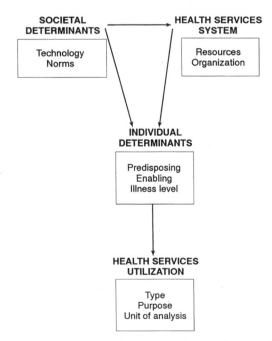

Figure 2. Andersen and Newman utilization framework. From Andersen and Newman (1973).

nents to be more responsive to societal and policy changes affecting health care, as well as to more fully reflect the increasing complexity of health care services delivery (Andersen & Newman, 1973). The expanded model integrated and elaborated Andersen's original model (Andersen, 1968), previous applications of the model to dental services utilization (Newman, 1971; Newman & Anderson, 1972), and a systems perspective developed by Andersen and his colleagues as a basis for comparing medical care use in Sweden and the United States (Andersen, Smedby, & Anderson, 1970).

Independent Variables

The unit of analysis implicit in the revised framework was individuals rather than families. The predisposing, enabling, and need predictors in the original model were incorporated as the principal *individual determinants* of health services utilization.

The revised framework characterizes illness according to perceived and evaluated need, rather than "illness" and "response," as in the original model. The indicators of "response" in Andersen's initial formulation (seeing a doctor for symptoms, regular physical examinations) may be more accurately viewed as dimensions, rather than predictors, of utilization. The distinction between perceived and evaluated need acknowledges that the need for care may be assessed subjectively by the patient (e.g., in terms of symptoms or function) or clinically evaluated by health care providers (on the basis of clinical tests and diagnoses).

The Andersen and Newman framework breaks out *societal determinants* (technology and norms), as well as *health services system* features (resources and organization), as important aggregate determinants of individuals' health-care-seeking behavior.

Technological developments and trends cited as affecting individuals' patterns of care seeking include the rapid decline of infectious diseases due to improvements in sanitation, immuniza-

tion, and antibiotics; the development of anesthesia and asepsis for surgical and other inpatient procedures; and the emergence of psychotropic drugs to treat mental illness. Examples of influential societal norms include shifting births from the home to the hospital and more recently to homelike birthing centers, the value of providing care for the seriously mentally or physically disabled in the least restrictive environment, and the dominance of "individual rights" (including rights to medical care) in formulating health policy.

The *health services system* component of the expanded model denotes the arrangements made for the potential rendering of care to consumers. It includes both the volume and distribution of services (resources) and the access to and structure of mechanisms for individuals entering and moving through the system (organization).

Dependent Variables

The expanded model also delineates a multi-faceted concept of utilization. The *type* of utilization was acknowledged in Andersen's original model and refers to the category of service rendered (e.g., physician's, dentist's, or other practitioner's services; hospital or long-term care admissions; prescription; medical equipment). The *purpose* refers to the reason care was sought: for health maintenance in the absence of no or minor symptoms (primary care), for the diagnosis or treatment of illness in the interest of returning to a previous state of well-being (secondary care), or rehabilitation or maintenance in the case of a long-term health problem (tertiary care). Another reason for rendering care is the maintenance or custodial care of medically fragile or dependent adults or children, in which the patient's personal as well as medical care needs are met. The *unit of analysis* refers to measures of (1) contact, based on whether the service was received during a particular time period (e.g., proportion seeing a physician within the last year); (2) volume, the total units of service received during that period (e.g., mean number of visits in a year for those seeing a physician); or (3) episode of illness based on the patterns of providers, referrals, and continuity of care for a given disease occurrence.

These dimensions are not mutually exclusive. A single utilization indicator may in fact be descriptive of a number of different dimensions. The "proportion seeing a physician in the year for a particular symptom" reflects, for example, the type, purpose, and time interval of utilization. In choosing a relevant utilization indicator, it is important to consider the precise dimension(s) one is interested in examining and what measures best operationalize it. Further, the process of selecting the appropriate models and variables for predicting or explaining utilization should be guided by their relevance to the particular dimension(s) of utilization being considered.

Causal Pathways

The expanded model hypothesizes that societal determinants affect individual determinants both directly and indirectly through the health services system. Individual determinants have the most immediate influence on people's decisions about the use of services. Andersen and Newman acknowledged, however, that the postulated causal links between the societal factors and resulting utilization behavior can only be inferred, since the data, methods, and theory that govern their influence are not well developed (Andersen & Newman, 1973, p. 100). The influences of the health services system on individuals' predisposing, enabling, and need characteristics pose an array of questions regarding the impact of health policy changes (e.g., funding personnel training or redistribution programs or innovative modes of service delivery) on individuals' propensity and ability to obtain care.

Generalizability

Andersen and Newman extended and applied Andersen's initial formulation of an approach to measuring the equity of the distribu-

tion of health services. They reiterated that the equity goal would attempt to maximize the role played by need and need-related demographic factors (age, gender) and minimize the role played by enabling factors (resource availability) and other predisposing factors (social structure and belief) in influencing the distribution of services. Efforts should also be made to evaluate the intervention potential of the various predictors on the basis of their mutability (susceptibility to change by health policy), as well as the empirically documented strength of the causal connections and interactions between the hypothesized predictors of use.

EXPANDED BEHAVIORAL MODEL: ADAY AND ANDERSEN ACCESS FRAMEWORK

The Aday and Andersen access framework, which drew directly on the Andersen and Newman model, was developed to guide the first national survey of access to medical care in the United States, conducted in 1975 by the Center for Health Administration Studies (formerly the Health Information Foundation) and the National Opinion Research Center at the University of Chicago, with support from the Robert Wood Johnson Foundation (see Figure 3). It provided a systematic basis for assessing the performance of major governmental and private (particularly foundation) programs in enhancing access to medical care in the United States (Aday & Andersen, 1974, 1975, 1981; Aday, Andersen, & Fleming, 1980).

Independent Variables

Health policy replaced societal norms in the Andersen and Newman model as the starting point for the consideration of the predictors of the utilization of and satisfaction with medical care. Utilization, particularly as it might indicate the population's or a subgroup's access to medical care, is often evaluated in a political context.

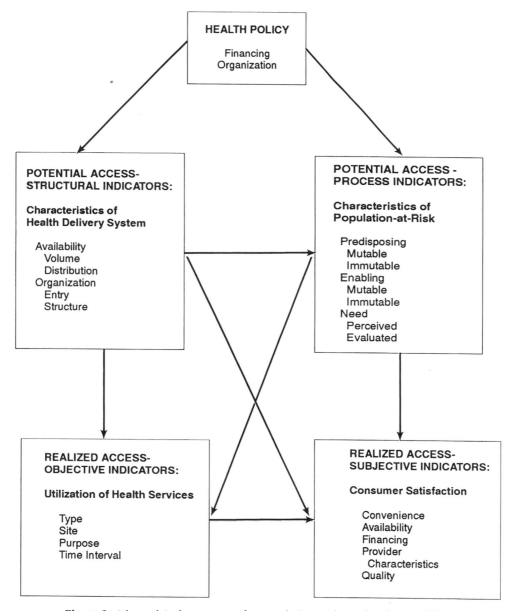

Figure 3. Aday and Andersen access framework. From Aday and Andersen (1981).

For example, major health care financing (e.g., Medicare and Medicaid) and organization programs (e.g., community health center or outreach arrangements) have been concerned with improving the ability of target groups to obtain care when it is needed. It is the effect of *health policy* on altering the utilization of and access to medical care that health policy makers and administrators often seek to evaluate.

The *characteristics of the health services*

system are, in general, those specified in the Andersen and Newman utilization framework. In the revised model, however, the "resources" dimension is translated into "availability" (which more directly reflects the types of measures used to operationalize this component) and the "access" subdimension of "organization" into "entry" (to more clearly distinguish it as a subcomponent of the broader access concept).

The *characteristics of the population-at-risk* are the predisposing, enabling, and need components in Andersen's original behavioral model of health services utilization. Those characteristics that are biological or social givens, such as age, gender, race, and place of residence, are termed *immutable*. Health policy cannot directly alter these attributes, but they define target groups at greater risk of illness or poorer access to care. The more manipulable beliefs and enabling variables, such as insurance coverage, are characteristics that health policy seeks to change in order to affect these groups' access to care. They are *mutable*, or alterable by health policy.

These predictors may be viewed as structural and process indicators of *potential* access, i.e., the probability that services will be obtained.

Dependent Variables

In the expanded behavioral model, applied to measuring the concept of access, the principal indicators of *realized* access were objective measures of health services utilization, as well as subjective assessments by consumers of their actual utilization experiences. Realized access indicators are essentially reflections of the extent to which the system and population characteristics actually predict whether or not or how much care is sought and how satisfied potential or actual consumers are with the medical care system.

The revised access framework adds *site* as another dimension of utilization, referring to the place where services were received, which might be an inpatient setting (e.g., short-term hospital stay, mental institution, nursing home), an ambulatory setting (e.g., hospital outpatient depart-

ment or emergency room, physician's office, health maintenance organization [HMO], public health clinic, community health center, free-standing emergency center), or the patient's home. It is particularly important to distinguish this dimension of utilization, given that many of the access-oriented program interventions are in fact intended to alter the patterns of sites in which services are sought (e.g., shifting care from hospital emergency rooms to community-based primary care group practices). The "unit of analysis" in the Andersen and Newman model is translated to "time interval" in the access framework, to more accurately reflect the temporal dimension implied in indicators of the contact, volume, and continuity of service utilization.

The addition of the *consumer satisfaction* outcome acknowledges the importance of directly incorporating patients' subjective experiences of care seeking in evaluating their access to care. Satisfaction may be evaluated by patients specifically, at a given facility or in terms of their particular experiences, or in general by the public, with respect to their perceptions of the performance of the medical care system as a whole. Both have been used as subjective assessments of the performance of the medical care system with respect to access.

Causal Pathways

The hypothesized relationships among the components are indicated by the arrows in the framework (see Figure 3). Health policy may be seen as directly affecting characteristics of the delivery system (such as increasing the supply of physicians in an area), or programs may be directed to changing characteristics of the population at risk either directly (by providing insurance coverage or linkage with a regular provider) or indirectly through the delivery system (such as establishing satellite clinics to reduce the time area residents must travel to obtain care).

The delivery system may in turn directly affect utilization patterns and the satisfaction of consumers with the system. These effects are determined by the structure itself (lower hospitalization rates among members of staff-model HMOs) and not necessarily mediated by the characteristics of potential users (enrollees). The characteristics of the population (attitudes toward medical care) may also directly affect use and satisfaction independent of system properties.

The arrow between utilization and satisfaction suggests that the type of provider seen, the location and purpose of the visit, and the number and continuity of visits are all likely to influence consumers' satisfaction with their experience of care seeking.

Generalizability

The Aday and Andersen access framework has been applied extensively in evaluating the extent to which services are equitably distributed. It has been used, for example, to operationalize the need-based norm of equity introduced by Andersen, as well as other explicit norms of fairness for distributing scarce health care resources (freedom of choice, similar treatment, decent basic minimum, cost-effectiveness) (Aday & Andersen, 1981; Aday, Begley, Lairson, & Slater, 1993).

EMPIRICAL APPLICATIONS OF THE MODEL

Andersen's model and the successive adaptations of it have been used to guide the design and conduct of large-scale international, national, and local surveys and related program evaluations conducted by Andersen and his colleagues. It has also been widely applied by other investigators to explain and predict a variety of health care utilization behaviors. The major types of empirical applications of the model are highlighted here.

Andersen and Colleagues

As mentioned, Andersen formulated the original behavioral model to provide guidance for the analyses of a 1964 national survey of families' health care utilization and expenditures (Andersen, 1968; Andersen & Anderson, 1967). In 1970, Andersen directed a second national survey, in which he applied the model once again, with a focus on extending and developing its potential for empirically evaluating the equity of the United States health care system on the basis of the relative contributions of various (predisposing, enabling, and need) predictors to explaining individuals' utilization of services (Andersen, Greeley, Kravits, & Anderson, 1972; Andersen, Kravits, Anderson, & Daley, 1973; Andersen, Kravits, & Anderson, 1975; Andersen, Lion, & Anderson, 1976). During this same period, Newman modified and used the framework in a nationwide study of dental services utilization (Andersen & Newman, 1973; Newman, 1971; Newman & Anderson, 1972).

The mid-1970s saw the further adaptation of the Andersen and Newman framework to the study of access. The 1975 national access survey, supported by the Johnson Foundation, developed and implemented the Aday and Andersen access framework (Aday & Andersen, 1975; Aday et al., 1980). Andersen and his colleagues subsequently applied the framework to the secondary analyses of a 1982 national survey supported by the foundation, and the framework continued to provide implicit guidance for subsequent national studies conducted by the Robert Wood Johnson Foundation in collaboration with Lou Harris and Associates (Aday, Fleming, & Andersen, 1984; Andersen, Aday, Lyttle, Cornelius, & Chen, 1987).

Andersen also introduced and adapted his model for cross-national comparative research on utilization. He used it most directly in comparing the utilization patterns and equity of the United States and Swedish health care systems in the early 1970s, and later in a multicountry World Health Organization International Collaborative Study of Dental Manpower Systems in Relation to Oral Health Status that involved the conduct of national surveys of dental health and use, as well as assessments of the availability and organization of dental care services in the study countries

(Andersen, 1976; Andersen & Chen, 1989; Andersen et al., 1970).

In the mid-1980s, Andersen and his colleagues utilized the expanded access framework in two large-scale national evaluations of programs supported by the Robert Wood Johnson Foundation to improve the delivery of primary health care services. The Access Evaluation of the Community Hospital Program involved baseline and follow-up personal interview surveys in 12 of more than 50 communities in which the foundation had funded community hospitals to develop primary care–oriented group practice arrangements (Aday, Andersen, Loevy, & Kremer, 1985). The Municipal Health Services Program Access Evaluation in 5 cities received foundation support to improve the design of primary care service delivery in their public health care systems (Fleming & Andersen, 1986). Both studies involved extensive interviews to gather data on the target population's utilization and access experiences.

Other Investigators

The model has also been used in a wide variety of other health services utilization studies (Aday & Eichhorn, 1972; Maurana, Eichhorn, & Lonnquist, 1981; Muller, 1986). It has been most widely applied in research on use of services by the elderly. In addition to research on general health services utilization (physician and hospital), studies on care-seeking behavior of the elderly have sought, for example, to explore the predictors of nursing home admissions and lengths of stay, use of in-home nursing and nurse's aides, other formal and informal helpers, social services, adult day care, and dental services (Arling, 1985; Conrad, Hughes, & Wang, 1992; Coulton & Frost, 1982; Counte & Glandon, 1991; Evashwick, Rowe, Diehr, & Branch, 1984; Eve, 1988; Freedman, 1993; Jette, Branch, Sleeper, Feldman, & Sullivan, 1992; Miller & McFall, 1991; Mutran & Ferraro, 1988; Rabiner, 1992; Rosner, Namazi, & Wykle, 1988; Wan, 1989).

Wolinsky and Bass and their colleagues, in particular, have been key contributors to the

critical evaluation and application of the model to studying use of services by the elderly (Bass & Noelker, 1987; Bass, Looman, & Ehrlich, 1992; Wolinsky, 1978; Wolinsky & Coe, 1984; Wolinsky & Johnson, 1991; Wolinsky et al., 1989; Wolinsky, Johnson, & Fitzgerald, 1992). Their research has not only provided valuable conceptual and empirical contributions to understanding older adults' health care–seeking behaviors, but also suggestions for modifying and strengthening the validity and generalizability of the framework itself. (Critiques and modifications of the model suggested by these investigators and others will be discussed in the section that follows).

The model has been helpful as well in identifying the utilization patterns of other subgroups, such as male and female veterans, American Indians, African-Americans, Hispanics, immigrants and refugees, the homeless, and adolescents and children, among others (Gilbert, Branch, & Longmate, 1992, 1993; Gilbert, Branch, & Orav, 1990; Guendelman, 1991; Kelley, Perloff, Morris, & Liu, 1992; Padgett, Patrick, Burns, & Schlesinger, 1994; Padgett, Struening, & Andrews, 1990; Romeis, Gillespie, Virgo, & Thorman, 1991; White-Means & Thornton, 1989; Wolinsky et al., 1989).

It has not been limited to studying traditional types of medical care (physician and hospital) and dentist service utilization, but has also been broadly applied in predicting the utilization of prescription and nonprescription drugs, dental sealants, mental health, substance abuse, rehabilitation, post-disaster health clinic, and social services (Aubin, Potvin, Béland, & Pineault, 1994; Cafferata & Meyers, 1990; Freeman et al., 1992; Harada, Sofaer, & Kominski, 1993; Leaf et al., 1988; Nichol, McCombs, Johnson, Spacapan, & Sclar, 1992; Padgett et al., 1990, 1994; Portes, Kyle, & Eaton, 1992; Selwitz, Colley, & Rozier, 1992).

In addition to Andersen's significant applications of the model in his cross-national comparative studies, it has been utilized by other investigators in examining predictors of health services utilization and access in developing countries as well as in other developed countries (Fosu, 1989; Keith & Wickrama, 1990; Kempen & Suurmeijer, 1991; Subedi, 1989).

CRITIQUES OF THE MODELS: RESEARCH AND METHODOLOGICAL ISSUES

A number of criticisms have been offered of Andersen's original and expanded models; these criticisms may be seen as being both informed by and extending the research agenda his framework has essentially served to define. The criticisms are broadly related to the definition and measurement of the major predictors (1) and indicators (2) of health services utilization, (3) the specification and testing of their hypothesized relationships, and (4) the robustness and generalizability of findings based on the models.

Independent Variables

The criticisms of the major predictors of utilization in Andersen's behavioral model relate primarily to (1) the validity of approaches to measuring the major study concepts, (2) the need to add other variables or dimensions to adequately capture relevant predictors, and (3) the inadequate capture of possible interactions between variables in specifying the model (Mechanic, 1979; Rundall, 1981; Tanner, Cockerham, & Spaeth, 1983; Wolinsky, 1978).

Criticisms of the validity of the study concepts concern how the predisposing, enabling, and need characteristics, as well as the system-level characteristics, are measured in the original and expanded models, as well as other large-scale quantitative studies based on the models. Mechanic (1979) argued, for example, that (1) measures of perceived need actually incorporate concepts of psychological distress that may be influenced by life events as well as physical illness, but are not interpreted as such in large-scale quantitative studies; (2) aggregate system-level resource availability indicators for large areas do not adequately capture the immediate experiences of individuals in their local communities; and (3) large-scale multivariate surveys fail to adequately model and measure patient decision making regarding care seeking.

Because of the range of variables and differing levels of analysis included, it is difficult to gather data to test the complete model (Becker & Maiman, 1983; Wolinsky, 1978). Its flexibility is evidenced, however, by investigators' frequent additions of other domains of predictors relevant to the particular type of utilization behavior they are exploring. For example, there has been extensive research applying the model to the utilization of various services by the elderly that argues for considering the role that kin play in influencing their care-seeking behavior, directly incorporating characteristics of the caregivers of the elderly (e.g., breaking out their predisposing, enabling, and need characteristics), or adding stress and social support, among other variables, as factors that predispose use (Bass & Noelker, 1987; Coulton & Frost, 1982; Counte & Glandon, 1991; Freedman, 1993; Mutran & Ferraro, 1988).

Other investigators have pointed out the utility of adding pharmacy consulting characteristics in explaining changes in over-the-counter medication purchases (Nichol et al., 1992), contextual factors related to refugees' prior use of mental health facilities (Portes et al., 1992), hearing impairment as a factor that predisposes to general health services utilization (Kurz, Haddock, VanWinkle, & Wang, 1991), and factors more directly relevant to predicting the use of dental services, e.g., dentate status, importance placed on oral health, and current source of dental care (Gilbert et al., 1990, 1992, 1993).

Another major criticism is that the predictors should be more appropriately considered as interacting, rather than as having separate (independent, additive, or main) effects. The impact of the hypothesized predictors may be different, for example, for groups of different age, gender, race, ethnicity, or income, or those with selected types of physical or cognitive impairment (Arling, 1985; Bass et al., 1992; Cafferata & Meyers, 1990; Coulton & Frost, 1982; Mutran & Ferraro, 1988; Ronis & Harrison, 1988; Rundall, 1981; White-Means & Thornton, 1989; Wolinsky, 1978; Wolinsky et al., 1989).

Dependent Variables

As mentioned, the framework has been applied to explaining a diverse array of utilization behaviors. Special consideration should be given to specifying accurately and appropriately the type, site, purpose, and time interval of utilization in measuring a given type of service (e.g., mammography screening, psychotropic drug use, rehabilitation services or mental health services use). An important extension of existing utilization research would be to explore more systematically the interrelationships (or trade-offs) between different types of service utilization (e.g., ambulatory versus inpatient, community-based versus nursing home care) (Wan, 1989; Wolinsky & Johnson, 1991). Researchers have also pointed out the importance of evaluating the distribution of the utilization variable and adjusting it as needed (through logarithmic or other transformations) to better meet the statistical assumptions (normality) of a given analytical technique (multiple linear regression) (Wolinsky & Coe, 1984).

Causal Pathways

There is a need to identify and test more fully the array of causal relationships implied in the original and expanded models. Analyses based on cross-sectional surveys do not provide a powerful approach to examining these hypothesized relationships. Research based on panel or longitudinal study designs afford a more direct opportunity to evaluate the temporal influence of various factors that influence utilization (such as nursing home placement among the elderly) (Counte & Glandon, 1991; Eve, 1988; Freedman, 1993; Gilbert et al., 1990; Miller & McFall, 1991; Rabiner, 1992). A number of studies have formulated variations on the original models, or have attempted to more fully test the hypothesized causal pathways, using path analysis or simultaneous equation modeling, or have incorporated both approaches (Aubin et al., 1994; Counte & Glandon, 1991; Gilbert et al., 1990; Harada et al., 1993; Miller & Champion, 1993; Mutran & Ferraro, 1988; Patrick, Stein, Porta, Porter, & Ricketts, 1988; Shortell et al., 1977; Siddharthan, 1991; Wolinsky, 1978; Yeatts, Crow, & Folts, 1992).

Generalizability

Major criticisms of the empirical research based on the model are that it tends to explain a very small percentage of the overall variation in utilization and that need remains a dominant predictor. These results have called into question the framework's overall predictive and explanatory capacity (Mechanic, 1979; Wolinsky, 1978). Many of the methodological considerations just reviewed (efforts to improve the measurement of study variables, adding other explanatory variables or dimensions to the framework, more accurately modeling the relationships between variables, and transforming relevant predictor or utilization variables or both) represent efforts to address these deficiencies.

Summary

In summary, various factors may determine who ultimately obtains care. Substantial progress has been made in measuring and specifying the relationships among these different factors. Andersen's model provides an integrative framework for considering many of these factors and their interrelationships. More focused studies are required, however, to model the causal relationships and internal processes associated with individual patients' decisions to seek care.

A FURTHER EXTENSION OF THE MODEL: A FRAMEWORK FOR EVALUATING MEDICAL CARE SYSTEM PERFORMANCE

An unexamined assumption during the period of initial development and application of the behavioral model was that it was desirable for individuals to seek access to and utilize medical care services because their doing so would enhance their prospects of maintaining or improving their health. This assumption has come to be increasingly examined and challenged, however, in the context of evaluating the effectiveness and efficiency of the United States medical care system. In this final section, these and related health policy issues are reviewed in the context of their implications for an expanded framework and set of indicators for evaluating the performance of the medical care system (see also Aday [1993a], on which the following discussion is based).

Andersen signaled these developments in a 1976 article elaborating the application of his model to cross-national comparisons of health systems (Andersen, 1976, p. 35):

> Given the rapidly rising cost of health services and the need to make decisions about the relative allocation of resources to health services and other sectors of the economy, it becomes increasingly important to focus on the extent to which health services are achieving their expected goals (effectiveness) and on the manner in which resources are being used to reach this level of attainment (efficiency).

Writing during this same period, radical critics such as Illich (1975) and Carlson (1975) argued that Western medicine had reached its limits in improving people's health and that it now had the potential to do as much harm as good to those who came within its compass. During the same period, McKeown (1976) similarly argued, on the basis of patterns of mortality in Western nations over nearly a century, that most reductions in death rates could be better attributed to improvements in nutrition and hygiene than to medical care alone.

Canadian Lalonde's (1975) field concept, which formed the conceptual basis for the U.S. Surgeon General's *Healthy People* report in the mid-1970s, and was subsequently made manifest programmatically in the Year 1990 and Year 2000 Objectives for the Nation's Health, gave further expression to these simultaneous irreverent, provocative, and important inquiries (Public Health Service, 1979, 1990). The field concept considers human biology, environment, lifestyle,

and health care organization all as possible predictors of health and illness.

These investigations have in fact highlighted the greater importance of lifestyle and environmental factors, relative to biological factors or medical care, in ameliorating many of the major health problems that plague contemporary Western society (including the United States). Other social and medical care critics, such as Tesh (1988), in her book *Hidden Arguments: Political Ideology and Disease Prevention Policy*, and Beauchamp (1988) in the United States, Evans and Stoddart (1990) of Canada, and the White and Black reports in England (Day & Klein, 1989; Gray, 1982), among others (Aday, 1993b), have looked more deeply into the social–structural origins of the variations in health risks and related health outcomes associated with varying access to social and economic resources as a function of age, gender, race, or social class in the United States as well as in other societies.

This *population-oriented view* of the determinants of people's health has been most widely heard and adopted in policy and practice in the public health field, rather than the medical care and associated health services research communities, in the United States. The current emphasis on medical outcomes research has highlighted the question of the extent to which medical care is effective. It may be seen, however, to fit within the context of a *clinically oriented* view of the role of medical care in promoting *individuals'* health and well-being (Aday et al., 1993).

Work on developing empirical indicators of access to personal medical care services, embodied in the deliberations of the Institute of Medicine (IOM) Committee on Monitoring Access to Personal Health Services, may similarly be seen as fitting more directly into the clinically oriented view of the role of personal health services in enhancing *individuals' medical care outcomes*—not the broader public health–oriented perspective on the determinants of a *population's health* (Institute of Medicine, 1993). Nonetheless, the IOM committee's work does seek, much more than in the past, to bring to the surface and illuminate *clinical effectiveness* norms in the formulation of recommended *access to medical care* indicators.

Over the past 25 years, there has been considerable interest in the multiplicity of factors reported to define access, such as the availability and organization of medical care providers and resources; the geographic, attitudinal, financial, and organizational barriers that individuals confront in seeking services; and the rates of actual utilization and satisfaction descriptive of the "outcomes" of the care-seeking experience.

The Aday and Andersen access framework (Figure 3), based on Andersen's original behavioral model, attempted to capture and examine the relative importance of an array of empirical predictors and indicators of access to medical care (Aday et al., 1980). This framework has been used in three principal types of research related to the access objective: descriptive, analytical, and evaluative research.

Descriptive research focuses on profiling access in terms of the potential and realized access indicators (such as number and distribution of medical providers, percentage of the population with insurance coverage or a regular source of care, proportion having seen a doctor or dentist in the past year, and mean number of visits for those who did) and in documenting and examining subgroup variation according to these indicators.

Analytical research is directed more toward understanding *why* some groups have better access than others through examining the role of potential access measures (system and population characteristics) in predicting the groups' actual rates of utilization or satisfaction with medical care.

Evaluative research is concerned with assessing how well policies, programs, and services developed and implemented on the basis of previous descriptive and analytical research have done in accomplishing the equity-of-access objective. These studies rely primarily on quasi-experimental evaluation designs to assess program or policy outcomes (Aday et al., 1993).

The access framework just reviewed has guided a great deal of the descriptive and ana-

lytical research surrounding equity of access to medical care. Underlying the application of that framework in assessing equity is the value judgment that the system would be deemed to be fair if need-based criteria, rather than resources (such as insurance coverage or income), are the main determinants of whether or not or how much care is sought.

Subgroup disparities (e.g., by income, race or ethnicity, or insurance coverage) in the use of services relative to underlying need would therefore be minimized in an equitable system. Access indicators developed within the context of this perspective on equity have focused on overall estimates and subgroup variations in the use of what were deemed to be necessary primary prevention–oriented, as well as illness-related, services: "the utilization of medical care services relative to need" (Aday et al., 1980).

Primary prevention–oriented measures include indicators of the trimester in which prenatal care was sought or the number of visits during pregnancy, as well as having a general physical exam, Pap smear, or breast exam in a given period of time.

Illness-related indicators that have been used directly in applying the Aday and Andersen framework to evaluating equity of access to medical care include the use/disability and symptoms/response ratios (Aday et al., 1980). The use/disability ratio is the ratio of the number of total physician visits reported by subgroups of interest to the total number of days of limited activity due to illness they reported during the year. Widely varying rates of overall utilization relative to disability were deemed to be indicative of an inequitable distribution of services relative to experienced need. Similarly, the symptoms/response ratio compared the proportion of people in a given age group who actually contacted a physician for a set of symptoms with the proportion a panel of physicians thought should see them, to assess the extent to which services that were deemed to be needed services were actually obtained.

The current and evolving concept of access to medical care summarized in Figure 4 builds

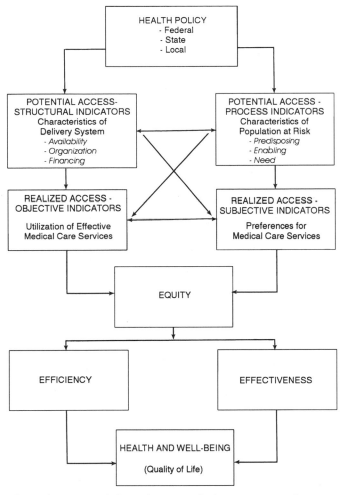

Figure 4. Framework for evaluating medical care system performance.

upon, extends, and modifies the perspective provided by the Aday and Andersen access framework and the associated use-relative-to-need approach to measuring equity (Aday et al., 1993; Weissman & Epstein, 1993).

In the original formulation, health status was viewed principally as a *predictor* of health services utilization. In the emerging conceptualization, it is viewed, significantly and additionally, as an implicit or explicit *outcome* of the medical care–seeking process.

Further, the choice of indicators of the use of *medical care* services in general or relative

to some generalized conception of underlying "need" has also been tempered and focused in the context of this question: "A difference might be made by readier access to what services?" In other words, what types of medical care does it make the most sense to enhance *utilization* of, because those services are most likely to be *effective* in improving *health*?

In this reconceptualization of access, there is more of an explicit focus on the bottom line: enhancing the health and quality of life of individuals by providing access to specific medical care services. Further, the goal of equity of access to medical care becomes a *means* toward this end, not simply an end in itself; in the latter case, the efficacious outcomes of seeking and receiving care are theoretically assumed rather than empirically evaluated.

Further, subjective measures of realized access, such as patient satisfaction, remain important evaluative yardsticks in assessing the performance of the medical care system. This subjective dimension is more directly expressed, however, in effectiveness-oriented considerations of patient preferences (or utilities) for different functional or longevity outcomes that are likely to be associated with alternative treatment procedures. There is an effort in both medical care outcomes research and applied clinical decision-making sciences to more explicitly invite patients to consider the risks and benefits associated with treatment options and to be full partners in choosing among these options.

Effectiveness, efficiency, and equity, then, all become guiding norms or prerequisites in ultimately ensuring the health and well-being of those to whom medical care services are directed; in this approach (Aday et al., 1993):

- *Effectiveness* refers to the benefits of medical care measured by improvements in health.
- *Efficiency* relates these health improvements to the resources required to produce them.
- *Equity* assesses whether the benefits and burdens of medical care are fairly distributed.

Contemporary considerations of *equity* of access to medical care explicitly embrace both effectiveness and efficiency norms.

The definition of equity, based on the revised framework (Figure 4), focuses on "the utilization of *effective and appropriate* medical care services *to improve health outcomes*," as well as the minimization of subgroup disparities in the extent to which this goal is achieved.

"Effective" care refers to services that are likely to result in health improvements. "Appropriate" care refers to those services that are most timely or fitting for achieving this objective. For example, penicillin may be an *effective* intervention to treat syphilis. *Appropriate* care to deal with congenital syphilis (i.e., syphilis in newborns) would concentrate, however, on the administration of penicillin to affected mothers prior to delivery to *prevent* its transmission in utero or during delivery, rather than administration after delivery to an affected newborn, in whom it could have been averted through appropriate prenatal care.

Efficiency research attempts to quantify the cost-effectiveness or cost-benefit of these or other procedures in assessing the extent to which finite public, private, or personal resources should be invested in assuring access to those procedures or services.

The IOM Committee on Monitoring Access to Personal Health Care Services, in its final report, *Access to Health Care in America* (Institute of Medicine, 1993), pointed out that the indicators selected to measure explicit access-related objectives should consider both (1) what health outcomes access was intended to affect and (2) what types of utilization would be most appropriate to enhance those outcomes. Its aim was to specify a core set of indicators that could comprise a monitoring system for evaluating the state of the nation's performance with respect to access, much as the Year 2000 guidelines provide for monitoring the nation's health (see Table 1).

A number of the access indicators recommended by the IOM committee on access do in fact mirror those used to measure the Year 2000 Health Objectives (Public Health Service, 1990). The committee considered what may be once again broadly characterized as primary prevention-oriented or illness-related access indicators and objectives. A number of the more prevention-oriented utilization indicators are similar to those highlighted in earlier generations of access studies. In selecting both relevant utilization and outcomes-oriented measures, however, the IOM committee identified those preventive services that were most likely to be effective in achieving specific health outcome objectives. The full IOM report provides more details on the methods of constructing these indicators, as well as national

Table 1. Access Indicators Recommended by the Institute of Medicine Committee on Monitoring Access to Personal Health Care Services[a]

Prevention-related

Objective 1. Promoting successful birth outcomes
Utilization indicators
    Adequacy of prenatal care
Health outcomes
    Infant mortality
    Low birthweight
    Congenital syphilis

Objective 2. Reducing the incidence of vaccine-preventable childhood diseases
Utilization indicators
    Immunization rates
Health outcomes
    Incidence of preventable childhood communicable diseases (diphtheria, measles, mumps, pertussis, polio, rubella, and tetanus)

Objective 3. Early detection and diagnosis of treatable diseases
Utilization indicators
    Breast and cervical cancer screening
Health outcomes
    Incidence of late-stage breast and cervical cancers

Illness-related

Objective 4. Reducing the effects of chronic diseases and prolonging life
Utilization indicators
    Chronic disease follow-up care
    Use of high-cost discretionary care (those that rely on the judgment of the physicians who provide first-contact care, who may or may not refer the patient for specialized procedures, such as hip/joint replacement, breast reconstruction after mastectomy, pacemaker insertion, coronary artery bypass surgery, or coronary angioplasty)
Health outcomes
    Avoidable hospitalizations for chronic diseases (admissions that might not have occurred had the patient received effective, timely, and continuous ambulatory medical care for the condition, such as angina, asthma, grand mal status, chronic obstructive pulmonary disease, congestive heart failure, convulsions, diabetes, hypoglycemia, or hypertension)
    Access-related excess mortality (i.e., between-group differences in death rates for diseases that can be managed by medical care, such as between blacks and whites, that remain after statistical adjustments for differing physiological and behavioral risk factors are made)

Objective 5. Reducing morbidity and pain through timely and appropriate treatment
Utilization indicators
    Acute illness-related medical care
Health outcomes
    Avoidable hospitalizations for acute conditions (such as bacterial pneumonia, cellulitis, dehydration as primary diagnosis, gastroenteritis, kidney/urinary infection, severe ear, nose, and throat infections, skin graft with cellullitis)

[a]Adapted from Institute of Medicine (1993).

data for the United States as a whole and age, sex, race, income, and education subgroups for which information is available.

In summary, the emerging conceptualization of access explicitly views health status as a desired *outcome* as well as a *predictor* of access to medical care. The new generation of access measures have their progenitors in those indicators that assumed that the use of services relative to need was desirable in improving health outcomes. These measures, in turn, have spun off others that examine, rather than presuppose, these assumptions, and persist in raising the important and provocative questions: "To *what* services should access be assured and (perhaps *most* important) *why*?"

Andersen's behavioral model of health services utilization, and the expanded frameworks based upon it, have provided and will continue to provide a defining foundation for the conduct of health services utilization and access research. The successive adaptations of the model on the part of its originator and his colleagues (including the expanded access framework introduced here), as well as the flexibility evidenced in its being adapted and applied in explaining a diverse array of health care–seeking behaviors, amply attest to its enduring usefulness *and* relevance.

REFERENCES

Aday, L. (1993a). Access to what and why? Toward a new generation of access indicators. *Proceedings of the Public Health Conference on Records and Statistics* (pp. 410–415). Washington, DC: U.S. Government Printing Office.

Aday, L. (1993b). *At risk in America: The health and health care needs of vulnerable populations in the United States*. San Francisco: Jossey-Bass.

Aday, L., & Andersen, R. (1974). A framework for the study of access to medical care. *Health Services Research, 9*, 208–220.

Aday, L., & Andersen, R. (1975). *Development of indices of access to medical care*. Ann Arbor, MI: Health Administration Press.

Aday, L., & Andersen, R. (1981). Equity of access to medical care: A conceptual and empirical overview. *Medical Care, 19*, 4–27.

Aday, L., Andersen, R., & Fleming, G. (1980). *Health care in the U.S.: Equitable for whom?* Beverly Hills, CA: Sage.

Aday, L., Andersen, R., Loevy, S., & Kremer, B. (1985). *Hospital–physician sponsored primary care: Marketing and impact*. Ann Arbor, MI: Health Administration Press.

Aday, L., Begley, C., Lairson, D., & Slater, C. (1993). *Evaluating the medical care system: Effectiveness, efficiency, and equity*. Ann Arbor, MI: Health Administration Press.

Aday, L., & Eichhorn, R. (1972). *The utilization of health services: Indices and correlates—A research bibliography*. DHEW Publication No. (HSM) 73-3003. Washington, DC: U.S. Government Printing Office.

Aday, L., Fleming, G., & Andersen, R. (1984). *Access to medical care in the U.S.: Who has it, who doesn't*. Chicago: Pluribus Press.

Andersen, R. (1968). *A behavioral model of families' use of health services*. Research Series No. 25. Chicago: Center for Health Administration Studies, University of Chicago.

Andersen, R. (1976). A framework for cross-national comparisons of health services systems. In M. Pflanz & E. Schach (Eds.), *Cross-national sociomedical research: Concepts, methods, practice* (pp. 25–35), Stuttgart, Germany: Georg Thieme.

Andersen, R., Aday, L., Lyttle, C., Cornelius, J., & Chen, M. (1987). *Ambulatory care and insurance coverage in an era of constraint*. Chicago: Pluribus Press.

Andersen, R., & Anderson, O. (1967). *A decade of health services: Social survey trends in use and expenditure*. Chicago: University of Chicago Press.

Andersen, R., & Chen, M. (1989). *Determinants of oral health status: An international comparison*. Chicago: Center for Health Administration Services, University of Chicago.

Andersen, R., Kravits, J., Anderson, O. W., & Daley, J. (1973). *Expenditures for personal health services—National trends and variations: 1953–1970*. DHEW Publication No. (HRA) 74-3105. Washington, DC: U.S. Government Printing Office.

Andersen, R., Greeley, R. M., Kravits, J., & Anderson, O. W. (1972). *Health service use—National trends and variations: 1953–1971*. DHEW Publication No. (HSM) 73-3004. Washington, DC: U.S. Government Printing Office.

Andersen, R., Kravits, J., & Anderson, O. (1975). *Equity in health services: Empirical analyses in social policy*. Boston: Ballinger.

Andersen, R., Lion, J., & Anderson, O. (1976). *Two decades of health services: Social survey trends in use and expenditure*. Boston: Ballinger.

Andersen, R., & Newman, J. (1973). Societal and individual determinants of medical care utilization in the United States. *Milbank Memorial Fund Quarterly, 51*, 95–124.

Andersen, R., Smedby, B., & Anderson, O. (1970). *Medical care use in Sweden and the United States—A comparative analysis of systems and behavior*. Research Series No. 27. Chicago: Center for Health Administration Studies, University of Chicago.

Arling, G. (1985). Interaction effects in a multivariate model of physician visits by older people. *Medical Care, 23*, 361–371.

Aubin, J., Potvin, L., Béland, F., & Pineault, R. (1994). Utilization of a specialized clinic following an ecological accident. *Medical Care, 32*, 1-14.

Bass, D., Looman, W., & Ehrlich, P. (1992). Predicting the volume of health and social services: Integrating cognitive impairment into the modified Andersen framework. *Gerontologist, 32*, 33-43.

Bass, D., & Noelker, L. (1987). The influence of family caregivers on elder's use of in-home services: An expanded conceptual framework. *Journal of Health and Social Behavior, 28*, 184-196.

Beauchamp, D. (1988). *The health of the republic: Epidemics, medicine, and moralism as challenges to democracy.* Philadelphia: Temple University Press.

Becker, M., & Maiman, L. (1983). Models of health-related behavior. In D. Mechanic (Ed.), *Handbook of health, health care and the health professions* (pp. 539-568). New York: Free Press.

Cafferata, G., & Meyers, S. (1990). Pathways to psychotropic drugs: Understanding the basis of gender differences. *Medical Care, 28*, 285-300.

Carlson, R. (1975). *The end of medicine.* New York: Wiley.

Conrad, K., Hughes, S., & Wang, S. (1992). Program factors that influence utilization of adult day care. *Health Services Research, 27*, 481-502.

Coulton, C., & Frost, A. (1982). Use of social and health services by the elderly. *Journal of Health and Social Behavior, 23*, 330-339.

Counte, M., & Glandon, G. (1991). A panel study of life stress, social support, and the health services utilization of older persons. *Medical Care, 29*, 348-361.

Day, P., & Klein, R. (1989). The politics of modernization: Britain's national health service in the 1980s. *Milbank Quarterly, 67*, 1-34.

Evans, R., & Stoddart, G. (1990). Producing health, consuming health care. *Social Science and Medicine, 31*, 1347-1363.

Evashwick, C., Rowe, G., Diehr, P., & Branch, L. (1984). Factors explaining the use of health care services by the elderly. *Health Services Research, 19*, 357-382.

Eve, S. (1988). A longitudinal study of use of health care services among older women. *Journal of Gerontology, 43*, M31-M39.

Fleming, G., & Andersen, R. (1986). *Can access be improved while controlling costs?* Chicago: Pluribus Press.

Fosu, G. (1989). Access to health care in urban areas of developing societies. *Journal of Health and Social Behavior, 30*, 398-411.

Freedman, V. (1993). Kin and nursing home lengths of stay: A backward recurrence time approach. *Journal of Health and Social Behavior, 34*, 138-152.

Freeman, D., Alegría, M., Vera, M., Muñoz, C., Robles, R., Jiménez, A., Calderón, J., & Peña, M. (1992). A receiver operating characteristic (ROC) curve analysis of a model of mental health services use by Puerto Rican poor. *Medical Care, 30*, 1142-1153.

Gilbert, G., Branch, L., & Longmate, J. (1992). Eligible veterans' choice between VA-covered and non-VA-covered dental care. *Journal of Public Health Dentistry, 52*, 277-287.

Gilbert, G., Branch, L., & Longmate, J. (1993). Dental care use by U.S. veterans eligible for VA care. *Social Science and Medicine, 36*, 361-370.

Gilbert, G., Branch, L., & Orav, J. (1990). Predictors of older adults' longitudinal dental care use: Ten year results. *Medical Care, 28*, 1165-1180.

Gray A. (1982). Inequalities in health: The Black Report—A summary and comment. *International Journal of Health Services, 12*, 349-380.

Guendelman, S. (1991). Health care users residing on the Mexican border: What factors determine choice of the U.S. or Mexican health care system? *Medical Care, 29*, 419-429.

Harada, N., Sofaer, S., & Kominski, G. (1993). Functional status outcomes in rehabilitation: Implications for prospective payment. *Medical Care, 31*, 345-357.

Illich, I. (1975). *Medical nemesis.* London: M. Boyars.

Institute of Medicine. (1993). *Access to health care in America.* Washington, DC: National Academy Press.

Jette, A., Branch, L., Sleeper, L., Feldman, H., & Sullivan, L. (1992). High-risk profiles for nursing home admission. *Gerontologist, 32*, 634-640.

Keith, P., & Wickrama, K. (1990). Use and evaluation of health services by women in a developing country: Is age important? *Gerontologist, 30*, 262-268.

Kelley, M., Perloff, J., Morris, N., & Liu, W. (1992). Primary care arrangements and access to care among African-American women in three Chicago communities. *Women and Health, 18*, 91-106.

Kempen, G., & Suurmeijer, T. P. (1991). Professional home care for the elderly: An application of the Andersen-Newman model in the Netherlands. *Social Science and Medicine, 33*, 1081-1089.

Kurz, R., Haddock, C., VanWinkle, D., & Wang, G. (1991). The effects of hearing impairment on health services utilization. *Medical Care, 29*, 878-889.

Lalonde, M. (1975). *A new perspective on the health of Canadians.* Ottawa: Information Canada.

Leaf, R., Bruce, M., Tischler, G., Freeman, D., Weissman, M., & Myers, J. (1988). Factors affecting the utilization of specialty and general medical mental health services. *Medical Care, 26*, 9-26.

Maurana, C., Eichhorn, R., & Lonnquist, L. (1981). *The use of health services: Indices and correlates—A research bibliography.* Rockville, MD: National Center for Health Services Research.

McKeown, T. (1976). *The role of medicine: Dream, mirage, or nemesis?* London: Nuffield Provincial Hospitals Trust.

Mechanic, D. (1979). Correlates of physician utilization: Why do multivariate studies of physician utilization find trivial psychosocial and organizational effects? *Journal of Health and Social Behavior, 20*, 387-396.

Miller, A., & Champion, V. (1993). Mammography in women > 50 years of age: Predisposing and enabling characteristics. *Cancer Nursing, 16,* 260–269.

Miller, B., & McFall, S. (1991). The effect of caregiver's burden on change in frail older person's use of formal helpers. *Journal of Health and Social Behavior, 32,* 165–179.

Muller, C. (1986). Review of twenty years of research on medical care utilization. *Health Services Research, 21,* 129–144.

Mutran, E., & Ferraro, K. (1988). Medical need and use of services among older men and women. *Journal of Gerontology, 43,* S162–171.

Newman, J. (1971). *The utilization of dental services.* Unpublished doctoral dissertation. Emory University, Atlanta, GA.

Newman, J., & Anderson, O. (1972). *Patterns of dental service utilization in the United States: A nationwide social survey.* Research Series No. 30. Chicago: Center for Health Administration Studies, University of Chicago.

Nichol, M., McCombs, J., Johnson, K., Spacapan, S., & Sclar, D. (1992). The effects of consultation on over-the-counter medication purchasing decisions. *Medical Care, 30,* 989–1003.

Padgett, D., Patrick, C., Burns, B., & Schlesinger, H. (1994). Ethnicity and the use of outpatient mental health services in a national insured population. *American Journal of Public Health, 84,* 222–226.

Padgett, D., Struening, E., & Andrews, H. (1990). Factors affecting the use of medical, mental health, alcohol, and drug treatment services by homeless adults. *Medical Care, 28,* 805–821.

Patrick, D., Stein, J., Porta, M., Porter, C., & Ricketts, T. (1988). Poverty, health services, and health status in rural America. *Milbank Quarterly, 66,* 105–136.

Portes, A., Kyle, D., & Eaton, W. (1992). Mental illness and help-seeking behavior among Mariel Cuban and Haitian refugees in South Florida. *Journal of Health and Social Behavior, 33,* 283–298.

Public Health Service. (1979). *Healthy people: The Surgeon General's report on health promotion and disease prevention.* DHEW-PHS Publication No. 79-55071. Washington, DC: U.S. Government Printing Office.

Public Health Service. (1990). *Healthy people 2000: National health promotion and disease prevention objectives: Full report, with commentary.* DHHS Publication No. PHS 91-50212. Washington, DC: U.S. Government Printing Office.

Rabiner, D. (1992). The relationship between program participation, use of formal in-home care, and satisfaction with care in an elderly population. *Gerontologist, 32,* 805–812.

Romeis, J., Gillespie, K., Virgo, K., & Thorman, K. (1991). Female veterans' and nonveterans' use of health care services. *Medical Care, 29,* 932–936.

Ronis, D., & Harrison, K. (1988). Statistical interactions in studies of physician utilization: Promise and pitfalls. *Medical Care, 26,* 361–372.

Rosner, T., Namazi, K., & Wykle, M. (1988). Physician use among the old-old: Factors affecting variability. *Medical Care, 26,* 982–991.

Rundall, T. (1981). A suggestion for improving the behavioral model of physician utilization. *Journal of Health and Social Behavior, 22,* 103–104.

Selwitz, R., Colley, B., & Rozier, R. (1992). Factors associated with parental acceptance of dental sealants. *Journal of Public Health Dentistry, 52,* 137–145.

Shortell, S., Richardson, W., LoGerfo, J., Diehr, P., Weaver, B., & Green, K. (1977). The relationships among dimensions of health services in two provider systems: A causal model approach. *Journal of Health and Social Behavior, 18,* 139–159.

Siddharthan, K. (1991). Evaluation of behavioral demand models of consumer choice in health care. *Evaluation Review, 15,* 455–470.

Subedi, J. (1989). Modern health services and health care behavior: A survey in Kathmandu, Nepal. *Journal of Health and Social Behavior, 30,* 412–420.

Tanner, J., Cockerham, W., & Spaeth, J. (1983). Predicting physician utilization. *Medical Care, 21,* 360–369.

Tesh, S. (1988). *Hidden arguments: Political ideology and disease prevention policy.* New Brunswick, NJ: Rutgers University Press.

Wan, T. (1989). The effect of managed care on health services use by dually eligible elders. *Medical Care, 27,* 983–1001.

Weissman, J., & Epstein, A. (1993). The insurance gap: Does it make a difference? *Annual Review of Public Health, 14,* 243–270.

White-Means, S., & Thornton, M. (1989). Nonemergency visits to hospital emergency rooms: A comparison of blacks and whites. *Milbank Quarterly, 67,* 35–56.

Wolinsky, F. (1978). Assessing the effects of predisposing, enabling, and illness-morbidity characteristics on health service utilization. *Journal of Health and Social Behavior, 19,* 384–396.

Wolinsky, F., Aguirre, B. E., Fan, L-J., Keith, V.M., Arnold, C. L., Niederhauer, J.C., & Dietrich, K. (1989). Ethnic differences in the demand for physician and hospital utilization among older adults in major American cities: Conspicuous evidence of considerable inequalities. *Milbank Quarterly, 67,* 412–448.

Wolinsky, F., & Coe, R. (1984). Physician and hospital utilization among noninstitutionalized elderly adults: An analysis of the Health Interview Survey. *Journal of Gerontology, 39,* 334–341.

Wolinsky, F., & Johnson, R. (1991). The use of health services by older adults. *Journal of Gerontology, 46,* S345–357.

Wolinsky, F., Johnson, R., & Fitzgerald, J. (1992). Falling, health status, and the use of health services. *Medical Care, 30,* 587–597.

Yeatts, D., Crow, T., & Folts, E. (1992). Service use among low-income minority elderly: Strategies for overcoming barriers. *Gerontologist, 32,* 24–32.

III

FAMILY DETERMINANTS

The family is presumed to be important in the acquisition and support of health behavior and would be a fertile area for health behavior research, yet relatively few empirical studies have explored how, and to what degree, the family serves as such a determinant. The literature relating the family to health and medical care is rich with studies that demonstrate the family's critical role as the social unit within which illness occurs and is treated; it is also rich with analyses of family activities and family involvement with illness, care seeking, and "becoming a patient" (e.g., Akamatsu, Stephens, Hobfoll, & Crowther, 1992; Litman, 1974). But reviews of the literature reveal no appreciable body of research on the family as a determinant of health behavior (e.g., Baranowski & Nader, 1985; Campbell, 1978; Gochman, 1985, 1992a,b; Sallis & Nader, 1988) and confirm that little is known about how family structure, internal processes, or child-rearing practices affect the health beliefs and actions of children and other family members.

The way in which a family links to the larger social system appears to be one variable that does consistently predict selected health behaviors. Considerable research (e.g., Geertsen, Klauber, Rindflesh, Kane, & Gray, 1975; Suchman, 1965/1972) has shown how the social integration of the family into the community affects health behaviors such as utilization of services. In a study of Philippine villagers (Friede, Waternaux, Guyer, DeJesus, & Filipp, 1985), parents who had greater involvement in the lives of their community were more likely to have their children immunized. Yet family structure and process themselves were not focal points of most such studies.

For convenience, research on family determinants can be discussed under three headings: child and adolescent health behaviors, adult health behaviors, and the family as a unit.

CHILD AND ADOLESCENT HEALTH BEHAVIORS

Health Cognitions

One of the earliest of the few extant studies of how family factors determine children's health-related cognitions is Campbell's (1975) demonstration that although mothers and children used the same signs and symptoms as a basis for attributing illness, there was no specific linkage within individual mother–child pairs; i.e., an individual mother's tendency to attribute illness did not predict her child's tendency to attribute illness. Campbell (1978) also observed that maternal valuing of self-direction in children is linked to children's being more inclined to communicate to parents that they are sick, while maternal valuing of self-assertiveness (in contrast to being attentive to others) reduces this inclination.

Dielman et al. (1982) did not find strong relationships between parental health beliefs and children's health beliefs. Blaxter and Paterson's (1982) examination of three generations of Scot-

173

ish families—children, mothers, and grand-mothers—found that while some of the grand-mothers' advice on health-related child care in-fluenced the mothers' behavior, there was less such influence than might have been expected; that contraception patterns between the two older generations were different; and that there was little intergenerational similarity in attitudes toward health and health services.

Adolescents' health-related knowledge seems not to be related in consistent ways to the family health histories. For example, the existence of somatic disorders in families did not consistently predict adolescents' understanding of medical terms and the accuracy of their health informa-tion (Hastrup, Phillips, Vullo, Kang, & Slomka, 1992). In contrast, Carandang, Folkins, Hines, and Steward (1979) presented interesting evi-dence, within a Piagetian framework, that the stresses associated with the presence of a child with diabetes in a family have a negative effect on the ability of the child's siblings to conceptualize the causes and treatment of illness.

In Chapter 10, Gochman provides an over-view of the relationships between family charac-teristics and a range of health cognitions.

Risk Behaviors

Selected family characteristics have been re-lated to risk behaviors. Turner, Irwin, Tschann, and Millstein (1993) observed in early adoles-cents that parental granting of autonomy was linked to lower likelihoods of initiation of sexual intercourse and that emotional detachment from parents was linked to greater likelihood of smok-ing and of using alcohol and other drugs. Parental safety attitudes and use of seat belts were found to be linked to pedestrian and bicycle injuries in children (Pless, Verrault, & Tenina, 1989) and thus possibly to the children's incautiousness or risk taking.

Lifestyle and Health Care Behaviors

In Chapter 9, Baranowski uses a develop-mental framework to provide a careful and sys-

tematic analysis of family factors in eating and nutritional behaviors. In Chapter 11, Tinsley ex-amines in a more focused way the particular role of the mother as a socializing agent in the emer-gence of health behaviors and in creating a health-promoting environment within the family household. Both Baranowski and Tinsley de-velop their analyses within frameworks of social learning and cognitive learning theories.

ADULT HEALTH BEHAVIORS

There has also been little work done on the family as a determinant of adult health beliefs and health behaviors. Longitudinal observations (Lau, Quadrel, & Hartman, 1990) suggested that paren-tal health beliefs and behaviors have an apprecia-ble impact on the emergence in young adult college students of lifestyle-related behaviors, such as exercise, diet, smoking, use of seat belts, and alcohol consumption. Conversely, the poten-tial role of adolescents as gatekeepers of health information has also been demonstrated (Nader et al., 1982), a finding that raises important ques-tions about the multidirectionality of the deter-minants of health behavior within the family.

The nature of spousal relationships has some relevance for selected health behaviors. Horwitz (1978) showed that characteristics of the husband–wife dyadic relationship are related to informal help-seeking behaviors, i.e., consult-ing with relatives and friends. Persons whose marital relationships were characterized as con-flicted were more likely to engage in active infor-mal help seeking for emotional problems among relatives and friends than were those whose mari-tal relationships were supportive and sympa-thetic. Spousal support was also found to be related to acceptance of medication in coronary disease prevention (Doherty, Schrott, Metcalf, & Iasiello-Vailas, 1983).

Although nearly all research on health care use has typically focused on individuals, Weimer, Hatcher, and Gould (1983) observed that family factors in utilization are beginning to be identi-fied. One emerging conceptual framework that encourages consideration of the family as a unit of health service use is the Moos Family Environment Scale, the employment of which revealed that families that are high users of clinical services tend to be less satisfied with physicians and more likely to use tranquilizers (Weimer et al., 1983) than families low in use of clinical services. Another conceptual framework, the Family Utilization Index (Schor, Starfield, Stidley, & Hankin, 1987), permits construction of average use rates for families based on comparisons of individual member use rates for different types of care.

Patterns of family and household medicine use have also been found to predict individual use of nonprescription medication. Individuals living in households with higher rates of use of nonprescription medicines by other household members were more likely to use these medicines themselves (Jackson, Smith, Sharpe, Freeman, & Hy, 1982).

THE FAMILY AS A UNIT: CONCEPTUAL ISSUES

A major obstacle to research lies in the failure to conceptualize the family qua family. Often, as has been noted (e.g., Gochman, 1985), research reports with the word "family" in their titles use a characteristic of one of the parents, such as mother's education, as a major variable, but do not consider the family as a total unit. While such studies can have considerable value in broadening understanding of health behavior, they do not shed light on how the family *as a unit* acts as a determinant.

In Chapter 9, Baranowski expands on this point in his discussion of "emergent characteristics" of families.

The Energized Family

Pratt's (1976) seminal work on the "energized" family remains one of the most important of the few efforts to conceptualize the family as a social system and to relate variables derived from this conceptualization to health behavior. Members of Pratt's "energized" family demonstrate regular interaction with one another, maintain contacts with the community to advance their interests, and attempt to cope and to master their lives. Such families show fluidity in internal organization, a sharing of power, flexibility in role relationships, and concern for and support of the growth of family members (Pratt, 1976, pp. 3–4). Pratt provides evidence that "energized" families can promote sound health practices (Pratt, 1976), and that "developmental" child-rearing practices, i.e., those that demonstrate use of reasons, rewards, and the granting of autonomy, are more likely to lead to apropriate health behaviors in children than methods that are based on punishment and discipline" (Pratt, 1973).

Consumerism

The consumerist impact on families in relation to health and illness can be seen in conceptualizations of families as decision-making units. There is evidence (Monroe, 1993) that families that engage in negotiating, information seeking, and consideration of alternatives are more likely to select a prepaid health plan than an insurance plan.

Familism

"Familism," the *presumed* inclination of immigrant or ethnic groups to rely excessively on the family and to distrust the social world beyond the family, has often been assumed to be a barrier to the development of appropriate health behaviors. Its impact on health behaviors, however, is neither empirically clear nor consistent. For example, despite such assumptions, among a Mexican-American sample, familism was not a barrier to use of biomedical services and was a positive factor in use of prenatal services (Hoppe & Heller, 1975). Moreover, familism was found to have a positive impact on acceptance of mammography among Mexican-American women; those women who were "least acculturated"— i.e., least removed from traditional Mexican family attitudes—were the ones most likely to have had a mammogram (Suarez, 1994).

Emerging Conceptual Models

The concepts of "intrafamilial transmission," denoting the degree of shared health cognitions within a family, and "interfamily consensus," denoting the degree of shared cognitions in randomly selected pairs (Susman, Hersh, Nannis, Strope, & Woodruff, 1982), may become important assessment tools in studying family determinants of a range of health behaviors. Similarly, the concept of "family aggregation" (e.g., Sallis & Nader, 1988), denoting intrafamilial similarities in health behavior, may also prove to be a valuable methodological tool. Baranowski discusses the synonymous concept of "family concordance" in Chapter 9.

The conceptual framework of the "household production of health," generated by health behavior research in developing countries, denotes the active and complex role of family units in the healing of sickness and in the preservation of health, as opposed to the passive role traditionally assigned to them (Harkness & Super, 1994). Within this framework, the concept of the "developmental niche" builds on anthropological, psychological, and biological models and evidence and focuses on the physical and social setting in which a child lives, the culturally regulated customs of child care, and the cognitive perspectives of the caretakers. The concept sensitizes health behavior researchers to the specific contexts in which children acquire knowledge about health and illness as well as to how children and their families adapt to illness and disease (Harkness & Super, 1994).

REFERENCES

Akamatsu, T. J., Stephens, M. A. P., Hobfoll, S. E., & Crowther, J. H. (Eds.). (1992). *Family health psychology*. Washington, DC: Hemisphere.

Baranowski, T., & Nader, P. R. (1985). Family health behavior. In D. C. Turk & R. D. Kerns (Eds.), *Health, illness, and families: A life-span perspective* (pp. 51-80). New York: Wiley.

Blaxter, M., & Paterson, E. (1982). *Mothers and daughters: A three-generational study of health attitudes and behaviour*. London: Heinemann.

Campbell, J. D. (1975). Attribution of illness: Another double standard. *Journal of Health and Social Behavior, 16*, 114-126.

Campbell, J. D. (1978). The child in the sick role: Contributions of age, sex, parental status, and parental values. *Journal of Health and Social Behavior, 19*, 35-51.

Carandang, M. L. A., Folkins, C. H., Hines, P. A., & Steward, M. S. (1979). The role of cognitive level and sibling illness in children's conceptualization of illness. *American Journal of Orthopsychiatry, 49*, 474-481.

Dielman, T. E., Leech, S., Becker, M. H., Rosenstock, I. M., Horvath, W. J., & Radius, S. M. (1982). Parental and child health beliefs and behavior. *Health Education Quarterly, 9*, 60-77.

Doherty, W. J., Schrott, H. G., Metcalf, L., & Iasiello-Vailas, L. (1983). Effect of spouse support and health beliefs on medication adherence. *Journal of Family Practice, 17*, 837-841.

Friede, A., Waternaux, C., Guyer, B., De Jesus, A., & Filipp, L. C. (1985). An epidemiological assessment of immunization programme participation in the Philippines. *International Journal of Epidemiology, 14*, 135-142.

Geertsen, R., Klauber, M. R., Rindflesh, M., Kane, R. L., & Gray, R. (1975). A re-examination of Suchman's views on social factors in health care utilization. *Journal of Health and Social Behavior, 16*, 226-237.

Gochman, D. S. (1985). Family determinants of children's concepts of health and illness. In D. C. Turk & R. D. Kerns (Eds.), *Health, illness, and families: A life-span perspective* (pp. 23-50). New York: Wiley.

Gochman, D. S. (1992a). Health cognitions in families. In T. J. Akamatsu, M. A. P. Stephens, S. E. Hobfoll, & J. H. Crowther (Eds.), *Family health psychology* (pp. 23-43). Washington: Hemisphere.

Gochman, D. S. (1992b). Here's looking at you, kid! New ways of viewing the development of health cognition. In E. J. Susman, L. V. Feagans, & W. J. Ray (Eds.), *Emotion, cognition, health, and development in children and adolescents* (pp. 9-23). Hillsdale, NJ: Erlbaum.

Harkness, S., & Super, C. M. (1994). The developmental niche: A theoretical framework for analyzing the household production of health. *Social Science and Medicine, 38*, 217-226.

Hastrup, J. L., Phillips, S. M., Vullo, K., Kang, G., & Slomka, L. (1992). Adolescents' knowledge of medical terminology and family health history. *Health Psychology, 11*, 41-47.

Hoppe, S. K., & Heller, P. L. (1975). Alienation, familism and the utilization of health services by Mexican Americans. *Journal of Health and Social Behavior, 16*, 304-314.

Horwitz, A. (1978). Family, kin, and friend networks in psychiatric help-seeking. *Social Science and Medicine, 12,* 297-304.

Jackson, J. D., Smith, M. C., Sharpe, T. R., Freeman, R. A., & Hy, R. (1982). An investigation of prescribed and non-prescribed medicine use behavior within the household context. *Social Science and Medicine, 16,* 2009-2015.

Lau, R. R., Quadrel, M. J., & Hartman, K. A. (1990). Development and change of young adults' preventive health beliefs and behavior: Influence from parents and peers. *Journal of Health and Social Behavior, 31,* 240-259.

Litman, T. J. (1974). The family as a basic unit in health and medical care: A social-behavioral overview. *Social Science and Medicine, 8,* 495-519.

Monroe, P. A. (1993). Family health care decision making. *Journal of Family and Economic Issues, 14*(1), 7-25.

Nader, P. R., Perry, C., Maccoby, N., Solomon, D., Killen, J., Telch, M., & Alexander, J. K. (1982). Adolescent perceptions of family health behavior: A tenth grade educational activity to increase family awareness of a community cardiovascular risk reduction program. *Journal of School Health, 52,* 372-377.

Pless, I. B., Verrault, R., & Tenina, S. (1989). A case-control study of pedestrian and bicyclist injuries in childhood. *American Journal of Public health, 79,* 885-998.

Pratt, L. (1973). Child rearing methods and children's health behavior. *Journal of Health and Social Behavior, 14,* 61-69.

Pratt, L. (1976). *Family structure and effective health behav-ior: The energized family.* Boston: Houghton-Mifflin.

Sallis, J. F., & Nader, P. R. (1988). Family determinants of health behavior. In D. S. Gochman (Ed.), *Health behavior: Emerging research perspectives* (pp. 107-124). New York: Plenum Press.

Schor, E., Starfield, B., Stidley, C., & Hankin, J. (1987). Family health: Utilization and effects of family membership. *Medical Care, 25,* 616-626.

Suarez, L. (1994). Pap smear and mammogram screening in Mexican-American women: The effects of acculturation. *American Journal of Public Health, 84,* 742-764.

Suchman, E. A. (1965/1972). Stages of illness and medical care. In E. G. Jaco (Ed.), *Patients, physicians and illness: A sourcebook in behavioral science and health* (2nd ed.) (pp. 155-171). New York: Free Press. [Reprinted from *Journal of Health and Human Behavior*, 1965, *6,* 114-128.]

Susman, E. J., Hersh, S. P., Nannis, E. D., Strope, B. E., & Woodruff, P. J. (1982). Conceptions of cancer: The perspectives of child and adolescent patients and their families. *Journal of Pediatric Psychology, 7,* 253-261.

Turner, R. A., Irwin, C. E., Jr., Tschann, J. M., & Millstein, S. G. (1993). Autonomy, relatedness, and the initiation of health risk behaviors in early adolescence. *Health Psychology, 12,* 200-208.

Weimer, S. R., Hatcher, C., & Gould, E. (1983). Family characteristics in high and low health care utilization. *General Hospital Psychiatry, 5,* 55-61.

9

Families and Health Actions

Tom Baranowski

OVERVIEW

Domains of Interest

Family determinants have been investigated in a broad variety of health behaviors, including— but not limited to—substance use (Denton & Kampfe, 1994), use of health care services (Tinsley, 1992), exercise (Lau, Quadrell, & Hartman, 1990), and smoking (Moreno et al., 1994). There have been numerous advances since the report of a 1981 conference concluded that knowledge about family influences on health behaviors was in its infancy and could provide little guidance to researchers (Bruhn & Parcel, 1982).

To provide a more thorough treatment of family determinants, this chapter focuses on dietary practices. While others have investigated the role of food in maintaining family functioning (Coughenour, 1972), this chapter focuses on family influences on food consumption. Heavy emphasis is placed on parent–child influences, but spousal effects are discussed as well.

Tom Baranowski • Department of Behavioral Sciences, M. D. Anderson Cancer Center, University of Texas at Houston, Houston, Texas 77030.

Handbook of Health Behavior Research I: Personal and Social Determinants, edited by David S. Gochman. Plenum Press, New York, 1997.

Diet is an initiator or contributor to a broad variety of diseases, including heart disease (Simon, 1992), cancer (Toniolo, Riboli, Shore, & Pasternack, 1994), diabetes (Kumanyika & Ewart, 1990), and even mental health (Aschheim, 1993). Diet and physical activity are obvious contributors to a primary risk factor for poor health: obesity (Bar-Or & Baranowski, 1994). Diet involves common behaviors that are performed several times a day, a characteristic that facilitates its examination. Thus, in regard to cancer or heart disease, of particular interest are those dietary behaviors that are associated with fat intake (e.g., ingestion of meat, dairy products, spreads) and antioxidants (e.g., ingestion of fruits and vegetables high in α-tocopherol) and methods of preparation that affect those nutrients (e.g., deep fat frying, boiling). In regard to obesity, the behavior of interest involves the amount of calories consumed, the sources of those calories, and the rapidity with which the calories are consumed. Cross-cutting these conditions are family factors related to food purchase.

This chapter also employs a developmental perspective that segments the population into reasonably homogeneous developmental groups who face common life span issues and who are at comparable levels in their skills for dealing with tasks and challenges.

Social Cognitive Theory

Social cognitive theory has been proposed as a conceptual framework for organizing and understanding the literature on family-related effects on health behavior (e.g., physical activity [Taylor, Baranowski, & Sallis, 1995]). A key construct in social cognitive theory is *reciprocal determinism*, which maintains that characteristics of the person, the person's behavior, and the environment are in constant interaction and that the influences operate in both directions.

Within social cognitive theory, key characteristics of the person include outcome expectations, expectancies, self-efficacy, and skills. Outcome expectations and expectancies are motivational variables concerning what consequences a person believes will occur as a result of performing a particular behavior (expectations) (Domel et al., 1995) and whether the outcomes are desirable (expectancies): The person performs that behavior to achieve those anticipated desired outcomes. Preferences for foods can be thought of as proximal outcome expectations: the pleasing tastes of foods to be consumed.

In order to perform a behavior, one must have the component skills. When a person learns a behavior, the person learns these skills. Whether the person performs the behavior in a future situation depends in part on the person's skills and on motivational factors, e.g., outcome expectations. For example, to make a particular dish, a person must know how to perform all the necessary recipe steps (i.e., the steps are the component skills). Whether the person makes the recipe depends on the skills, motivational factors in regard to these foods and recipes, and environmental factors, e.g., availability of the foods in the home. One set of skills of particular interest in social cognitive theory is self-regulatory skills, i.e., being able to control or change one's behavior. This ability includes the component abilities of setting goals for behavior change that one can reasonably achieve, monitoring behavior in regard to those goals, exerting the effort and skills to achieve the change, and

rewarding oneself (intrinsically or extrinsically) when one achieves the goal.

Self-efficacy is a motivation-related construct and denotes a person's confidence in being able to perform a particular behavior (Domel et al., 1996). Self-efficacy includes confidence both in having the skills to perform the behavior and in being able to overcome the barriers to performing the behavior (Baranowski, 1990).

Environmental components of interest include the foods that are available, as well as social support (Sallis, Grossman, Pinski, Patterson, & Nader, 1987), rewards or incentives (Curry, Wagner, & Grothaus, 1991), and barriers to performing particular behaviors. Members of the family are parts of each others' social environment, and thereby extend the model of reciprocal determinism to include each member of the family in a common environment. Furthermore, parents may "model" behaviors for a child (Bandura, 1972), thereby hastening the child's learning of the skills to perform the behavior and enhancing the child's motivation when the child sees the parent rewarded for the behavior (e.g., enjoying the taste). This process is represented in Figure 1, the model of family reciprocal determinism.

The dynamic character of this model can be highlighted by examplifying each path of influence in the model (see Table 1). As one example, parental behavior can affect the child's environment by establishing or eliminating barriers to consumption, making selected foods available in the home, making certain foods more readily accessible (e.g., providing cut carrot sticks in a glass of water at the front of a shelf in the refrigerator), and enhancing access to certain kinds of foods outside the home (e.g., selecting a fast food restaurant that has certain desired foods). Parental behavior can directly affect the child's behavior, skills, cognition, or affect through modeling of or persuading to desired dietary behaviors, rewarding of desired behaviors, ignoring or punishing undesired behaviors, and employing authoritative parenting procedures to help the child build general self-control skills (R. W. Jackson, McDaniel, & Rao, 1994).

Table 1. Social Cognitive Constructs and Linkages in the Model of Family Reciprocal Determinism

Construct categories	Constructs
Environmental/situational factors	Physical environment
	Cultural environment
	Distal social environment
	Proximal social environment
Cognition	Outcome expectations
	Self-efficacy
	Situation
Affect	Preferences
	Outcome expectancies
Behavior	Skills
	Actions

Other-focused linkages	Examples
Parent behavior → Child environment → Child behavior, skills, cognition, affect	Parent purchasing child's favorite fruit for child's future consumption.
Parent behavior → Child behavior, skills, cognition, affect	Parent encouraging child to eat more fruits and vegetables by emphasizing things the child likes about fruits and vegetables.
Child behavior → Parent environment → parent behavior, skills, cognition, affect	Child writing parents' favorite fruit and vegetables on the grocery shopping list.
Child behavior → Parent behavior, skills, cognition, affect	Child persuading parent of ability to make favorite vegetable dish.

Self-focused linkages	Examples
Parent behavior → Parent environment → parent behavior, skills, cognition, affect	Parent not purchasing high-fat foods so they are not available in the environment for consumption.
Child behavior → Child environment → child behavior, skills, cognition, affect	Child pre-preparing carrot sticks so they will be avilable in the refrigerator for future consumption.

The child's environment can shape the child's behavior by easily yielding to or resisting the child's attempts to secure certain foods and providing rewards or punishments for the child's behaviors. The child, in turn, can affect the parent's food environment by asking to go to certain fast food restaurants, hiding undesired foods in the home, or asking that certain foods be, or not be, bought (Nader et al., 1982). The child can also affect the parent's behavior, skills, cognition, and affect through providing information, rewards (e.g., saying nice things, cooperative behaviors), and punishments (e.g., resistance or uncooperative behaviors) (e.g., Knight & Grantham-McGregor, 1985).

The family environment also shapes the parents' behavior, skills, cognition, and affect by providing the resources to facilitate the purchase, preparation, or consumption of selected foods (e.g., level of income, proximity to stores providing desired foods), easily yielding to or resisting the parents' attempts to secure, prepare, or consume the selected foods (barriers), or providing social supports for change. The parents can obviously manipulate their own environment to affect their behavior (e.g., by not purchasing certain kinds of food so they cannot be consumed), as can the children (e.g., by asking to go to restaurants that serve foods they prefer).

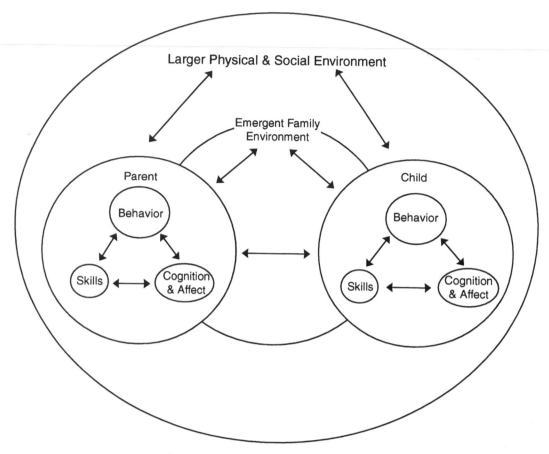

Figure 1. Family reciprocal determinism.

Emergent Characteristics of the Family

While the family reciprocal determinism model provides important conceptual tools for analyzing family factors in regard to health behaviors in general, and diet in particular, the study of the family poses a number of problems as well. First, it is hard to identify what constitutes a family. Baranowski, Dworkin, Dunn, Nader, and Brown (1986) identified nine generic combinations of people across three generations to characterize those who were included in only 113 groups of people who called themselves families.

Furthermore, the most common structures varied by ethnic group. Also, the reciprocal nature of many of the relationships is hard to delineate, even in longitudinal research.

The concept of family suggests that the family is something more than the sum of its parts, i.e., that it demonstrates emergent characteristics. Investigators have studied many emergent characteristics of families, e.g., family cohesion (Moos, 1974), family adaptation (D. H. Olson et al., 1983), and family support (Sallis et al., 1987). Because the family can act as a unit, family members can compensate for the strengths or weaknesses of other family members in response to events. For example, one family member may have the skills or resources to purchase or prepare certain foods that the family member desiring the food may not have. When external events are overwhelming, e.g., loss of a job, the whole family may suffer financially or emotionally, even though individual members may have sufficient individual resources to cope with the problem. Within a broad social structure, families have important responsibilities including obtaining resources and spending them wisely for self-maintenance and safety, attention to raising children who are physically, cognitively, and emotionally healthy, and cognitive and emotional support for enhancing each member's development. Furthermore, family units vary in levels of expressed affection (overt and covert), priorities or values, child-rearing skills, and numerous characteristics. These diverse characteristics emerge from the way people think of a family, their role in the family, and how they act together as a unit.

These emergent characteristics reflect in part the pattern of the many behaviors in which the family members engage with one another and in part the concepts that each member uses to characterize and understand the family unit. People's behaviors reflect their concepts of their family. Some family members at times may create idealized notions of the family and strive toward those ideals, while some respond to their perceptions of what others are willing or not willing to do in the family. Within the social cognitive model, when an individual identifies a situation as involving family-related phenomena, then family-related concepts, e.g., family outcome expectations, are activated for use. The relationships between emergent family characteristics and social cognitive variables need to be delineated.

The family unit, as well as each of the actors, acts within a broader social environment. An attempt was made in Figure 1 to depict this situation by characterizing the emergent family environment and the larger social environment as a pair of concentric circles. Within the domain of diet and family, it is not clear what the most important emergent characteristics of the family are, how the family behaviors and other factors lead to these set of emergent characteristics, or how the emergent characteristics enhance or constrain dietary behavior. Nor is it clear to what extent emergent family characteristics are genetically determined (Plomin, Reiss, Hetherington, & Howe, 1994). Despite these inadequacies in available knowledge, this chapter assumes that diet is related to chronic disease and health promotion and emphasizes family-related determinants of consumption.

Chapter 16 in Volume IV of this *Handbook* reviews the literature on the relevance of health behavior knowledge to health promotion programs focused on families.

FAMILY INFLUENCES ON DIET AND NUTRITION

Genetics of Family Influences

While there has developed an appreciable understanding of genetic influences on health (Slyper & Schechtman, 1994) and some understanding of genetic influences on health-related behaviors (Rose, 1995), family influences on health behaviors have usually been considered volitional and changeable on the part of family members. Behavioral genetic research, however, has revealed genetic components to some family influences. Model-fitting analyses demonstrated that 30% of the variance in the perceived adequacy of social support was genetically determined (Bergeman, Plomin, Pedersen, McClearn, & Nesselroade, 1990). Some 18–53% of the variance in parental behavior toward children could be accounted for by genetic factors (D. Pérusse, Neale, Heath, & Eaves, 1994; Plomin et al., 1994). While all the details and mechanisms of genetic influence need to be clarified, these analyses indicate that genetic factors account for a potion of family interactions. In part, these findings mean that social behavior is less volitional than previously thought and may mean that some of these parent-child behaviors are particularly resistant to change. Mechanisms of genetic influence must be delineated, a process that may temper consideration of how to use the accumulating data to improve the human condition.

Familial Concordance for Diet

The degree to which family members consume the same kinds of foods or not is called *familial concordance for diet*. High levels of concordance would indicate that families should be considered the appropriate units for analysis and intervention, since an attempt to change diet in one family member may require changes in all family members. Low levels of concordance, revealing individual freedom in selection and preparation of foods, would indicate that individuals should be the unit of analysis and intervention. Kolonel and Lee (1981) reported modest to moderate intraclass correlations between spouses for the frequency of consumption of foods, ranging from 0.33 for beef to 0.55 for pork and for rice. This result indicates that spouses influence each other's consumption, but they do not eat identically.

Concordance in the dietary habits of parents and children is ordinarily assessed by a Pearson correlation coefficient across pairs of people focusing on one nutrient or food group. Table 2 presents representative correlations in regard to total calorie consumption for four pairings of family members in four published studies. The

values are low to moderate. Caution must be used in interpreting this table, since the values come from different studies reflecting different approaches to dietary assessment, different samples (ethnicity, age, region of country, socioeconomic status), and different analyses. Despite these caveats, there is remarkable congruence across rows in the table.

Since mothers often play a more nurturing role in the family, exert greater control over foods coming into the home and over preparation, and are more likely to be present during meals, one might expect greater concordance between mothers' and children's consumption. Similarly, one might surmise that since older children assert more independence from the family, including eating away from home, parent-child concordance would be higher for younger than for older children. In a study comparing total calorie consumption by African-American and white families in Cincinnati, Laskarzewski et al. (1980) demonstrated a significant relationship between mothers and their children, but not between fathers and their children, and substantially higher values for African-American parents and their children than for white families. In a study among white families in Framingham, Oliveria et al. (1992) reported substantially higher correlations for mother-child than for father-child pairs, for most nutrients, for both daughters and sons. In a study comparing Californian Anglo- and Mexican-American families, Patterson, Rupp, Sallis, Atkins, and Nader (1988) demonstrated

Table 2. Concordance in Consumption of Total Calories for Four Pairings of Family Members in Four Studies

| Family pairs | Patterson et al. (1988) | | Laskarzewski et al. (1980) Mixed | Oliveria et al. (1992) Euro-American | Pérusse et al. (1994) Canadian |
	Euro-American	Mexican-American			
Father-mother	0.44	0.28	—	0.39	0.37
Father-child	0.05	−0.19	—	0.16	—
Mother-child	0.35	0.21	0.25	0.17	0.25
Sibling-sibling	0.48	0.38	—	—	0.23

consistently higher concordance between white parents (father or mother) and their younger children than between parents and their older children, and higher concordance between Mexican-American parents (father or mother) and their older children than between parents and their younger children. Mexican-American mothers tended to have higher concordance than Mexican-American fathers for younger and older children. Ethnic group differences in the extent to which families shared meals might account for the differences in correlations. These authors reported that Mexican-American families were much more likely to eat breakfast and lunch with their children, while Anglo-American families were more likely to eat dinner with their children. The patterns were comparable by gender, except that Mexican-American mothers were most likely to eat breakfast with their children. Patterns of snacking were not reported.

In a longitudinal study with young children of both African- and Euro-American heritage in Augusta, Georgia, Lipis (1992) reported higher correlations across a variety of foods for mothers and children than for fathers and children, higher mother–daughter than mother–son correlations, more food items increasing in concordance over time for mother–daughter pairs, and more food items decreasing in concordance over time for mother–son pairs. No ethnic differences were reported.

It is possible that some of the parent–child concordance in food consumption could be accounted for by a genetic predisposition to consume or prefer certain foods (e.g., genetically determined preference for sweetness). While mothers and fathers generally liked the same foods, no such preference concordance was obtained with their college-age children; mothers and fathers tended to rank similarly the importance of good cooking, preference for exotic foods, and culinary knowledge, but parent–child pairs obtained concordance only on the rank of cooking; there was no concordance in spousal or parent–child pairs as to the importance of eating (Rozin, Fallon, & Mandell, 1984). Shared levels of

disgust for certain foods were highest for mother–father pairs, but similar relationships were obtained in parent–child pairs (Rozin et al., 1984). In a design comparing biological and nonbiological parent–child pairs, L. Pérusse et al. (1988) demonstrated no genetic influence on total energy consumption, but 50% of the variance was accounted for by home environment effects. Alternatively, in a study comparing mono- and dizygotic twins, Falciglia and Norton (1994) found evidence for genetic effects in preferences for a limited number of foods, but presented no data on consumption. The authors hypothesized that the genetic effect was mediated by a known genetically determined sensitivity to bitterness in food (Krondl, Coleman, Wade, & Miller, 1983). Birch (1980) demonstrated that correlations between children and randomly selected other adults in their community in ratings of preference for selected foods were almost as high as the correlations between children and their parents, suggesting that preferences for foods are shared socially in homogeneous communities. In a large study of biological and nonbiologically related families of children aged 4–11 years, Hartz, Giefer, and Rimm (1977) estimated that about 11% of the variability in obesity was related to genetic factors and between 32% and 39% was due to family environment factors.

One may conclude from these analyses that there is evidence for familial concordance in dietary preferences and consumption. The concordance is in general relatively low, and it varies by the nutrients or foods analyzed and by family role (mother, father), ethnicity, and age of the children. Portions of this concordance may be accounted for by genetic predispositions, cultural patterns in preference and consumption, common availability of food in the home, and shared meals. None of these studies assessed the role of socioeconomic status. It is likely that in homes with higher income levels, the family can afford to stock different kinds of the same category of foods (thereby catering to the preferences of individual family members) and can permit more individual freedom in whether, how often, and where families can dine out (which permits different family selections). These shared and non-shared environments can have substantial impacts on concordance. Further research will elucidate the proportion of concordance accounted for by these various influences.

Families do not overwhelmingly determine the diet behaviors of their members, but there is sufficient evidence for behavior change programs to consider the influences of family members. Lack of concordance would not necessarily indicate that families have no influence on children's diets. Families may have different standards for what should be eaten by parents and by children, or parents may influence part of the children's diet (e.g., dinners at home), for which the children may compensate in other parts of their diet (e.g., lunches at school, snacks in the company of friends).

FOOD PURCHASE AND AVAILABILITY

The obvious fact that children cannot eat foods that are not available for consumption, either at home or elsewhere, prompts recognition that eating at home entails a chain of events that begins with the availability of food in a neighborhood, progresses through selection of a grocery store, selection of food in the store, purchase of food in the store, availability in the home, pre-preparation of the item at home (if necessary), preparation of the dish, and distribution in the family, and ends with selection and consumption at the table (Campbell & Desjardins, 1989). Similarly, eating away from home involves selection of a family or fast food restaurant, selection from the menu, ordering of the items, preparation of the items (usually by the cook), and consumption. Since the child has more options when eating out (e.g., can select the restaurant, the food, the method of preparation), the child probably has more influence and independence at those eating events. A growing body of research has been conducted on family influences at each step in the chain of food availability.

Availability in a Neighborhood

Sallis, Nader, Rupp, Atkins, and Wilson (1986) surveyed neighborhoods around elementary schools and demonstrated that some neighborhoods had no food stores and some neighborhoods had many. The availability of health-related foods (low-fat and low-sodium) varied substantially, with supermarkets offering 78% of items on a prespecified list of such foods and neighborhood groceries, convenience stores, and health food stores offering 35%, 16%, and 29% of the items, respectively. Heart-healthy foods were most likely to be available in middle-class neighborhoods. Thus, heart-healthy foods were not generally available, but were more widely available in larger stores and in middle-class neighborhoods.

Local food availability is often beyond a family's control and may induce changes in the family's use of food. McDonald, Sigman, Espinosa, and Neimann (1994) assessed the effects of a temporary food shortage in Kenya. During the food shortage, parents decreased their own food consumption and that of their school-aged children, but not of the toddlers, resulting in a weight-for-age decline for the schoolchildren and parents, but not for the toddlers. The food shortage appeared to exacerbate a natural decline in the caring and holding behaviors of the mothers for the toddlers, but had no effect on the mothers' talking to toddlers or responding to toddler's vocalization behaviors. Thus, changes in availability have consequences for families' health, management of consumption, and interpersonal interactions.

Store Selection

Since there is differential availability of health-related foods (Sallis et al., 1986), factors that affect store selection can have implications for the healthfulness of the foods purchased and consumed. In 1987 (Food Marketing Institute, 1987), 55% of households reported that they visited only one supermarket each week; 37%, two different supermarkets each week; 8%, three supermarkets; and 2%, four or more. These data reveal habitual use of a single supermarket by a majority of households. In this study, 29% of households reported making one visit per week to the supermarket; 32%, two visits; 21%, three visits; 8%, four visits; 3%, five visits; 4%, six or more visits; and 1%, one visit every 2 weeks. Thus, although households tend to shop at one store, they tend to make multiple visits to that store during the course of a week. Given the Sallis et al. (1986) results, this pattern of store selection bodes well for the availability of heart-healthy foods.

When purchasing take-out meals to be eaten at home, 43% of households reported selecting a fast food restaurant, 38% the carryout section of a restaurant, 10% the carryout section of a supermarket, and 2% some other place. A much higher percentage of larger households reported selecting a fast food restaurant, while a higher percentage of smaller households reported the carryout section of a supermarket or some other place (Food Marketing Institute, 1987). This pattern does not bode well for the availability of heart-healthy foods when families buy meals for consumption at home. Brinberg and Durand (1983) reported negative influences from parents and peers in children's selecting fast food restaurants, with parents being more influential than peers. Nutrition education programs can point out how families can maximize their selection of more healthful items at supermarkets and fast food restaurants and which of these establishments are more likely to offer a more healthful menu.

Food Selection in the Store

Selection of foods in the store is the primary determinant of availability at home. Married couples vary by stages in the family life cycle (Schafer & Keith, 1981) from young married couples with one child all the way to married senior couples with no children remaining at home. While the spouses' preferences were always most important and the children's preferences second most important in selection of food, the importance of others (parents, relatives, friends, and neighbors) declined as stages advanced (Schafer & Keith, 1981).

Working women assumed at least five different perspectives when making food choices for their families with young children (Kirk & Gillespie, 1990), including: nutritionist, manager/organizer of time and people, family economist, meaning creator (to enhance meaningful family interactions at mealtimes), and family diplomat (to forestall undesirable forms of family interaction). Working mothers experienced guilt in their attempts to fulfill their own expectations in regard to those perspectives. The influences of these perspectives or guilt on selection in the store were not explored.

The more people in a family, the greater need there is for nurturance from parents, with correspondingly less time for other activities. In the Food Marketing Institute (1987) study, 39% of households reported that it is very important and 41% that it is somewhat important to save time while shopping in the supermarket. The percentages in these importance categories tended to increase as the number of family members increased and were greater for families with children versus those with no children. In 1987, 54% of households reported being very concerned about the nutritional content of foods purchased and 31% were very concerned about the nutritional content of foods when eating out (Food Marketing Institute, 1987). There was virtually no difference between households with and without children on either variable. Shoppers ranked cost, nutrition, quality, and convenience as the most important factors affecting selection, in that order (Fox, Linsenmeyer, & Kohn, 1984). Shoppers who ranked nutrition high spent *less* money on food than persons with other priorities. Contrary to standard theory, wherein purchasers are seen as selecting items for which they have a predisposition, the purchaser is in constant interaction with the environment, responding to the many environmental cues (Phillips & Bradshaw, 1993). Thus, many families are interested in the nutritional quality of their food, even when they are concerned about cost. Families can be influenced in the store in their purchases, but require simple, credible, straightforward messages, since they do not want to leisurely consider detailed dietary information on food labels.

Children can influence food selections, and their influence appears to be increasing. In the 1960s, up to a third of children were reported to influence the selection of breakfast foods and snack foods, but much lower percentages were reported for selecting noon and evening meal foods (Eppright, Fox, Fryer, Lamkin, & Vivian, 1969). In this study, 58% of mothers reported considering a child's preferences in selecting and preparing foods. In the 1990s, 74% of 4th- to 8th-grade children reported influencing what they ate for snacks; 65%, what they ate for breakfast; 46%, lunch; and 8%, dinner (International Food Information Council, 1992). Sommer, Wynes, & Brinkley (1992) demonstrated that shoppers in groups (often with children) purchased more than shoppers alone. Children were twice as likely as parents to initiate a purchase of breakfast cereal in the store and parents were more likely to agree to a child's requests or demands (Atkin, 1978). There was substantial variability in the frequency of children's requests for differing food items, with high frequency for foods most frequently desired by children (snacks, candy, breakfast cereal) (Ward & Wackman, 1972). While the frequency of requests did not generally increase with age of the child, there was a tendency for the mothers to yield to influence attempts as the age of the child increased (Ward & Wackman, 1972). Teenage children were most influential in the initiation stage of the consideration of purchase of a breakfast cereal, but were second to the mother in the search, evaluation, and final decision stages (Belch, Belch, & Ceresino, 1985). Teenagers reported greater influence on minor grocery trips (i.e., shopping for a few items), in single-parent families, and for female teenagers (Talpade, Beatty, & Trilokekar-Talpade, 1993).

Teenagers' preceptions of their influence were higher than their parents' perceptions.

From in-store observations, most parents appeared to enjoy shopping with their children. Younger children (5 years of age or younger) tended to ride in the cart, point at foods, become physically involved with the product (through touch), and want to learn the names of many objects, and were more likely to have their food choices rejected by the parent. Older children (6 years old or older) tended to be team players with the parent in the shopping process, reading marketing stimuli in the store and showing signs of preplanning at home (e.g., in use of shopping lists, coupons) (Rust, 1993). On food shopping trips, however, children accompanied mothers only 15% of the time and fathers only 8% of the time (Polegato, 1994).

Nutrition education programs with children can capitalize on their influence in the food selection process. If children can be trained to ask for more healthful foods (Baranowski et al., 1993), then more would be purchased for consumption. This "asking behavior" could include simple requests for breakfasts and snacks, plus putting items on a shopping list, going shopping for more healthful foods and helping select them, asking to go to fast food restaurants that offer more healthful foods, and selecting more healthful foods off the fast food menus (Baranowski et al., 1993).

Purchase

Marketing data (Food Marketing Institute, 1987) revealed that the weekly grocery expenditures per person in the household declined as the number of people in the house increased. Similarly, families with children spent less per person than families without children. (There are many potential explanations for this finding, including the possibility that in older, more financially established families, children had already left the home.) Lower-income families were concerned about their expenditure of funds in general, and some mothers tightly controlled the amount spent on food (Campbell & Desjardins, 1989). Mothers concerned about cost more tightly controlled their food finances than carefully planned their food selections. Many of the mothers were not aware of what they spent on food. In a small group of lower-income families, men retained tight control of finances including food, which limited the women's ability to influence what was bought and consumed (Wilson, 1988). More than half of all children got a formal allowance, and 36% of that money went for food, snacks, and beverages ("Kids' allowances," 1993, Nov. 28). Nutrition education programs must point to less expensive, but just as tasty, ways of selecting nutritious meals.

Availability in the Home

The primary determinant of whether children ate a food was whether the parent served it (Michela & Contento, 1986). Snacks at home, where one would expect more healthful snacks to be available, were more likely to be nutritious than those eaten elsewhere (Gillespie, 1983). Undernourished inner city children were less likely than well-nourished children of comparable socioeconomic status to have available "basic" foods that required preparation by an adult at home and more likely to have foods that were of low nutritional value (Karp et al., 1984). Thus, even though lower-income families had less money available for foods, they selected foods with lower nutritional value.

Elementary students' consumption of fruits and vegetables was low in part because the parents did not keep these foods at home (Baranowski et al., 1993). Some of the parents reported that they did not like fruits and vegetables themselves, and so would not serve them to their children. The availability of fruits and vegetables in the home was a function of socioeconomic status, with middle- and upper-class families having ample fruits and vegetables at home (Kirby, Baranowski, Reynolds, Bishop, & Binkley, 1995). Lower-class families were concerned about the perishability of fresh fruits and vegetables and about spending money on foods that were not consumed. In a structured telephone interview, however, Hearn, Baranowski, and Baranowski, (1997) demonstrated no difference in availability of fruits and vegetables by socioeconomic status.

Pre-preparation and Accessibility

If a parent wants a child to eat a specific food for a snack, e.g., raw carrot sticks, pre-preparation may be necessary, i.e., cleaning and cutting the carrots, putting them in a glass of water to keep them moist, and setting the glass in the refrigerator within easy sight and reach. Pre-preparation of the snack food thus makes it easily accessible to the child. Kirby et al. (1995) reported that upper-middle-class families were likely to do this, but not lower-class families. Due to the latchkey phenomenon, children reported becoming increasingly responsible for the preparation of all their meals and snacks (International Food Information Council, 1992). No families reported pre-preparing vegetables so children could use them to make a dish when they were responsible for making their own meals (Kirby et al., 1995).

Preparation

The manner of food preparation (e.g., addition of fat and sodium) has implications for health. Convenience foods tend to be high in fat and sodium. Wives working outside the home felt less responsibility than housewives for serving nutritious meals to their family and were less interested in garnering praise from the family for cooking (R. W. Jackson et al., 1985). Mothers of undernourished inner city children were less likely to regularly prepare meals at home (Karp et al., 1984). In one study, 83% of children reported making their own snacks, 80% their own breakfast, 73% their own lunch, and 38% their own dinner (International Food Information Council, 1992). Recipes and other suggestions for improving the nutritional qualities of food must be kept very simple and safe and consume little time, both for the benefit of busy parents and for the training of their children. More attention needs to be given to training children to prepare more healthful snacks and meals when they become responsible for food preparation.

Food Distribution in the Home

In the United States, the prevalent image is that food is available in the home for general family consumption somehow in proportion to each family member's needs or wants. Food is generally plentiful in the United States, requiring little or no rationing. Research in less developed countries, which more commonly experience poverty and hunger, has revealed that food may be distributed to family members on the basis of other considerations. One study revealed two polar opposite rules for intrafamily distribution of food: (1) the "contribution" rule: Give more food to those members of the family who make the biggest contribution, e.g., working husbands; and (2) the "needs" rule: Give more food to those family members who need it most (as based on visual indicators of growth and starvation) (Engle & Nieves, 1993a,b). In this study, 35% of respondents endorsed an equal distribution of food, 29% endorsed more food to the parents, 16% endorsed more food to the husband than to the wife, and 20% endorsed giving more to the children. Such distribution rules can induce starvation in some circumstances (Haaga & Mason, 1987) and can wreak havoc with charitable organizations' food distribution programs that target specific members of a family. For example, children targeted for food supplementation were receiving no more food than their siblings or controls (Engle & Nieves, 1993b).

Haaga and Mason (1987) reviewed the literature that indicated that maldistribution of food in the family had consequences for the growth and health of young children. Maldistribution also has been reported in regard to females, adolescents, and senior citizens. Investigators in the United States may seek evidence for such patterns in lower-income or recent immigrant populations, in which food may be scarce and rationing of some nature may be necessary or habitual. Evidence for distributional rules may also be sought in families with children experiencing failure to thrive. The effects of emergent family characteristics or outcome expectations on these distribution rules provide an important issue for investigation.

Consumption

Dinner meals are highly patterned rituals, with families engaging in similar behaviors from day to day (Dreyer & Dreyer, 1973). In one study, 53% of households reported always eating dinner together as a family (Food Marketing Institute, 1987), 48% reported always eating the main course together, and 20% reported usually eating the main course together. As the size of the household increased, there were small increases in the percentages that always or usually ate together, up to a household size of four, after which the percentages declined, perhaps revealing the difficulties in arranging so many different schedules. In another study, 54% of 4th- to 8th-grade children reported eating meals with their family every day, and an additional 35% reported doing so 3–5 times per week (International Food Information Council, 1992). Family interaction patterns during meals are discussed in the section that follows.

This review clearly indicates that there are many steps between availability of foods in a neighborhood and consumption in the household or restaurant. The factors that influence these steps appear to vary, providing many opportunities for intervention, but also providing many links in a chain that need to be considered when proposing change. For example, simply increasing vegetable purchases in the store may not result in increased consumption, if the vegetables are not prepared to suit the preferences of the family members. More systematic research using social cognitive theory should elucidate the influences at each step in regard to consumption of healthier foods.

DEVELOPMENTAL PHASES

The issues concerning what people should be eating and the influences on their consumption vary by developmental stage from infancy to older ages.

Infancy (First Year of Life)

Many factors influence growth in the first year of life; prominent among them is infant diet. The primary feeding issue facing a family of an infant is whether and how long to breast-feed. Breast-feeding provides nutrients uniquely formulated for the human infant (Heinig, Nommsen, Peerson, Lonnerdahl, & Dewey, 1993) and has been encouraged as the sole form of feeding for the first 6 months of life (American Dietetic Association, 1986; Nutrition Committee, 1978). The *Healthy People 2000: National Health Promotion and Disease Prevention Objectives* (U.S. Department of Health and Human Services, 1991) set this national objective (No. 2.11): "Increase to at least 75 percent the proportion of mothers who breastfeed their babies in the early postpartum period and to at least 50 percent the proportion who continue breastfeeding until their babies are 5 to 6 months old" (p. 123). In 1988, the Department estimated that 54% were breast-feeding at discharge and 21% at 5–6 months.

In a lower-income triethnic sample, ethnicity was the primary predictor of who initiated breast-feeding, with African-American mothers least likely to breast-feed (9.2%), Euro-American mothers most likely (43.5%), and Mexican-American mothers in between (22.6%) (Rassin et al., 1984). Similar percentages were obtained in a later study (Bee, Baranowski, Rassin, Richardson, & Mikrut, 1991), and greater likelihood of breast-feeding was associated with increasing socioeconomic status among Euro-Americans, but with decreasing socioeconomic status among African-Americans. A variety of explanations for the ethnic group differences have been proposed (Rassin, Richardson, & Baranowski, 1986). Baranowski et al. (1983) demonstrated that the levels of social support for breast-feeding from several of the mother's social role partners (i.e., male partner, mother, grandmother, best friend, children) were highly associated with breast-feeding among Euro-American mothers, but not among African-American or Mexican-American mothers. The primary source of support varied by ethnic group, with husbands being most important among Euro-Americans, mothers among Mexican-Americans, and best friends among African-Americans (Baranowski et al., 1983).

Outcome expectations have also been related to breast-feeding (Baranowski, Rassin, Richardson, Bee, & Brown, 1986; Baranowski, Rassin, et al., 1990). Personal inconveniences, benefits for the infant, and physical inconveniences were the most important outcome expectation predictors of breast-feeding among Euro-Americans, in that order; personal inconveniences were a weaker influence among African-Americans and Mexican-Americans (Baranowski, Rassin, et al., 1986). A later study revealed that the benefits of breast-feeding for the mother were the primary predictor of breast-feeding (Baranowski, Rassin, et al., 1990). The perceived benefits for the mother were equally high among Mexican-American and Euro-American mothers and were significantly higher than among African-Americans.

In a study of mothers along the United States border with Mexico (Rassin et al., 1993, 1994), an ethnicity-related variable, acculturation to American society, was the major predictor of breast-feeding. Mothers who showed high acculturation levels, however, were the least likely to breast-feed (Rassin et al., 1993), suggesting that Mexican-American mothers were acculturating to a lower socioeconomic status norm to the detriment of their children. Acculturation was a predictor of the selection of breast-feeding at 3 months prior to delivery, right after delivery, and within 3 weeks after delivery, with more acculturated mothers less likely to select breast-feeding at all times (Rassin et al., 1994).

In another study, ethnicity was a major determinant of the initiation of breast-feeding, but no demographic characteristics predicted duration of breast-feeding (Brodwick, Baranowski, & Rassin, 1989). Only 15% of participants in this sample breast-fed for at least 4 months and started solids only at 4 months or later. Commercially available cereals and fruit juices were the most common nonmilk foods that were introduced early. Depression, lower socioeconomic status, younger age, and lower educational attainment were the primary personal predictors of termination of breast-feeding (Cooper, Murray, & Stein, 1993). Health sector practices (e.g., health professionals suggesting introducing formula) and food industry factors (e.g., receiving a free sample of formula) also were primary negative determinants of the duration of breast-feeding (Adair, Popkin, & Guilkey, 1993).

While the primary value of breast-feeding may be that it provides the infant with nutrients in a form or combination most likely to meet human needs for growth (Heinig et al., 1993), there are nurturant or mental health benefits for the child and mother as well. Using observational methods, Ainsworth and Bell (1969) elucidated nine different patterns in how mothers breast-fed their infants, including as variables the timing of feedings, the amount of milk ingested, the mother's handling of child preferences for solids, and the mother's pacing of the rate of intake. Their analyses revealed that these categories of infant-feeding practices were systematically related to the amount of infant crying during infancy, the relationship of the mother to the child, and the child's exploratory behavior in a strange situation at 12 months of age. In general, mothers who were more responsive to the baby's rhythms, signals, pacings, and preferences had children who cried less and demonstrated more exploratory behavior. These mothers had a better relationship with their child. Characteristics of mother's and infant's feeding behavior predicted growth in the first month of life (Pollitt, Gilmore, & Valcarel, 1978; Pollitt & Wirtz, 1981). Babies who were small for gestational age were more likely to exhibit negative interaction patterns during feeding, which then predisposed them to growth failure (Mullen, Coll, Vohr, Muriel, & Oh, 1988). Children whose mothers were not responsive to

their patterns were more likely to have lower achievement and lower emotional health in both the 1st and 2nd grades (Egeland, Pianta, & O'Brien, 1993). Some authors have suggested that breast-feeding promotes the "bonding" of mothers to infants, but more recent literature (Eyer, 1994) disputes the validity of this finding.

Implications for Intervention. What infants eat and how mothers present it can have a substantial impact on the future physical, cognitive, and emotional growth and health of children, even into their adult years. Since the United States is well below the levels proposed in the national objectives, efforts to encourage breast-feeding are important among all mothers, and particular encouragement must be given to African-American and acculturated Mexican-American mothers. Enhancing social support for breast-feeding and emphasizing the perceived beneficial effects for mothers and their children seem to be promising procedures to increase the numbers of mothers initiating breast-feeding. The food industry and medical disincentives for breast-feeding need to be stopped. Mothers starting to breast-feed need to be encouraged, or even trained, to be responsive to the patterns and preferences of their children.

Further Research. Much needs to be learned about the details of social support for breast-feeding: What procedures under what circumstances are perceived as being most supportive? How can one encourage such support? From whom would mothers be most receptive to support? The characteristics of mothers' infant-feeding practices and their relationships to later physical, mental, and emotional growth need to be firmly established.

Toddlers (1–2 Years of Age)

Children are more likely to eat foods they prefer (Birch, 1980; Domel, Baranowski, Davis, Leonard, et al., 1993). Some have asserted that there is a critical period wherein preferences for foods are developed in the first 2 years of life

(Breckenridge & Murphy, 1969). Toddlers were more likely to ask to eat an unfamiliar food than were 4-year-olds, more likely to eat an unfamiliar food offered by an unfamiliar adult, and even more likely to eat one offered by a parent (Harper & Sanders, 1975). A social effect on acceptance of an unfamiliar food was detected at both ages, but less so among the older children. Thus, the toddler years may be a critical period for encouraging preferences for more healthful foods.

In this age period, children develop the skills for volitional behavior, including establishing a goal, paying attention to standards, self-monitoring those activities, and stopping upon completion of a task or attainment of a goal (Bullock & Lutkenhaus, 1988). Thus, there is a transition from heavy dependence on parents to independent action. There has been some concern that obesity may begin at the earliest ages (Birch & Johnson, 1994), and self-control over food consumption is an issue in the onset of obesity (Costanzo & Woody, 1985).

Further Research. Verifying whether a critical period exists in the toddler years for establishing food preferences and, if it does, determining the limits of this period (in terms of time and types of foods) are important research issues. If verified, programs should be established and evaluated to encourage parents of toddlers to establish children's preferences for more healthful foods. A major issue in the evaluation would be whether children who learn to like more foods also become obese. The processes in the development of self-control over food consumption and how families influence toddler dietary practices in this age need to be addressed.

Preschoolers (3–5 Years of Age)

All children need to consume sufficient calories and other nutrients to ensure their optimal growth and health. Since clinical malnutrition and abnormally slow growth are not common problems in the United States, the focus on children's diet is shifting away from a concern for growth. Cardiovascular disease (CVD) has been

detected among children (Velican & Velican, 1980), CVD risk factors track among children (Burke et al., 1987) and into the adult years (Mahoney, Lauer, Lee, & Clarke, 1991), and diet tracks among children (Stein, Shea, Basch, Contento, & Zybert, 1991) and into the adult years (Kelder, Perry, Klepp, & Lytle, 1994). As a result, there is an interest in arresting CVD processes, disrupting the tracking of CVD risk factors, and establishing healthful dietary patterns and preferences among children that will protect them from CVD in their adult years (Berenson, Srinivasan, Weber, & Wattigney, 1991). Thus, this literature is moving from a focus on adequate nutrients for childhood growth to prevention of later adult chronic disease. For CVD and cancer prevention purposes, this literature often focuses on reducing dietary fat, cholesterol, and calories and increasing consumption of fruits, vegetables, and dietary fiber (Surgeon General, 1988).

Behavior. Most families in a large Midwest sample could afford to provide an adequate diet for their preschool children, but reported a number of problems (Eppright et al., 1969). The mothers reported inadequate consumption of vegetables and fruit; 24% of the children disliked vegetables by 3 years of age. The mothers were concerned that their children were not consuming a sufficient variety of foods (35.8%) and were eating too many sweets (20.7%). More than half of 3-year-olds had always or sometimes participated in a broad variety of food-related activities, with 82% reporting sometimes or always helping set the table, 79% involved in making baked goods, and 72% serving themselves from a container (Anliker, Laus, Samonds, & Beal, 1992). Thus, even preschoolers were frequently involved in many aspects of food selection, preparation, and service, but consumed inadequate amounts of fruits and vegetables.

Environment. Family income is an important characteristic of the home environment, affecting the quantity and quality of various foods available in the home. Families eligible for the Women's, Infants', and Children's (WIC) program had higher percentages of children with low consumption of energy, vitamin C, and iron (three of the five targeted nutrients) (J. E. Brown & Tiernan, 1986). WIC supplementation reduced the percentage of children with low iron intake.

Television is a major component of a family's environment. The Nielsen report (A. C. Nielsen Co., 1989) estimated that 2- to 5-year-olds spent an average of 27 hours and 49 minutes watching TV per week. Robertson (1979) reported complex patterns of association between exposure to TV and requests for advertised products by children. Clancy-Hepburn (1974) documented that mothers who were well informed about nutrition had children who made fewer requests for advertised foods and who consumed less of them. Several studies (Dietz & Gortmaker, 1985; Gortmaker, Dietz, & Cheung, 1990; Locard et al., 1992), but not all (Robinson et al., 1993), supported the hypothesis that children who watch more TV are more likely to be obese. While parents can to some extent control access to TV, more than a third of families set no limits (Bernard-Bonnin, Gilbert, Rousseau, Masson, & Maheux, 1991), and 22% reported using TV as a "safe distraction," which substantially increased the children's viewing time (Taras, Sallis, Nader, & Nelson, 1990). TV could affect adiposity through four paths (Dietz & Strasburger, 1991): what and how much children eat while watching TV (Taras, Sallis, Patterson, Nader, & Nelson, 1989), what and how much children eat at other times as influenced by TV commercials and programming (Taras et al., 1989), taking the place of physical activity that could have been engaged in during the time TV was being watched (DuRant, Baranowski, Johnson, & Thompson, 1994, 1995), and reductions in resting metabolic rates during TV watching (Klesges, Shelton & Klesges, 1993).

Low family income has been associated with many health problems, and inadequate diet appears to be one of the mediating variables. There is a need to determine whether low-income families purchase foods low in nutrition because of low nutritional or food knowledge or low cost (lower-cost foods are sometimes less nutritious) or because they are maximizing outcome expectations (e.g., taste) in their lives. While TV has in many ways enhanced the quality of many lives, it also appears to enhance certain conditions that predispose to chronic disease, especially lower physical activity and poorer diet. The role of TV in diet needs more attention in terms of its direct effects (e.g., through advertising) and indirect effects (e.g., through displacement of other activities) on diet and adiposity, how these effects vary by types of families, and how knowledge of the effects might be used to reach parents and children together to improve diet.

Family Characteristics. How families interact with preschool children in regard to food can affect the children's food-related knowledge, preferences, and consumption. Fathers were not involved with children in food selection or preparation, but the husband's preferences were the most common determinant of the mother's selection and preparation of foods (Eppright et al., 1969). Foods were often used for nonnutritional purposes: rewards for good behavior (23%), food deprivation as a punishment (10%), and food provision as a pacifier (29%). Sweets were the most commonly used foods for rewards and punishments. Also in this study, 75% of mothers reported child reluctance to eat at mealtimes (Eppright et al., 1969); mothers' responses included: ignore (46%), punish or deny (18%), force or demand (16%), reason or coax (15%), substitute a liked food (4%), and threaten or bribe (1%). Birch, Marlin, and Rotter, (1984) demonstrated that using rewards (physical or social) decreased the preference for the targeted foods.

Parents who spoke to their preschool children about nutrition, and spoke in more specific detail about nutrition, had children with greater nutrition knowledge (Anliker, Laus, Samonds, & Beal, 1990). Among obese Mexican-American mothers of 4- to 8-year-old children (Olvera-Ezzell, Power, & Cousins, 1990), mother's education was positively correlated with the amount of healthy foods served, use of reasoning to encourage consumption, prohibitions concerning unhealthy foods, inquiring what the child eats away from home, and preparing what the child likes, and negatively correlated with the frequency of serving foods at the table. In the Anliker et al. (1992) study, 3-year-old children with greater control over the selections of foods and the amounts of food served were more aware of the role of foods in the energy balance equation. Highly permissive families were least likely to allow 3-year-old children control over the selection of foods (Anliker et al., 1992). Mothers who selected foods for their preschool children to consume based on considerations of health (rather than taste or other considerations) had more nutrition knowledge and had children who ate more healthful diets (fewer calories, lower fat, and more vitamin A).

M. Lewis and Feiring (1982) reported an observational study of interactions during a family meal among families with 3-year-old children. Information seeking was the most common function performed during a meal. Requests for information were most common from parents to children and declined dramatically as the size of the family increased. The frequency of father's caregiving increased, however, as family size increased. The authors concluded that the mother's primary role during the meal was to maintain contact among the family as a unit concerning activities at other times. In a similar study, Beals (1993) reported that mothers made more utterances (42.9%) than children (32.2%) or fathers (14.2%) during meals, and about 15% of these utterances involved explanations. Children who experienced more explanatory talk during meals at 3 or 4 years of age had larger vocabularies and could tell better stories at age 5.

Negative interactions also occur during meals. Heptinstall et al. (1987) reported that 4-year-olds (from a lower-class community) below the 10th percentile for height and weight were not smaller at birth and did not consume fewer calories (in fact consumed more kilocalories per kilogram body weight) than other matched children. These growth-challenged children did experience, however, a broad variety of adverse family influences during a mealtime, including more negative affect, more instructions, and more parental indifference or anxiety. Among 4- to 8-year-old children of obese Mexican-American mothers (Olvera-Ezzell et al., 1990), mother's use of threats or bribes was least likely to meet with compliance on the part of the child and most likely to result in being ignored or resisted. In a follow-up study among obese Mexican-American mothers of 4- to 8-year-old children, age of the child was inversely associated with whether a parent encouraged eating, and both external locus of control and level of acculturation were associated with the use of questions, commands, and aggravators in promoting or discouraging eating (Cousins, Power, & Olvera-Ezzell, 1993). Alternative parenting strategies for control of eating were correlated with children's knowledge of food practices (Cousins, Power, & Olvera-Ezzell, 1994). These findings were interpreted to support the internalization model of development of prosocial behavior.

The family meal involves preschoolers in a complex social event wherein the mother attempts to address a number of important family agendas, including the child's general consumption of foods, within a larger framework of family relationship maintenance issues. Families characterized by more conversation at meals and particularly more food explanations to the child, and families who minimized child selections, appeared to have children with more healthful dietary practices and better cognitive outcomes. Families characterized by indifference or negative family meal interactions had more child resistance to healthful eating and poorer growth outcomes. Given the paucity of such research, more work is needed to clarify all these relationships, especially within the larger context of general family functioning.

Elementary-School Years

Characteristics of Age. With respect to elementary-school children, there also has been a transition from concern for adequate nutrition for growth and development to concern for adult chronic disease prevention. In addition, children entering daylong kindergarten or elementary school make a dramatic break from the family's dietary practices and influences: New influences are exerted on the foods available, the methods of preparation, and what is said by peers and adults during the snacks and meals. One would expect to see dramatic shifts in what children eat and in influences on their consumption, with reciprocal effects on what is happening in the family.

Environment. The children in the family can be considered as competitors for all resources, including the available food in the household. Within this framework, only children were most likely to be obese (least competition), and those with four or more siblings had less than optimal nutritional status (Jacoby, Altman, Cook, Holland, & Elliott, 1975). Only children ate more protein, but less carbohydrate, with no difference in fat or total calories. The lack of difference in fat consumption coupled with their greater likelihood of being obese suggests that only children may engage in less physical activity. Another study, however, showed no relationship between number of children in the family and the quality of the diet (Touliatos, Lindholm, Wenberg, & Ryan, 1984). Widowed mothers were more likely to have obese children than married or divorced mothers (Jacoby et al., 1975). While income was not related (Jacoby et al., 1975; Touliatos et al., 1984), children whose mothers were employed tended to have more nutritious diets (Touliatos et al., 1984), perhaps reflecting mothers' higher education levels or revealing mothers' guilt reactions to their absence from the home. The possible competing influences of number of consumers (e.g., children), level of resources (e.g., income), and parent education on the quality of the diet must be disentangled in future research.

Family Characteristics. Among lower-income African-American mothers, 32% defined health for their elementary-school children as

including primarily nutrition (Reis, 1992). Mothers and fathers of elementary-school children reported frequently discussing diet and nutrition topics with their family (Gillespie & Achterberg, 1989), such discussion being more common for mothers and for better-educated parents. Only a small percentage of the variance in children's snack frequency or breakfast frequency was predicted by parents' corresponding beliefs and behaviors (Dielman et al., 1982). Elementary-school children's health beliefs were virtually unpredictable using parental beliefs and behaviors as predictors (Dielman et al., 1982). Mothers who felt that "eating too much" caused harm tended to have elementary-school children who believed otherwise (Reis, 1992). These relationships are not what would be predicted from the model of family reciprocal determinism.

There are limited data concerning family influences on dietary practices among elementary-school children. The inability to predict children's food beliefs from parents' food beliefs may reflect the new peer and adult influences from school. In light of the vast array of new influences on children's food environment and behavior, it would be important to learn how children interact in regard to food at snack times and mealtimes soon after the beginning of the school year, how these interactions stabilize over time, and how they in turn affect children's ensuing preferences and consumption and their food-related interactions at home. Perhaps this time of change provides an opportunity for teachers, either through what they say or how they control peer interactions, to positively influence children's dietary practices. Perhaps interventions with families can enhance positive changes and blunt negative changes that occur at this time.

Adolescence

Characteristics of Age. Adolescence is a period of personal turmoil in which children are establishing a foundation for their adulthood. Children experience puberty with its hormonal maelstrom, become increasingly responsive to peer influences, and begin the process of separating from their families. While parents and children share many values and parent–adolescent relationships are not inherently stormy, conflict increases at this age (Crockett & Petersen, 1993). Thirty seven and a half percent of adolescents rated their satisfaction with their families as low (Nader et al., 1982). At least half of adolescents reported that their major methods for coping with stress were listening to music, spending time with friends, and watching TV (Nader et al., 1982), emphasizing peer and individual, rather than family, coping efforts.

Environment. Adolescents missing one or both parents are more likely to be overweight (Nolte, Smith, & O'Rourke, 1983). Parents' health behaviors and their attempts to influence their children's behavior were primary determinants of college students' consumption of breakfast, eating nutritious meals, and frequency of skipping meals (Lau et al., 1990). Thus, parental influences may be reasserting themselves after having weakened in the elementary years. There is a paucity of data on family influences on adolescents' diet (Sallis, 1993).

Eating Disorders. Early adolescence is the usual time of onset of the eating disorders anorexia nervosa and bulimia, especially among girls. Anorexia is the underconsumption of calories usually associated with an intense fear of becoming fat, distortion of self-image, and preoccupation with weight loss. Bulimia is the consumption of adequate calories, but purging or eliminating of a meal soon after it is consumed. These disorders are often comorbid. There has been much interest in the role of the family in the onset of these behavioral disorders. Some of these studies have measured the disorder; others have measured attitudes and behaviors associated with the disorder.

Mothers of anorexic–bulimic children tended more often to have fed the children on schedule rather than on demand when they were infants and to have introduced solid foods earlier

than mothers of normal adolescents, but there were no differences in breast-feeding, bottle-feeding, or change in formula (Steiner, Smith, Rosenkranz, & Litt, 1991). These mothers, however, treated the nonanorexic siblings in the same way. Thus, infant feeding practices may influence predisposed children to experience eating disorders, but the predisposing factors are not known.

In a nonclinical sample of 10th-grade health education students, no variables on a family functioning scale were related to a measure associated with anorexia (Gibbs, 1986). In a study comparing clinically diagnosed anorexic–bulimics with normal controls, the anorexic–bulimics and their parents reported more conflict and isolation and less organization and support (Humphrey, 1986). Another study comparing clinically diagnosed anorexic–bulimics with normals found the opposite: The clinical group reported lower disagreement between parents and children, an indication of conflict avoidance, and more stability in their family organization, an indication of rigidity (Kog & Vandereycken, 1989). In a larger sample of clinically diagnosed anorexic–bulimics, no differences in family functioning were found between the clinical groups and a normative population (Thienemann & Steiner, 1990). Families in which one or both parents abuse alcohol or other drugs are clearly dysfunctional (Reich, Earls, & Powell, 1988). In a large survey of middle and high school students ($N = 36,254$ students in 7th–12th grades), children who reported that one or both parents abused alcohol or other drugs were more likely to report each of seven risk factors for disordered eating (Chandry, Harris, Blum, & Resnick, 1994).

It is not clear from these results whether family factors are implicated in the etiology of eating disorders. The studies varied by country, measure of family functioning, sample size, and important other characteristics. The studies using measures of family functioning with larger samples tended to show no relationship. The small differences obtained in the Chandry et al. (1994) study could be due to small response biases among children of alcoholics. Clearly, more research is warranted.

Adulthood

The adult years encompass a broad range of developmental stages (Schafer & Keith, 1981). A common event in the adult years is getting married, thereby forming the family unit. Thus, this section emphasizes spousal relationships in regard to food. A review of studies of determinants of fat and cholesterol intake (Stafleu, de Graaf, van Staveren, & Schroots, 1991/2) revealed the importance of perceived social norms, obviously including family members.

Family Characteristics. Adults, particularly men, appeared to eat better when both partners were involved in food purchasing and preparation. Among husbands, influence of the spouse and a concern for the health of other family members were the most important influences on their dietary quality (Schafer, 1978). Among wives, however, classes, personal preferences, and using information from the media were the most important. Among married seniors, husbands had better diets when they were involved in selecting foods to buy and in the shopping; wives had better diets when husbands were involved in food decisions (Schafer & Keith, 1982).

The quality of the marital relationship also affected dietary intake. Husbands, and especially wives, who scored high on the family cohesion scale were likely to have better diets, while the relationships of other family functioning characteristics to diet were more varied and tended to differ by gender (Kintner, Boss, & Johnson, 1981). Wives had poorer diets when they were dissatisfied with their marriage (Schafer & Keith, 1982).

One aspect of a positive marital relationship is social support. Use of a measure of family support for heart-healthy eating generated a Family-Healthy-Diet-Encouragement Scale, scores on which were related to healthier eating, and an orthogonal Family-Healthy-Diet-Sabotage Scale

that was not related to healthier eating (Sallis et al., 1987). Women reported higher family encouragement, and Anglo-Americans reported higher family sabotage. Social support from family and friends for eating low-fat foods was among the strongest predictors of dietary fat (Glanz et al., 1993). Within 3 months of a heart attack, the spouse of the victim assumed a major share of the household responsibilities (including food-related responsibilities), and this share increased further at 12 months. Family consumption of and positive attitudes toward milk tended to affect personal milk consumption as mediated by a more positive attitude toward milk among undergraduates and as mediated by more positive attitude and behavioral modeling among adults (C. J. Lewis, Sims, & Shannon, 1989).

Yetley, Yetley, and Aquirre (1981) reported that family role relationships even among traditional Mexican-American families were more egalitarian than expected. Consistent with this finding, husbands to whom a meal they did not like was served most often reported eating the meal and requesting that it not be served again (as opposed to coercing a change in the wife's behavior), and the wives most often acceded to the request (Schafer & Bohlen, 1977).

Adults appeared to eat better when they had a positive family relationship, including social support for healthy eating, and when both partners were involved in food purchase or selection. How family members relate to one another in regard to food may not reflect our stereotyped notions. Whether these relationships are true of all stages in the family life cycle and why positive family relationships are important need to be elucidated. For example, couples with more positive relationships might eat better because of such factors as concern for one another's well-being expressed as concern for diet, more brainpower focused on in-store food purchases, more support at home or at restaurants for better eating, and less subversion of healthful eating practices. Documenting differences in these relationships by socioeconomic status, ethnic group, and other characteristics would be valuable as well.

Family and Obesity

Obesity is the point on the continuum of body adiposity (amount of body fat) at which health problems are likely to develop. The role of parent influences on the development of obesity has generated substantial research interest. Among 3- or 4-year-old children, those with one or both parents overweight were significantly more likely to increase their weight over a 1-year period than those with neither parent overweight (Eck, Klesges, Hanson, & Slawson, 1992). These differences occurred despite no difference in total calories consumed and marginally ($p < 0.06$) lower energy expended. The authors attributed the differential weight gain to higher levels of dietary fat consumed. Clearly, genetics plays a role in the etiology of obesity (Stunkard et al., 1986), as do culture (P. J. Brown, 1991) and socioeconomic status (Sobal & Stunkard, 1989). Some, reflecting clinical insights, have proposed a role for family in the psychosocial component of obesity (Satter, 1986).

Some of the earliest work in this area was psychoanalytical (Loader, 1985). Bruch (1973), a leader of this school of thought, suggested that there were several etiologies of obesity: constitutional (i.e., genetic), reactive (i.e., overeating in response to perceived stress), and developmental (i.e., starting in childhood, reflecting parenting disorders). The developmental form reflected a deficiency in a person's self-awareness of body states (including hunger), which in turn was due to parents' not responding appropriately to an infant's signaling of bodily needs. In this case, the child associates feelings of hunger with a variety of emotional states, which are resolved with food. Attempts to verify these hypothesized relationships empirically have generally not met with success (Loader, 1985). When Bruch's ideas were operationalized within a more behavioristic focus with college students and their mothers, no relationships were obtained between student adiposity and scales measuring the use of food in reward, punishment, soothing, and affection (Rogers, Canady, & Wentworth, 1980).

Behavioristic approaches have been shown to be useful in predicting adiposity among toddlers. Among children 12–30 months of age, Klesges et al. (1983) found that the number of parental offers of food and parental encouragements to eat were highly positively related to the children's relative weight. Klesges, Malott, Boschee, and Weber (1986) replicated these findings with children 22–46 months of age. Among slightly older children, self-control issues appeared to take precedence. In a controlled laboratory study, Klesges, Stein, Eck, Isbell, and Klesges (1991) found that when 4- to 7-year-old children knew their mother would review lunch selections, the children selected food lower in sugar (than when no parental review was announced); parents modified the children's selections to be lower in total calories, saturated fatty acids, and sodium, primarily by removing foods considered to be low in nutrition. There were no differences in these findings by adiposity status of the parent or the child. Klesges et al. (1992) concluded that childhood obesity was not a function of family psychosocial factors.

Using a more social–psychological perspective, Costanzo and Woody (1985) proposed that children become obese due to a parenting syndrome. In particular, they proposed that parents are always looking for signs of deviance and excellence in their children. A parent who perceives early signs of excess adiposity initiates a parenting style that attempts to carefully regulate or control the child's food consumption. This controlling style both inhibits the child's opportunity to develop self-regulation skills in regard to eating and expresses a serious parental concern about adiposity. As a result, the child never learns to self-regulate eating and internalizes the parents' concern and negative affect about the child's eating and obesity. Partial support for these ideas is provided by the findings that mothers interact less frequently and less positively with obese children (Drabman, Cordra, Hammer, Jarvie, & Horton, 1979; C. M. Olson, Pringle, & Schoenwetter, 1976).

Since it is not clear at this time in the biological literature whether obesity is a problem of metabolism, overeating, underactivity, or some combination of these factors (Stunkard, 1980), efforts to determine the precise role of the family in the etiology of obesity may be premature.

FINAL COMMENTS: RESEARCH AND METHODOLOGICAL ISSUES

Families influence dietary practices in many different and complex ways, with important implications for health and disease. While interventions to help families effectively change diet to improve health are an ultimate goal, more research is needed to delineate all the avenues and the extent of family influences on diet. This research should provide better targets and mechanisms for change.

This review reveals that there really is *not* an extensive literature on family influences on diet. What can be said about diet at different developmental stages is limited by the literature available at each stage. Most of this research is unsystematic, i.e., one-time studies, rather than series of studies systematically conducted to capitalize or clarify earlier work. Much of this work is atheoretical, not benefiting from the conceptualization and linkages to other work based on similar theory. The model of family reciprocal determinism provides a useful theoretical framework for structuring this research. A focus on emergent family characteristics will permit analyzing social learning mechanisms within different types of families.

Much of this literature is cross-sectional, minimizing the ability to draw causal inferences. Small samples are common and perhaps provide insufficient power to detect relationships. American society is in turmoil, with many changes over time in family structures and relationships among family members (Hamburg, 1994). What can be said about families and diet at one time may not be true of them at another time.

Measurement is a chronic problem in dietary research (Baranowski & Simons-Morton,

1991). Due to intraindividual (day-to-day) variability in dietary practices, many days of assessment are needed to obtain reliable estimates of habitual consumption. Much of the research pays little attention to this issue, and there is enormous variety in the types of dietary variables used, e.g., actual consumption of foods or nutrients, consumption compared to some standard, interpretations of adequacy of consumption, whether or not meals were eaten, or preferences for foods. Furthermore, a substantial portion of this research employs qualitative research methods that emphasize the attentiveness, skills, and interpretations of the qualitative researchers. This variability in the type and quality of measurement decreases our ability to compare results and may account for some of the apparent inconsistencies across studies.

The ability to design effective interventions to encourage more healthful eating among families requires a more systematic and comprehensive understanding of how families influence consumption. At least two health education leaders have stated our need to develop theories of the problem (Burdine & McLeroy, 1992) or theories of the behavior (McLeroy et al., 1993). It is hoped that this review provides a theoretical structure that will enhance the ability of future researchers to better design research on the relationships among family and diet. What is learned in this behavioral arena may also enhance understanding of family influences on other health-related behaviors.

REFERENCES

Adair, L., Popkin, B. M., & Guilkey, D. K. (1993). The duration of breastfeeding: How is it affected by biological, socio-demographic, health sector, and food industry factors? *Demography, 30,* 63–80.

Ainsworth, M. D. S., & Bell, S. M. (1969). Some contemporary patterns of mother–infant interaction in the feeding situation. In A. Ambrose (Ed.), *Stimulation in early infancy* (pp. 133–170). New York: Academic Press.

American Dietetic Association. (1986). Position of the American Dietetic Association: Promotion of breastfeeding. *Journal of the American Dietetic Association, 78,* 1580–1582.

Anliker, J. A., Laus, M. J., Samonds, K. W., & Beal, V. A. (1990). Parental messages and the nutrition awareness of preschool children. *Journal of Nutrition Education, 22,* 24-29.

Anliker, J. A., Laus, M. J., Samonds, K. W., & Beal, V. A. (1992). Mothers' reports of their three-year-old children's control over foods and involvement in food-related activities. *Journal of Nutrition Education, 24,* 285-291.

Aschheim, E. (1993). Dietary control of psychosis. *Medical Hypotheses, 41,* 327-328.

Atkin, C. K. (1978). Observation of parent-child interaction in supermarket decision-making. *Journal of Marketing, 42,* 41-45.

Bandura, A. (1972). *Psychological modeling.* New York: Aldine, Atherton.

Baranowski, T. (1990). Reciprocal determinism at the stages of behavior change: An integration of community, personal and behavioral perspectives. *International Quarterly of Community Health Education, 10,* 297-327.

Baranowski, T. (1992-1993). Beliefs as motivational influences at stages in behavior change. *International Quarterly of Community Health Education, 13,* 3-29.

Baranowski, T., Bee, D., Rassin, D., Richardson, J. D., Brown, J., Guenther, N., & Nader, P. R. (1983). Social support, social influence, ethnicity and the breastfeeding decision. *Social Science and Medicine, 17,* 1599-1611.

Baranowski, T., Domel, S., Gould, R., Baranowski, J., Leonard, S., Treiber, F., & Mullis, R. (1993). Increasing fruit and vegetable consumption among 4th and 5th grade students: Results from focus groups using reciprocal determinism. *Journal of Nutrition Education, 25,* 114-120.

Baranowski, T., Dworkin, R. J., Dunn, J. K., Nader, P. R., & Brown, J. (1986). Reliability of two measures of family functioning. *Family Perspective, 20,* 353-364.

Baranowski, T., Henske, J., Simons-Morton, B., Palmer, J., Hooks, P., Tiernan, K., & Dunn, J. K. (1990). Dietary change for CVD prevention among black-American families. *Health Education Research, 5,* 433-443.

Baranowski, T., Rassin, D., Harrison, J. A., Bryan, G., Henske, J., & Puhl, J. (1990). Infant feeding practices and childhood stature in three ethnic groups. *American Journal of Human Biology, 2,* 283-290.

Baranowski, T., Rassin, D., Richardson, J. C., Bee, D., & Brown, J. (1986). Attitudes toward breastfeeding. *Journal of Developmental and Behavioral Pediatrics, 7,* 367-372.

Baranowski, T., & Simons-Morton, B. G. (1991). Children's physical activity and dietary assessment: Measurement issues. *Journal of School Health, 61,* 195-197.

Bar-Or, O., & Baranowski, T. (1994). Physical activity, obesity and adiposity among adolescents. *Pediatric Exercise Science, 6,* 348-360.

Beals, D. E. (1993). Explanatory talk in low-income families' mealtime conversations. *Applied Psycholinguistics, 14,* 489-513.

Bee, D., Baranowski, T., Rassin, D., Richardson, J., & Mikrut, W. (1991). Breastfeeding initiation in a tri-ethnic population: Demographic correlates. *American Journal of Diseases of Children, 145,* 306-309.

Belch, G. E., Belch, M. A., & Ceresino, G. (1985). Parental and teenage child influences in family decision making. *Journal of Business Research, 13,* 163-176.

Berenson, G., Srinivasan, S., Webber, L., & Wattigney, W. (1991). Coronary heart disease as a pediatric disorder. *Progress in Cardiology, 4,* 127-139.

Bergeman, C. S., Plomin, R., Pedersen, N. L., McClearn, G. E., & Nesselroade, J. R. (1990). Genetic and environmental influences on social support: The Swedish Adoption/Twin Study of Aging. *Journal of Gerontology, 45,* 101-106.

Bernard-Bonnin, A.-C., Gilbert, S., Rousseau, E., Masson, P., & Maheux, B. (1991). Television and the 3- to 10-year old child. *Pediatrics, 88,* 48-54.

Birch, L. L. (1980). The relationship between children's food preferences and those of their parents. *Journal of Nutrition Education, 12,* 14-18.

Birch, L. L., & Johnson, S. L. (1994). Appetite control in children. In J. D. Fernstrom & G. D. Miller (Eds.), *Appetite and body weight regulation: Sugar, fat and macronutrient substitutes* (pp. 5-15). Boca Raton, FL: CRC Press.

Birch, L. L., Marlin, D. W., & Rotter, J. W. (1984). Eating as the "means" activity in a contingency: Effects on young children's food preference. *Child Development, 55,* 431-439.

Breckenridge, M. A., & Murphy, M. N. (1969). *Growth and development of the young child.* Philadelphia: W. B. Saunders.

Brinberg, D., & Durand, J. (1983). Eating at fast-food restaurants: An analysis using two behavioral intention models. *Journal of Applied Social Psychology, 13,* 459-472.

Brodwick, M., Baranowski, T., & Rassin, D. (1989). Infant feeding patterns in three ethnic groups. *Journal of the American Dietetic Association, 89,* 1129-1132.

Brown, J. E., & Tiernan, P. (1986). Effect of income and WIC on the dietary intake of preschoolers: Results of a preliminary study. *Journal of the American Dietetic Association, 86,* 1189-1191.

Brown, P. J. (1991). Culture and the evolution of obesity. *Human Nature, 2,* 31-57.

Bruch, H. (1973). *Eating disorders.* New York: Basic Books.

Bruhn, J. G., & Parcel, G. S. (1982). Current knowledge about the health behavior of young children: A conference summary. *Health Education Quarterly, 9,* 142-166.

Bullock, M., & Lutkenhaus, P. (1988). The development of volitional behavior in the toddler years. *Child Development, 59,* 664-674.

Burdine, J. N., & McLeroy, K. R. (1992). Practitioner's use of theory: Examples from a workgroup. *Health Education Quarterly, 19,* 331-340.

Burke, G. L., Voors, A. N., Shear, C. L., Webber, L. S., Smoak, C. G., Cresanta, J. L., & Berenson, G. S. (1987). Cardiovascular risk factors from birth to 7 years of age: The Bogalusa

Heart Study—Blood Pressure. *Pediatrics, 80*(Supplement), 784-788.

Campbell, C. C., & Desjardins, E. (1989). A model and research approach for studying the management of limited food resources by low income families. *Journal of Nutrition Education, 21,* 162-171.

Chandry, J. M., Harris, L., Blum, R. W., & Resnick, M. D. (1994). Disordered eating among adolescents whose parents misuse alcohol: Protective and risk factors. *International Journal of the Addictions, 29,* 505-516.

Clancy-Hepburn, K. (1974). Children's behavior responses to TV food advertisements. *Journal of Nutrition Education, 6,* 93-96.

Cooper, P. J., Murray, L., & Stein, A. (1993). Psychosocial factors associated with the early termination of breastfeeding. *Journal of Psychosomatic Research, 37,* 171-176.

Costanzo, P. R., & Woody, E. Z. (1985). Domain-specific parenting styles and their impact on the child's development of particular deviance: The example of obesity proneness. *Journal of Social and Clinical Psychology, 3,* 425-445.

Coughenour, M. C. (1972). Functional aspects of food consumption activity and family life cycle stages. *Journal of Marriage and the Family, 34,* 656-664.

Cousins, J. H., Power, T. G., & Olvera-Ezzell, N. (1993). Mexican-American mothers' socialization strategies: Effects of education, acculturation, and health locus of control. *Journal of Experimental Child Psychology, 55,* 258-276.

Cousins, J. H., Power, T. G., & Olvera-Ezzell, N. (1994). *Effects of maternal socialization strategies on children's nutrition knowledge.* Paper presented to the Society of Behavioral Medicine.

Crockett, L. J., & Petersen, A. C. (1993). Adolescent development: Health risks and opportunities for health promotion. In S. G. Millstein, A. C. Petersen, & E. D. Nightingale (Eds.), *Promoting the health of adolescents* (pp. 13-37). New York: Oxford University Press.

Curry, S. J., Wagner, E. H., & Grothaus, L. C. (1991). Evaluation of intrinsic and extrinsic motivation interventions with a self-help smoking cessation program. *Journal of Consulting and Clinical Psychology, 59,* 318-324.

Denton, R. E., & Kampfe, C. M. (1994). The relationship between family variables and adolescent substance abuse: A literature review. *Adolescence, 29,* 475-495.

Dielman, T. E., Leech, S., Becker, M. H., Rosenstock, I. M., Horvath, W. J., & Radius, S. M. (1982). Parental and child health beliefs and behavior. *Health Education Quarterly, 9,* 156-173.

Dietz, W. H., & Gortmaker, S. L. (1985). Do we fatten our children at the television set? Obesity and television viewing in children and adolescents. *Pediatrics, 75,* 807-812.

Dietz, W. H., & Strasburger, V. C. (1991). Children, adolescents and television. *Current Problems in Pediatrics, 21,* 8-31.

Domel, S. B., Baranowski, T., Davis, H., Leonard, S. B., Riley, P., & Baranowski, J. (1993). Measuring fruit and vegetable preferences among fourth and fifth grade students. *Preventive Medicine, 22,* 866-879.

Domel, S. B., Baranowski, T., Davis, H. C., Thompson, W. O., Leonard, S. B., Riley, P., & Baranowski, J. (1995). A measure of outcome expectations for fruit and vegetable consumption among fourth and fifth grade children: Reliability and validity. *Health Education Research: Theory and Practice, 10,* 65-72.

Domel, S., Baranowski, T., Davis, H., Thompson, W. O., Leonard, S. B., Riley, P., Baranowski, J., Dudovitz, B., & Smyth, M. (1993). Development and evaluation of a school intervention to increase fruit and vegetable consumption among 4th and 5th grade students. *Journal of Nutrition Education, 25,* 345-349.

Domel, S. B., Baranowski, T., Davis, H. C., Thompson, W. O., Leonard, S. B., Vignati, P. R., & Baranowski, J. (1996). Psychosocial predictors of fruit and vegetable consumption among elementary school children. *Health Education Research, 11,* 299-308.

Drabman, R. S., Cordna, G. D., Hammer, D., Jarvie, G. J., & Horton, W. (1979). Developmental trends in eating rates of normal and overweight preschool children. *Child Development, 50,* 211-220.

Dreyer, C. A., & Dreyer, A. S. (1973). Family dinnertime as a unique behavior habitat. *Family Process,* 291-301.

DuRant, R., Baranowski, T., Johnson, M., & Thompson, W. O. (1994). The relationship among television watching, physical activity and body composition in young children. *Pediatrics, 94,* 449-455.

DuRant, R. H., Baranowski, T., Johnson, M., & Thompson, W. O. (1996). The relationship among television watching, physical activity and body composition of 5, 6, or 7 year old children. *Pediatric Exercise Science, 8,* 15-26.

Eck, L. H., Klesges, R. C., Hanson, C. L., & Slawson, D. (1992). Children at familial risk for obesity: An examination of dietary intake, physical activity and weight status. *International Journal of Obesity, 16,* 71-78.

Egeland, B., Pianta, R., & O'Brien, M. A. (1993). Mental intrusiveness in infancy and child maladaptation in early school years. *Development and Psychopathology, 5,* 359-370.

Engle, P. L., & Nieves, I. (1993a). Intra-household food distribution among Guatemalan families in a supplementary feeding programme: Mothers' perceptions. *Food and Nutrition Bulletin, 14,* 314-322.

Engle, P. L., & Nieves, I. (1993b). Intrahousehold food distribution among Guatemalan families in a supplementary feeding program: Behavior patterns. *Social Science and Medicine, 36,* 1605-1612.

Eppright, E. S., Fox, H. M., Fryer, B. A., Lamkin, G. H., & Vivian, V. M. (1969). Eating behavior of preschool children. *Journal of Nutrition Education, 6,* 16-19.

Eyer, D. E. (1994). Mother-infant bonding, a scientific fiction. *Human Nature, 5,* 69-94.

Falciglia, G. A., & Norton, P. A. (1994). Evidence for a genetic influence on preference for some foods. *Journal of the American Dietetic Association, 94,* 154–158.

Food Marketing Institute. (1987). *Trends, 1987: Consumer attitudes and the supermarket.* Washington, DC: Food Marketing Institute.

Fox, H., Linsenmeyer, B., & Kohn, H. (1984). Influence of food purchases on nutritional adequacy of diets in Lincoln, Nebraska. *Nutrition Reports International, 30,* 1385–1393.

Gibbs, R. E. (1986). Social factors in exaggerated eating behavior among high school students. *International Journal of Eating Disorders, 5,* 1103–1107.

Gillespie, A. (1983). Assessing snacking behavior of children. *Ecology of Food and Nutrition, 13,* 167–172.

Gillespie, A. H., & Achterberg, C. L. (1989). Comparison of family interaction patterns related to food and nutrition. *Journal of the American Dietetic Association, 89,* 509–512.

Glanz, K., Kristal, A. R., Sorensen, G., Palombo, R., Heimendinger, J., & Probart, C. (1993). Development and validation of measures of psychosocial factors influencing fat- and fiber-related dietary behavior. *Preventive Medicine, 22,* 373–387.

Gortmaker, S. L., Dietz, W. H., & Cheung, L. W. (1990). Inactivity, diet, and the fattening of America. *Journal of the American Dietetic Association, 90,* 1247–1252, 1255.

Haaga, J. G., & Mason, J. B. (1987). Food distribution within the family: Evidence and implications for research and programmes. *Food Policy,* 146–160.

Hamburg, B. A. (1994). *Children and families in a changing world: Challenges and opportunities.* Austin, TX: Hogg Foundation.

Harper, L. V., & Sanders, K. M. (1975). The effect of adults' eating on young children's acceptance of unfamiliar foods. *Journal of Experimental Child Psychology, 20,* 206–214.

Hartz, A., Giefer, E., & Rimm, A. A. (1977). Relative importance of the effect of family environment and heredity on obesity. *Annals of Human Genetics (London), 41,* 185–192.

Hearn, M., Baranowski, T., & Baranowski, J. (1997). Availability and accessibility of fruits and vegetables and their consumption among families in two ethnic groups. *Journal of Health Education.*

Heinig, M. J., Nommsen, L. A., Peerson, J. M., Lonnerdal, B., & Dewey, K. B. (1993). Energy and protein intakes of breast-fed and formula-fed infants during the first year of life and their association with growth velocity: The DARLING study. *American Journal of Clinical Nutrition, 58,* 152–161.

Heptinstall, E., Puckering, C., Skuse, D., Start, K., Zur-Szpiro, S., & Dowdney, L. (1987). Nutrition and mealtime behavior in families of growth-retarded children. *Human Nutrition: Applied Nutrition, 41A,* 390–402.

Humphrey, L. L. (1986). Family relations in bulimic–anorexic

and nondistressed families. *International Journal of Eating Disorders, 5,* 223–232.

International Food Information Council. (1992). How children are making food choices. *IFIC Review.*

Jackson, C., Bee-Gates, D. J., & Henriksen, L. (1994). Authoritative parenting, child competencies and initiation of cigarette smoking. *Health Education Quarterly, 21,* 103–116.

Jackson, R. W., McDaniel, S. W., & Rao, C. P. (1985). Food shopping and preparation: Psychographic differences of working wives and housewives. *Journal of Consumer Research, 11,* 110–113.

Jacoby, A., Altman, D. G., Cook, J., Holland, W. W., & Elliott, A. (1975). Influence of some social and environmental factors on the nutrient intake and nutritional status of school children. *British Journal of Preventive and Social Medicine, 29,* 116–120.

Karp, R., Snyder, E., Fairorth, J., Nelson, M., Solimano, G., Acker, W., Greene, G., & Krehl, W. A. (1984). Parental behavior and the availability of foods among undernourished inner-city children. *Journal of Family Practice, 18,* 731–735.

Kelder, S. D., Perry, C. L., Klepp, K. I., & Lytle, L. L. (1994). Longitudinal tracking of adolescent smoking, physical activity, and food choice behaviors. *American Journal of Public Health, 84,* 1121–1126.

Kids' allowances. (1993, Nov. 28). *The Atlanta Journal-Constitution,* p. D5.

Kintner, M., Boss, P. G., & Johnson, N. (1981). The relationship between dysfunctional family environments and family member food intake. *Journal of Marriage and the Family, 43,* 633–641.

Kirby, S., Baranowski, T., Reynolds, K., Taylor, G., & Binkley, D. (1995). Children's fruit and vegetable intake: Socioeconomic, adult child, regional and urban–rural influences. *Journal of Nutrition Education, 27,* 261–271.

Kirk, M. C., & Gillespie, A. H. (1990). Factors affecting food choices of working mothers with young families. *Journal of Nutrition Education, 22,* 161–168.

Klesges, R. C., Coates, T. J., Brown, G., Sturgeon-Tillisch, J., Moldenhauer-Klesges, L. M., Holzer, B., Woolfrey, J., & Vollmer, J. (1983). Parental influences on children's eating behavior and relative weight. *Journal of Applied Behavior Analysis, 16,* 371–378.

Klesges, R. C., Haddock, C. K., Stein, R. J., Klesges, L. M., Eck, L. H., & Hanson, C. L. (1992). Relationship between psychosocial functioning and body fat in preschool children: A longitudinal investigation. *Journal of Consulting and Clinical Psychology, 60.*

Klesges, R. C., Malott, J. M., Boschee, P. F., & Weber, J. M. (1986). The effects of parental influences on children's food intake, physical activity and relative weight. *International Journal of Eating Disorders, 5,* 335–346.

Klesges, R. C., Stein, R. J., Eck, L. H., Isbell, T. R., & Klesges, L. M. (1991). Parental influence on food selection in young children and its relationships to childhood obesity. *American Journal of Clinical Nutrition*, *53*, 859–864.

Knight, J., & Grantham-McGregor, S. (1985). Using primary-school children to improve child-rearing practices in rural Jamaica. *Child: Care, Health and Development*, *11*, 81–90.

Kog, E., & Vandereycken, W. (1989). Family interactions in eating disorder patients and normal controls. *International Journal of Eating Disorders*, *8*, 11–23.

Kolonel, L. N., & Lee, J. (1981). Husband–wife correspondence in smoking, drinking, and dietary habits. *American Journal of Clinical Nutrition*, *34*, 99–104.

Krondl, M., Coleman, P., Wade, J., & Milner, J. (1983). A twin study examining the genetic influence on food selection. *Human Nutrition, Applied Nutrition*, *37A*, 189–198.

Kumanyika, S. K., & Ewart, C. K. (1990). Theoretical and baseline considerations for diet and weight control of diabetes among blacks. *Diabetes Care*, *13*, 1154–1162.

Laskarzewski, P., Morrison, J. A., Khoury, P., Kelly, K., Glatfelter, L., Larsen, R., & Glueck, C. J. (1980). Parent–child nutrient intake interrelationships in school children ages 6 to 19: The Princeton School District Study. *American Journal of Clinical Nutrition*, *33*, 2350–2355.

Lau, R. R., Quadrell, M. J., & Hartman, K. A. (1990). Development and change of young adults' preventive health beliefs and behavior: Influence from parents and peers. *Journal of Health and Social Behavior*, *31*, 240–259.

Lewis, C. J., Sims, L. S., & Shannon, B. (1989). Examination of specific nutrition/health behaviors using a social cognitive model. *Journal of the American Dietetic Association*, *89*, 194–202.

Lewis, M., & Feiring, C. (1982). Some American families at dinner. In L. M. Laosa & I. E. Siegel (Eds.), *Families as learning environments for children* (pp. 115–145). New York: Plenum Press.

Lipis, P. H. (1992). *Food preferences among parents and their children: A longitudinal study*. MPH thesis. Emory University School of Public Health, Atlanta, GA.

Loader, P. J. (1985). Childhood obesity: The family perspective. *International Journal of Eating Disorders*, *4*, 211–225.

Locard, E., Mamelle, N., Billette, A., Miginiac, M., Munoz, F., & Rey, S. (1992). Risk factors of obesity in a five year old population: Parental versus environmental factors. *International Journal of Obesity*, *16*, 721–729.

Mahoney, L. T., Lauer, R. M., Lee, J., & Clarke, W. R. (1991). Factors affecting tracking of coronary heart disease risk factors in children: The Muscatine Study. *Annals of the New York Academy of Sciences*, *623*, 120–132.

McDonald, M. A., Sigman, M., Espinosa, M. P., & Neimann, C. G. (1994). Impact of a temporary food shortage on children and their mothers. *Child Development*, *65*, 404–415.

McLeroy, K. R., Steckler, A. B., Simons-Morton, B., Goodman, R. M., Gottlieb, M., & Burdine, J. N. (1993). Social science theory in health education: Time for a new model? *Health Education Research: Theory and Practice*, *8*, 305–312.

Michela, J. L., & Contento, I. R. (1986). Cognitive, motivational, social, and environmental influences on children's food choices. *Health Psychology*, *5*, 209–230.

Moos, R. H. (1974). *Family Environment Scale*. Palo Alto, CA: Consulting Psychologists Press.

Moreno, C., Larriado-Laborin, R., Sallis, J. F., Elder, J. P., de Moor, C., Castro, F. G., & Deosaransingh, K. (1994). Parental influences to smoke in Latino youth. *Preventive Medicine*, *23*, 48–53.

Mullen, M. K., Coll, C. G., Vohr, B. R., Muriel, A. C., & Oh, W. (1988). Mother–infant feeding interaction in full-term small-for-gestational-age infants. *Journal of Pediatrics*, *112*, 143–148.

Nader, P. R., Baranowski, T., Vanderpool, N. A., Dunn, J. K., Dworkin, R., & Ray L. (1983). The Family Health Project: Cardiovascular risk reduction education for children and parents. *Journal of Developmental and Behavioral Pediatrics*, *4*, 3–10.

Nader, P. R., Perry, C., Maccoby, N., Solomon, D., Killen, J., Telch, M., & Alexander, J. K. (1982). Adolescent perceptions of family health behavior: A tenth grade educational activity to increase family awareness of a community cardiovascular risk reduction program. *Journal of School Health*, *52*, 372–377.

A. C. Nielsen Co. (1989). *Nielsen Report on Television 1989*. Northbrook, IL: Nielsen Media Research.

Nolte, A. E., Smith, B. J., & O'Rourke, T. (1983). The relationship between health risk attitudes and behaviors and parental presence. *Journal of School Health*, *53*, 234–240.

Nutrition Committee of the Canadian Paediatric Society and the Committee on Nutrition of the American Academy of Pediatrics. (1978). Breastfeeding: A commentary in celebration of the international year of the child. *Pediatrics*, *62*, 591–592.

Oliveria, S. A., Ellison, R. C., Moore, L. L., Gillman, M. W., Garrahie, E. J., & Singer, M. R. (1992). Parent–child relationships in nutrient intake: The Framingham Children's Study. *American Journal of Clinical Nutrition*, *56*, 593–598.

Olson, C. M., Pringle, D. J., & Schoenwetter, C. D. (1976). Parent–child interaction: Its relation to growth and weight. *Journal of Nutrition Education*, *8*, 67–70.

Olson, D. H., McCubbin, H. I., Barnes, H. L., Larson, A. S., Muxen, M. J., & Wilson, M. A. (1983). *Families: What makes them work*. Beverly Hills, CA: Sage.

Olvera-Ezzell, N., Power, T. G., & Cousins, J. H. (1990). Maternal socialization of children's eating habits: Strategies used by obese Mexican-American mothers. *Child Development*, *61*, 395–400.

Patterson, T. L., Rupp, J. W., Sallis, J. F., Atkins, C. J., & Nader, P. R. (1988). Aggregation of dietary calories, fats, and sodium in Mexican-American and Anglo families. *American Journal of Preventive Medicine*, *4*, 75–82.

Perry, C., Baranowski, T., & Parcel, G. (1990). How individuals, environments and health behavior interact: Social learning theory. In K. Glanz, F. M. Lewis, & B. K. Rimer

(Eds.), *Health behavior and health education: Theory, research and practice* (pp. 161–186). San Francisco: Jossey-Bass.

Pérusse, D., Neale, M. C., Heath, A. C., & Eaves, L. J. (1994). Human parental behavior: Evidence for genetic influence and potential implication for gene-culture transmission. *Behavior Genetics, 24,* 327–335.

Pérusse, L., Tremblay, A., Leblanc, C., Cloninger, C. R., Reich, T., Rice, J., & Bouchard, C. (1988). Familial resemblance in energy intake: Contribution of genetic and environmental factors. *American Journal of Clinical Nutrition, 47,* 629–635.

Phillips, H., & Bradshaw, R. (1993). How customers actually shop: Customer interaction with the point of sale. *Journal of the Market Research Society, 35,* 51–62.

Plomin, R., Reiss, D., Hetherington, E. M., & Howe, G. W. (1994). Nature and nurture: Genetic contributions to measures of the family environment. *Developmental Psychology, 30,* 32–43.

Polegato, R. (1994). The role of family members in food shopping: Implications for retailers and manufacturers. *Journal of Food Products Marketing, 2,* 3–15.

Pollit, E., Gilmore, M., & Valcarel, M. (1978). Early mother-infant interaction and somatic growth. *Early Human Development, 1,* 325–329.

Pollitt, E., & Wirtz, S. (1981). Mother–infant feeding interaction and weight gain in the first month of life. *Journal of the American Dietetic Association, 78,* 596–601.

Rassin, D. K., Markides, K. S., Baranowski, T., Bee, D. E., Richardson, C. J., Mikrut, W. D., & Winkler, A. (1993). Acculturation and breastfeeding on the United States-Mexican border. *American Journal of Medicine Sciences, 306,* 28–34.

Rassin, D. K., Markides, K. S., Baranowski, T., Richardson, C. J., Mikrut, W. D., & Bee, D. E. (1994). Acculturation and the initiation of breastfeeding. *Journal of Clinical Epidemiology, 47,* 739–746.

Rassin, D., Richardson, C. J., & Baranowski, T. (1986). Ethnic determinants of lactation in a population of mothers in the United States. In M. Hamosh & A. S. Goldman (Eds.), *Human lactation 2: Effect of maternal environmental factors* (pp. 69–81). New York: Plenum Press.

Rassin, D., Richardson, C. J., Baranowski, T., Nader, P. R., Guenther, N., Bee, D., & Brown, J. (1984). Incidence of breastfeeding in a lower socio-economic group of mothers in the United States: Ethnic patterns. *Pediatrics, 73,* 132–137.

Reich, W., Earls, F., & Powell, J. (1988). A comparison of the home and social environments of children of alcoholic and non-alcoholic parents. *British Journal of the Addictions, 83,* 831–839.

Reis, J. (1992). *Mothers' teaching about health: A descriptive study of low income black mothers and their children.* Paper presented to the Annual Meeting of the American Public Health Association.

Robertson, T. S. (1979). Parental mediation of television advertising effects. *Journal of Communication, 29,* 12–25.

Robinson, T. N., Hammer, L. D., Killen, J. D., Kraemer, H. C., Wilson, D. M., Hayward, C., & Taylor, C. B. (1993). Does television viewing increase obesity and reduce physical activity? Cross-sectional and longitudinal analyses among adolesent girls. *Pediatrics, 91,* 273–280.

Rogers, C. S., Canady, H., & Wentworth, J. (1980). Obesity, child-feeding attitudes, and reactive eating: An intergenerational study. *Home Economics Research Journal, 8,* 173–183.

Rose, R. J. (1995). Genes and human behavior. *Annual Review of Psychology, 46,* 625–654.

Rozin, P., Fallon, A., & Mandell, R. (1984). Family resemblance in attitudes to foods. *Developmental Psychology, 20,* 309–314.

Rust, L. (1993). Observations: How to reach children in stores: Marketing tactics grounded in observational research. *Journal of Advertising Research, 33,* 67–72.

Sallis, J. F. (1993). Promoting healthful diet and physical activity. In S. G. Millstein, A. C. Petersen, & E. D. Nightingale (Eds.), *Promoting the health of adolescents* (pp. 209–241). New York: Oxford University Press.

Sallis, J. F., Grossman, R. M., Pinski, R. B., Patterson, T. L., & Nader, P. R. (1987). The development of scales to measure social support for diet and exercise behaviors. *Preventive Medicine, 16,* 825–836.

Sallis, J. F., Nader, P. R., Rupp, J. W., Atkins, C. J., & Wilson, W. C. (1986). San Diego surveyed for heart healthy foods and exercise facilities. *Public Health Reports, 101,* 216–219.

Satter, E. M. (1986). The feeding relationship. *Journal of the American Dietetic Association, 86,* 352–356.

Schafer, R. B. (1978). Factors affecting food behavior and the quality of husbands' and wives' diets. *Journal of the American Dietetic Association, 72,* 138–143.

Schafer, R. B., & Bohlen, J. M. (1977). Exchange of conjugal power in the control of family food consumption. *Home Economics Research Journal, 6,* 1–10.

Schafer, R. B., & Keith, P. M. (1981). Influences on food decisions across the family life cycle. *Journal of the American Dietetic Association, 78,* 144–148.

Schafer, R. B., & Keith, P. M. (1982). Social psychological factors in the dietary quality of married and single elderly. *Journal of the American Dietetic Association, 81,* 30–34.

Simon, J. A. (1992). Vitamin C and cardiovascular disease: A review. *Journal of the American College of Nutrition, 11,* 107–125.

Slyper, A., & Schechtman, G. (1994). Coronary artery disease risk factors from a genetic and developmental perspective. *Archives of Internal Medicine, 154,* 633–638.

Sobal, J., & Stunkard, A. J. (1989). Socioeconomic status and obesity: A review of the literature. *Psychological Bulletin, 105,* 260–275.

Sommer, R., Wynes, M., & Brinkley, G. (1992). Social facilitation effects in shopping behavior. *Environment and Behavior, 24,* 285–297.

Stafleu, A., de Graaf, C., van Staveren, W. A., & Schroots, J. J. (1991/2). A review of selected studies assessing social-psychological determinants of fat and cholesterol intake. *Food Quality and Preference, 3*, 183–200.

Stein, A. D., Shea, S., Basch, C. E., Contento, I. R., & Zybert, P. (1991). Variability and tracking of nutrient intakes of preschool children based on multiple administrations of the 24-hour dietary recall. *American Journal of Epidemiology, 134*, 1427–1437.

Steiner, H., Smith, C., Rosenkranz, R. T., & Litt, I. (1991). The early care and feeding of anorexics. *Child Psychiatry and Human Development, 21*, 163–167.

Stunkard, A. J. (Ed.). (1980). *Obesity*. Philadelphia: W. B. Saunders.

Stunkard, A. J., Sorensen, T. I. A., Hanis, C., Teasdale, T. W., Chakraborty, R., Schull, W. J., & Schulsinger, F. (1986). An adoption study of human obesity. *New England Journal of Medicine, 314*, 193–198.

Surgeon General. (1988). *The Surgeon General's report on nutrition and health*. DHHS (PHS) Publication No. 88-50210. Washington, DC: U.S. Government Printing Office.

Talpade, S., Beatty, S. E., and Trilokekar-Talpade, M. (1993). Teenager influence on family grocery purchases: Conceptualization and empirical analysis. *Journal of Food Products Marketing, 1*, 25–47.

Taras, H. L., Sallis, J. F., Nader, P. R., & Nelson, J. (1990). Children's television-viewing habits and the family environment. *American Journal of Diseases of Children, 144*, 357–359.

Taras, H. L., Sallis, J. F., Patterson, T. L., Nader, P. R., & Nelson, J. A. (1990). Television's influence on children's diet and physical activity. *Developmental and Behavioral Pediatrics, 10*, 176–180.

Taylor, W., Baranowski, T., & Sallis, J. (1995). Family determinants of childhood physical activity: A social cognitive model. In R. K. Dishman (Ed.), *Exercise adherence: Its impact on public health* (pp. 319–342). Champaign, IL: Human Kinetics Publishers.

Thienemann, M., & Steiner, H. (1990). *Family environment in eating disordered adolescents*. Paper presented at the Annual Meeting of the Northern California Psychiatric Society.

Tinsley, B. J. (1992). Multiple influences on the acquisition and socialization of children's health attitudes and behavior: An integrative review. *Child Development, 63*, 1043–1069.

Toniolo, P., Riboli, E., Shore, R. E., & Pasternack, B. S. (1994). Consumption of meat, animal products, protein, and fat and risk of breast cancer: A prospective cohort study in New York. *Epidemiology, 5*, 391–397.

Touliatos, J., Lindholm, B. W., Wenberg, M. F., & Ryan, M. (1984). Family and child correlates of nutrition knowledge and dietary quality in 10-13 year olds. *Journal of School Health, 54*, 247–249.

U.S. Department of Health and Human Services. (1991). *Healthy people 2000: National health promotion and disease prevention objectives*. DHHS Publication No. (PHS) 91-50212. Washington, DC: U.S. Government Printing Office.

Velican, D., & Velican, C. (1980). Atherosclerotic involvement of the coronary arteries of adolescents and young adults. *Atherosclerosis, 36*, 449–460.

Ward, S., & Wackman, D. B. (1972). Children's purchase influence attempts and parental yielding. *Journal of Marketing Research, 9*, 316–319.

Wilson, G. (1988). Family food systems, preventive health and dietary change: A policy to increase the health divide. *Journal of Social Policy, 18*, 167–185.

Yetley, E. A., Yetley, M. J., & Aquirre, B. (1981). Family role structure and food-related roles in Mexican-American families. *Journal of Nutrition Education, 13*(Supplement), S96–S101.

10

Family Health Cognitions

David S. Gochman

THE DOMAIN
OF HEALTH COGNITIONS

The term *cognition* denotes the "personal thought processes that serve as frames of reference for organizing and evaluating experiences. Beliefs, expectations, perceptions, values, motives, and attitudes all provide the person with ways of filtering, interpreting, understanding, and predicting events" (Gochman, 1988b, p. 21). The term *health cognitions* refers to beliefs, expectations, perceptions, values, motives, and attitudes that provide frames of reference for organizing and evaluating health, illness, disease, and sickness regardless of whether those cognitions have demonstrable empirical linkages with health status and regardless of whether they are objectively valid.

The domain of this chapter, family health cognitions, comprises those health cognitions that have relevance for a family. Such cognitions include beliefs and perceptions about illnesses and health procedures involving a family member and behavioral expectations for a family or

David S. Gochman • Kent School of Social Work, University of Louisville, Louisville, Kentucky 40292.

Handbook of Health Behavior Research I: Personal and Social Determinants, edited by David S. Gochman. Plenum Press, New York, 1997.

one of its members in relation to maintaining health or avoiding or coping with illness. To maintain a focus on the family, the chapter does not discuss those cognitions either in children and adolescents or in cohorts of persons identified as parents, mothers, or fathers that have no reference to family.

The chapter begins with a review of what is known about health cognitions of family members, parental role dimensions related to health cognitions, and the impact of family health cognitions on health actions, i.e., how such cognitions determine or relate to health activities. The chapter continues with a discussion of what is known about family determinants of children's health cognitions, identifies research and methodological issues, and concludes with an agenda for future research.

FAMILY HEALTH COGNITIONS

Discussion and evaluation of work on health cognitions of family members through the early 1980s are available elsewhere (e.g., Baranowski & Nader, 1985; Gochman, 1985, 1988a). More recent studies can be organized around beliefs about conditions and treatment (e.g., beliefs about the causes of cancer or asthma), role dimensions (e.g., a mother's involvement in work activity), and the impact of cognitions on other behaviors (e.g., parent's illness beliefs upon immunizations).

Beliefs about Conditions and Interventions

Cognitions related to conditions and treatment include general beliefs related to health and illness, as well as beliefs about specific conditions. The specific conditions discussed are cancer, asthma, and diarrhea. The interventions are oral rehydration therapy (discussed along with diarrhea) and immunizations. (Although a later section deals explicitly with the impact of family health cognitions, i.e., with the way they determine other health actions, material in this section combines description with some data on impact, since the nature of the literature makes it more sensible to do this.)

Beliefs about Health and Illness. The illness of a hospitalized child generates parental perceptions of uncertainty. These perceptions contain ambiguity, lack of clarity, lack of information, and unpredictabilty (Mishel, 1983), which result from the novelty and complexity of medical technology, inadequate communication from physicians and nurses, and unknown prognoses. Parents who judged their child to be more seriously ill were observed to have higher levels of perceived uncertainty than those who judged their child to be less seriously ill (Mishel, 1983).

Families vary greatly in their responses to illness, reflecting the degree of "fit" between the demands of an illness, particularly chronic illness, and a family's history, traditions, values, rituals, and resources (Jacobs, 1992). Family perceptions of whether the illness is a burden or an invasion reflect the predictability, disability, and stigma of the illness, as well as its intrusion on the family's autonomous functioning, role structures, space and generational boundaries, and communication (Jacobs, 1992).

Complementing these relatively complex conceptual structures is a simple narrative of how Zulu mothers define their children's health (Craig & Albino, 1982). Interview data revealed that their criteria for health were eating and playing behaviors, a sick baby being one who does not eat or play.

Cancer. Parents of children with acute lymphoblastic leukemia were found to have many theories of the cause of the disease. For example, interview data from an Australian sample revealed that more than half believed that it was environmentally determined; other parents believed that a previous infection caused it (McWhirter & Kirk, 1986).

In Saudi Arabia, where cancer is perceived as a "sly disease," commonly thought to be fatal, and considered to be a taboo subject, most parents of children with cancer had an adequate, "biomedically valid" understanding about their child's cancer (Bahakim, 1987). They also believed, however, that the future, i.e., the prognosis, was "in the hands of Allah" and thus took few initiatives in finding out more about treatment alternatives. Given these findings, Bahakim (1987) urged health professionals providing care for this population to take initiatives themselves in suggesting treatment procedures to parents.

Asthma. Having a child with an asthmatic condition does not necessarily have an appreciable impact on parental health beliefs. The parents of asthmatic children in an Australian sample differed from controls only in having higher levels of belief in an allergic etiology for the condition (Spykerboer, Donnelly, & Thong, 1986). They also had less negative, less pessimistic views of asthma (Donnelly, Donnelly, & Thong, 1987). The two groups of parents did not differ on other variables, and two thirds of both groups had surprisingly high levels of knowledge about asthma.

Diarrhea and Oral Rehydration Therapy. High morbidity and mortality rates from diarrhea in developing countries have stimulated efforts to understand parental beliefs about this condition in the hopes of increasing acceptance of therapies and thus of decreasing the toll from diarrhea. A number of these studies have focused on oral rehydration therapy (ORT). Interviews with a random sample of Haitian mothers showed that despite a diversity of beliefs about diarrhea, its causes, etiology, and treatment, more than two thirds of the respondents were knowledgeable about the therapy, and these respondents tended to be more urban than rural (Coreil & Genece, 1988). Although knowledge of ORT was not directly related to whether it was used, it was related to using it in the recommended way, as well as to delay in starting the therapy; mothers who were knowledgeable about ORT waited until sufficient water loss had occurred before they initiated ORT. The interviews further revealed that folk beliefs about diarrhea may be less potent than had been thought and did not uniformly dictate use or nonuse of ORT.

Folk beliefs often allow for contradictions and inconsistencies. For instance, mothers in Swaziland who were patients of traditional healers generally shared the traditional healers' beliefs that diarrhea is caused by sorcery or ancestral displeasure (Green, 1985). A minority, however, would nevertheless take a child to a clinic first, and then to the traditional healer if the clinic treatment was ineffective. Mothers responding to a survey in Ethiopia similarly held "supernatural" beliefs. Many of them believed that diarrhea was caused by the "will of God" or sorcery (Sircar & Dagnow, 1988). Despite such beliefs, more than two thirds of these mothers used modern medical care and ORT. In contrast, mothers in rural Pakistan revealed in interviews that they believed diarrhea was a natural condition that did not require treatment (Mull & Mull, 1988).

Immunizations. Cognitions related to immunization are a critical area for study because there are inappropriately low levels of children's immunizations in both developed and developing countries. For example, interviews in Gazankulu, South Africa, showed that most mothers consider measles to be natural and "essential for

the normal development of their children" (Ijsselmuiden, 1983, p. 361). Yet these mothers seek the "injection" primarily because they believe it to hasten the rash, the early appearance of which they believe is related to a better outcome. They apparently favor vaccination even though they do not understand it and do not perceive it in terms of prevention. In Ghana, mothers who perceive that the effects of childhood diseases are not very severe and who perceive no benefits in immunization are less likely to participate in measles, tuberculosis, and polio immunizations than mothers who perceive greater severity and greater benefits (Fosu, 1991). Moreover, mothers who have higher levels of beliefs in external control or luck are *more* likely to participate in tuberculosis immunization programs than mothers with higher levels of internal control. Fosu (1991) suggested that this tendency may be related to the strong sanctions against people with communicable diseases like tuberculosis and leprosy in traditional societies, the inference being that higher levels of concern about these sanctions may be associated with belief in external forces and luck. Fosu also noted how perceptions of a child's health status were also related to participation in immunization programs; mothers who perceived their child's health as poor tended to stay away, possibly perceiving no preventive benefits for a child who was already sick or believing that the immunization might worsen the child's condition.

Parental beliefs about the efficacy of immunizations were also found to be unrelated to immunization of the children of Philippine villagers (Friede, Waternaux, Guyer, De Jesus, & Filipp, 1985). Parents who were more active in the communal life of their villages, however, were more likely to have their children immunized. The importance of "valid" cognitions as determinants of health actions is thus open to question.

Paradoxically, some of the more negative assessments of immunizations are found in developed countries. Many mothers, in a random sample in the outskirts of Milan, believed that children must get measles and pertussis as part of their natural development (Profeta, Lecchi, De-Donato, & Fraizzoli, 1989). Complementing this finding, more than a quarter of a random sample of Irish parents would not have their children vaccinated against measles; a number of them believed that the natural illness was better than the vaccine (Sze-Tho & Gill, 1982). These observations suggest that health professionals need to know more about what a target population actually perceives or believes rather than simply making assumptions about such beliefs. Such knowledge may lead toward increasing acceptance of these procedures.

Parental Role Dimensions

Role dimensions related to family health cognitions embrace both the broader and more traditional aspects of parental roles, such as the work role of the mother, and newer role conceptions, such as the role of parents as health educators. There are few studies reported in this area, but these studies are more often derived from conceptual frameworks than are studies in other areas.

Role dimensions relevant to mothers' beliefs about the quality of health services, and to their perceptions of a child's illness and needs for treatment, were examined in a field study in which single, working Canadian mothers were interviewed (Semchuk & Eakin, 1989). Concepts such as role conflict—between the roles of "good mother" (nurturing responsibilities) and "good worker" (work responsibilities)—and role flexibility (ability to alter schedules to meet emergencies) were found to be related to health cognitions. Mothers who experienced greater conflict between these roles tended to perceive their children's illnesses as more stressful than mothers who experienced less conflict. Those with little role flexibility used services they perceived as less "trusted," such as hospital emergency rooms, while those with greater role flexibility used services that were more "trusted," such as family physicians and pediatricians. Maternal working conditions can thus be seen to be

related to whether a child's condition is perceived as a crisis and to what type of care will be sought.

An injury belief model (Peterson, Farmer, & Kashani, 1990) integrated variables such as a child's injury history, how much parents worried about injuries, their expectatons that the child would be injured, and their beliefs that injuries were preventable. Parents' knowledge about safety skills, their beliefs in their own competence to teach these skills, their confidence in the efficacy of their efforts to teach these skills, and their beliefs that teaching safety skills can prevent injury were found to be effective predictors of the degree of parental teaching about injury prevention (Peterson et al., 1990).

Impact of Cognitions

The impact of of family health cognitions can be considered in terms of use of services, personal health actions, children's health behaviors, and health policies. Much of the work in this area is derived from the health belief model (e.g., Kirscht, 1988) or models of locus of control (e.g., Lau, 1988). These are two major conceptual frameworks for predicting health actions from health cognitions. The health belief model (from which the injury belief model discussed earlier is derived) emphasizes the role of a cluster of cognitions: perceptions of vulnerability to health problems, perceptions of the severity or seriousness of those problems, perceptions of the efficacy of actions taken to prevent or control these problems, and perceptions of barriers and costs in taking such actions. These perceptions are used to predict a variety of preventive, illness, and sick role behaviors such as getting routine medical checkups and acceptance of medical regimens (e.g., Kirscht, 1988; Strecher, Champion, & Rosenstock, Chapter 4, in this volume).

Locus of control models (e.g., Reich, Erdal, & Zautra, Chapter 5, in this volume) emphasize how persons perceive themselves as being in control over events in their lives (internal locus of control) as opposed to perceiving that things that happen to them are capricious or subject to control by others (external locus of control). By itself, the locus of control concept has been less consistent in explaining health activities (e.g., Lau, 1988) than the health belief model.

Use of Services. High agreement was observed between parents' and physician's perceptions of levels of urgency in relation to use of pediatric emergency services by a representative cross section of patients admitted to the Emergency Department at Minneapolis Children's Medical Center (Braunstein, Abanobi, & Goldhagen, 1987). Other data obtained in the self-administered questionnaire and structured interviews of this study indicated, however, that there was also agreement that most visits to such services were not urgent. Use of the emergency service was apparently not determined by a parental perception of pediatric medical emergency.

In contrast, parents' beliefs in the efficacy of therapy for otitis media (middle ear infection) and their general health motivation were related to their appointment keeping for their children with otitis media in a walk-in clinic at Children's Hospital in Philadelphia (Casey, Rosen, Glowasky, & Ludwig, 1985). Furthermore, a sample of mothers of infants from both low-income and middle-income families demonstrated that mothers who believed in their own control over their children's health were more likely to take their children for timely well-baby examinations and to have their children immunized (Tinsley & Holtgrave, 1989). On the basis of the Parental Health Beliefs scales, which were designed to examine mothers' perceptions of internal control with respect to their children's health, and mothers' beliefs that chance or powerful others affected their children's health, this study also showed that degrees of belief in chance or powerful others did not predict these examination and immunization outcomes. Somewhat in contrast, whereas mothers' perceptions of their children's health status predicted use of a prepaid pediatric service, other maternal cognitions, such as health locus of control, attitudes toward

health providers, and satisfaction with pediatric care, bore no relationship to use of the service (Horwitz, Morgenstern, & Berkman, 1988)

In a study of health belief model variables in a high-risk population, mothers' health cognitions, such as their beliefs in their children's susceptibility to health problems, in the severity of those problems, and in the benefits and effectiveness of well-baby services services, did not predict use of well-baby services as such. These factors did predict, however, having a child immunized (Kviz, Dawkins, & Ervin, 1985). Beliefs in the efficacy of the immunizations were found to be the most important predictors.

A survey of Iowa parents' attitudes toward dental disease in preschool children revealed that 89% did not think that preschoolers would have dental problems and thus did not see the need for preschool dental care (Walker, Beck, & Jakobsen, 1984). Finally, observations of a sample of mothers in Scotland showed the existence of skeptical beliefs concerning proprietary medicines, together with varied attitudes about the role of pharmacists. These cognitions often led to use of the pharmacist as an alternative to the physician or as a first step toward later physician use in primary health care for children with minor complaints (Cunningham-Burley & MacLean, 1987)

Although cultural factors are implicit in some of the preceding discussions of cognitions about diarrhea, cancer, and immunizations in developing countries, the issue of cultural differences was not addressed directly. Few studies do so. In a study that did deal explicitly with cultural differences as such, Canadian families from English backgrounds were found to emphasize "normalization" of a child with a disability, i.e., they preferred that the child not stand out as being different. They were thus more likely to accept advice from health professionals that encouraged rehabilitation. In contrast, Canadian families from Chinese backgrounds apparently accepted the nonnormality on its own terms and emphasized the child's "contentment" or "happiness," thus risking a clash with health professionals who wanted to "push" the disabled child and did not want to accept the child's differences. These families were less inclined to perceive the benefits of rehabilitation (Anderson & Chung, 1982).

Personal Health Actions. A survey of a random sample of Maryland parents with children under 5 found that the best predictors of intention to use car safety seats were parental beliefs about the children's comfort and resistance and about wasting time (Gielen, Eriksen, Daltroy, & Rost, 1984). Use of child restraints in automobiles was found to be linked to adult beliefs about their relative benefits and costs, in a questionnaire survey of occupants of motor vehicles in Australia (Webb, Sanson-Fisher, & Bowman, 1988). Parents who used a restraint were more likely to believe they could afford one, that restraints were a safety factor, and that they could prevent injuries, and less likely to believe that restraints were a nuisance or bother. Parents of unrestrained children were more likely to believe they could prevent injuries by carrying their children on their laps.

Children's Health Behaviors. Parental beliefs were related to fluoride tablet use in a sample of Swedish preschool children (Widenheim, 1982). When parents believed that swallowing the tablets was dangerous, their children were likely not to take them. Overall, parents weigh the benefits that health educators emphasize but also consider costs that are based on both personal experience and unwarranted assumptions.

Mothers' beliefs about dental health seemed to be unrelated either to their children's toothbrushing behavior or preventive dental visits (Chen, 1986) or to their children's use of fluoride tablets in a Danish sample (Friis-Hasche et al., 1984). Mothers' beliefs about the seriousness of dental disease, however, did predict children's flossing behaviors (Chen, 1986). It was suggested (Chen, 1986) that although mothers rarely communicate beliefs orally to children, or influence them through "cognitive mediation," mothers' behaviors may be more visible to children and thus more a determinant of the children's behavior.

Health Policy. About 90% of mothers surveyed in New Zealand held strong positive attitudes about legislating the use of car seat restraints and mandating pool fencing, yet fewer than half believed in legislating fluoridation (Fergusson, Horwood, & Shannon, 1983). One reason for this paradox is that the community surveyed had strong antifluoridation sentiments.

In a study with more experimental manipulation than most of those reported in this chapter, a sample of socially deprived mothers of nursery-school children in Scotland were asked about attitudes toward a hypothetical vaccine as well as their attitudes toward tooth loss and preventive care (Kay & Blinkhorn, 1989). Levels of the vaccine's effectiveness and safety were systematically varied throughout the sample. Variation in the vaccine's risk was found to have a greater impact on its acceptability than variation in the degree of protection it afforded. Moreover, mothers had more positive attitudes toward a vaccine than to fluoridation, suggesting that parents want to have a role in determining their children's own health future. The data also revealed a skepticism about biomedical technology.

Summary

Although a few of the studies reviewed reflect conceptual frameworks or derive from hypotheses, the far greater number do not. While one can abstract to some degree from their findings, generalizations are at best limited.

Studies that dealt with beliefs about health and illness revealed an appreciable amount of diversity within cultural and subcultural groups, as well as complexity and heterogeneity. In developed, industrialized societies as well as in less industrialized, developing ones, family cognitions about diseases reflect interwinings of folk beliefs with beliefs that are congruent with, or derived from, biomedical technology. Moreover, the existence of folk beliefs is not necessarily a barrier toward acceptance of scientific, biomedically valid technologies.

There is little convincing evidence that family health cognitions have important impacts on use of health services, personal health actions, or health policy. Moreover, neither of the two basic conceptual models that underlie much research on family health cognitions—the health belief model and the locus of control model—has proven to be an unequivocally strong predictor of health actions.

FAMILY DETERMINANTS OF CHILDREN'S HEALTH COGNITIONS

While the family is presumed to be a major determinant of health cognitions, literature reviews (e.g., Bush & Iannotti, 1990; Lau, Quadrel, & Hartman, 1990) continue to affirm earlier assessments (e.g., Baranowski & Nader, 1985; Gochman, 1985, 1988c) that knowledge about relationships between family characteristics and children's health cognitions is virtually nonexistent. Baranowski and Nader (1985) described this relationship as "almost ignored" (p. 53). Whatever knowledge of such intergenerational linkages is available can be discussed under headings of parent characteristics and child cognitions and parent cognitions and child cognitions.

Parent Characteristics and Child Cognitions

Father's occupation was related to the validity of youngsters' beliefs about heart disease and nutrition in a Texas sample (Burdine, Chen, Gottlieb, Peterson, & Vacalis, 1984). Students whose fathers had professional or managerial positions scored highest in nutritional knowledge.

Parents' smoking behaviors generally were found to have no effect on children's beliefs about smoking, with the exception that those whose parents smoked were more likely to disagree that smoking "stops you feeling tired" or "makes you out of breath" and more likely to agree that smoking makes your teeth yellow (Eiser, Walsh, & Eiser, 1986). In contrast to parental beliefs, however, parents' smoking behaviors did have impact on youngsters maintaining nonsmoking, once they self-initiated smoking cessa-

tion (Hansen, Collins, Johnson, & Graham, 1985). In addition, parental attitudes toward smoking and their smoking behaviors have an interactive effect on the likelihood that their youngsters would smoke (Newman & Ward, 1989). When parents themselves smoked, their negative attitudes toward smoking—as these attitudes were perceived by their children—had significant impact on increasing adolescent nonsmoking. The adolescent children of nonsmoking parents with indifferent attitudes were about as likely to smoke as those of smoking parents who disapproved of smoking. Parental cognitions in this case were more important predictors of adolescent smoking than was parental behavior.

Intactness of family structure, as measured by the presence of both parents in a home, in comparison to the absence of at least one parent, was related to youngsters' expectations that parents would be upset if they smoked, that smoking was a health problem, and that they would ask permission to smoke (Nolte, Smith, & O'Rourke, 1983). Moreover, parental presence decreased the likelihood of youngsters' believing that friends and family enjoyed smoking.

The importance of intact family structure, along with family characteristics such as parental intellectual ability and socialization techniques, was found to have an impact on children's illness orientations, such as the "correctness" of their beliefs about illness and doctors and their faking of illness (Lau & Klepper, 1988). Brokenness of families, families' use of punishment as a socialization technique, and lower parental intellectual ability were observed to be determinants of less appropriate illness orientations in children. Moreover, the children's self-esteem was found to be the important mediating linkage between these family factors and such illness orientations.

Parent Cognitions and Child Cognitions

Beliefs about Health and Illness. Linkages were observed between caregiver and child cognitions in relation to concerns about illness, attributions of illness, perceptions of vulnerability, perceptions of severity, health locus of control, and attitudes toward health-related risk behaviors among schoolchildren in the District of Columbia; no linkages were observed, however, for perceptions of health status, medicine use, or the perceived medical and nonmedical benefits of medicine use (Bush & Iannotti, 1988). Moreover, while the youngsters' cognitions were observed to be relatively stable, older childrens' beliefs were closer to the beliefs of their caregivers than were the beliefs of younger children on several variables, suggesting a possible, albeit weak, developmental effect.

Parents' beliefs about the efficacy of exercise, diet, nonconsumption of alcohol, and seat belt usage were appreciably related to the beliefs of their university-student children (Lau et al., 1990). Further, health education priorities of pupils in urban, coeducational black, Indian, and white primary schools in Pretoria and Cape Town, South Africa, were found to be related to those of their parents and teachers (Ross & Van der Merwe, 1983).

On the other hand, no relationship between mothers' and children's beliefs was observed for any dimension of the Parcel and Meyer Health Locus of Control scale (Perrin & Shapiro, 1985). Mothers of children with chronic conditions, however, were lower on internality and higher in beliefs about powerful others than mothers of healthy children. No linkages were observed in a Texas sample between parents' nutritional beliefs and children's beliefs (Touliatos, Lindholm, Wenberg, & Ryan, 1984).

Specific Conditions and Interventions. A group of New Zealand female anorexia nervosa patients and their mothers had more positive evaluations of sickness and pain and more negative evaluations of thinness than did a control, nonpatient–mother group (Hall & Brown, 1983). Although this study did not directly relate mother and daughter cognitions, it pointed to familial similarities in beliefs related to anoretic conditions.

More direct mother–daughter linkages were observed in other studies. Females with idiopathic scoliosis evaluated other people with scoliosis similarly to the way their mothers evaluated them (Kahanovitz & Weiser, 1989). Mothers and daughters were also observed to have relatively similar beliefs about menstruation (Stolzman, 1986). Daughters, however, were more similar to their friends on some of the menstrual attitudes and beliefs than they were to their mothers, suggesting the importance of social and peer influences on these cognitions.

Somewhat in contrast, Scottish families showed less intergenerational influence than might have been expected. Data from three generations—children, mothers, and grandmothers—showed that grandmothers' cognitions regarding health-related child care influenced maternal behavior to a minimal degree and that there was little intergenerational similarity in cognitions related to health and use of health services (Blaxter & Paterson, 1982).

Asthmatic children and their mothers in a large western Pennsylvania metropolitan area were found to have significantly similar perceptions of prognosis, level of chest pain, and breathing difficulty related to asthmatic attacks, but the study found no intergenerational relationships with respect to thoughts about threats of asthma to the children's lives (Khampalikit, 1983). Children and mothers were found to have similar but more moderately linked beliefs about impact of asthma on social life.

High levels of "intrafamilial transmission," a concept denoting the degree to which a family member and a child or adolescent with cancer have similar cancer-related conceptions, were found among children and adolescents with cancer as well as a family member (usually the mother). High degrees of intrafamilial correlation were observed for knowledge about cancer, for expectations of a future that generated enthusiasm, for levels of reality in perceptions of the future, and for expectations about resumption of social activities on leaving the hospital (Susman et al., 1982).

The only positive linkage found in a sample

of obese youngsters and their parents was between parental and child beliefs about the threat of obesity (Uzark, Becker, Dielman, Rocchini, & Katch, 1988). Negative linkages were found between the children's beliefs about the threat of obesity and parents' perceptions of personal control and between the children's perception of personal control over weight and parents' perceptions of barriers or difficulty in weight reduction. Children believed that they had less control to the degree that their parents perceived greater difficulty in managing weight. Parents' and children's attributions of obesity were related in four cases, lack of exercise, family problems, nervous tension, and medical problems, but they were not related in seven other areas.

Yet linkages were not generally observed between parents' and their children's perceptions of seriousness, susceptibility, and efficacy in relation to dental disease and its treatment, except for beliefs in luck, fate, or chance (Cipes, 1985). Parents who believed that dental disease was serious, however, had children who believed in the efficacy of tooth brushing. Moreover, very little correlation was found between parents' own perceptions and their perceptions of parallel beliefs in their child.

In contrast to these reports of linkages— albeit sometimes modest linkages—between parent and child cognitions, significant disparities were found between the perceptions of pediatric outpatients at a tumor institute and those of their parents about the amount of choice available in relation to tests and treatment, the helpfulness of additional information, and the effects on the condition of alcohol, smoking, and drugs (Levenson, Copeland, Morrow, Pfefferbaum, & Silberberg, 1983). Parents nearly always attributed greater importance to these dimensions than did their children.

Summary

Relatively few studies have attempted to demonstrate relationships between health cognitions and other family characteristics or between specific cognitions and others. As a result, there is only spotty evidence pointing to any such relationships. Health cognitions in families can be seen to have only very limited relationships either to parental characteristics, to health actions, or to one another. To the degree that these limited findings permit generalizations, family intactness, i.e., the presence of both parents (caretakers) in a family, is one characteristic that has some importance in determining youngster's health cognitions, particularly those related to smoking (Nolte et al., 1983) and more general beliefs about health and illness (Lau & Klepper, 1988). Otherwise, no consistent patterns or coherent relationships are observed.

Sallis and Nader (1988) noted the paucity of documentation of mechanisms of family influence. Moreover, Dielman, Leech, Becker, Rosenstock, and Horvath (1982), noting that studies relating parents' and youngsters' health beliefs have been "relatively rare," were unable in their own investigation to demonstrate any relationships. They asserted, "Child health beliefs are scarcely influenced by parental characteristics" (p. 63). In the intervening years, there has been insufficient study either to confirm or to refute their assertion.

RESEARCH AND METHODOLOGICAL ISSUES

Evaluation of Knowledge

Lack of a Coherent Corpus. At the mid-1990s, knowledge about family cognitions permits little meaningful generalization. The preceding narrative is a "laundry list"—a pastiche rather than a mosaic. The lack of a coherent corpus of research precludes even a pedestrian evaluation, except in the most superficial terms, of method, nature, size of sample, and such. In terms of a sociology of knowledge (e.g., Hayes-Bautista, 1978), at the mid-1990s, data-based knowledge of family health cognitions is lacking in depth, coherence, and organization. It reflects minimal effort at broadening samples and, with a few notable exceptions (e.g., Bush & Iannotti, 1990; Lau et al., 1990), rare focused replications that build upon prior research or specific theoretical or conceptual models.

The research presented here still is largely exploratory, descriptive, and essentially atheoretical and nonconceptual. Although relationships have been shown to exist between some parental cognitions and use of selected health services for children, very little can be said about parental cognitions and child health behaviors or child health cognitions. Even in areas in which some knowledge exists, there is an urgent need for systematic expansion. There remains a consensus that little is known about health cognitions in families (e.g., Bush & Iannotti, 1988; Lau et al., 1990) or about the mechanisms by which they are transmitted among family members (e.g., Sallis & Nader, 1988).

Clinical or Applied Characteristics.   Much of this research appears to be driven by clinical or applied interests, e.g., the need to assess, develop, or improve service delivery (e.g., Walker et al., 1984). These concerns are legitimate and important, but they do not lead to systematic development of a coherent body of knowledge.

Promising Concepts and Directions

A small number of systematic studies on cognitions about specific conditions, particularly asthma and cancer (e.g., Perrin & Shapiro, 1985; Susman et al., 1982), offer promise of movement toward an increase in consistent, coherent understanding of how families perceive and evaluate these conditions and their treatment. Equally important from the perspective of increasing generalizable knowledge, a small number of research programs (e.g., Bush & Iannotti, 1988; Lau & Klepper, 1988; Lau et al., 1990) are moving toward complex and thoughtful integrations of conceptual frameworks and away from single-model approaches, such as the health belief model or the locus of control model.

Simultaneously, there is movement toward testing hypotheses with greater specificity that compare the relative merits of conceptual models. Lau et al. (1990) proposed the *enduring family socialization* model, which suggests that health cognitions are learned within the family during childhood, that parents have primary influence on these cognitions, and that the cognitions remain stable throughout adulthood. They also propose a complementary yet contrasting *lifelong openness* model, which suggests that health cognitions are influenced by several socialization agents and change throughout the life cycle. Each of these models integrates developmental concepts, such as life cycle and socialization within the family, with health behavior concepts. Longitudinal data provide limited support for each of these models and have led to the development of a *windows of vulnerability* model that suggests that parental influence will continue unless and until the youngster experiences other potent socializing agents during critical developmental periods (Lau et al., 1990).

The concept of *consumerism* in family decision making, referring to family cognitions involving physician authority, skepticism of medicine in general as well as of physicians' competence, and physician altruism, had been expected to be related to care-seeking decisions, particularly to decisions to enter HMOs. Data, however, did not show such a linkage (Monroe, 1993).

Conceptualization of the Family

It is possible that the lack of a coherent body of knowledge reflects an unfortunate combination of inadequate conceptualizations of the family, together with a very small number of studies conducted in this area. Research has seldom looked at the family as an entity or unit, i.e., as a social group or social system. More often than not, research has considered the family solely in terms of some personal or demographic characteristic of one or both parents or in terms of its size.

Family Health Culture: Do Family Health Cognitions Exist? Black (1985) used the concept of *family health culture* to refer to the unique combination of family experiences, beliefs, perceptions of symptoms, and reactions to them, which apparently influences the way in which families seek care or treatment for their children. At the same time, Black raised questions about whether such family health cultures are homogeneous. Jacobs's (1992) clinical observations of family responses to illness imply a degree of normativeness within families about values and about beliefs regarding family history, ritual, and traditions, but nonclinical data about such normativeness are scarce.

It is likely that even within the family unit, mothers, fathers, and children have different beliefs and attitudes. It may not matter how one conceptualizes the family if there is no consensus about health-related cognitions within a family unit. The absence of observed intergenerational linkages may be accounted for less by the manner of inquiry than by the nature of the phenomenon. In the absence of any body of rigorous data, it is premature to conjecture on the question of family health culture.

Measurement Issues

There are few widely accepted standardized instruments used in family health behavior research. Promising approaches to measuring (and conceptualizing) the family as a social unit have begun to appear in the literature. Focusing on family use of health services, a Family Utilization Index (Schor, Starfield, Stidley, & Hankin, 1987) takes rates of individual family members' use of different types of care—acute, chronic, psychiatric, and nonillness care—to construct average usage rates for families. This index is then used to determine variability in usage both within and between families. Individual usage can then be examined to see how much of it is determined by family patterns or norms. The index may be seen as a paradigm for assessing the degree to which

cognitions within a family are consistent, i.e., normative.

The concept of *intrafamilial transmission*, referring to the degree of shared or similar conceptions about cancer within a family, and a related concept, *interfamily consensus*, referring to the degree of such shared conceptions in randomly selected pairs (Susman et al., 1982), can be used to develop measures of the degree of family consensus on cognitions related to other conditions, as well as to a broader range of health issues. Sallis and Nader (1988) proposed the concept of *family aggregation* to denote intrafamilial similarities in health variables compared to nonfamily similarities. This concept has also become the basis for correlational assessment of family consensus.

AN AGENDA FOR FUTURE RESEARCH

A future research agenda for health cognitions in families would assign priority to exploring the origins and development of health cognitions, sharpening the conceptualization of the family, and approaching the topic from a perspective that emphasizes basic research.

Origins and Development of Health Cognitions

Literature reviews summarizing and evaluating the increasing body of work on health cognitions in young populations (e.g., Burbach & Peterson, 1986; Gochman, 1985, 1992; Kalnins & Love, 1982; Lau & Klepper, 1988) confirmed that nearly all of this work has been conducted without reference to family context. Virtually nothing is known of the determinants even of those cognitions such as perceived vulnerability and locus of control that have been most frequently studied in younger populations. An enormous gap thus exists in knowledge about the determinants of these health cognitions, particularly those determinants that involve the family.

Coupled with the need for greater knowl-

edge and understanding about the origins of
health cognitions is the need for greater knowledge and understanding about how they develop, about their developmental changes, and
about possible differential patterns related to
other personal, family, and social characteristics.
The dearth of well-conducted, rigorous research
in this area has been noted repeatedly (e.g., Bush
& Iannotti, 1988; Gochman, 1985, 1988a,c, 1992;
Kalnins & Love, 1982; Lau & Klepper, 1988).

Questions arise about the importance of a
range of family factors, including, but not limited
to, parental health cognitions, family size, structure, role relationships, methods of child rearing,
access to resources, health history, and linkages
to the larger community. Moreover, the relative
importance of family factors in the origins and
development of such cognitions needs to be
compared with the impact of friendship and peer
groups, social relationships, and societal and cultural values and institutions. Basic research into
the origins of family health cognitions and how
they develop is thus a major challenge for the
future and leads directly to the second area identified for future research—the family conceptualized as a social unit.

The Family as a Social Unit

Future research into health cognitions should
examine the family in terms of its characteristics
as an integral social unit. Important family characteristics such as role structure, norms, values,
and patterns of communication are critical areas
for future investigation. Pratt's (1976) conception of the *energized family* is one of the few
extant conceptual models that consider the family in this way, and studies based on her model, or
similarly coherent ones, are sorely needed. The
energized family is one in which members demonstrate regular interaction with one another and
attempt to cope and to master their lives. Energized families show fluidity in internal organization, sharing of power, flexibility in role relationships, and concern for and support of the growth
of family members (Pratt, 1976, pp. 3–4).

The Family and Larger Social Units. Energized families also maintain contacts with the
community to advance the interests of their
members. Family linkages with larger social units
such as friendship networks, and the community
and its institutions, had been a focus for research
through the early 1980s (reviewed elsewhere
[e.g., Gochman, 1985]), much of which related
family use of health services and other overt
health behaviors—health cognitions among
them—to characteristics of communities and society. Finding such community linkages to be
related to immunizations (Friede et al., 1985)
reaffirms the need to look beyond the family itself
for increasing understanding of a range of health-
related behavior. The family needs to be conceptualized as an integral social unit embedded in a
context of other such units.

Health Cognitions in Families as a Basic Research Focus

Laudable pragmatic objectives underlie almost all of the studies discussed in this chapter
and a good deal of other research on health-
related behaviors. These objectives include—but
are not limited to—increasing timely use of
a health service, increasing population immu-
nities, reducing family distress caused by illness,
raising consciousness about care and treatment,
reducing individual behaviors that are risk factors for illness, and making health educational
programs more effective. When such pragmatic
objectives are the primary driving forces in the
research process, however, they are likely to impede the development of data that lend themselves to generalizations, to building a body of
scientific knowledge, and to answering basic research questions.

One way of increasing the likelihood that
future research, including the research agenda
suggested in this section, will be scientifically
valuable, i.e., that it will generate a body of
knowledge that has depth, coherence, and organization and that broadens understanding and
increases generalizability, is to adopt a *health*

behavior research perspective. Such a perspective (e.g., Gochman, 1992) would begin with the premise that health cognitions in families are *interesting in their own right* and are inherently worthy of serious scientific investigation—and therefore ought to be the focus of some *basic* scientific activity. Basic health behavior research would thus complement research on risk-factor behavior and research on health interventions and programs. Health cognitions would then be looked upon in terms of their interrelationships, as well as how they are determined by a variety of diverse personal and social processes. The primary focus of research must be the behaviors—in this case family health-related cognitions—not the treatment or the health promotion package or the marketing attempt or the health education program; the behaviors, rather than the technology; the basics, rather than the applications.

SUMMARY

This chapter has identified some beginnings in understanding health cognitions in families and has evaluated existing knowledge in this area. Important future research directions have been suggested, particularly around the origins and development of health cognitions and the conceptualization of and role of the family. A "health behavior" perspective, emphasizing both basic research and interdisciplinary efforts, offers maximum promise of increasing knowledge of family health cognitions and of remedying gaps in this knowledge.

AUTHOR'S NOTE. This chapter represents a revision and reorganization of an earlier version that appeared under the title "Health Cognitions in Families" in *Family Health Psychology*, pp. 23–43, edited by T. J. Akamatsu, M. A. P. Stephens, S. E. Hobfoll, and J. H. Crowther and published by Hemisphere Press, a member of the Taylor & Francis Group, 1101 Vermont Avenue, N.W., Suite 200, Washington, D.C. 20005-3521, in 1992. Pas-

sages from that work are reproduced with the publisher's permission. All rights reserved.

REFERENCES

Anderson, J., & Chung, J. (1982). Culture and illness: Parents preceptions [sic] of their child's long term illness. *Nursing Papers, 14*, 40–52.

Bahakim, H. M. (1987). Muslim parents' perception of and attitude towards cancer. *Annals of Tropical Paediatrics, 7*, 22–26.

Baranowski, T., & Nader, P. R. (1985). Family health behavior, In D. C. Turk & R. D. Kerns (Eds.), *Health illness and families: A life-span perspective* (pp. 51–80). New York: Wiley.

Black, N. (1985). The "health culture" of families as an influence on the use of surgery for glue ear: A case–control study. *International Journal of Epidemiology, 14*, 594–599.

Blaxter, M., & Paterson, K. (1982) *Mothers and daughters: A three-generational study of health attitudes and behavior.* London: Heinemann.

Braunstein, J., Abanobi, O. C., & Goldhagen, J. L. (1987). Parental perception of urgency and utilization of pediatric emergency services. *Family Practice Research Journal, 6*, 130–137.

Burbach, D. J., & Peterson, L. (1986). Children's concepts of physical illness: A review and critique of the cognitive-developmental literature. *Health Psychology, 5*, 307–325.

Burdine, J. N., Chen, M. S., Gottlieb, N. H., Peterson, F. L., & Vacalis, T. D. (1984). The effects of ethnicity, sex and father's occupation on heart health knowledge and nutrition behavior of school childen: The Texas Youth Health Awareness Survey. *Journal of School Health, 54*, 87–90.

Bush, P. J., & Iannotti, R. J. (1988). Origins and stability of children's health beliefs relative to medicine use. *Social Science and Medicine, 27*, 345–352.

Bush, P. J., & Iannotti, R. J. (1990). A children's health belief model. *Medical Care, 28*, 69–86.

Casey, R., Rosen, B., Glowasky, A., & Ludwig, S. (1985). An intervention to improve follow-up of patients with otitis media. *Clinical Pediatrics, 24*, 149–152.

Chen, M.-S. (1986). Children's preventive dental behavior in relation to their mothers' socioeconomic status, health beliefs and dental behaviors. *Journal of Dentistry for Children, 53*, 105–109.

Cipes, M. H. (1985). Self-management versus parental involvement to increase children's compliance with home flouride mouthrinsing. *Pediatric Dentistry, 7*, 111–118.

Coreil, J., & Genece, E. (1988). Adoption of oral rehydration therapy among Haitian mothers. *Social Science and Medicine, 27*, 87–96.

Craig, A. P., & Albino, R. C. (1982). Urban Zulu mothers' views on the health and health care of their infants. *South African Medical Journal, 63*, 571–572.

Cunningham-Burley, S., & MacLean, U. (1987). The role of the chemist in primary health care for children with minor complaints. *Social Science and Medicine, 24*, 371–377.

Dielman, T. E., Leech, S. L., Becker, M. H., Rosenstock, I. M., & Horvath, W. J. (1982). Parental and child health beliefs and behavior. In D. S. Gochman & G. S. Parcel (Eds.), Children's health beliefs and health behaviors. *Health Education Quarterly, 9*, 60–77.

Donnelly, J. E., Donnelly, W. J., & Thong, Y. H. (1987). Parental peceptions and attitudes toward asthma and its treatment: A controlled study. *Social Science and Medicine, 24*, 431–437.

Eiser, C., Walsh, S., & Eiser J. R. (1986). Young childen's understanding of smoking. *Addictive Behaviors, 11*, 119–123.

Fergusson, D. M., Horwood, L. J., & Shannon, F. T. (1983). Attitudes of mothers of five-year-old children to compulsory child health provisions. *New Zealand Medical Journal, 96*, 338–340.

Fosu, G. B. (1991). Maternal influences on preventive health behavior in children. *International Quarterly of Community Health Education, 12*(1), 1–19.

Friede, A., Waternaux, C., Guyer, B., De Jesus, A., & Filipp, L. C. (1985). An epidemiological assessment of immunization programme participation in the Philippines. *International Journal of Epidemiology, 14*, 135–142.

Friis-Hasche, E., Bergmann, J., Wenzel, A., Thylstrup, A., Pedersen K., & Petersen, P. E. (1984). Dental health status and attitudes to dental care in families participating in a Danish flouride tablet program. *Community Dentistry and Oral Epidemiology, 12*, 303–307.

Gielen, A. C., Eriksen, M. P., Daltroy, L. H., & Rost, K. (1984). Factors associated with the use of child restraint devices. *Health Education Quarterly, 11*, 195–206.

Gochman, D. S. (1985). Family determinants of children's concepts of health and illness. In D. C. Turk & R. D. Kerns (Eds.), *Health, illness, and families: A life-span perspective* (pp. 23–50). New York: Wiley.

Gochman, D. S. (1988a). Assessing children's health concepts. In P. Karoly & C. May (Eds.), *Handbook of child health assessment: Biopsychosocial perspectives* (pp. 332–356). New York: Wiley.

Gochman, D. S. (Ed.) (1988b). *Health behavior: Emerging research perspectives*. New York: Plenum Press.

Gochman, D. S. (1988c). Health behavior: Present and future. In D. S. Gochman (Ed.), *Health behavior: Emerging research perspectives* (pp. 409–424). New York: Plenum Press.

Gochman, D. S. (1992). Here's looking at you kid! New ways of viewing the development of health cognitions. In E. J. Susman, L. V. Feagans, & W. J. Ray (Eds.), *Emotion, cognition, health and development in children and adolescents* (pp. 9–23). Hillsdale, NJ: Erlbaum.

Green, E. C. (1985). Traditional healers, mothers and childhood diarrheal disease in Swaziland: The interface of anthropology and health education. *Social Science and Medicine, 20*, 277–285.

Hall, A., & Brown, L. B. (1983). A comparison of the attitudes of young anorexia nervosa patients and non-patients with those of their mothers. *British Journal of Medical Psychology, 56*, 39–48.

Hansen, W. B., Collins, L. M., Johnson, C. A., & Graham, J. W. (1985). Self-initated smoking cessation among high school students. *Addictive Behaviors, 10*, 265–271.

Hayes-Bautista, D. E. (1978). Chicano patients and medical practitioners: A sociology of knowledge paradigm of lay-professional interaction. *Social Science and Medicine, 12*, 83–90.

Horwitz, S. M., Morgenstern, H., & Berkman, L. F. (1988). Factors affecting pediatric preventive care utilization in a prepaid group practice. *Pediatrician, 15*, 112–118.

Ijsselmuiden, C. B. (1983). Beliefs and practices concerning measles in Gazankulu. *South African Medical Journal, 63*, 360–362.

Jacobs, J. (1992). Understanding family factors that shape the impact of chronic illness. In T. J. Akamatsu, M. A. P. Stephens, S. E. Hobfoll, & J. H. Crowther (Eds.), *Family health psychology* (pp. 111–127). Washington, DC: Hemisphere.

Kahanovitz, N., & Weiser, S. (1989). The psychological impact of idiopathic scoliosis on the adolescent female: A preliminary multi-center study. *Spine, 14*, 483–485.

Kalnins, I., & Love, R. (1982). Children's concepts of health and illness—and implications for health education: An overview. In D. S. Gochman & G. S. Parcel (Eds.), Children's health beliefs and health behaviors. *Health Education Quarterly, 9*, 8–19.

Kay, E. J., & Blinkhorn, A. S. (1989). A study of mothers' attitudes towards the prevention of caries with particular reference to flouridation and vaccination. *Community Dental Health, 6*, 357–363.

Khampalikit, S. (1983). The interrelationships between the asthmatic child's depdency behavior, his perception of his illness, and his mother's perception of his illness. *Maternal-Child Nursing Journal, 12*, 221–296.

Kirscht, J. P. (1988). The health belief model and predictions of health actions. In D. S. Gochman (Ed.), *Health behavior: Emerging research perspectives* (pp. 27–41). New York: Plenum Press.

Kviz, F. J., Dawkins, C. E., & Ervin, N. E. (1985). Mothers' health beliefs and use of well-baby services among a high-risk population. *Research in Nursing and Health, 8*, 381–387.

Lau, R. R. (1988). Beliefs about control and health behavior. In D. S. Gochman (Ed.), *Health behavior: Emerging research perspectives* (pp. 43–63). New York: Plenum Press.

Lau, R. R., & Klepper, S. (1988). The development of illness orientations in children aged 6 through 12. *Journal of Health and Social Behavior, 29*, 149–168.

Lau, R. R., Quadrel, M. J., & Hartman, K. A. (1990). Development and change of young adults' preventive health beliefs and behavior: Influence from parents and peers. *Journal of Health and Social Behavior, 31,* 240-259.

Levenson, P. M., Copeland, D. R., Morrow, J. R., Pfefferbaum, B., & Silberberg, Y. (1983). Disparities in disease-related perceptions of adolescent cancer patients and their parents. *Journal of Pediatric Psychology, 8,* 33-45.

McWhirter, W. R., & Kirk, D. (1986). What causes childhood leukaemia? *Medical Journal of Australia, 145,* 314-316.

Mishel, M. H. (1983). Parents' perception of uncertainty concerning their hospitalized child. *Nursing Research, 32,* 324-330.

Monroe, P. A. (1993). Family health care decision making. *Journal of Family and Economic Issues, 14*(1), 7-25.

Mull, J. D., & Mull, D. S. (1988). Mothers' concepts of childhood diarrhea in rural Pakistan: What ORT program planners should know. *Social Science and Medicine, 27,* 53-67.

Newman, I. M., & Ward, J. M. (1989). The influence of parental attitude and behavior on early adolescent cigarette-smoking. *Journal of School Health, 59,* 150-152.

Nolte, A. E., Smith, B. J., & O'Rourke, T. (1983). The relationship between health risk attitudes and behaviors and parental presence. *Journal of School Health, 53,* 234-240.

Perrin, E. C., & Shapiro, E. (1985). Health locus of control beliefs of healthy children, children with a chronic physical illness, and their mothers. *Journal of Pediatrics, 107,* 627-633.

Peterson, L., Farmer, J., & Kashani, J. H. (1990). Parental injury prevention endeavors: A function of health beliefs? *Health Psychology, 9,* 177-191.

Pratt, L. (1976). *Family structure and effective health behavior: The energized family.* Boston: Houghton-Mifflin.

Profeta, M. L., Lecchi, G. M., DeDonato, S., & Fraizzoli, G. (1989). Inchièsta sulla applicazióne delle vaccinazióni contro la pertósse e contro il morbillo in una città dell'hinterland Milanese. *Annali de Igiène, Medicina Preventiva e de Communità, 1,* 1173-1184 [English summary].

Ross, M. H., & Van der Merwe, G. J. (1983). Health interests of schoolchildren, parents and teachers and their application to health education in primary schools. *Central African Journal of Medicine, 29,* 185-188.

Sallis, J. F., & Nader, P. R. (1988). Family determinants of health behavior. In D. S. Gochman (Ed.), *Health behavior: Emerging research perspectives* (pp. 107-124). New York: Plenum Press.

Schor, E., Starfield, B., Stidley, C., & Hankin, J. (1987). Family health: Utilization and effects of family membership. *Medical Care, 25,* 616-626.

Semchuck, K. M., & Eakin, J. M. (1989). Children's health and illness behaviour: The single working mother's perspective. *Canadian Journal of Public Health, 80,* 346-350.

Sircar, B. K., & Dagnow, M. B. (1988). Beliefs and practices related to diarrhoeal diseases among mothers in Gondar Region, Ethiopia. *Tropical and Geographical Medicine, 40,* 259-263.

Spykerboer, J. E., Donnelly, W. J., & Thong, Y. H. (1986). Parental knowledge and misconceptions about asthma: A controlled study. *Social Science and Medicine, 22,* 553-558.

Stoltzman, S. M. (1986). Menstrual attitudes, beliefs, and symptom experiences of adolescent females, their peers, and their mothers. *Health Care for Women International, 22,* 97-114.

Susman, E. J., Hersh, S. P., Nannis, E. D., Strope, B. E., Woodruff, P. J., Pizzo, P. A., & Levine, A. S. (1982). Conceptions of cancer: The perspectives of child and adolescent patients and their families. *Journal of Pediatric Psychology, 7,* 253-261.

Sze-Tho, R., & Gill, D. G. (1982). Measles virus and vaccination—A survey of parental attitudes. *Irish Medical Journal, 75,* 250-251.

Tinsley, B. J., & Holtgrave, D. R. (1989). Maternal health locus of control beliefs, utilization of childhood preventive health services, and infant health. *Journal of Dvelopmental and Behavioral Pediatrics, 10,* 236-241.

Touliatos, J., Lindholm, B. W., Wenberg, M. F., & Ryan, M. (1984). Family and child correlates of nutrition knowledge and dietary quality in 10-13 year olds. *Journal of School Health, 54,* 247-249.

Uzark, K. C., Becker, M. H., Dielman, T. E., Rocchini, A. P., & Katch, V. (1988). Perceptions held by obese children and their parents: Implications for weight control intervention. *Health Education Quarterly, 15,* 185-198.

Walker, J. D., Beck, J. D., & Jakobsen, J. (1984). Parental attitudes and dental disease in preschool children in Iowa. *Journal of Dentistry for Children, 51,* 141-145.

Webb, G. R., Sanson-Fisher, R. W., & Bowman, J. A. (1988). Psychosocial factors related to parental restraint of preschool chldren in motor vehicles. *Accident Analysis and Prevention, 20,* 87-94.

Widenheim, J. (1982). A time-related study of intake pattern of flouride tablets among Swedish preschoolchildren and parental attitudes. *Community Dentistry and Oral Epidemiology, 10,* 296-300.

11

Maternal Influences on Children's Health Behavior

Barbara J. Tinsley

Many health problems have their origins and potential solutions in behaviors developed in early childhood, in the context of families (Alexander, 1992). Parents are responsible for promoting children's wellness and ameliorating their illness, and parents provide the context within which children begin to develop patterns of health behavior (Tinsley, 1992b; Tinsley & Lees, 1995). An emerging focus of research on children's health is centered on how families socialize child health behavior and thereby affect child health status (Tinsley, 1992b; Tinsley & Lees, 1995). A variety of parental socialization antecedents have been identified as potential or demonstrated markers of both concurrent and predictive child health behavior and outcomes. These antecedents include many variables ranging from sociodemographic factors (e.g., social class, ethnicity), structural factors (e.g., family size, ordinal position), and systems characteristics (e.g., mother–child interaction patterns). This research area is

characterized, however, by a major limitation: insufficient attention to the delineation of the mechanisms by which these factors influence child health behavior and outcomes.

MOTHERS AS THE PRIMARY FAMILIAL HEALTH INFLUENCE ON CHILDREN

Mothers have assumed a dominant and pivotal role in performing health-related activities for all family members and for young children in particular (Carpenter, 1990). Studies suggest that although fathers are making modest gains in participating in child care in general (Parke, 1996), mothers continue to be assigned child health care responsibilities in the division of household labor. Several studies suggest that a substantial cause of women's work absenteeism is caregiving for ill children (Carpenter, 1990); women report losing about three times as many work hours as men for this task. Mothers have also been demonstrated to take greater responsibility for family health (Hibbard & Pope, 1983). In a study of the extent to which members of almost 700 families with children had similar and interrelated health behavior, Schor, Starfield, Stidley,

Barbara J. Tinsley • Department of Psychology, University of California, Riverside, California 92521.

Handbook of Health Behavior Research I: Personal and Social Determinants, edited by David S. Gochman. Plenum Press, New York, 1997.

and Hankin (1987) found that while overall rates of use of health services by children were affected by the utilization rates of both parents, the effect of the mother was 2.3 times that of the father, and only mothers' utilization rates significantly influenced children's rates of visits for non-illness care.

Other studies suggest that women play a predominant role in establishing health behavior of their children, decision making concerning health services utilization, delivering children for pediatric care, and providing home nursing care for ill children (Carpenter, 1990). Mothers appear to engage in most of the needs assessment and access to formal medical services for children, and in addition usually take their children to obtain these services (Aday & Eichhorn, 1973). Carpenter (1990, p. 1214) suggested, eloquently: "Women are the principal brokers or arrangers of health services for their children.... The assignment of family health responsibilities to the female in her role as ... mother ... is deeply rooted in cultural norms. These activities are seen as an integral part of the maternal and nurturant role women are expected to assume within the family structure." This chapter will therefore examine the multiple ways in which mothers influence their children's health behaviors and health outcomes.

MECHANISMS INVOLVED IN MATERNAL SOCIALIZATION OF CHILD HEALTH

Child health attitudes and behavior are socialized by mothers through a variety of mechanisms, including maternal health attitudes and expectations, modeling and reinforcement, maternal control practices, maternal supervision and monitoring of child health activities, and maternal establishment, training, and enforcement of household health-related rules.

Maternal Health Beliefs

A major way in which mothers influence children's health behavior is related to mothers' attitudes toward health. Studies of mothers' attitudes and beliefs concerning their children's health suggest that these attitudes and beliefs are important factors in mothers' health behavior on behalf of their children and their socialization of children's health behavior. Mothers' beliefs and behavior may be transmitted unintentionally to their children, or they may be transferred in the context of training children to engage in health behavior (Lau, Quadrel, & Hartman, 1990). Lau et al. (1990) found that mothers influenced their children either indirectly through the transmission of health beliefs or directly through explicit training for four different areas of health behavior: exercise, diet, alcohol use, and seat belt use.

In an investigation of the relation between the health beliefs of mothers and their children, Dielman et al. (1982) found that mothers' and children's perceptions of seriousness of and susceptibility to disease were significantly linked. Mothers' health attitudes, however, are a somewhat indirect influence on children's preventive health behavior because they usually function via their influence on mothers' behavior, rather than by direct communication to the child (Dielman et al., 1982).

Another area in which mothers' health attitudes appear to significantly affect children's health is in regard to medication. Maiman, Becker, and Katlic (1986) found that mothers' perceptions concerning their children's susceptibility to health problems and the effectiveness of non-prescription medications were related to possessing and using a greater number of categories of medication. In addition, possession and use of over-the-counter medications were also positively associated with mothers' perceptions that their families had more illnesses and with their perceptions of control. Similarly, Bush and Iannotti (1988) found moderate agreement between mothers and their elementary-school children in terms of their health beliefs concerning medicine use. Later interviews of a subset of these children and mothers revealed stability across a 3-year interval.

Mothers' beliefs about health affect mothers' health behavior not only on behalf of abled children, but also on behalf of disabled children. Affleck and his colleagues studied how mothers' beliefs about children's disabilities affect maternal behavior. Results of these studies indicated that mothers who blame others for their children's developmental disabilities are more likely to have caregiving problems and to be less sensitive to their children than mothers who accept at least partial responsibility for their children's condition (Affleck, McGrade, Allen, & McQueeney, 1985).

Another area in which mothers' beliefs about child health appear to be very powerful in determining mothers' health behavior on behalf of their children is injury prevention. L. Peterson, Farmer, and Kashani (1990) utilized a health belief model to predict parental teaching of safety skills and unintentional injury prevention. Results indicated that the more parents felt they knew about safety, the more confident they felt about intervening to prevent children's injuries. In turn, parents who perceived interventions to be effective in preventing childhood injuries reported more attempts at teaching their children to avoid behavior that would render them susceptible to injury. While these data are not related to actual childhood injury levels, they suggest further avenues for investigating the relations between maternal health beliefs, maternal health behavior on behalf of children, and child health behavior.

Tinsley completed a series of studies investigating the relations among maternal attitudes concerning the control mothers perceive with respect to their children's health, utilization of prenatal or childhood preventive health services, and child health (Tinsley & Holtgrave, 1989). The results of these studies suggested that mothers' perception of their control over their children's perinatal and pediatric outcomes is related to their use of prenatal and pediatric services, which in turn relates to child health outcomes. Specifically, mothers' belief in their control of their infants' health was positively related to utilization of prenatal and pediatric care, and children who received this care had better perinatal and pediatric health status. Studies of other types

of maternal health beliefs, focused on the value mothers place on their children's health and the subsequent effect these attitudes have on maternal behavior, also demonstrated that maternal health beliefs can be expressed in maternal health behavior on behalf of children. Tinsley (1995) found that the value mothers placed on their children's health was a significant factor in women's use of prenatal health services. In this study, women who placed the highest value on health obtained prenatal health services with the greatest reliability and conformance with their physicians' recommended schedule for prenatal health visits.

Mothers from different cultures may have varying beliefs about the causes of wellness and illness and transmit these beliefs to their children. Euro-American mothers often reflect a direct scientific cause-and-effect relationship between biological problems and child development. The views of mothers of other ethnicities often place a strong emphasis on fate, bad luck, sins of parents, foods the mother eats, or evil spirits as the causative factors in health status (Hanson, Lynch, & Wayman, 1990). These views affect the ways in which child health is viewed within families and cultures and the types of health services utilization mothers are willing to address on behalf of their children's health. For example, in an interview study of Mexican mothers of handicapped infants, Gault (1990) found that 93% of the mothers attributed the child's handicap to the mothers' experiencing a "big fright" during pregnancy.

Other research confirms that health-related stereotypes are culturally related and transmitted from mother to child. Hall, Cousins, and Power (1991) found significant concordance in the judgments of weight-related physical attractiveness in obese and normal-weight Mexican-American mothers and their 7- to 12-year-old daughters. Several studies have suggested similar parent–child socialization of preference for body builds (Adams, Hicken, & Salehi, 1988). Thus, although there is solid evidence that mothers' health beliefs influence their health behavior on behalf of their children, the mechanisms through which this influence is exerted are not well explored.

Fiese and Sameroff (1989) identified a number of family beliefs that affect child health, which they term the *family code*. They defined the family code as a system of family definitions that are used as guidelines for the family's behavior, and it includes family paradigms (core assumptions, convictions, or beliefs that each family member holds), family stories and myths, and family rituals (Reiss, 1989). As indicated, maternal beliefs about children's health have a substantial impact on maternal health behavior on behalf of their children and, in turn, children's health outcomes. Family stories and myths can illuminate how individual family members, or the family group as a whole, interpret and manage health-related experiences and events (Tinsley, Reisch, & Phillips, 1997). For example, a mother who believes that her children have fewer colds than other children because "angels are protecting them" presents a different opportunity for the pediatrician to provide anticipatory guidance than a mother who recounts her numerous and continuing efforts to protect her children from infectious disease through good nutrition and hygiene. Finally, family rituals appear to provide, at least in some cases, some buffering from the negative aspects of a family member's poor health. Wertlieb, Hauser, and Jacobson (1986) found that maintaining regular routines and engaging in social and recreational activities as a family helped to avoid behavioral problems in families with a diabetic child. These findings provide strong support for the ways in which maternal beliefs, in the context of the family, affect child health symptom perception and health services usage.

Child Rearing: A Pathway between Maternal Beliefs and Behavior

One pathway through which similarity in the health beliefs of mother and child may occur is through parental child-rearing behavior. The classic study relating parent child-rearing behavior to child health behavior was undertaken by Pratt (1973). This interview investigation of 273 families (mother, father, 9- to 13-year-old child)

involved assessing the relations between child-rearing styles and child health behaviors (e.g., tooth brushing, exercise, nutrition). Pratt identified a particular style of parenting, which she termed the *energized family*, as being related to the highest levels of child health practices. The parents in these "energized families" permitted their children a high degree of autonomy and used reasoning rather than punishment as a disciplinary strategy. Although most of the correlations were low, Pratt reported that child-rearing practices have a significant effect on children's health behavior, even when the parents' own health behaviors are controlled. Parental attitudes that recognized the child as an individual and fostered the child's assumption of responsibility were associated with positive health behavior in children (tooth brushing, sleep habits, exercise, nutritional practices, and refraining from smoking). In contrast, children raised in families with an autocratic child-rearing style were not as likely to practice such behavior. The study was weakened by reliance on the children's perceptions of their parents' child-rearing practices even when evidence from the parents themselves was available. Moreover, the contribution of mothers' child-rearing practices independent of fathers' child-rearing practices was not examined.

Four more recent studies confirm these relations between general maternal child-rearing practices and child health behavior. Lau and Klepper (1989), in a study of the illness orientations of 6- to 12-year-old children, examined parents' child-rearing practices. Parental punishment and control (i.e., frequency of spanking, frequency of isolation, parents' strictness, and the importance of discipline to parents) were found to influence children's self-esteem, approaching statistical significance. In turn, child self-esteem was a significant predictor of children's illness orientation.

Further validation of this work is found cross-ethnically as well. A series of studies of nutrition-related motivational strategies of Mexican-American mothers of 4- to 8-year-old children indicated that serving and helping children with their food was associated with food consumption compliance, and threats and bribes were negatively associated with consumption of healthful food (see Birch, Marlin, & Rotter, 1984; Olvera-Ezzell, Power, & Cousins, 1990).

Finally, a study by Lees and Tinsley (1997) provided additional evidence for the link between maternal child-rearing practices and child health behavior. In this study, mothers' parenting behavior and child health behavior were assessed in a sample of 70 preschool children. Results indicated that warm, nurturant mothers (those who gave higher than average amounts of verbal praise, hugs, and kisses as rewards for good behavior) had children who were more independent in a variety of health behaviors, such as tooth brushing, hand washing, exercising, going to bed at a regular time, and avoiding risk by staying away from poisons, as reported by parents. Additional results suggested that children whose mothers reported using monetary rewards and granting special privileges for good behavior had a tendency to make fewer nutritious food choices, as reported by their preschool teachers, than mothers who chose to use warmth and nurturance as strategies for encouraging good behavior in their children. In addition, mothers' general beliefs about child rearing were related to some of their children's safety behaviors. For example, parents who believed that children should get more discipline than they usually receive reported that their children showed less independence in seat belt use, whereas mothers who believed that parents should be more flexible with children reported that their children exercised more independence. These findings seemed to indicate some relations between maternal orientations toward more child-oriented mothering styles and autonomous healthy behaving by their children, with a corresponding possible relation between authoritarian mothering and less independence in risk-preventive behaviors of children.

In support of Pratt's findings about the value of rewarding children for their good behavior, the Lees and Tinsley study found that the total time mothers reported using rewards for good behavior related to children's independence in taking naps and keeping regular bedtimes. Use of rewards was also related to less risky behavior as reported by preschool teachers. These studies, considered together, suggest that non-health-specific maternal child-rearing behavior affects child health behavior and illustrate the potential of this path from maternal attitudes to maternal behavior to child health behavior.

Together, these studies provide support for the hypothesis of mother–child transmission of health attitudes. Additional longitudinal work is necessary to clarify these relations.

Modeling and Reinforcement

Social learning theory focuses on the role of observational learning and reinforcement in childhood socialization (Bandura, 1971, 1989). The acquisition of internal health values and overt health behavior determined by maternal role models is well documented in the child health behavior literature. Mothers who behave in health-enhancing or health-destructive ways are teaching these behaviors to their children. Children may learn and adopt similar behavior strategies by emulating and imitating the health-related behavior of their mothers.

Research suggests that modeling of health behavior is the most effective technique for socializing children's health behavior (Lau et al., 1990). The strongest support for the modeling effects of mothers on children's health behavior comes from United States and British studies of the relations between mothers' and children's smoking behavior (Doherty & Allen, 1994; Shute, Pierre, & Lubell, 1981). These studies suggest that having a mother who models smoking strongly increases the chances that a child will smoke and, conversely, that mothers who do not smoke are equally if not more likely to have a child who does not smoke (Nolte, Smith, & O'Rourke, 1983). Other examples of health behavior that appear, on the basis of studies of Euro-American children, to be taught to children at least partially by maternal modeling include using seat belts in a moving car (Lau et al., 1990; A. F. Williams, 1972), eating behavior (Dielman et al., 1982; Lau et al., 1990), exercise (Lau et al., 1990; Moore et al., 1991; Sallis et al., 1992), alcohol use (Lau et al., 1990), and Type A behavior patterns (Forgays & Forgays, 1991).

Research with non-Euro-American samples on maternal modeling of health behavior as a factor in children's health socialization is somewhat consistent with these findings. In studies of the maternal socialization of Latino children's eating habits, Olvera-Ezzell et al. (1990) found that while mothers did report using modeling as a socialization technique for influencing their children's mealtime behavior, this technique was reportedly used much less often than other techniques such as threats, bribes, and punishments, and nondirectives such as suggestions, questions, and offering choices. Thus, although modeling appears to be a significant mechanism for understanding the relations between mothers' and children's health behavior, there appear to be cultural differences in maternal health socialization strategies.

Investigators have begun to examine the role of modeling and reinforcement in childhood health socialization more closely. Dunn-Geier, McGrath, Rourke, Latter, and D'Astous (1986) found that adolescents who did not cope well with chronic pain, in comparison to adolescents who did, had mothers who were more likely to demonstrate behavior that discouraged adolescents' efforts at coping with an exercise task. Others found that mothers who maintained positive environments for their children's pain, and created observational opportunities for their children with respect to pain, had children who reported more pain (Osborne, Hatcher, & Richtsmeier, 1989; Rickard, 1988; J. O. Robinson, Alverez, & Dodge, 1990). Still other research suggests a maternal basis for children's sick role behavior. Walker and Zeman (1992), in a study of parents' responses to their children's illness behavior, found that mothers encouraged their children's illness behavior more than fathers. Furthermore, the results of this study indicated that mothers reported that they encouraged illness

behavior related to gastrointestinal symptoms more than cold symptoms. These studies underscored the effectiveness of maternal modeling and reinforcement of children's health behavior.

A significant area of research related to maternal modeling and reinforcement effects on child health behavior is concerned with maternal influences on children's coping with medical procedures. Researchers in this area have explored a variety of questions related to maternal competence in facilitating children's health treatment. Bush and his colleagues (Bush & Cockrell, 1987; Bush, Melamed, Shearas, & Greenbaum, 1986) have studied maternal influences on children's fear and coping during outpatient pediatric medical visits. These studies suggest that a variety of behaviors including maternal use of distraction and low rates of ignoring are associated with lower child distress and increased levels of child prosocial behavior. Mothers' self-report of positive reinforcement was associated with better child adjustment, and poorer child adjustment was related to punishment. Several maternal behaviors were related to child distress during these procedures, including maternal agitation and reassurance. Euro-American mothers were much more likely than African-American or Haitian mothers to report using modeling in dealing with their children during fearful pediatric situations such as injections (Reyes, Routh, Jean-Gilles, Sanfilippo, & Fawcett, 1991). Melamed (1993), in a review of maternal influences on children's coping with medical procedures, suggested that much more research in this area is needed, in order to sort out the definition of maternal competence in these situations and the developmental trajectories of maternal influences on child competence during medical events.

ESTABLISHING A HEALTH-PROMOTING CHILD-REARING ENVIRONMENT

Mothers influence their children's health in yet another way, by providing an environment that enables or constrains child health behavior and status. This perspective on mothers' health behavior on behalf of their children, however, has not been researched very broadly. Four main although slightly overlapping issues have been the foci of this line of research: mothers' socioeconomic status, mothers' impact on the emotional climate of children's lives, the impact of mothers' own health on children's health, and the effect of mothers' supervision on children's health.

Mothers' Socioeconomic Status

Mothers' demographic status, specifically socioeconomic status, has traditionally been the focus of efforts to describe and predict mothers' impact on their children's health. Social class, however, is not an explanatory variable, and in most cases merely describes mothers and children who vary in health attitudes, behavior, and actual health. In this chapter, in contrast to its traditional use, social class is being conceptualized as a proxy for a broad set of environmental characteristics, including access to preventive health care and maternal education, that may be associated with the extent to which children's health socialization occurs in health-enhancing conditions.

Mothers and children of higher social classes usually experience better health services access and utilization, as well as better health. Although the mechanisms by which social class affects health are poorly understood (Adler et al., 1994), maternal socioeconomic variables such as education, occupation, and income are clearly associated with children's health status. These factors strongly influence aspects of the health environment in which children develop, including such aspects as mother–child interaction (e.g., maternal teaching strategies, disciplinary tactics), maternal beliefs and attitudes, physical attributes (space, crowding, cleanliness, noise), organization, regularity and predictability of schedules and caregiving, and the availability of food, materials, and other resources (Aylward, 1992). Several researchers have investigated the relation

between environment and health, most notably Sameroff (Sameroff & Chandler, 1975; Sameroff, Seifer, Barocas, et al., 1987). Results of these studies confirm that single environmental risk factors have smaller effects on health and development, while the accumulation of risk factors produces geometric increases in childhood morbidity (Aylward, 1992). Moreover, the transactional model advanced by Sameroff and Chandler (1975) suggests that children engage in constant adaptive reorganizing, in the contexts of their environments. Poor environments compromise children's developmental progress, while more favorable environments facilitate childhood resiliency and better outcomes. By this view, children learn about health during their interactions with their mothers, who are in most cases their primary socialization agents during infancy and early childhood. From this perspective, therefore, the role the mother plays in structuring and maintaining a health-enhancing or health-deleterious environment for her child, as a function of her socioeconomic status, is a focus of mothers' impact on children's health (Fiese & Sameroff, 1989).

Utilization of childhood preventive and ameliorative health services, as well as childhood morbidity, are not distributed randomly; a number of studies have shown that mothers living in environments characterized by high levels of stress and low levels of support are poor utilizers of health services, especially well-child visits (Children's Defense Fund, 1988). Low-income mothers take their children to pediatricians or primary care providers, dentists, and immunization providers less often than higher-income mothers (Rosenstock & Kirscht, 1980). Even when health services are designed specifically for low-income families, those mothers within low-income groups with higher education levels and nontargeted mothers who normally use services utilize the services at a higher rate than the targeted low-income mothers with lower levels of education (Elinson, Henshaw, & Cohen, 1976).

Research in the domains of maternal social class and children's health finds that lower socioeconomic status is related to lower levels of knowledge about health, less positive health-related attitudes, less stoicism when ill, and less healthy life-style practices, in both mothers and children (Campbell, 1978). Socioeconomic status, however, is a descriptive variable, rather than an explanatory variable, and also covaries with several factors known to influence health behavior, including family income and maternal education, which appear to be strongly related to utilization of childhood health services and child health. For example, several papers from the National Health Examination Survey examined the utility of various family demographic variables as predictors of child health (Shakato, Edwards, & Grossman, 1980). The results of these studies suggested that the number of years of parents' education, especially that of the mother, was the best predictor of child health status.

Mothers' Impact on Children's Emotional Climate

Some research has examined the relations between family process variables and children's health. The foundation of this research is the concept of the family as the "breeding ground for somatic complaints" (Fiese & Sameroff, 1989, p. 294). For example, Minuchin et al. (1975) described how children's physical symptoms can be related to family interaction characterized as enmeshed, overprotective, and rigid. Some years later, Walker and Greene (1987) demonstrated that children who perceive their families as low in cohesion report more physical symptoms than those with high family cohesion.

In our study of preschool children and their parents (Lees & Tinsley, 1997), a variety of characteristics of children's family dynamics were significantly related to mothers' and teachers' reporting of children's health behavior. For example, more cohesion in the family was associated with children's independent compliance with regular bedtimes. Perhaps children in cohesive families feel particularly motivated to comply with household health rules. Another finding from this study

suggested that as reports of family conflict increase, mothers characterized children as demonstrating less selecting of nutritious snacks and less independent use of seat belts. These findings might be explained as a function of parental energy in conflictful families; perhaps family energy is being spent on conflict and not on teaching children independence of or responsibility for behavior. Alternatively, it is possible that child contentiousness about use of seat belts may be one source of family conflict (Tinsley & Lees, 1995). One child behavior, frequent selection of healthful food, related to two somewhat associated family characteristics: a moral–religious emphasis in the family and utilizing control as a method of system maintenance. Perhaps children in families characterized by these dimensions select healthy foods to maintain order by "doing the right thing."

Thus, it appears that characteristics of family interaction and dynamics are associated with children's health-related behavior, as measured independently by teachers and mothers. Again, the mechanisms of this association are unexplored, but provide fruitful areas for future research on the development of children's health behavior in the family context.

Another area of inquiry that focuses on the links between mother–child interaction and child health is research that relates the quality of mother–child relationships with children's health status. O'Leary (1990), in an in-depth review of the relations between stress, emotion, and immune function, suggested that emotional experience, including affect regulation, appears to be an immunological mediator of health. Feeney and Ryan (1994) demonstrated that one such indicator of emotional experience, mother–child attachment quality, affects child health. Early family experiences of illness, mother–child attachment style (secure, avoidant, anxious/ambivalent), and three health outcomes (symptom reporting, health services utilization, and health status) were assessed in a sample of college freshman. Findings confirmed that parent–child attachment style was related to maternal responses to subjects' early childhood illness. Specifically, avoidant attachment was negatively related to parental overindulgence during childhood illness and negatively related to parental responsiveness. Anxious/ambivalent attachment was positively related to reported parental overindulgence, and avoidant attachment was inversely linked with later visits to health care professionals. The results of this study suggest important implications of the influence of mother–child relationships on physical well-being, and specifically highlight the relation between child affect regulation, as a function of mother–child interaction, and later health behavior and outcomes.

A related avenue of research has considered the impact of maternal anxiety on children's health behavior and health status. Three effects of maternal anxiety on child health behavior and health status have been identified: the effects of maternal anxiety on child behavior during medical procedures, the impact of maternal anxiety on utilization of health care services, and the influence of maternal anxiety on childhood minor illness. In a study of children's fear and coping during medical examinations, Bush et al. (1986) found that high maternal state and trait anxiety was related to poor ratings of children's handling of previous medical experience. Additionally, mothers who were agitated provided less information and ignored their children more, which the authors interpreted to suggest that maternal anxiety was associated with a pattern of mothering during medical events that is characterized by less effectiveness and more disorganization.

Consistent with earlier research in this area (Campion & Gabriel, 1985; Roghmann & Haggerty, 1973), Goldman and Owen (1994), in an investigation of the relation between maternal trait anxiety and mothers' utilization of pediatric services for their infants, found that mothers' reports of anxiety during pregnancy predicted increased use of pediatric acute care visits during infancy. In interpreting these results, Goldman and Owen suggested that highly anxious mothers may be hypervigilant for health problems in their

children and more predisposed to consult formal health institutions to determine the etiology of the problems. These findings become even more interesting when considered in light of data from Richtsmeier and Hatcher (1994) that suggest that highly anxious parents appear to have poorer understanding of their children's condition following their interaction with their children's pediatricians. Together, these studies suggest that maternal anxiety about children's health is a negative factor in a variety of ways in its influence on child health behavior and status.

Mothers' Health

A relatively new area of research is emerging that examines the effect of mothers' health status on childhood health. Virtually all mothers are afflicted with minor acute illnesses periodically while rearing their children, and many mothers experience chronic illness; more than 10 million adults under the age of 45 years suffer limitation of activity associated with chronic illness (Benson & Marano, 1994). Most researchers who study familial socialization of childhood health behavior and outcomes ignore this aspect of mothers' influence on their children's health (Drotar, 1994). Investigators are becoming increasingly aware, however, of the effects of such maternal health behavior as cigarette smoking on both childhood behavior (e.g., childhood cigarette smoking, as discussed earlier) and child health (e.g., the deleterious effects of secondhand smoke) (Leftwich & Collins, 1994). In fact, evidence suggests striking effects of mothers' smoking during pregnancy on daughters' smoking behavior. Kandel, Wu, and Davies (1994) found that mothers' smoking during pregnancy increased the probability that daughters would initiate smoking and continue to smoke during adolescence. These researchers hypothesized that nicotine or other associated substances from cigarettes predispose fetal nervous systems for subsequent addictive behavior during later life.

In a comprehensive study of the effect of maternal physical symptomatology and health services utilization on children, Stein and New-comb (1994) found that mothers' reporting of a large number of major health problems in the past 4 years was a predictor of more psychosomatic complaints in their children, than in the children of mothers who did not report such problems. While the cross-sectional nature of this study did not permit questions of causality to be answered, the results suggested either a social learning or a biological predisposition explanation. Regardless, these data indicate the salience of mothers' health status and behavior for child health behavior.

Parmelee (1986, 1993) argued for examining the specific ways in which mothers socialize their children concerning how to respond to recurring minor illness. Parmelee suggested that as children become ill with minor contagious acute illnesses, and transmit them to their parents, the children are provided repetitive opportunities to observe and participate in the care of their mothers, who are experiencing what they have experienced. Parmelee believes that these shared personal illness experiences help children develop an understanding of the feelings of others and that they are an important beneficial aspect of children's social growth experience, in addition to providing models of sick role behavior. Very young children are quite capable of empathic behavior (Zahn-Waxler, Radke-Yarrow, & King, 1979), and in combination with the saliency of physical symptomatology for young children (Bretherton & Beeghly, 1982), mothers' minor illnesses provide a potent learning resource for childhood socialization (Parmelee, 1986).

Mothers' Supervision of Children

Investigations of maternal monitoring of children have been primarily focused on delinquency and risky behavior as outcomes. It may be useful, however, to conceptualize risky behavior as a health behavior and to consider how mothers' monitoring of childhood activities affects childhood risk. Two areas will be highlighted in this

discussion: maternal monitoring of children's behavior in general and, more specifically, maternal monitoring of children's television viewing. In a thoughtful discussion of maternal monitoring of children's whereabouts, activities, and companions, Ladd, Le Sieur, and Profilet (1993) concluded that the absence of maternal monitoring is associated with childhood maladjustment. Research on samples of delinquent adolescents has found that mothers engage in less monitoring and supervision of these children's activiites, and significant relations have been established between inadequate maternal monitoring and children's petty crime, rule breaking, poor academic performance, poor school conduct, and general antisocial behavior (Crouter, MacDermid, McHale, & Perry-Jenkins, 1990; Patterson & Stouthamer-Loeber, 1984). Although the empirical link to childhood health outcomes has yet to be found these behaviors that are related to less than adequate maternal monitoring are associated with such health outcomes as unintentional injuries and are therefore important to consider as significant childhood health behaviors affected by maternal behavior. Empirical attention should be focused on the pathways through which maternal monitoring of childhood activities and behavior affect child health behavior and outcomes. One area of maternal supervision of children's behavior, however, has been closely examined: mothers' supervision of childhood television viewing.

Mothers' Supervision of Children's Television Viewing. Mothers regulate children's television viewing, at least in early childhood, in several respects, including the quantity and the subject matter of programming they permit their children to watch. Both of these aspects of maternal television regulation appear to have consequences for children's health. With respect to the content of permitted programming, there are two well-researched aspects: the influence on children of television food and medicine advertising. A close reading of this literature suggests that television appears to highly influence children's nutrition, but has surprisingly little influence on children's use of medicines.

Long-term exposure to commercials for low-nutrition foods (i.e., foods high in sugar or fat or both) has a significant influence on children's eating behavior (Liebert & Sprafkin, 1988). Content analyses of children's television have demonstrated that commercials for low-nutrition food products (a risk factor in a number of diseases and dental problems) comprise approximately 80% of television advertising directed at children (Barcus, 1987). Studies suggest that these commercials substantially affect the attitudes and behaviors of children with respect to nutrition and food selection. Representative studies have determined that young children (4 to 7 years old) do not understand that sugary foods are detrimental to health, nor are disclosure portions of these commercials (e.g., cautions that sugary cereals should be part of a balanced breakfast) effective (Liebert & Sprafkin, 1988). Furthermore, information about food and eating on television is not restricted to commercials; studies indicate that there are more food-related references in programming than in commercials (Kaufman, 1980). Other research indicates that eating, drinking, or talking about food occurs more than 9 times per hour in prime time and weekend daytime programming (Gerbner, Gross, Morgan, & Signorielli, 1981). Snacking represented 39% of the portrayals of eating during these time periods, with representations of healthful snacking virtually absent. Studies indicate that television characters are usually happy in the presence of food, yet food is usually not used to satisfy hunger in television programming. Instead, it is used to bribe others or to facilitate social interactions (Kaufman, 1980).

Television consistently presents characters who are thin; 88% of all television characters are thin or average in body build (Kaufman, 1980). Ironically, however, the nutritional products and behaviors most heavily advertised on television promote obesity (Strasburger, 1992).

Studies of children's actual food selection as influenced by television commercials underscore the potency of televisions' impact on this type of child health behavior. Experimental studies of exposure to commercials of low-nutrition foods revealed that children choose more low-nutrition and fewer high-nutrition foods (Gorn & Greenberg, 1982), especially boys (Jeffrey, McClerran, & Fox, 1982). Field studies of the relation between children's television viewing and nutritional status yielded similar findings: a linear relation between television viewing and poor nutritional habits and nutrition misconceptions (e.g., of what is a healthy breakfast, of food from fast food restaurants as nutritious) (Signorielli & Lears, 1992).

Pronutritional advertising is less successful in modifying behavior; nutrition knowledge increases, but consumption patterns do not change (P. E. Peterson, Jeffrey, Bridgewater, & Dawson, 1984). Combining pronutritional programming with positive evaluative comments by an adult coviewer, however, such as the child's mother, can be effective in reducing 3- to 6-year-old children's consumption of low-nutrition foods (Galst, 1980). Together, these studies suggest, at least, the powerful potential of mothers' permitting their children to watch nutrition-related television advertising.

A second issue in mothers' patterns of supervising children's television viewing is that of programming that depicts substance use and commercials for medicine. Although very little medical television advertising is aimed at child audiences, children see many commercials for medicines (Liebert & Sprafkin, 1988). Research on child viewing of medicine commercials has focused on licit and illicit substance use. Moderate to weak relations between children's viewing of commercials for medicine and their requests for and use of these drugs have been found (Liebert & Sprafkin, 1988; Rossiter & Robertson, 1980). In light, however, of the high rates of self-medication by young children (Iannotti & Bush, 1992) with both over-the-counter and prescription medicines, even modest relations between television viewing of medicine commercials and use of these medicines are important. Children's use of illicit drugs does not appear to be affected by viewing of commercials for licit drugs (Milovsky, Pekowsky, & Stipp, 1975–1976).

A related impact of mothers' monitoring of children's television viewing on children's health behavior is concerned with the ability of media such as television to suggest to children that risky behaviors, like substance use, are socially acceptable and that the health consequences for engaging in these behaviors are probabilistically based. In light of young children's self-perceived invulnerability to negative health outcomes (Gochman, 1987), the media's tendency to publicize individuals who "beat the odds" can be construed as further encouragement for children to engage in risk-taking (Bruhn & Cordova, 1977).

Mothers' decisions to permit children's television viewing has another type of effect on children's health behavior, beyond program influence. Television has been demonstrated to alter time use and activity choices in children (Robinson, 1972; Strasburger, 1992). A survey by *Prevention* magazine (1994) found that while children spent approximately 18 hours a week watching television (equal to the waking hours in 2 months per year), parents reported that 66% of children get 20 minutes of strenuous exercise at least 3 times per week. Williams and Handford (1986) found that the number of sports activities (i.e., health-promoting exercise) engaged in by adolescents markedly decreased after the introduction of television into the community. The consequences of these shifts are illustrated in a study (Hei & Gold, 1990) that found that children who watched television 2–4 hours a day had dramatically higher cholesterol levels than children who watched television less than 2 hours per day, probably mediated by insufficient exercise and television-related snacking on high-fat foods. The number of hours spent watching television is a strong predictor of adolescent obesity, with the prevalence increasing 2% for each hour viewed above the norm (Dietz & Gortmaker, 1985).

These impacts of maternal monitoring of television viewing may derive from its substitu-

tion for a more health-promoting type of recreational activity, portrayal of poor nutritional behavior, advertising of low-nutrition products, or some combination of all of these (Strasburger, 1992). Moreover, the issue of the direction of effects is still open as well; obese children may be less likely to play actively and therefore to watch television more.

In summary, mothers' regulation of children's television viewing appears to have significant effects on several aspects of children's health-related attitudes and behavior.

MOTHERS' ESTABLISHMENT, TRAINING, AND ENFORCEMENT OF CHILD HEALTH BEHAVIOR

The emergence of young children's ability to control and regulate their own health behavior is a very important aspect of maternal socialization of children's health behavior. Researchers who study childhood behavioral socialization believe that children's ability to self-regulate develops as a function of their emerging abilities to engage in behavior that they understand to be approved as a result of their caregivers' transmission of standards of behavior (Gralinski & Kopp, 1993; Maccoby, 1984). Research in childhood socialization has focused on a number of factors that influence the effectiveness of maternal socialization of children, including factors that mediate its effectiveness (e.g., maternal responsiveness, warmth, control [Baumrind, 1973]).

Other research has examined the nature of mothers' rules, as communicated to their children through the socialization process, and how these rules change with children's development. LeVine (1974) posited that socialization is first aimed at protecting children and later at promoting family and cultural standards. Two decades later, Gralinski and Kopp (1993), in a longitudinal study of mothers' rules for everyday standards of behavior, demonstrated that mothers' earliest socialization efforts are focused on ensuring children's safety, and as children age (18–30 months), mothers move their socialization attention to other issues, including children's self-care. Finally, by the time children are 3½ years old, mothers elaborate on previously established rules and combine categories of rules about self-care and social norms (e.g., you must be dressed before you go outdoors). Other findings from this study suggested that safety rules are very important to mothers. Interestingly, very young children's compliance with mothers' safety rules is highly advanced, in contrast to children's compliance with other categories of mothers' rules. These findings suggest the early and sustained salience of safety rules for both mothers and children and highlight the importance of further research focused on the description of the developmental pathways associated with mothers' socialization of health and safety rules.

With respect to the impact of mothers' direct training and enforcement of children's health behavior, research suggests that mothers explicitly attempt to train their children in health behavior and that this training is an important channel through which mothers socialize their children's behavior (Lau et al., 1990).

Sexuality Training

One health-related area in which mothers explicitly train children is sexuality. Fraley, Nelson, Wolf, and Lozoff (1991) asked a sample of 117 mothers of preschool children what words for genitals they used with their children. Results indicated that preschool children were not likely to be given standard anatomical genital terms, although many children received "colorful and colloquial expressions" (p. 301). Girls were less likely than boys to have labels for their own genitals, but were more likely to be taught names for boys' genitals by their mothers. Other studies of mother–child communication about sexuality confirm that mothers are the predominant agents of sexual socialization for boys and girls, but more so for girls (Nolin & Petersen, 1992).

Mother–daughter communication about sexuality appears to be more wide-ranging than mother–son sexuality communication, with these gender differences most pronounced for discussions about sexuality focused on factual and moral topics, which are the types of communications most likely to transmit information and values (Nolin & Petersen, 1992). Mother–child communication about sexuality appears to make a difference; Fox and Inazu (1980) found that frequency of mother–daughter communication about sexuality is linked to knowledge of birth control and responsible sexual behavior in adolescence.

In the era of AIDS, maternal socialization of childhood sexual knowledge has become a critical aspect of health socialization. Sigelman, Derenowski, Mullaney, and Siders (1993) examined mothers' propensity to discuss AIDS with their children in grades 1–12. Although previous research had suggested that children learn more about AIDS from television than from their parents (Fassler, McQueen, Duncan, & Copeland, 1990; McElreath & Roberts, 1992), findings indicated that frequency of mother–child communication about AIDS was positively associated with children's level of knowledge about AIDS.

Negative Effects

Maternal training of child health behavior is not always successful, however, and in fact may produce negative effects. For example, Johnson & Birch (1994) found that mothers who attempt to protect their children from obesity may create children who do not know how to stop eating when they have had enough. The study of 77 children ages 3–5 found that those with the most body fat had the most "controlling" mothers concerning the amount of food eaten. The more control the mother reported using to manage her child's eating behavior, the less food self-regulation the child demonstrated. In contrast, children whose mothers allowed them to be most spontaneous about food (e.g., eating when they were hungry and not necessarily being forced to finish all the food given them) displayed a natural instinct for regulating their own food intake.

These findings appear to hold cross-culturally as well, as demonstrated in a Japanese study in which mothers of young adolescent girls were found, as reported by mothers and daughters, to contribute to their daughters' eating disorder tendencies through control and monitoring (Mukai, 1993). Another study that focused on the role of parents in children's physical activity found that parental encouragements to be active played no role in 4th-graders' activity level (Sallis et al., 1992).

CONCLUSIONS: METHODOLOGICAL AND RESEARCH ISSUES

Theoretically, the findings from this area of research promise to increase understanding of maternal health socialization and of parental socialization more generally. Within an applied perspective, this research has the potential to improve the effectiveness of maternal health training of children, thereby positively affecting the health status of children as they age and develop.

It appears that mothers are very powerful socializers of their children's health behavior. As portrayed in this chapter, maternal health socialization is accomplished both directly and indirectly. Further research is needed to disentangle mothers' multiple influences and their mediators in order to understand children's health in the context of maternal socialization. Moreover, additional investigation is necessary to elucidate more carefully the mechanisms by which mothers teach their children to behave in a salutary manner and the contexts that facilitate this teaching.

Several other issues remain to be investigated. First, the various maternal influences on children's health have been treated independently, but in reality probably operate together in producing their effects. The ways in which these various influences combine is an issue that needs more research. Second, the links between maternal beliefs and behavior need to be examined

more closely. Specifically, the conditions under which beliefs translate into maternal action need to be specified. Third, the way in which maternal health practices change as a function of the developmental level of the child requires more attention. Perhaps modeling and reinforcement are more common with younger children and other less direct forms of influence are more salient for older children. Fourth, the issue of direction of effects should be studied. It is assumed that parents influence their children's behavior, but the role of child characteristics in shaping maternal behaviors needs attention as well. Fifth, more systematic research on how cultural background alters both maternal beliefs and behavior is needed. Finally, almost no attention has been directed to how patterns of secular changes in health care delivery alter mothers' health behavior on behalf of their children.

REFERENCES

Adams, G. R., Hicken, M., & Salehi, M. (1988). Socialization of the physical attractiveness stereotype: Parental expectations and verbal behaviors. *International Journal of Psychology, 23*, 137–149.

Aday, L., & Eichhorn, R. (1973). *The utilization of health services and correlates: A research bibliography*. DHEW Publication No. (HSM) 73-3003. Rockville, MD: National Center for Health Services Research and Development.

Adler, N. E., Boyce, T., Chesney, M. A., Cohen, S., Folkman, S., Kahn, R. L., & Syme, S. L. (1994). Socioeconomic status and health. *American Psychologist, 49*, 15–24.

Affleck, G., McGrade, B. J., Allen, D. A., & McQueeney, M. (1985). Mothers' beliefs about behavioral causes for their developmentally disabled infant's condition: What do they signify? *Journal of Pediatric Psychology, 10*, 293–303.

Alexander, D. F. (1992). Research challenges in children's health behavior. Presidential Citation Address, American Psychological Association, August.

Aylward, G. P. (1992). The relationship between environmental risk and developmental outcome. *Developmental and Behavioral Pediatrics, 13*, 222–229.

Bandura, A. (1971). *Social learning theory*. New York: General Learning Press.

Bandura, A. (1989). Social cognitive theory. In R. Vasta (Ed.), *Annals of child development* (pp. 1–60). Greenwich, CT: JAI Press.

Barcus, F. E. (1987). *Food advertising on children's televi-*

sion: An analysis of appeals and nutritional content. Newtonville, MA: Action for Children's Television.

Baumrind, D. (1973). The development of instrumental competence through socialization. In A. Pick (Ed.), *Minnesota symposia on child psychology: Vol. 7* (pp. 3–46). Minneapolis: University of Minnesota Press.

Benson, V., & Marano, M. (1994). Current estimates from the National Health Interview Survey. *National Center for Health Statistics, Vital and Health Statistics.* Series 10, No. 189. Washington, DC: U.S. Government Printing Office.

Birch, L. L., Marlin, D. W., & Rotter, J. (1984). Eating as the "means" activity in a contingency: Effects on young children's food preference. *Child Development, 55,* 431–439.

Bretherton, I., & Beeghly, M. (1982). Talking about internal states: The acquisition of an explicit theory of mind. *Developmental Psychology, 18,* 906–921.

Bruhn, J. G., & Cordova, F. D. (1977). A developmental approach to learning wellness behavior: Infancy to early adolescence. *Health Values, 1,* 246–254.

Bush, J. P., & Cockrell, C. S. (1987). Maternal factors predicting parenting behaviors in the pediatric clinic. *Journal of Pediatric Psychology, 12,* 505–518.

Bush, J. P., & Iannotti, R. J. (1988). Origins and stability of children's health beliefs relative to medicine use. *Social Science and Medicine, 27,* 345–352.

Bush, J. P., Melamed, B. G., Sheras, P. L., & Greenbaum, P. E. (1986). Mother–child patterns of coping with anticipatory medical stress. *Health Psychology, 5,* 137–157.

Campbell, J. D. (1975). Illness is a point of view: The development of children's concepts of illness. *Child Development, 46,* 92–100.

Campbell, J. D. (1978). The child in the sick role: Contributions of age, sex, parental status and parental values. *Journal of Health and Social Behavior, 19,* 35–51.

Campion, P. D., & Gabriel, J. (1985). Illness behavior in mothers with young children. *Social Science and Medicine, 20,* 325–330.

Carpenter, E. S. (1990). Children's health care and the changing role of women. *Medical Care, 28,* 1208–1218.

Children's Defense Fund (1988). *A call for action to make our nation safe for children: A briefing book on the status of American children in 1988.* Washington, DC: Children's Defense Fund.

Crouter, A. C., MacDermid, S. M., McHale, S. M., & Perry-Jenkins, M. (1990). Parental monitoring and perceptions of children's school performance and conduct in dual- and single-earner families. *Developmental Psychology, 26,* 649–657.

Dielman, T. E., Leech, S., Becker, M. H., Rosenstock, I. M., Horvath, W. J., & Radius, S. M. (1982). Parental and child health beliefs and behavior. *Health Education Quarterly, 9,* 63–77.

Dietz, W. H., & Gortmaker, S. L. (1985). Do we fatten our children at the television set? Obesity and television viewing in children and adolescents. *Pediatrics, 75,* 807–812.

Doherty, W. J., & Allen, W. (1994). Family functioning and parental smoking as predictors of adolescent cigarette use: A six-year prospective study. *Journal of Family Psychology, 8,* 347–353.

Drotar, D. (1994). Impact of parental health problems on children: Concepts, methods, and unanswered questions. *Journal of Pediatric Psychology, 19,* 525–536.

Dunn-Geier, B. J., McGrath, P. J., Rourke, B. P., Latter, J., & D'Astous, J. (1986). Adolescent chronic pain: The ability to cope. *Pain, 26,* 23–32.

Elinson, J., Henshaw, S., & Cohen, S. (1976). Responses by a low-income population to a multiphasic screening program: A sociological analysis. *Preventive Medicine, 5,* 414–424.

Fassler, D., McQueen, K., Duncan, P., & Copeland, L. (1990). Children's perceptions of AIDS. *Journal of the American Academy of Child and Adolescent Psychiatry, 29,* 459–462.

Feeney, J. A., & Ryan, S. M. (1994). Attachment style and affect regulation: Relationships with health behavior and family experiences of illness in a student sample. *Health Psychology, 13,* 334–345.

Fiese, B. H., & Sameroff, A. J. (1989). Family context in pediatric psychology: A transactional perspective. *Journal of Pediatric Psychology, 14,* 293–314.

Forgays, D. K., & Forgays, D. G. (1991). Type A behavior within families: Parents and older adolescent children. *Journal of Behavioral Medicine, 14,* 325–339.

Fox, G. L., & Inazu, J. K. (1980). Patterns and outcomes of mother–daughter communication about sexuality. *Journal of Social Issues, 36,* 7–29.

Fraley, M. C., Nelson, E. C., Wolf, A. W., & Lozoff, B. (1991). Early genital naming. *Developmental and Behavioral Pediatrics, 12,* 301–304.

Galst, J. P. (1980). Television food commercials and pronutritional public service announcements as determinants of young children's snack choices. *Child Development, 51,* 935–938.

Gault, A. R. (1990). Mexican immigrant parents and the education of their handicapped children: Factors that influence parent involvement. *Dissertation Abstracts Int'l, 50* (n7-A), 1865–1866.

Gerbner, G., Gross, L., Morgan, M., & Signorielli, N. (1981). *Aging with television commercials: Images on television commercials and dramatic programming, 1977–1979.* Unpublished manuscript. Annenberg School of Communication, Philadelphia: University of Pennsylvania.

Gochman, D. S. (1987). *Youngsters' health cognitions: Cross-sectional and longitudinal analyses.* Louisville, KY: Health Behavior Systems.

Goldman, S. L., & Owen, M. T. (1994). The impact of parental trait anxiety on the utilization of health care services in infancy: A prospective study. *Journal of Pediatric Psychology, 19,* 369–381.

Gorn, G. J., & Greenberg, M. E. (1982). Behavioral evidence of the effects of televised food messages on children. *Journal of Consumer Research, 9,* 200–205.

Gralinski, G. H., & Kopp, C. B. (1993). Everyday rules for behavior: Mothers' requests to young children. *Developmental Psychology, 29,* 573–584.

Hall, S. K., Cousins, J. H., & Power, T. G. (1991). Self-concept and perceptions of attractiveness and body size among Mexican-American mothers and daughters. *International Journal of Obesity, 15,* 567–575.

Hanson, M. J., Lynch, E. W., & Wayman, K. I. (1990). Honoring the cultural diversity of families when gathering data. *Topics in Early Childhood Special Education, 10,* 112–131.

Hei, T. K., & Gold, V. (1990). The effect of television viewing on children's cholesterol levels. Paper presented at the annual meeting of the American Heart Association, Dallas.

Henggeler, S. W., Cohen, R., Edwards, J. J., Summerville, M. B., & Ray, G. E. (1991). Family stress as a link in the association between television viewing and achievement. *Child Study Journal, 21,* 1–10.

Hibbard, J. H., & Pope, C. R. (1983). Gender roles, illness orientation and use of medical services. *Social Science and Medicine, 17,* 129–137.

Iannotti, R. J., & Bush, J. P. (1992). The development of autonomy in children's health behaviors. In E. J. Susman, L. V. Feagans, & W. J. Ray (Eds.), *Emotion cognition, health and development in children and adolescents*. Hillsdale, NJ: Erlbaum.

Jeffrey, D. B., McClerran, R. W., & Fox, D. T. (1982). The development of children's eating habits: The role of television commercials. *Health Education Quarterly, 9,* 78–93.

Johnson, S. L., & Birch, L. L. (1994). Parents' and children's adiposity and eating style. *Pediatrics, 94,* 653–661.

Kandel, D. B., Wu, P., & Davies, M. (1994). Maternal smoking during pregnancy and smoking by adolescent daughters. *American Journal of Public Health, 84,* 1407–1413.

Kaufman, L. (1980). Prime time nutrition. *Journal of Communication, 30,* 37–46.

Ladd, G. W., Le Sieur, K. D., & Profilet, S. M. (1993). Direct parental influences on young children's peer relations. In S. Duck (Ed.), *Learning about relationships* (pp. 152–183). Newbury Park, CA: Sage.

Lau, R. R., & Klepper, S. (1989). The development of illness orientations in children aged 6–12. *Journal of Health and Social Behavior, 29,* 149–168.

Lau, R. R., Quadrel, M. J., & Hartman, K. A. (1990). Development and change of young adults' preventive health beliefs and behavior: Influence from parents and peers. *Journal of Health and Social Behavior, 31,* 240–259.

Lees, N. B., & Tinsley, B. J. (1997). *Maternal child-rearing practices as a factor in preschool children's health and safety behavior.* Manuscript submitted for publication.

Leftwich, M. J. T., & Collins, F. L., Jr. (1994). Parental smoking, depression, and child development: Persistent and unanswered questions. *Journal of Pediatric Psychology, 19,* 557–570.

LeVine, R. A. (1974). Parental goals: A cross-cultural view. *Teachers College Record, 76,* 226–239.

Liebert, R. M., & Sprafkin, J. (1988). *The early window: Effects of television on children and youth* (3rd ed.). New York: Pergamon Press.

Maccoby, E. E. (1984). Socialization and developmental change. *Child Development, 55,* 317–328.

Maiman, L. A., Becker, M. H., & Katlic, A. W. (1986). Correlates of mothers' use of medications for their children. *Social Science and Medicine, 22,* 41–51.

McElreath, L. H., & Roberts, M. C. (1992). Perceptions of acquired immune deficiency syndrome by children and their parents. *Journal of Pediatric Psychology, 17,* 477–490.

Melamed, B. (1993). Parental influences on children's coping: A review of "Putting the family back in the child." *Behaviour Research and Therapy, 31,* 239–247.

Milovsky, J. R., Pekowsky, B., & Stipp, H. (1975–1976). TV drug advertising and proprietary and illicit drug use among boys. *Public Opinion Quarterly, 39,* 457–481.

Minuchin, S., Baker, L., Rosman, B. L., Liebman, R., Milman, L., & Todd, T. C. (1975). A conceptual model of psychosomatic illness in children. *Archives of General Psychiatry, 32,* 1031–1038.

Moore, L. L., Lombardi, D. A., White, M. J., Campbell, J. L., Oliveria, S. A., & Ellison, R. C. (1991). Influence of parents' physical activity levels on activity levels of young children. *Journal of Pediatrics, 118,* 215–219.

Mukai, T. (1993). *Socialization of eating attitudes and weight preoccupation among Japanese girls: Maternal and peer influences.* Paper presented at the biennial meeting of the Society for Research in Child Development, New Orleans, March.

Nolin, M. J., & Petersen, K. K. (1992). Gender differences in parent–child communication about sexuality. *Journal of Adolescent Research, 7,* 59–79.

Nolte, A. E., Smith, B. J., & O'Rourke, T. (1983). The relationship between health risk attitudes and behaviors and parental presence. *Journal of School Health, 53,* 234–240.

O'Leary, A. (1990). Stress, emotion, and human immune function. *Psychological Bulletin, 108,* 363–382.

Olvera-Ezzell, N., Power, T. G., & Cousins, J. H. (1990). Maternal socialization of children's eating habits: Strategies used by obese Mexican-American mothers. *Child Development, 61,* 395–400.

Osborne, R. B., Hatcher, J. W., & Richtsmeier, A. J. (1989). The role of social modeling in unexplained pediatric pain. *Journal of Pediatric Psychology, 14,* 43–61.

Parke, R. D. (1996). *Fatherhood.* Boston: Harvard University Press.

Parke, R. D., & Tinsley, B. J. (1987). Family interaction in infancy. In J. D. Osofsky (Ed.), *Handbook of infant development* (2nd ed.) (pp. 579–641). New York: Wiley.

Parmelee, A. H., Jr. (1986). Children's illnesses: Their beneficial effects on behavioral development. *Child Development, 57,* 1–10.

Parmelee, A. H., Jr. (1993). Children's illnesses and normal behavioral development: The role of caregivers. In *Zero to three* (pp. 2–3). Madison, WI: National Center for Clinical Infant Programs.

Patterson, G. R., & Stouthamer-Loeber, M. (1984). The correlation of family management practices and delinquency. *Child Development, 55,* 1299–1307.

Peterson, L., Farmer, J., & Kashani, J. H. (1990). Parental injury prevention endeavors: A function of health beliefs? *Health Psychology, 9,* 177–191.

Peterson, P. E., Jeffrey, D. G., Bridgewater, C. A., & Dawson, B. (1984). How pronutrition television programming affects children's dietary habits. *Developmental Psychology, 20,* 55–63.

Pratt, L. (1973). Child-rearing methods and children's health behavior. *Journal of Health and Social Behavior, 14,* 61–69.

Prevention magazine. (1994). *Children's Health Index.* Emmaus, PA: Rodale Press.

Reiss, D. (1989). The represented and practicing family: Contrasting visions of family continuity. In A. J. Sameroff & R. N. Emde (Eds.), *Relationship disorders in early development: A developmental approach.* New York: Basic Books.

Reyes, M. B., Routh, D. K., Jean-Gilles, M. M., Sanfilippo, M. D., & Fawcett, N. (1991). Ethnic differences in parenting children in fearful situations. *Journal of Pediatric Psychology, 16,* 717–726.

Richtsmeier, A. J., & Hatcher, J. W. (1994). Parental anxiety and minor illness. *Developmental and Behavioral Pediatrics, 15,* 14–19.

Rickard, K. (1988). The occurrence of maladaptive health-related behaviors and teacher-related conduct problems in children of chronic low back pain patients. *Journal of Behavioral Medicine, 11,* 107–116.

Robinson, J. O., Alverez, J. H., & Dodge, J. A. (1990). Life events and family history in children with recurrent abdominal pain. *Journal of Psychosomatic Research, 34,* 171–181.

Robinson, J. P. (1972). Television's impact on everyday life: Some cross-national evidence. In E. A. Rubinstein, G. A. Comstock, & J. P. Murray (Eds.), *Television and social behavior: Vol. 4. Television in day-to-day life: Patterns of use.* Washington, DC: U.S. Government Printing Office.

Roghmann, K. J., & Haggerty, R. J. (1973). Daily stress, illness, and use of health services in young families. *Pediatrics Research, 7,* 520–526.

Rosenstock, I. M., & Kirscht, J. P. (1980). Why people seek health care. In G. L. Stone, F. Cohen, & N. E. Adler (Eds.), *Health psychology—A handbook* (pp. 161–188). San Francisco: Jossey-Bass.

Rossiter, J. R., & Robertson, T. S. (1980). Children's dispositions toward proprietary drugs and the role of television drug advertising. *Public Opinion Quarterly, 44,* 316–329.

Sallis, J. F., Alcaraz, J. E., McKenzie, T. L., Hovell, M. F., Kolody, B., & Nader, P. R. (1992). Parental behavior in relation to physical activity and fitness in 9-year-old children. *American Journal of Diseases of Children, 146,* 1383–1388.

Sameroff, A. J., & Chandler, M. J. (1975). Reproductive risk and the continuum of caretaking casualty. In F. D. Horowitz, M. Hetherington, S. Scarr-Salapatek, & G. Sigel (Eds.), *Review of child development research: Vol. 4* (pp. 187–244). Chicago: University of Chicago Press.

Sameroff, A. J., Seifer, R., Barocas, R., et al. (1987). Intelligence quotient scores of 4-year-old children: Social-environmental risk factors. *Pediatrics, 79,* 343–349.

Schor, E., Starfield, B., Stidley, C., & Hankin, J. (1987). Family health: Utilization and effects of family membership. *Medical Care, 25,* 616–626.

Shakato, R., Edwards, L., & Grossman, M. (1980, February). *An exploration of the dynamic relationship between health and cognitive development in adolescence.* National Bureau of Economic Research Working Paper No. 454. Washington, DC: NBER.

Shute, R., Pierre, R., & Lubell, E. (1981). Smoking awareness and practices of urban pre-school and first grade children. *Journal of School Health, 5,* 347–351.

Sigelman, C. K., Derenowski, E. B., Mullaney, H. A., & Siders, A. T. (1993). Parents' contributions to knowledge and attitudes regarding AIDS. *Journal of Pediatric Psychology, 18,* 221–235.

Signorielli, N., & Lears, M. (1992). Television and children's conceptions of nutrition: Unhealthy messages. *Health Communication, 4,* 245–257.

Stein, J. A., & Newcomb, M. D. (1994). Children's internalizing and externalizing behaviors and maternal health problems. *Journal of Pediatric Psychology, 19,* 571–594.

Strasburger, V. C. (1992). Children, adolescents, and television. *Pediatrics in Review, 13,* 144–151.

Tinsley, B. J. (1992a). The influence of familial and interpersonal factors on children's development and associated cardiovascular risk. In H. S. Friedman (Ed.), *Hostility, coping, and health.* Washington, DC: American Psychological Association.

Tinsley, B. J. (1992b). Multiple influences on the acquisition and socialization of children's health attitudes and behavior: An integrative review. *Child Development, 63,* 1043–1069.

Tinsley, B. J. (1995). *The value placed on children's health as a predictor of women's use of prenatal health services.* Unpublished manuscript.

Tinsley, B. J., & Holtgrave, D. R. (1989). Parental health beliefs, utilization of childhood preventive health services, and infant health. *Journal of Developmental and Behavioral Pediatrics, 10,* 236–241.

Tinsley, B. J., & Lees, N. B. (1995). Health promotion for parents. In M. H. Bornstein (Ed.), *Handbook of parenting: Vol. 4, Part 2.* Hillsdale, NJ: Erlbaum.

Tinsley, B. J., Reisch, L., & Phillips, G. (1997). Manuscript submitted for publication.

Walker, L. S., & Greene, J. W. (1987). Life events, psychosocial resources, and psychophysiological symptoms in adolescents. *Journal of Clinical Child Psychology, 16,* 29–36.

Walker, L. S., & Zeman, J. L. (1992). Parental response to child illness behavior. *Journal of Pediatric Psychology, 17,* 49–71.

Wertlieb, D., Hauser, S. T., & Jacobson, A. M. (1986). Adaptation to diabetes: Behavior symptoms and family context. *Journal of Pediatric Psychology, 11,* 463–479.

Williams, A. F. (1972). Factors associated with seat belt use in families. *Journal of Safety Research, 4,* 133–138.

Williams, T. H., & Handford, A. G. (1986). Television and other leisure activities. In T. H. Williams (Ed.), *The impact of television: A natural experiment in three communities.* Orlando, FL: Academic Press.

Zahn-Waxler, C., Radke-Yarrow, M., & King, R. A. (1979). Child rearing and children's prosocial initiations toward victims of distress. *Child Development, 50,* 319–330.

IV
SOCIAL DETERMINANTS

An appreciable literature exists relating social factors to mortality, to incidence and prevalence (morbidity) of diseases, to accessibility and availability of care, and to other dimensions of health (e.g., Cockerham, 1995, chaps. 2 & 3; Mechanic, 1979, chaps. 5–7; Syme & Berkman, 1986; Wolinsky, 1988, chaps. 1–2). In contrast, rigorous research on the social determinants of health behavior reflecting clear conceptualizations of the social factors is less abundant. Much research that has been labeled, indexed, or given the key word "social" or "sociocultural" or "sociopsychological" has dealt with demographic attributes of the person, i.e., age, gender, race, and other personal characteristics, rather than with variables that reflect interactions between persons and groups. A truly "social" literature, however, is emerging. Three major areas of research on the social determinants of health behavior are those that deal with social structures, social roles, and social movements.

SOCIAL STRUCTURE DETERMINANTS

Two major focal points subsume much of the research on how social structure affects health behavior: group characteristics, including group membership, group norms, social status or stratification, and lifestyle; and network characteristics, including social ties or linkages.

Group Characteristics

Group Membership and Norms. Suchman's (1965/1972) investigation of the dimension of social group organization and the utilization of health services has had a pronounced heuristic impact on medical sociology as well as on health behavior research. Suchman's work integrated demography, family structure, and social status in an attempt to use group characteristics to predict utilization of services as well as attitudes toward scientific medicine. He concluded that the degree of "parochialism" or "cosmopolitanism" of family backgrounds influenced patterns of beliefs about illness and medical care and ultimately affected patterns of utilization. Suchman's studies have generated both considerable research and an appreciable amount of controversy.

Subsequent investigations have shown the need to revise Suchman's conclusions. Geertsen (1988) presented a precis and assessment of Suchman's model, and a reexamination of its validity in the face of new data, suggesting an alternate model that takes into account the content of specific social and subcultural beliefs and values relevant to health and modern medicine. In Chapter 13, Geertsen further elaborates on how group structures affect use of services.

In a complementary approach to group characteristics, Greenley and Mechanic's (1976) examination of reference groups in relation to

241

seeking care for personal problems revealed that college students who sought counseling from members of the clergy were more oriented to the traditional student culture, while those who used outpatient psychiatric facilities for personal problems were more oriented to the student "counterculture."

The importance of reference groups for health behavior is perhaps greatest in the emergence of risk behaviors in adolescents. The effect of peer pressure on the initiation of adolescent smoking behavior is well documented, as is the complexity of its impact (e.g., Castro, Maddahian, Newcomb, & Bentler, 1987). How group pressure operates in conjunction with self-esteem and other personal characteristics in relation to adolelescent smoking, alcohol use, and sexual risk behavior is becoming more clearly understood (e.g., Dolcini & Adler, 1994).

Social Status and Stratification. The stratification patterns of American and other societies have become the bases for numerous investigations of health behavior. Koos's (1954) large-scale study of health and illness in "Regionville" is an early analysis of how social status is related to the interpretation of signs of illness. The definition of social class or socioeconomic status, however, has been the subject of much debate. To define class or status solely in terms of any—or any combination—of the factors of income, money, and property would make it a "personal" rather than a "social" characteristic. Among the earliest systematic investigators of stratification in American society, Warner (e.g., 1949) demonstrated that class or status was multifaceted, that it reflected education, occupation, lifestyle, and mobility in addition to income and property, and that it reflected not only objective measures of these factors but also social appraisals or evaluations. Yet many attempts to relate socioeconomic position to health behaviors have employed overly simplistic measures that reflect individual income, educational, and occupational levels in some additive fashion. Most studies, if well-conceived and properly conducted, have re-

vealed little if any relationship between income and health behaviors (e.g., Rundall & Wheeler, 1979). Neighbors (1984) urged a thoughtful reconsideration of how income is used in analyses of health behavior research data. Moreover, Allen (1970) cautioned against making inappropriate assumptions about the true beliefs and values of poor persons and about overgeneralizing from the "culture of poverty."

In contrast to any simplistic approach, Coburn and Pope (1974), using a measure of socioeconomic status that reflected income, occupation, and education, together with measures of six variables such as social participation, work self-direction, and powerlessness/planfulness that were thought to reflect "lifestyle" factors that would go beyond personal attributes and that would help account for the effects of socioeconomic status, found that education, income, and social participation were positively related to making preventive dental visits and obtaining vaccinations for polio. Moreover, the relationship between socioeconomic status and having routine preventive physical examinations was curvilinear, with those lowest and highest in socioeconomic status making more such visits than those in the middle socioeconomic ranges. The research raised questions about the overall predictive value of socioeconomic status; social participation was considered to be the most predictive of the explanatory variables. Questions about the value of socioeconomic status as determinants of health beliefs also arise in the work of Moody and Gray (1972)—who observed that it was a less valuable predictor of preventive behavior than was social integration—and in the work of Suchman (1965/1972) and Gochman (1975).

Lifestyle. Badura's (1984) analysis of the behavioral factors in illness led to an attempt to integrate the varied and diverse personal characteristics that underlie behaviors that place people at risk for diseases into a discussion of the concept of "lifestyle" as it relates to health and illness. Badura's model considered stressful experiences in conjunction with personality variables, particularly self-concept and emotional equilibrium. Badura developed a critical analysis of the term "lifestyle" and pointed to the need to clarify its meaning. Bruhn (1988) identified a number of behaviors that relate to health risks and discussed them in relation to lifestyle, paying particular attention to the way in which lifestyle is acquired. Although lifestyle is often thought of as a personal characteristic, it is appropriately considered as a social one as well. Concerns for fitness and for appearing to be fit are linked to the concept of the "social self," advanced by Mead (1934 [cited in Glassner, 1989]) and reflect an ideology consistent with a postindustrial society, consumerism, and decreasing faith in medical technology (Glassner, 1989).

Cockerham, Lueschen, Kunz, and Spaeth (1986) employed a concept of group status that is related to the "esteem a person is accorded by other people" (p. 4) and thus represents a social appraisal. Persons who had low group status perceived a greater number of symptoms as requiring medical care, and were more likely to have made physician's visits for those symptoms, than persons who had higher group status. More important, however, was the finding that group status did not otherwise appreciably relate to healthful lifestyles. Cockerham and his associates advanced the concept of "culture of medicine" to replace the "culture of poverty" concept as a way of looking at those few social group differences that were observed. In Chapter 12, Cockerham elaborates on the relationship between social characteristics and lifestyles.

Among other studies of social stratification, or social status, or social class, M. H. Miller (1973) observed that upper- and middle-class persons were more likely to consult only with a spouse before seeking professional care for cancer symptoms, but that there were no class differences in informal consultations with medically knowledgeable persons. Moreover, socioeconomic status was found to be inversely related to taking lay advice. Osborn (1973) found that social ranking was directly related to positive self-evaluations of health status, but that the influence of rank on

these evalations was greatest among those with no reported chronic conditions.

Pflanz, Basler, and Schwoon (1977) reported that among adult German males—but not among females—there was a greater use of tranquilizing drugs among those in the upper and upper-middle classes than in the lower class. This difference, however, could not be accounted for by social participation or any other of several social characteristics. In an Indian study, Ramachandran and Shastri (1983) were unable to relate occupational status to choice of source of medical care. Verbrugge (1978) was unable to find that socioeconomic status was related to being among the "early accepters" or "new users" of contraceptive methods for family planning.

Social Networks

In both the Ramachandran and Shastri (1983) study and the Verbrugge (1978) study, the absence of socioeconomic status effects was complemented by observations of the importance of social networks and informal social contacts. For example, Ramachandran and Shastri observed that decisions to seek medical care at specific sites were often influenced by the location of relatives near such sites. Verbrugge noted the importance of certain communicator characteristics of the "early accepters" as effective transmitters of information, advice, and influence throughout informal networks of their relatives, friends, and neighbors. It is the interactions among such informal social contacts—the degree to which persons participate in a variety of social interaction processes—that comprise the essence of research on social networks.

Moody and Gray (1972), using Suchman's model, provided one of the earliest demonstrations of the important role played by social interaction, in contrast to socioeconomic status, in predictions of mothers' having their children participate in oral polio immunization. Mothers who had higher levels of social integration, i.e., higher rates of participating in community activities, and lower levels of alienation were more likely to have their children participate in the immunization program than mothers who had lower levels of social integration and higher levels of alienation. These relationships were found, in general, to be independent of socio-economic status.

Pilisuk and Froland (1978) noted how circles of "intimates" have replaced families in urbanized and mobile societies, pointed out the value of such social support networks in the area of health and illness, and outlined a model of network analysis. Wallston, Alagna, DeVellis, and DeVellis (1983), in the context of reviewing the literature on social support and physical health, identified how social supports are related to adherence to medication regimens and to self-management programs. Levy's (1983, 1986) reviews of the literature on social support and compliance clearly identified some major problems in the definition and description of social support as well as the methodological problems inherent in much of this research. Hammer (1983) examined the relationships between social networks, health status, buffering of stresses, and health behaviors and concluded that while social networks may mediate health status through their effects on health behaviors, their impact on health status cannot be accounted for solely through this mediation. Jacobson (1986) called attention to the need to examine the timing of support and to characterize the type of support more specifically. Neighbors and Jackson (1984) identified patterns of illness behavior in the black community in relation to differential use of informal networks and professional help. Women were more likely to use informal networks than men, persons with physical problems were less likely to use *only* informal networks than persons with emotional problems, and use of these informal networks for physical problems was likely to result in decisions to seek professional care.

Ritter (1988) distinguished between social support and social networks, calling attention to the need for greater precision and clarity in dealing with these concepts. He related social networks and social support to health beliefs, utiliza-

tion of services, and health-promoting behaviors and presented a model to account for the influence of social networks.

Data on the effects of social networks and support are equivocal. There is inconsistency in the way they are defined and measured. Critical treatments of social networks are provided by Hibbard (1985); by Turner and Marino (1994); by Stewart (1989), who analyzes social support in relation to five different conceptual frameworks; by Heitzmann and Kaplan's (1988) evaluation of 23 methods of assessing social support; and in Undén and Orth-Gomér's (1989) report on the reliability and validity of an Interview Schedule for Social Interaction.

Broadhead, Gehlbach, DeGruy, and Kaplan (1989), among others, made the important distinction between *functional* support, which refers to what the supportive relationship provides (e.g., emotional, informational, instrumental support), and *structural* support, which refers to the quantitative aspects of the social network (e.g., size, frequency of interaction). They also examined the differential impacts of emotional and instrumental support and the interactions between these types of support and gender. Shumaker and Hill (1991) critiqued support concepts and demonstrated some important gender differences in the composition and impact of support. The differential impact of social support on chronic, embarrassing, and life-threatening conditions was demonstrated by Martin, Davis, Baron, Suls, and Blanchard (1994). In Chapter 13, Geertsen additionally discusses the impact of social networks on use of services in relation to different ethnic groupings.

The importance of social integration is also evidenced in Langlie's (1977) analysis of health belief model variables and preventive behaviors. Langlie dealt not only with social group characteristics, but also with patterns of family and social interaction, and made an important conceptual and empirical distinction between "indirect risk" and "direct risk" preventive health behaviors. Other ways in which the breadth of social networks and support systems influence health behaviors are pointed out in Finlayson's (1976) observations that women whose husbands had more successful recoveries from heart attacks had wider social contacts than those whose husbands had less sucessful recoveries; in Baranowski et al.'s (1983) observations of the differential influence on breast-feeding of specific members of a mother's network, depending on ethnicity; in Calnan's (1983) observations in Britain that in the case of sudden illnesses or accidents away from home, decisions to seek medical care are made more quickly when others are consulted than when no one is consulted; in Frankel and Nuttall's (1984) findings in a Canadian sample that social support becomes a significant predictor of use of physician services for persons experiencing high distress; and in Furstenberg and Davis's (1984) case history observations of older persons showing how conversations among older persons in which information was either sought or transmitted, or that led to help with daily tasks, also led to social support that reinforced health actions and use of health services.

SOCIAL ROLES

The concept of "role" provides a way of integrating the individual and society; of relating personal behavior to group or societal norms; of examining individual performances within the context of social expectations about those performances. Research on health behavior makes use of two critical role concepts: the sick role and gender-based roles.

Sick Role

Parsons's conception of the sick role (e.g., Parsons, 1951, 1972) has provided an important framework for understanding the behavior of sick persons in terms of role and role relationships in the context of the social system, particularly in relation to such traditional American values as achievement, autonomy, and produc-

tivity. By virtue of accepting the role, and by performing it appropriately, the incumbent in the sick role is temporarily allowed to demonstrate dependency and is relieved of performing other roles and tasks, i.e., is allowed to behave in ways that are contrary to the society's dominant values. Within the Parsonian framework, the "sick role" is only conditionally legitimate.

Twaddle's (1979) elaboration of the concept of sick role treats health and illnesses as statuses, with health having a higher value than illness. Health and illness are thus seen as the bases for social evaluations and consequently for social stratification. Twaddle further considers health as a norm and illness as deviance from this norm.

In a lively debate, Gallagher (1976/1979) systematically critiqued parts of Parsons's position, to which Parsons (1975 [sic]) developed a rejoinder. Arluke, Kennedy, and Kessler's (1979) literature review of research on the sick role showed that although little association exists within individual beliefs about the four major sick role dimensions, and while some economic and social factors are related to individual sick role dimensions, there is nonetheless consensus in the way people conceptualize the sick role. Questions have been raised about the "coherence" of the role's components and about its universality; data suggest that the dimensions are not empirically correlated (e.g., Segall, 1976). Despite both conceptual and empirical criticisms, the construct of "sick role" has been unquestionably heuristic and has generated research linking personal health behavior to the demands, expectations, status, and value systems of the social world.

Social class or socioeconomic status or both have been important variables in research related to the sick role. Britt (1975) observed that social class and sick role incumbency have a reciprocal relationship, mediated by the stresses that arise from the poor housing, crowding, and inadequate social conditions associated with low incomes. Occupying the sick role tends to reduce income and income-generating opportunities. These reductions, in turn, increase both stress and certain behaviors that may additionally decrease employability (e.g., reduction of job seeking) and thus increase the likelihood that occupation of the sick role will be continued.

Physicians are traditionally considered to be the legitimate gatekeepers of entry into the sick role. Field (1961/1972) described economic and political factors that affect physicians' behavior in relation to granting the sick role, i.e., to the certification or legitimization of illness. Dodier (1985) reported on how French physicians may vary in their moral evaluations of workers and how these evaluations affect their allowing workers to occupy the sick role.

The physicians' power to legitimate the sick role thus increases in importance as society becomes overmedicalized. The overmedicalizing of American society (e.g., Fox, 1977) is reflected in the medicalization of deviance, i.e., the selective labeling of nonnormative behaviors such as alcoholism and other behavioral problems as illnesses. How certain behavior problems have been labeled as illnesses, and how professionals employ sick role concepts in dealing with them, can be demonstrated in the research of Chalfant and Kurtz (1971) and Kurtz and Giacopassi (1975). Brown and Rawlinson's (1977) analysis of sick role incumbency after recovery from cardiac surgery showed that males more readily relinquish the sick role than females and thus pointed to the issue of gender and its relationship to health behavior.

In Chapter 14, Segall provides a mid-1990s perspective on the sick role, emphasizing its demedicalization and the distinctions between the patient role and the sick role. The revised sick role model incorporates social "others" into the role relationships either in addition to or instead of the physician.

Gender-Based Roles

A literature review does not reveal the level of intensity of sick role research in the years since the mid-1980s that characterized the previous 30- to 35-year period. Much of the sick role research since the mid-1980s, however, has focused on gender issues and gender differences. Gender has historically been an important basis for role differentiation within social systems, whether these systems be as small as the family or as large as a culture, although anthropologists have shown that there is little or no biological determinism that accounts for this differentiation (e.g., Mead, 1950). Nathanson (1975) and Harrison (1978) both provided seminal and critical analyses of the linkages between gender-based roles and health status. Nathanson noted higher morbidity rates among women as well as their higher rates of utilization of health services—independent of reproduction-related conditions—and identified hypotheses to provide a conceptual frame of reference for understanding the relationship between illness and the female role. In complementary fashion, Harrison's literature review indicated that there were health dangers inherent in the male role.

Harrison's work is anomalous. Generally, research into gender differences has focused on women—on their reportedly poorer health status relative to men and on their greater use of health services. The problem itself has often unknowingly been stated in sexist terms—i.e., of women's behaving inappropriately through *over*use—rather than in terms of men's inappropriate *under*use of health services or of the seeming reluctance of men to enter the sick-role when their doing so would in fact reflect appropriate adaptive coping mechanisms or problem-solving behavior.

The linkages between gender and health status are mediated in large measure by health behaviors, such as perceptions of health status, accepting the sick role, and utilizing appropriate health services. Horwitz (1977) has identified gender differences in discussing problems with others, women being more inclined to do so than men.

A body of research data is accumulating that looks critically at dimensions of gender roles to determine whether some common assumptions or hypotheses about these linkages are warranted. Verbrugge's (1985) critical review of such gender differences also provided an integration of different approaches to accounting for some of them, e.g., gender differences in biological risks, acquired risks, psychosocial aspects of symptoms and care, health-reporting behavior, and history of health care.

In Chapter 15, Waldron systematically explores gender differences in a number of health behaviors and relates these differences to social and cultural role patterns. Citing a large, well-controlled study in which gender differences in utilization of health services similar to those in United States samples were observed in Thailand (Fuller, Edwards, Sermsri, & Vorakitphokatorn, 1993), Waldron notes that in some non-Western cultures, in contrast, the gender differences in utilization of services are reversed: Males use health services more frequently than females!

Multiple Role, Fixed Role, Nurturant Role, and Other Role Hypotheses. The literature on gender-based differences in health behavior moved rapidly from the well-considered conceptualizations of Nathanson and Harrison to the testing of specific role-related hypotheses. Among the prominent models advanced as ways of explaining some of the gender differences in psychosocial aspects of symptoms and care are the multiple role, fixed role, and nurturant role hypotheses. Verbrugge (1983) systematically explored the "multiple role" hypothesis and showed that the combination of roles in which a person is involved (i.e., employee, spouse, parent) has no *special* effect on health or health behavior. While individual roles do have an impact on health and health behaviors, no additional interactive impact is observed for combinations of roles. Thus, data showing women's greater utilization of health services and drugs cannot be explained in terms of women's not engaging in multiple roles. Furthermore, when age and number of roles were controlled, gender differences in health diminished. Verbrugge reasoned, however, that ability to occupy roles such as that of spouse or parent, or to perform successfully as an em-

ployee, may itself require at least some minimal level of health status.

Marcus and Siegel's (1982) exploration of the fixed role hypothesis that women typically have fewer "fixed" role obligations to others (e.g., to employers) that would prevent them from seeking services revealed no gender differences in utilization of care for acute conditions and revealed that the gender differences in utilization observed for chronic conditions disappeared when role obligations were controlled. In other, related research, Marcus, Seeman, and Telesky (1983) showed that fixed role obligations were related to remaining in the sick role, but were not likely to explain adoption of the sick role. Moreover, they pointed out that the decision to adopt the sick role may itself be congruent with commitments to fulfilling a number of other role obligations in the long run.

Gove (1984a) proposed the "nurturant role" hypothesis as an alternative to the fixed role hypothesis to account for women's higher rates of illness. According to the nurturant role hypothesis, women's role as nurturer places them in a position where they have greater responsibilities than men for meeting the needs and demands made by others; these demands, in turn, are likely to draw attention to the women's own troubles, and the lack of structure of the nurturant role gives women more time to dwell upon those troubles. Marcus, Seeman, and Telesky (1984) and Gove (1984b) debated the relative merits of their hypotheses.

Hibbard and Pope (1983) showed that while females were more likely than males to report experiences of symptoms, there were no observable gender differences in acceptance of the sick role when ill. They further observed that women with greater role responsibilities used medical services more than women with fewer such responsibilities. Moreover, Hibbard and Pope reasoned from their data that the perceptual and behavioral aspects of illness operate differently in males and females, that the greatest gender differences occur in relation to perception of symptoms rather than in utilization behavior, and that role responsibilities may be related to differences in paying attention to or interpreting ambiguous symptoms—as opposed to serious or obvious symptoms. The complexity of their analyses enabled them to show, for example, that increased reports of symptoms were inversely related to adoption of the sick role among females. Hibbard and Pope clearly pointed out how difficult it is to compare males and females on role responsibilities, noting that it is difficult to control for the amount of time and attention that the genders give to any paticular role.

Caretaker, peacekeeper, teacher, and partner were among women's roles examined in the context of family life cycle and nutritional behavior by Devine and Olson (1992). The complexity of their interaction is seen in observations that the caretaker role can have both positive and negative impacts on a woman's personal nutritional care. Since caretaking involves responsibilities for the nutritional needs of the family, women in caretaking roles often focused on the needs of others, rather than on their own needs; yet such attention to others could provide support for their own nutritional care (Devine & Olson, 1992).

Women who occupied "traditional" roles (not employed outside the home and supported by men) and women who shared family financial responsibilities with men were found to have more Pap smears and breast examinations than women who occupied "nontraditional" roles (employed and carrying full family responsibilities alone) (Lutz, 1989). Women in "nontraditional" roles were more likely to have blood pressure screening. HMO participation did not increase preventive behaviors for traditional women, but did help somewhat in increasing the number of breast examinations for women who shared financial burdens and in increasing the number of blood pressure screenings for nontraditional women (Lutz, 1989).

Feminist Perspectives. Ross and Bird (1994, p. 162) noted: "National health statistics capture male health problems such as heart disease, cancer, and emphysema. Problems which women experience may be minor from a medical viewpoint, but they are not so in women's daily lives." There is emergent, however, a much-needed, complementary "feminist" perspective. For example, Chrisler (1993) noted the importance of a feminist perspective in looking at eating behaviors, placing these behaviors in the context of cultural norms of beauty and "fat oppression."

Moreover, while systematically collected data (Gabe & Calnan, 1989) indicated that the majority of women have positive views about life-saving technology, they also showed that women are dubious about technology in cancer research and treatment and have much less faith in technology's value in relation to "minor" illnesses and discomfort—the issues of concern to them. They believe that the treatments for these conditions, e.g., penicillin, drugs, are inappropriate. Gabe and Calnan (1989) cautioned against overgeneralizing about women's dependency, victimization, vulnerability to physician power, and other components of medicalization: "Women are not simply passive victims of such a process" (p. 230).

Kandrack, Grant, and Segall (1991) raised several important questions about the conceptual, methodological, and theoretical issues that frame questions about health status and health behavior, as well as about a feminist critique of parts of the scientific process that "finds" gender differences. Noting that many of the differences are insubstantial and that the studies that do not find differences do not get published, Kandrack et al. suggested that it is necessary to rethink the scientific paradigm for gender and health and to move away from merely uncovering differences and toward greater understanding of the social construction of gender relations.

SOCIAL MOVEMENTS: CONSUMERISM AND SELF-CARE

Although there have been diverse social movements related to health issues and health behavior (e.g., temperance, Christian Science, antifluoridation, the feminist health movement), two related social "movements" with special relevance for health behavior are consumerism and self-care. (The feminist health movement itself embraces both of these issues.) For social phenomena to be labeled as "social movements," they must involve an ideology, a sense of common purpose, a structure or institutionalization, and a course of strategy and action (e.g., Schiller & Levin, 1983). Temperance, Christian Science, consumerism, the feminist health movement, and consumerism all meet these criteria; as will be seen, whether self-care does is debatable. But both consumerism and self-care have had a considerable impact on the way in which relationships between the physician–professional and the patient–client–consumer are conceptualized.

Consumerism

One major model of consumerist analysis focuses on changes taking place in the power distribution of the physician–patient relationship (e.g., Haug, 1994; Lavin, Haug, Belgram, & Breslau, 1987), challenging physician authority and assigning a more assertive role to the patient. A complementary model looks beyond the physician–patient relationship to a broad range of information, attitudes, and behavioral expectations involving the purchase of health care (Hibbard & Weeks, 1987). In either case, interactions between persons and health care institutions are no longer viewed in traditional terms of an authoritative/authoritarian physician with a monopoly on knowledge dictating to a passive, accepting patient. Patients are increasingly viewed as consumers who engage in active information seeking to increase their own knowledge, who question physician authority, whose interactions with physicians are likely to include negotiations about diagnosis and treatment, and who make independent judgments about health care and illness.

Data support some shift toward consumerism in the population (Hibbard & Weeks, 1987), although the magnitutde of its impact is difficult to determine. Data also show some shift in medical students' own views toward a more consumerist perpsective (Lavin et al., 1987). Consumerism would also seem to meet the criteria for a social movement. It reflects an ideology and common purpose, it has several institutions or structures (e.g., *Consumers Union*, *Consumers Report*, various bureaus of consumer affairs), and it has resulted in the taking of action (consumer boycotts, actions for improved product safety). The extent to which consumerism is a determinant of health behavior, an outcome of other social and economic processes, or a combination of the two remains to be ascertained.

In Chapter 3, Volume II, of this *Handbook*, Haug provides a critical discussion of consumerism in the context of an analysis of physicians' power and health behavior.

Self-Care

Self-care is the most frequently observed form of primary health care, and the layperson's centrality in disease control and illness management has long been acknowledged (e.g., Levin, 1976). Self-care as a social phenomenon can be observed as a reflection of the "de-professionalization" that took place in the mid-1960s and resulted in social pressure to increase consumer participation and control over health care and in special programs to train consumers (Levin, 1976). Whether self-care meets the criteria for social movements, however, is questionable. Schiller and Levin (1983) raised serious questions about whether there is consensus around an ideology, a sense of common purpose, an organizational or institutional structure, or collective plans for social action. Whether or not self-care can legitimately be labeled as a social movement, it is an important conceptual framework in the area of social norms in relation to decisions about care seeking and treatment.

Self-care is manifest in much of the mid-1990s emphasis on self-regulation or self-management in chronic conditions. Lau introduced these processes in Chapter 3.

In Volume II, chapters by Clark (Chapter 8), Wysocki and Greco (Chapter 9), and Di Iorio (Chapter 11) are among those that highlight self-care in adherence to a broad range of regimens.

REFERENCES

Allen, V. L. (1970). Theoretical issues in poverty research. *Journal of Social Issues, 26,* 149–167.

Arluke, A., Kennedy, L., & Kessler, R. C. (1979). Reexamining the sick-role concept: An empirical assessment. *Journal of Health and Social Behavior, 20,* 30–36.

Badura, B. (1984). Life-style and health: Some remarks on different viewpoints. *Social Science and Medicine, 19,* 341–347.

Baranowski, T., Bee, D. E., Rassin, D. K., Richardson, C. J., Brown, J. P., Guenther, N., & Nader, P. R. (1983). Social support, social influence, ethnicity and the breastfeeding decision. *Social Science and Medicine, 21,* 1599–1611.

Britt, D. W. (1975). Social class and the sick role: Examining the issue of mutual influence. *Journal of Health and Social Behavior, 16,* 178–182.

Broadhead, W. E., Gehlbach, S. H., DeGruy, F. V., & Kaplan, B. H. (1989). Functional versus structural social support and health care utilization in a family medicine outpatient practice. *Medical Care, 27,* 221–233.

Brown, J. S., & Rawlinson, M. E. (1977). Sex differences in sick role rejection and in work performance following cardiac surgery. *Journal of Health and Social Behavior, 18,* 276–292.

Bruhn, J. G. (1988). Life style and health behavior. In D. S. Gochman (Ed.), *Health behavior: Emerging research perspectives* (pp. 71–86). New York: Plenum Press.

Calnan, M. (1983). Social networks and patterns of help-seeking behaviour. *Social Science and Medicine, 17,* 25–28.

Castro, F. G., Maddahian, E., Newcomb, M. D., & Bentler, P. M. (1987). A multivariate model of the determinants of cigarette smoking among adolescents. *Journal of Health and Social Behavior, 28,* 273–289.

Chalfant, H. P., & Kurtz, R. A. (1971). Alcoholics and the sick role: Assessments by social workers. *Journal of Health and Social Behavior, 12,* 66–72.

Chrisler, J. C. (1993). Feminist perspectives on weight loss therapy. *Journal of Training and Practice in Professional Psychology, 7*(1), 35–48.

Coburn, D., & Pope, C. R. (1974). Socioeconomic status and preventive health behaviour. *Journal of Health and Social Behavior, 15,* 67–78.

Cockerham, W. C. (Ed.). (1995). *Medical sociology* (6th ed.). Englewood Cliffs, NJ: Prentice-Hall.

Cockerham, W. C., Lueschen, G., Kunz, G., & Spaeth, J. L. (1986). Social stratification and self-management of health. *Journal of Health and Social Behavior, 27,* 1–14.

Devine, C. M., & Olson, C. M. (1992). Women's perceptions about the way social roles promote or constrain personal nutrition care. *Women and Health, 19*(1), 79–95.

Dodier, N. (1985). Social uses of illness at the workplace: Sick leave and moral evaluation. *Social Science and Medicine, 20,* 123–128.

Dolcini, M. M., & Adler, N. E. (1994). Perceived competencies, peer group affiliation, and risk behavior among early adolescents. *Health Psychology, 94,* 496–506.

Field, M. G. (1961/1972). The doctor–patient relationship in the perspective of "fee-for-service" and "third-party" medicine. In E. G. Jaco (Ed.), *Patients, physicians and illness: A sourcebook in behavioral science and health* (2nd ed., pp. 222–232). New York: Free Press. [Reprinted from *Journal of Health and Human Behavior, 2,* 252–262.]

Finlayson, A. (1976). Social networks as coping resources. *Social Science and Medicine, 10,* 97–103.

Fox, R. C. (1977). The medicalization and demedicalization of American society. In J. H. Knowles (Ed.), *Doing better and feeling worse: Health in the United States.* New York: Norton.

Frankel, B. G., & Nuttall, S. (1984). Illness behaviour: An exploration of determinants. *Social Science and Medicine, 19,* 147–155.

Fuller, T. D., Edwards, J. N., Sermsri, S., & Vorakitphokatorn, S. (1993). Gender and health: Some Asian evidence. *Journal of Health and Social Behavior, 34,* 252–271.

Furstenberg, A. L., & Davis, L. J. (1984). Lay consultation of older people. *Social Science and Medicine, 18,* 827–837.

Gabe, J., & Calnan, M. (1989). The limits of medicine: Women's perception of medical technology. *Social Science and Medicine, 28,* 223–231.

Gallagher, E. B. (1976/1979). Lines of reconstruction and extension in the Parsonian sociology of illness. In E. G. Jaco (Ed.), *Patients, physicians, and illness: A sourcebook in behavioral science and health* (3rd ed., pp. 162–183). New York: Free Press, (Reprinted from *Social Science and Medicine,* 1976, *10,* pp. 207–218.)

Geertsen, R. (1988). Social group characteristics and health behavior. In D. S. Gochman (Ed.), *Health behavior: Emerging research perspectives* (pp. 131–148). New York: Plenum Press.

Glassner, B. (1989). Fitness and the postmodern self. *Journal of Health and Social Behavior, 30,* 180–191.

Gochman, D. S. (1975). The measurement and development of dentally relevant motives. *Journal of Public Health Dentistry, 35,* 160–164.

Gove, W. R. (1984a). Gender differences in mental and physical illness: The effects of fixed roles and nurturant roles. *Social Science and Medicine, 19,* 77–91.

Gove, W. R. (1984b). On understanding illness, illness behavior, and reading what has been written: A reply to Marcus, Seeman and Telesky. *Social Science and Medicine, 19,* 88–91.

Greenley, J. R., & Mechanic, D. (1976). Social selection in seeking help for psychological problems. *Journal of Health and Social Behavior, 17*, 249-262.

Hammer, M. (1983). "Core" and "extended" social networks in relation to health and illness. *Social Science and Medicine, 17*, 405-411.

Harrison, J. (1978). Warning: The male sex role may be dangerous to your health. *Journal of Social Issues, 34*, 65-86.

Haug, M. R. (1994). Elderly patients, caregivers, and physicians: Theory and research on health care triads. *Journal of Health and Social Behavior, 35*, 1-12.

Heitzman, C. A., & Kaplan, R. M. (1988). Assessment of methods for measuring social support. *Health Psychology, 7*, 75-109.

Hibbard, J. H. (1985). Social ties and health status: An examination of moderating factors. *Health Education Quarterly, 12*, 23-34.

Hibbard, J. H., & Pope, C. R. (1983). Gender roles, illness orientation and use of medical services. *Social Science and Medicine, 17*, 129-137.

Hibbard, J. H., & Weeks, E. C. (1987). Consumerism in health care: Prevalance and predictors. *Medical Care, 25*, 1019-1032.

Horwitz, A. (1977). The pathways into psychiatric treatment: Some differences between men and women. *Journal of Health and Social Behavior, 18*, 169-178.

Jacobson, D. E. (1986). Types and timing of social support. *Journal of Health and Social Behavior, 27*, 250-264.

Kandrack, M.-A., Grant, K. R., & Segall, A. (1991). Gender differences in health related behaviour: Some unanswered questions. *Social Science and Medicine, 32*, 579-590.

Koos, E. L. (1954). *The health of Regionville: What the people thought and did about it.* New York: Columbia University Press.

Kurtz, R. A., & Giacopassi, D. J. (1975). Medical and social work students' perceptions of deviant conditions and sick role incumbency. *Social Science and Medicine, 9*, 249-255.

Langlie, J. K. (1977). Social networks, health beliefs, and preventive health behavior. *Journal of Health and Social Behavior, 18*, 244-260.

Lavin, B., Haug, M., Belgrave, L. L., & Breslau, N. (1987). Change in student physicians' views on authority relationships with patients. *Journal of Health and Social Behavior, 28*, 258-272.

Levin, L. S. (1976). The layperson as the primary health care practitioner. *Public Health Reports, 91*, 204-210.

Levy, R. L. (1983). Social support and compliance: A selective review and critique of treatment integrity and outcome measurement. *Social Science and Medicine, 18*, 1329-1338.

Levy, R. L. (1986). Social support and compliance: Salient methodological problems in compliance research. *Journal of Compliance in Health Care, 1*(2), 189-198.

Lutz, M. E. (1989). Women, work, and preventive health care: An exploratory study of the efficacy of HMO membership. *Women and Health, 15*(1), 21-33.

Marcus, A. C., Seeman, T. E., & Telesky, C. W. (1983). Sex differences in reports of illness and disability: A further test of the fixed role hypothesis. *Social Science and Medicine, 17*, 993-1002.

Marcus, A. C., Seeman, T. E., & Telesky, C. W. (1984). Teetering on the horns of a dilemma: Professor Gove's latest paper on sex differences in illness behavior. *Social Science and Medicine, 19*, 84-88.

Marcus, A. C., & Siegel, J. M. (1982). Sex differences in the use of physician services: A preliminary test of the fixed role hypothesis. *Journal of Health and Social Behavior, 23*, 186-197.

Martin, R., Davis, G. M., Baron, R. S., Suls, J., & Blanchard, E. B. (1994). Specificity in social support: Perceptions of helpful and unhelpful provider behaviors among irritable bowel syndrome, headache, and cancer patients. *Health Psychology, 13*, 432-439.

Mead, G. H. (1934). *Mind, self and society.* Chicago: University of Chicago Press.

Mead, M. (1950). *Sex and temperament in three primitive societies.* New York: Mentor.

Mechanic, D. (Ed.). (1979). *Medical sociology: A comprehensive text (2nd ed.).* New York: Free Press.

Miller, M. H. (1973). Seeking advice for cancer symptoms. *American Journal of Public Health, 63*, 955-961.

Moody, P. M., & Gray, R. M. (1972). Social class, social integration, and the use of preventive health services. In E. G. Jaco (Ed.), *Patients, physicians and illness: A sourcebook in behavioral science and health* (2nd ed., pp. 250-261). New York: Free Press.

Nathanson, C. A. (1975). Illness and the feminine role: A theoretical review. *Social Science and Medicine, 9*, 57-62.

Neighbors, H. W. (1984). Professional help use among black Americans: Implications for unmet need. *American Journal of Community Psychology, 12*, 551-566.

Neighbors, H. W., & Jackson, J. J. (1984). The use of informal and formal help: Four patterns of illness behavior in the black community. *American Journal of Community Psychology, 12*, 629-644.

Osborn, R. W. (1973). Social rank and self-health evaluation of older urban males. *Social Science and Medicine, 7*, 209-218.

Parsons, T. (1951). *The social system.* Glencoe, IL: Free Press.

Parsons, T. (1972). Definitions of health and illness in the light of American values and social structure. In E. G. Jaco (Ed.), *Patients, physicians and illness: A sourcebook in behavioral science and health* (2nd ed.) (pp. 97-117). New York: Free Press.

Parsons, T. (1975). The sick role and the role of the physician reconsidered. *Milbank Memorial Fund Quarterly/Health and Society, 53*(Summer), 257-278.

Pflanz, M., Basler, H.-D., & Schwoon, D. (1977). Use of tranquilizing drugs by a middle-aged population in a West

German city. *Journal of Health and Social Behavior, 18*, 194–205.

Pilisuk, M., & Froland, C. (1978). Kinship, social networks, social support and health. *Social Science and Medicine, 12B*, 273–280.

Ramachandran, H., & Shastri, G. S. (1983). Movement for medical treatment: A study in contact patterns of a rural population. *Social Science and Medicine, 17*, 177–187.

Ritter, C. (1988). Social supports, social networks, and health behaviors. In D. S. Gochman (Ed.), *Health behavior: Emerging research perspectives* (pp. 149–161). New York: Plenum Press.

Ross, C. E., & Bird, C. E. (1994). Sex, stratification and health lifestyle: Consequences for men's and women's perceived health. *Journal of Health and Social Behavior, 35*, 161–178.

Rundall, T. G., & Wheeler, J. R. C. (1979). The effect of income on use of preventive care: An evaluation of alternative explanations. *Journal of Health and Social Behavior, 20*, 397–406.

Schiller, P. L., & Levin, J. S. (1983). Is self-care a social movement? *Social Science and Medicine, 17*, 1343–1352.

Segall, A. (1976). Sociocultural variation in sick role behavioural expectations. *Social Science and Medicine, 10*, 47–51.

Shumaker, S. A., & Hill, D. R. (1991). Gender differences in social support and physical health. *Health Psychology, 10*, 102–111.

Stewart, M. J. (1989). Social support: Diverse theoretical perspectives. *Social Science and Medicine, 28*, 1275–1282.

Suchman, E. A. (1965/1972). Stages of illness and medical care. In E. G. Jaco (Ed.), *Patients, physicians and illness: A sourcebook in behavioral science and health* (2nd ed.,

pp. 155–171). New York: Free Press. [Reprinted from *Journal of Health and Human Behavior*, 1965, *6*, 114–128.]

Syme, S. L., & Berkman, L. F. (1976/1990). Social class, susceptibility, and sickness. In P. Conrad & R. Kern (Eds.), *The sociology of health and illness* (3rd ed., pp. 28–34). New York: St. Martin's. (Reprinted from *American Journal of Epidemiology*, 1976, *104*, 1–8).

Turner, R. J., & Marino, F. (1994). Social support and social structure: A descriptive epidemiology. *Journal of Health and Social Behavior, 35*, 193–212.

Twaddle, A. C. (1979). *Sickness behavior and the sick role*. Boston: G. K. Hall.

Undén, A.-L., & Orth-Gomér, K. (1989). Development of a social support instrument for use in population surveys. *Social Science and Medicine, 29*, 1387–1892.

Verbrugge, L. M. (1978). Peers as recruiters: Family planning communications of West Malaysian acceptors. *Journal of Health and Social Behavior, 19*, 51–68.

Verbrugge, L. M. (1983). Multiple roles and physical health of women and men. *Journal of Health and Social Behavior, 24*, 16–30.

Verbrugge, L. M. (1985). Gender and health: An update on hypotheses and evidence. *Journal of Health and Social Behavior, 26*, 156–182.

Wallston, B. S., Alagna, S. W., DeVellis, B. M., & DeVellis, R. F. (1983). Social support and physical health. *Health Psychology, 2*, 367–391.

Warner, W. L. (1949). *Democracy in Jonesville: A study of quality and inequality*. New York: Harper Brothers.

Wolinsky, F. D. (Ed.). (1988). *The sociology of health: Principles, practitioners, and issues* (2nd ed.). Belmont, CA: Wadsworth.

12

Lifestyles, Social Class, Demographic Characteristics, and Health Behavior

William C. Cockerham

The study of lifestyles is one of the most important new developments in health behavior research. Lifestyles are utilitarian social practices and ways of living adopted by individuals that reflect personal, group, and socioeconomic identities (Giddens, 1991). Modern lifestyles consist of self-selected forms of consumerism, involving particular choices in bodily dress and appearance, food, housing, automobiles, work habits, forms of leisure, and other types of status-oriented behavior. Increasing numbers of sociologists have found lifestyles to be particularly significant expressions of individual and collective behavior (Bourdieu, 1984; Giddens, 1991; Turner, 1988), while some have even argued that lifestyle situations are more important influences on behavior than social class position (Hradil, 1987).

Whether or not lifestyles have become stronger predictors of behavior than social class is not resolved, but clearly there is growing interest in researching lifestyles (Abel, 1991). The reason for this interest can be linked to the social change that is occurring in the late 20th century. As industrial society undergoes a transition to postindustrial or late modernity, the certainties and modes of living of the industrial age are being altered. Just as modernization dissolved the structure of feudal society and created the industrial age, modernization today is dissolving industrial society and another modernity is coming into being (Beck, 1992).

There is considerable disagreement about the exact nature and definition of postmodernity, but a common theme is that of an epochal shift, discontinuity, or break with modernity that is bringing with it new social conditions and principles (Baudrillard, 1988; Featherstone, 1991; Frisby, 1985; Smart, 1993). Smart (1993, p. 39) offered perhaps the best definition of this change to date: "The idea of postmodernity indicates a modification or change in the way(s) in which we experience and relate to modern thought, modern conditions, and modern forms of life, in short

William C. Cockerham • Department of Sociology, University of Alabama at Birmingham, Birmingham, Alabama 35294-3350.

Handbook of Health Behavior Research I: Personal and Social Determinants, edited by David S. Gochman. Plenum Press, New York, 1997.

to modernity." Smart suggests that since modernity itself is in a continuous state of flux and perpetually in motion, postmodernity is focused on transformations in society, culture, economics, technology, communications, and politics.

The irony surrounding modernization and its destruction of feudal society is that its success led to its own transformation by postmodern processes (Bauman, 1992; Beck, 1992). Life and thinking in modern societies have had to become more flexible in adjusting to social and economic changes occurring in a postmodern context. As Denzin (1991) points out, the terms *postmodern* and *postmodernity* encompass the form of social, cultural, and economic life under late capitalism. While postmodernity has other meanings in other contexts and disciplines, much of its sociological relevance lies in its depiction of the destabilization of accepted meanings and efforts to adjust to new realities in society after industrialization.

People are finding themselves subjected to evolving social circumstances with the potential for greater behavioral options and fewer constraints than in the past (Giddens, 1991; Smart, 1993). Consequently, the lifestyle choices that people make and the social processes that influence those choices are promoting lifestyles as a major area of sociological inquiry.

The focus of this chapter is upon health lifestyles. Decisions about whether or not to live in a healthful manner are common features of everyday life and constitute a major form of contemporary lifestyles. When it comes to health, lifestyles include forms of interaction with the medical profession for preventive care, such as physical checkups, but the majority of activities take place outside the health care delivery system. These activities typically consist of choices and practices, influenced by the individual's potential for realizing them, that range from brushing one's teeth and eating properly to relaxing at health spas. For most people, health lifestyles involve decisions about food, exercise, coping with stress, smoking, alcohol and drug use, risk of accidents, and physical appearance. In social

conditions of late or postmodernity, lifestyles can be a decisive factor in determining an individual's health status and life expectancy (Cockerham, 1995); therefore, while lifestyles are recognized as important determinants of behavior generally, health lifestyles are a particularly relevant form of health behavior.

Crawford (1984) explained why health lifestyles are particularly relevant. First, the general public has increasingly recognized that the major disease patterns have changed from infectious illnesses to chronic diseases—such as heart disease, cancer, and diabetes—that medicine cannot cure. Second, several health disorders, such as AIDS and tobacco-induced lung cancer, are caused by particular styles of living. Third, there have been public health campaigns emphasizing lifestyle change and individual responsibility for health. The result has been growing awareness that medical care is not always the automatic answer to dealing with threats to the health of individuals. Taking control over one's own health through adoption of a healthful lifestyle has also become a major option for many people. This discussion will begin with a Weberian definition of health lifestyles, followed by a discussion of health lifestyles as normative behavior, lifestyles and class distinctions (from the standpoint of Bourdieu), the late modern–postmodern context, and the spread of health lifestyles in Western society.

DEFINING HEALTH LIFESTYLES

The theoretical basis for understanding the lifestyle concept, including health lifestyles, begins with the work of German sociologist Max Weber (1864–1920). Among the classic theorists in sociology, Weber (1978) provided the deepest insight into what constitutes a lifestyle. Although his thoughts on lifestyles were a marginal aspect of his analysis of status and he did not discuss health lifestyles at all, Weber nonetheless provides the theoretical background for understanding the term *lifestyle*. Weber connected lifestyles with socioeconomic status by suggesting that status groups—aggregates of people with similar status, social class backgrounds, and political influence—originate through a sharing of lifestyles. That is, a specific style of life is expected from people who belong to a given status group. Even though lifestyles reflect individual identity, they primarily reflect the norms and values of particular groups. Lifestyles are therefore a collective rather than an individual phenomenon. When it comes to health, the discrete practices of individuals are more appropriately defined as self-care behaviors, while behaviors that form clusters of complex interactions between multiple social, psychological, and cultural factors are lifestyles (Dean, 1989).

Weber makes the further observation that lifestyles are not based on what a person produces, but on what a person consumes. This is an important point, because, as Baudrillard (1988) explains, consumption should not be interpreted primarily in relation to pleasure or satisfaction of needs, but as a mode of social activity by which individuals insert themselves into a consumer society. Consumption often requires education and effort, and in the process of consuming, a person is conforming to socially normative behavior and signals belonging to a certain stratum. Consumption, however, is not independent of production; rather, lifestyle differences between status groups are based on their relationship to a society's means of consumption, and not solely to the means of production as Marxist theory would suggest. The economic mode of production sets the basic parameters within which consumption occurs, but does not determine or even necessarily affect specific forms of consumption (Bocock, 1993), the reason being that the consumption of goods and services conveys a social identity of the consumer. Consumption can therefore be regarded as a set of social and cultural practices that *establish* differences between social groups, not merely as a means by which to *express* differences that already exist because of economic factors (Bocock, 1993, p. 64; Bourdieu, 1984).

Health lifestyles are grounded in consumption, because even though people who participate in a healthful lifestyle are producing good health, the aim of this activity is ultimately one of consumption. That is, people typically produce health in order to use it for some end, such as work, a longer life, enhanced enjoyment of their physical being, or a pleasing physical appearance (Cockerham, 1995; Cockerham, Abel, & Lüschen, 1993; d'Houtaud & Field, 1984). Studies of corporate exercise programs in the United States show, for example, that people participate in fitness activities not only because they want to stay in shape and lose weight, but also because they want to look better and socialize with friends (Conrad, 1988; Kotarba & Bentley, 1988). In other words, people exercise because they want to do something with their health. In France, other research found that health was conceptualized among the middle class as a state to be cultivated for enjoyment of life and among the lower class as a means of maintaining the capability to continue to work (d'Houtaud & Field, 1984). Consequently, health lifestyles serve the function of producing health for the purpose of using or consuming in some way.

The connection between lifestyles and socioeconomic status is not evident just in Weber's notion of consumption, but extends into his view of the structure of lifestyles. In the original German, Weber's work suggests that lifestyles have two basic components: life choices (*Lebensführung*) and life chances (*Lebenschancen*) (Cockerham et al., 1993). Life choices are the choices that people have in their selection of lifestyles and life chances are the probabilities of realizing those choices. Weber (1978) believed that choice is the major factor in the operationalization of a lifestyle; however, the actualization of choices is influenced by life chances. Dahrendorf (1979, p. 73) noted that while Weber is vague about what he means by life chances, the best interpretation is that life chances are "the crystallized probability of finding satisfaction for interests, wants and needs, thus the probability of the occurrence of events which bring about satisfaction." The probability of acquiring satisfaction is anchored in structural conditions that are largely economic—involving income, property, the opportunity for profit, and the like—but Dahrendorf suggested that the concept of life chances also includes rights, norms, and social relationships (the probability that others will respond in a certain manner). According to Dahrendorf, Weber does not consider life chances to be a matter of pure chance; rather, they are the chances people have in life because of their social situation. The overall thesis is that chance is socially determined and social structure is an arrangement of chances. Hence, lifestyles are not random behaviors unrelated to structure, but typically are deliberate choices influenced by life chances.

Consequently, Cockerham et al. (1993) pointed out that Weber's most important contribution to conceptualizing lifestyles in sociological terms is to place a dialectical capstone on the interplay of choice and structure in lifestyle determination. Choices and constraints interact to determine a distinctive lifestyle for individuals and groups. The identification of life chances as the opposite of life choices in Weber's lifestyle dialectic provides the theoretical key to conceptualizing the manner in which lifestyles are operationalized in the empirical world. It can be said that individuals have a range of freedom, yet not complete freedom, in choosing a lifestyle. That is, people are not entirely free in determining their lifestyle, but have the freedom to choose within the social constraints that apply to their situation in life. Lifestyle constraints are largely, but not entirely, socioeconomic in origin. The value of Weber's concept, therefore, is that it can account for the interplay of individual choice and structural constraints in operationalizing a lifestyle. Those who have the desire and the means may choose; those lacking in some way cannot choose so easily and may find their lifestyle determined more by circumstance than by choice.

Weber's overall contribution to understanding contemporary lifestyles is that lifestyles (1) are associated with status groups and are therefore principally a collective rather than an individual phenomenon; (2) represent patterns of consumption, not production; and (3) are formed by the dialectical interplay between life choices and life chances, with choice playing the greater role.

The following definition of health lifestyles is therefore suggested:

> Health lifestyles are collective patterns of health-related behavior based on choices from options available to people according to their life chances.

This definition incorporates the interplay of choice and chance, but omits the requirement that choices be voluntary. This requirement is omitted because of the possibility that individuals may be more or less coerced into choices by pressure from family, friends, health care providers, mass media campaigns, and their own socioeconomic circumstances.

HEALTH LIFESTYLE AS A NORMATIVE BEHAVIOR

The significance of living as healthful a lifestyle as possible is not a new concept. Early humans apparently recognized the cause-and-effect relationship of different activities and behaviors with respect to health, even though they may have lacked a scientific understanding of the situation (DuBos, 1959). Historical research by Green (1986) on health and fitness in the United States showed a long-term interest on the part of Americans to be healthy for a variety of reasons, including religion, patriotism, the potential for upward social mobility, and the association of health with ideas about success. The dominant American view was that health was an ideal end state that people should achieve.

What is new is the reawakened interest in health lifestyles that occurred in the mid-20th century because of the profound decline in infectious diseases and increase in chronic diseases associated with poor health behavior. Health professionals and the mass media have spread the message that healthy people need to avoid certain behaviors and adopt others as part of their daily routine if they want to maximize their life expectancy and remain healthy as long as possible. These adjurations are supported by ample evidence that a lack of exercise, diets high in fat and cholesterol, stress, smoking, obesity, alcohol and drug abuse, and exposure to chemical pollutants cause serious health problems and early deaths. It is also well known that lifestyles involving male homosexuality and intravenous drug use increase the risk of AIDS, while smoking is linked to lung cancer, alcoholism to cirrhosis of the liver, and high-fat diets to atherosclerosis and heart disease. Conversely, there is strong evidence that pursuing a health lifestyle can enhance one's health and life expectancy. Exercise has been found to reduce the risk of dying from heart disease, as have cessation of cigarette smoking, eating a more healthful diet, controlling one's weight, and coping satisfactorily with stress (Berkman & Breslow, 1983; Blair et al., 1989).

This situation suggests that the ever-increasing emergence of health lifestyles as a major form of normative behavior has the potential for crossing class boundaries. It was Weber's position that lifestyles can spread beyond the groups in which they originate (Bendix, 1960). The best example of this circumstance in Weber's work is his analysis of the spread of the Protestant ethic into the general culture of Western society. The origin of health lifestyles appears to be in the upper-middle class, since the current emphasis on exercise, sports, health diets, avoidance of smoking, and the like began with this group (Featherstone, 1987). Certainly the life chances that enhance participation in a health lifestyle are greatest among upper and upper-middle socioeconomic groups who have the resources to maintain a healthful way of life. Regardless of a person's socioeconomic position, however, an important feature of modern society appears to be the tendency of many people to adopt a health lifestyle within the limits of their life chances. If this be the case, it would suggest that health lifestyles are emerging as a normative pattern of behavior in

the population at large, rather than being restricted to one or two status groups.

LIFESTYLES AND CLASS DISTINCTIONS: BOURDIEU

The research literature on health lifestyles in sociology began to develop only in the mid-1980s as the extent of participation in such lifestyles in Western society became apparent. The focus in most studies to date has been on determining socioeconomic differences and similarities, with one body of research detailing variations between social classes and another noting growing similarities. The discussion on lifestyles has recently moved, however, from descriptive accounts of social behavior, notable in leisure research, to a more analytical and theory-oriented debate (Lüschen et al., 1995). One of the earliest and most theoretically influential studies is Bourdieu's (1984) well-known work *Distinction*. Utilizing survey research data collected during the 1960s and not published until several years later, Bourdieu examined class competition over cultural meanings and the role of culture in class reproduction in France. He constructed a general model of stratified lifestyles based on differing cultural tastes in art, music, food, dress, and the like organized into the following categories: legitimate, middlebrow, and popular. Bourdieu (1984, p. 173) defined *taste* as the capacity to materially or symbolically appropriate a given class of objects and practices as a set of distinctive preferences. Consequently, taste functions, in his view, to mediate the "elective affinity" between certain products and consumers in relation to social class.

Although Bourdieu did not focus on health lifestyles, he included an analysis of sports and food preferences in his study. He found that distinct class preferences existed in these areas. People in the professions, for example, preferred tennis, while the working class favored soccer. The working class was more attentive to notions of masculinity and the physical strength of males and also tended to choose foods that were cheap, nutritious, and abundant. The professions, in contrast, were more concerned about body forms and opted more for food that was light, tasty, and lower in calories. Bourdieu's principal interest, however, was not in describing class differences, but in describing how routine practices of individuals are influenced by the external structure of their social world and how these practices, in turn, contribute to the maintenance of that structure (Jenkins, 1992). Whereas class culture may influence food habits, those habits collectively help reproduce class culture when they are enacted.

This situation underlies Bourdieu's (1990, p. 53) concept of *habitus*, which he defined as "systems of durable, transposable dispositions, structured structures [sic] predisposed to operate as structuring structures, that is, as principles which generate and organize practices and representations that can be objectively adapted to their outcomes without presupposing a conscious aiming at ends or an express mastery of the operations necessary in order to attain them." In other words, social structures and conditions engender enduring personal orientations that are more or less routine, and when these orientations are acted upon, they tend to reproduce the structures from which they are derived.

Habitus provides a cognitive map of an individual's social world and the dispositions or "procedures to follow" appropriate for that person in a particular situation. As Bourdieu explains, the human mind is socially bounded and constructed within the limits of experience, upbringing, and training (Bourdieu & Wacquant, 1992). People are able to figure out their circumstances, but their perceptions are typically shaped by their social and economic conditions. "The *habitus*," stated Bourdieu (1990, p. 54), "... ensures the active presence of past experiences, which, deposited in each organism in the form of schemes of perception, thought and action, tend to guarantee the 'correctness' of practices and their constancy over time, more reliably than all formal rules and explicit norms." Habitus therefore channels behavior down paths that appear reasonable to the individual.

Although Bourdieu (Bourdieu & Wacquant, 1992, p. 135) rejected the notion that his scheme is overly deterministic (structures produce habitus, which determine practices, which reproduce structures), he nonetheless assigned a preference to structure in influencing behavior. According to Bourdieu, categories of perception and appreciation—the basis for self-determination—are themselves largely determined by upbringing and the reality of class circumstances. In his scheme, social practices are based upon both (1) the objective structures that define external constraints that affect interaction and (2) the immediate lived experience of agents that shape internal categories of perception and appreciation. While the two components are equally necessary, however, they are not equal, and Bourdieu awarded epistemological priority to objective conditions over subjectivist understanding (Wacquant, 1992, p. 11).

What this priority implies for understanding lifestyles is the strong influence of structure (i.e., life chances) on the habitus mind-set from which lifestyle choices are derived. This view suggests that selection of and participation in a particular lifestyle are affected by life chances to a much greater extent than allowed by Weber. Bourdieu's work indicates that lifestyle choices are not only constrained but also shaped by life chances. As Bourdieu (1984, p. 171) explained, lifestyles are produced as follows: (1) Objective conditions of existence combine with positions in the social structure to (2) produce the habitus, which consists of (3) a system of schemes generating classifiable practices and works and (4) a system of schemes of perception and appreciation (taste) that together produce (5) specific classifiable practices and works that (6) result in a lifestyle. Although individuals choose their lifestyles, they do not do so with complete free will, as the habitus predisposes them toward certain choices. They have the option to reject or modify these choices, but Bourdieu suggests that agents' choices are consistent with their habitus.

Choices also tend to reflect class position because persons in the same social class share the same habitus. Bourdieu (1990) pointed out that internalization of the same structures and common schemes of perception and appreciation produce the same or similar set of distinctive signs or tastes; consequently, there is a widespread sharing of a class-based world view.

While the habitus produces lifestyles, lifestyles themselves are viewed by Bourdieu as a system of classified and classifying practices involving differing tastes. These practices consist of particular forms of dress, food selection, music, art, sport, leisure activities, and the like—all of which express class distinctions. Lifestyles are viewed as systematic products of habitus that, perceived in their relations to the schemes of habitus, become sign systems that are socially qualified. Lifestyles therefore function as forms of cultural capital with symbolic values. In Bourdieu's view, the human body constitutes physical capital that is transformed into cultural capital as a consequence of class practices (Shilling, 1993; Turner, 1992). As Shilling (1993, p. 140) pointed out, dominant groups have the ability to define themselves and their lifestyles as superior, worthy of reward, and metaphorically and literally the embodiment of class.

It can therefore be argued that structure is the dominant aspect of Bourdieu's concept of lifestyles. The notion of "structure" suggests persistence, repetition, and self-maintenance; hence, habituation, or the tendency of lifestyles to become habitual, is a major feature of his perspective. Lifestyles not only reflect class differences in ways of living, but also reproduce them. Compared to Weber, whose ideas emphasize the voluntary nature of lifestyles. Bourdieu's approach is grounded more in the social support inherent in lifestyle selection. By virtue of being class-based, lifestyles, as unitary sets of tastes or distinctive preferences, are practices that are classified and supported not only by members of a given class, but also by members of other classes (Münch, 1994).

Health lifestyles vary strongly by social class,

and health practices are indeed class-bound in Bourdieu's study. His data, however, were collected prior to the emphasis on health lifestyles that appeared in the 1980s and do not account for changes that have since occurred in France. There have been reports of increased spending on personal health care items and a significant increase in participation in sport and exercise generally in French society (Ardagh, 1987). Herzlich and Pierret (1987) identified a shift in French thinking toward a norm of a "duty to be healthy." Herzlich and Pierret found that this norm is strongest in the middle class, but they provided accounts of less socially advantaged persons espousing the same orientation and implied that this norm is spreading in French society. They described health as a necessity for both society and the individual and as the means by which people achieve self-realization. "Today," they stated (Herzlich and Pierret, 1987, p. 231), "the 'right to health' implies that every individual must be made responsible for his or her health and must adopt rational behavior in dealing with the pathogenic effects of modern life." The most recent data from France show that health lifestyles are indeed expanding across class lines (Lüschen et al., 1995).

The finding that health lifestyles have possibly become more common in French society does not negate Bourdieu's theoretical perspective. Typically, the dispositions generated by habitus to behave in a certain way are consistent with the constraints set by society through experience and socialization; therefore, usual modes of behavior ordinarily occur. Yet Bourdieu (1990) pointed out that habitus is not a mechanical response to all situations. Rather, it is an open system of dispositions that are affected by experience in ways that can either reinforce or change behavior. The same habitus can generate different outcomes, even opposite outcomes, and people are able to orient themselves to dealing with new circumstances. Consequently, habitus has the potential to structure health lifestyle responses across social classes and at the same time maintain some variation between classes. An objective theoretical and empirical argument would suggest that it does function in this way.

THE SPREAD OF HEALTH LIFESTYLES

The author and his colleagues sought to determine whether lifestyles pertaining to the self-management of health had spread across class lines in American society (Cockerham, Lüschen, Kunz, & Spaeth, 1986a). Using data collected from a statewide sample of adults in Illinois, it was found that considerable similarity existed between socioeconomic groups in certain lifestyles involving appearance, food habits, physical exercise, smoking, and alcohol use. Exercise, for instance, emerged as a behavioral pattern that people from all social classes accepted as something a person should do and that most people say they attempt in some form, ranging from short walks to participation in sports. When it came to food habits, most people, regardless of their socioeconomic situation, attempted to obtain the best nutritional value in the food available to them, avoid chemical additives, and the like. This latter finding is supported by Blackburn's (1991) research in Great Britain, in which she found that low-income families spend a higher proportion of their total income on food and shop more efficiently for value and nutrients than higher-income families.

Subsequent research (Abel, Cockerham, Lüschen, & Kunz, 1989; Cockerham, Kunz, & Lueschen, 1988a,b; Cockerham, Lüschen, Kunz, & Spaeth, 1986b; Lueschen, Cockerham, & Kunz, 1987) compared the health lifestyles of Americans to those of Germans and found a distinct lack of difference between social classes, races, and occupational groups in health behavior. Although the quality of participation may vary, health lifestyles in these studies appeared to be widely accepted and practiced.

One study (Cockerham et al., 1988a) examined whether there were significant differences between people with comprehensive health care benefits provided by their government (Ger-

mans) and those who generally lack such coverage (Americans) in regard to participating in health lifestyles. Germany has an extensive system of national health insurance that covers 92% of the total population (the wealthiest are excluded and required to obtain private health insurance), while in the United States, only some 20% of the population — the aged and the poor — have government-sponsored health insurance through Medicare and Medicaid. The study sought to determine whether Americans, who do not have the security of a national health insurance program, work harder to stay healthy than Germans, who have their health care costs covered by a national health plan. The data showed a general lack of difference between Americans and Germans, as well as between social strata in the two countries, with respect to participation in health lifestyles. The more paternalistic German system of health insurance coverage did not appear to undermine personal incentives to stay physically fit in comparison to the American system.

This research would suggest that — at least in the United States and Germany — health lifestyles are spreading across class boundaries in a manner similar to that suggested by Weber for the Protestant ethic. This finding does not mean that everyone is trying to live in a healthful manner, but many people are, and those who are include persons in all social strata. Several other studies in the two countries supported this conclusion. For example, in the United States, Ransford (1986) found in a national sample that lower-class black adults were especially likely to adopt health-protective measures because of particular concern about heart disease. Well-educated whites were found to participate in health lifestyles because of a concern about their health in general. The result, however, was the same: Health behavior cut across class and racial lines. In Ohio, Harris and Guten (1979) found that practically all respondents in their survey did something to protect their health. Other research in South Carolina found a lack of socioeconomic differences in health practices in a sample of state government employees (Kronenfeld, Jackson, Davis, & Blair, 1988). Most respondents had made positive changes in their health habits.

In Germany, the pattern of participation in health lifestyles is becoming increasingly similar to that of the United States. The number of Germans involved in sport and exercise has risen substantially, diets have become more healthful, and smoking has declined (Lüschen, Cockerham, & Kunz, 1989; Scheuch, 1989). The most recent data from western Germany show a distinct lack of socioeconomic differences in health lifestyle behavior, thereby suggesting that healthful ways of living have become normative (Lüschen et al., 1995). This situation appears to be the case in many other West European countries as well. The Lüschen et al. (1995) study of health in the European Union found few or no differences among Germany, the Netherlands, Belgium, and France in health lifestyles. Although many respondents in this study reported unhealthful behavior, such as above-average alcoholic intake and heavy smoking, others were markedly health-conscious, and this group represented sizable proportions of people from all social strata. Consequently, social class was not highly significant.

The exception to the spread of health lifestyles in western Europe is Great Britain. A major survey of health behavior indicated that important differences persist between the classes in the things they do to stay healthy, with the upper and upper-middle classes tending to take much better care of themselves than the working class and the lower class (Blaxter, 1990). In this study, unhealthful living conditions stemming from poverty were a major barrier to good health, and those living in poverty were considered resistant to changes in lifestyles. Nevertheless, there is evidence from Britain that physical fitness activities are spreading, smoking is declining, and class differences in health lifestyles in the most affluent region, southern England, are lessening (Calnan, 1989; Featherstone, 1987; Reid, 1989).

On balance, it appears that health lifestyles are spreading in British society, but distinct social class differences remain. That they do is not too

surprising, because class divisions in Britain remain more rigid than in the United States and Germany (Reid, 1989). While the case cannot be made on the basis of the existing studies that health lifestyles have spread completely throughout Western society, such lifestyles do show signs of spreading across class boundaries. At least it appears that they are in the United States and much of western Europe. Clearly, more research is needed to determine national, regional, and global patterns of health lifestyles. An emphasis on healthful living, however, is an important part of late modernity. While it seems that persons in the upper and middle socioeconomic groups pursue this lifestyle more extensively, strong evidence is emerging that participation also involves members of the lower social strata.

THE LATE MODERN–POSTMODERN CONTEXT

Given the destabilization–deconstruction of industrial society in the late 20th century, health lifestyles provide one with greater self-control over one's body and quality of life (Glassner, 1989). The rationality underlying this development is what Weber (1978) referred to as "formal rationality." Formal rationality is the purposeful calculation of the most efficient means to achieve a goal. Weber made a major contribution to the development of social thought by explaining how formal rationality became the dominant mode of thinking in Western society and joined with the Protestant ethic to stimulate the rise of capitalism in the West. In the context of formal rationality, health is valued not so much as a substantive idealized state as for its ability to serve a practical function. In the late modern or postmodern situation, a distinctive feature in the health sphere, as suggested by Gallagher's (1988) work, is a more widespread and penetrating awareness of the value of health and individual efforts to achieve it.

This development suggests that health lifestyles will be particularly significant aspects of behavior in the fullest sense of postmodernity. Destabilization of industrial age norms and values suggests the potential for greater diversity in lifestyle options. Turner (1988, p. 75) argued that cultural styles become mixed, interwoven, and flexible in postmodern situations, thereby precluding clear maintenance of hierarchical distinctions and a standardization of lifestyles. Featherstone (1987) further observed that some lifestyles grounded in consumerism (namely, certain choices of clothes, leisure activities, consumer goods, and bodily dispositions) are not limited to specific status groups. Featherstone does not claim that this situation is evidence of a dramatic change in class structure. Instead he maintains, consistent with Bourdieu (1984), that this development is a new movement within the existing class hierarchy consisting of an expansion and legitimation of upper-middle-class lifestyles. On one hand, postmodern conditions promote uncertainty and diversity in lifestyle choices. On the other hand, they push people toward greater individual responsibility; i.e., they push people toward making choices. This evolution includes the norm that everybody has choices and should seek improvement, including better health, regardless of age and class origin. Hence, the potential for lifestyles becoming a stronger predictor of behavior than social class is increased with postmodernity.

DEMOGRAPHIC CHARACTERISTICS

As research on health lifestyles continues, a review of the literature in the United States and western Europe shows that the personal characteristics of those likely to be involved in such behavior are emerging (Cockerham, 1995; Lüschen et al., 1995). As the previous discussion suggests, people from the upper and upper-middle classes are most likely to pursue fitness activities, but this behavior stretches to a significant degree across all classes. The fundamental difference is that the extent and quality of participation are less the lower one is on the social

ladder. The bulk of the evidence from relatively recent studies conducted outside of Great Britain indicates that socioeconomic status is generally not a robust predictor of health lifestyle participation. When the three variables that constitute socioeconomic status are examined separately, education is a far stronger predictor of health behavior than either income or occupational status.

Age and Gender

Age and gender are also important in that older rather than younger persons and females more than males are more likely to participate in health lifestyles. People seem to take better care of themselves as they grow older in a number of behaviors, such as improved diet, more relaxation, and either abstinence or decreased use of tobacco and alcohol. Exercise, however, significantly declines at older ages, so one major health lifestyle practice is lost with age. As for gender, the clear and consistent pattern is one of females participating in health lifestyles to a much greater extent than males. One of the better studies in this regard is that of Ross and Bird (1994), who found that men are more likely than women to exercise strenuously and to walk, but are also more likely to smoke and be overweight. Other research shows that men are also more likely to consume alcohol (Cockerham et al., 1988a; Lüschen et al., 1995). Ross and Bird concluded that the access of men to the goods and services they receive because of their advantage in the labor market (higher salaries and greater leadership roles) may actually worsen their health, if their advantage is accompanied by smoking, high-fat foods, and passive leisure-time activities.

Race and Ethnicity

An area in need of greater attention is the relationship between health lifestyles and race. In the United States, the health of the African-American population, primarily that of males, has been declining (Cockerham, 1995; Otten, Teutsch, Williamson, & Marks, 1990). This development suggests that blacks have considerably less participation in health lifestyles than whites. Studies including race as an independent variable, however, show little difference between whites and members of minority groups generally (Cockerham et al., 1988b). Socioeconomic status appears to be a much stronger variable in predicting health lifestyles of racial/ethnic minorities in relation to the majority population. Research in western Europe shows that there is little or no difference according to nationality, but European studies typically do not include race as a focus in lifestyle research (Lüschen et al., 1995).

MAJOR RESEARCH AND METHODOLOGICAL ISSUES

While lifestyle research has become an increasingly important topic in the social sciences since Bourdieu (1984) published *Distinction*, a gap exists between theoretical concepts and measurement techniques. The crucial question for the researcher in selecting an appropriate analytical method is: What explicitly is it that lifestyle concepts are supposed to measure? As Abel (1991) explained, this question stresses the general issue of the transition between theory and methods or, more specifically, between theoretical validity and methods of statistical analysis. Most lifestyle studies to date, however, have failed to address this issue. The lifestyle concept is typically used to distinguish between groups of individuals by looking at their commonly shared behaviors and attitudes. For theoretical validity, lifestyle studies should therefore apply methods of statistical analysis that detect distinct groups of people on the basis of their lifestyle characteristics. Although lifestyles reflect an integration of specific social practices with potentially complex interrelationships, lifestyles usually follow a general pattern in specific groups. Consequently, methods that display this pattern are needed.

Abel (1991) suggested that cluster analysis is a useful method to determine lifestyle variations

because it separates cases (people), not variables, into distinct groups. Another promising method is correspondence analysis, which was utilized by Bourdieu (1984) in his seminal study. Correspondence analysis, a less well known method, is a descriptive and exploratory method capable of sorting a multiplicity of variables into dichotomous categories and has been primarily used in Europe (Greenacre & Blasius, 1994). The advantage of correspondence analysis is that it determines how categories of variables cluster in particular relationships and the strengths and weaknesses of these relationships. As a multidimensional scaling procedure for nominal scaled data, it uses as an input matrix the columns and rows of a table of contingency having two or more dimensions. Different categories of one variable (column variables), such as age, can be related to a multiplicity of descriptive variables (row variables), such as different health behaviors. Correspondence analysis has some similarities to factor analysis in that it produces a set of orthogonal vectors to locate different categories in a multidimensional space. In contrast to factor analysis, however, in which the main emphasis is on reducing complexity (combining different variables into one factor), the focus of correspondence analysis is to determine complexity. It does so by identifying a comprehensive pattern of the interrelationships among all categories of a set of variables simultaneously in the same space.

As a method to structure data and investigate similarities and differences between categories, correspondence analysis is also somewhat similar to cluster analysis. Though both methods have been employed in lifestyle research, there are some major differences. Compared to cluster analysis, which allows choices among different algorithms and numbers of clusters, the algorithm is fixed in correspondence analysis. This property helps to overcome the instability sometimes found in cluster analysis. Furthermore, the application of cluster analysis usually requires two steps to determine relations between sociodemographic variables, such as age and gender, and patterns of behavior. First, cluster analysis identifies different patterns of behavior; then, another method, loglinear regression analysis, relates these patterns to sociodemographic variables (Abel, 1991). In correspondence analysis, the relations between behavioral and sociodemographic variables are investigated in one step. Correspondence analysis may be superior to cluster analysis because it identifies complex patterns of behavior in relation to sociodemographic variables more efficiently and reduces the potential for instability in the results.

Correspondence analysis, however, is an exploratory technique. The goal of the method is to transform numerical information into a graphic display or plot, thereby facilitating the interpretation of the data (Greenacre & Blasius, 1994). Correspondence analysis is useful for describing data, viewing the structure of variables, and developing hypotheses. It is an initial step in analysis. Other techniques such as multiple regression or logistic regression can then be used to determine statistical significance.

The question of whether or not cluster analysis and correspondence analysis are optimal methods for assessing the manner in which lifestyle variables form clusters and identifying specific groups in the process awaits further research. Nevertheless, it is clear from the discussion in this chapter that theoretical developments in lifestyle research are moving ahead, and the development of appropriate methods needs to do likewise. Closing the gap between theory and method remains a major task for current research in the field.

SUMMARY

This chapter has reviewed the general literature on health lifestyles, including the theoretical work of Weber and Bourdieu. The chapter proposed defining health lifestyles as collective patterns of health-promoting behavior based on choices from options available to people according to their life chances. The trend in late modern–postmodern society suggests that health lifestyles are expanding across class boundaries and becoming a normative pattern of behavior. This development is relatively recent, but appears to be enduring as the social conditions accompanying the evolution out of the industrial age bring massive change. Health lifestyle research is still developing and promises to be a major area of inquiry in health behavior in the future.

REFERENCES

Abel, T. (1991). Measuring health lifestyles in a comparative analysis: Theoretical issues and empirical findings. *Social Science and Medicine, 32*, 899–908.

Abel, T., Cockerham, W. C., Lüschen, G., & Kunz, G. (1989). Health lifestyles and self-direction in employment among American men: A test of the spillover effect. *Social Science and Medicine, 28*, 1269–1274.

Ardagh, J. (1987). *France today*. London: Penguin.

Baudrillard, J. (1988). *Selected writings* (M. Poster, Ed.). Stanford, CA: Stanford University Press.

Bauman, Z. (1992). *Intimations of postmodernity*. London: Routledge.

Beck, U. (1992). *Risk society*, translated by M. Ritter. London: Sage.

Bendix, R. (1960). *Max Weber: An intellectual portrait*. New York: Doubleday.

Berkman, L. F., & Breslow, L. (1983). *Health and ways of living: The Alameda County study*. Fairlawn, NJ: Oxford University Press.

Blackburn, C. (1991). *Poverty and health*. Milton Keynes, UK: Open University Press.

Blair, S. N., Kohl, H. W., III, Paffenbarger, R. S., Clark, D. G., Cooper, K. H., & Gibbons, L. W. (1989). Physical fitness and all-cause mortality. *Journal of the American Medical Association, 262*, 2395–2401.

Blaxter, M. (1990). *Health and lifestyles*. London: Routledge.

Bocock, R. (1993). *Consumption*. London: Routledge.

Bourdieu, P. (1984). Distinction [translated by R. Nice]. Cambridge: Harvard University Press.

Bourdieu, P. (1990). *The logic of practice*. Stanford, CA: Stanford University Press.

Bourdieu, P., & Wacquant, J. D. (1992). *An invitation to reflexive sociology*. Chicago: University of Chicago Press.

Calnan, M. (1989). Control over health and patterns of health-related behavior. *Social Science and Medicine, 29*, 131–136.

Cockerham, W. C. (1995). *Medical sociology* (6th ed.). Englewood Cliffs, NJ: Prentice-Hall.

Cockerham, W. C., Abel, T., & Lüschen, G. (1993). Max Weber, formal rationality, and health lifestyles. *Sociological Quarterly, 34*, 413–435.

Cockerham, W. C., Kunz, G., & Lüschen, G. (1988a). Social

stratification and health lifestyles in two systems of health care delivery: A comparison of America and West Germany. *Journal of Health and Social Behavior, 29*, 113-126.

Cockerham, W. C., Kunz, G., & Lüschen, G. (1988b). Psychological distress, perceived health status, and physician utilization in America and West Germany. *Social Science and Medicine, 26*, 829-838.

Cockerham, W. C., Lüschen, G., Kunz, G., & Spaeth, J. L. (1986a). Social stratification and self-management of health. *Journal of Health and Social Behavior, 27*, 1-14.

Cockerham, W. C., Lüschen, G., Kunz, G., & Spaeth, J. L. (1986b). Symptoms, social stratification, and self-responsibility for health in the United States and West Germany. *Social Science and Medicine, 22*, 1263-1271.

Conrad, P. (1988). Health and fitness at work: A participant's perception. *Social Science and Medicine, 26*, 545-550.

Crawford, R. (1984). A cultural account of health: Control, release, and the social body. In J. McKinley (Ed.), *Issues in the political economy of health care* (pp. 60-103). New York: Tavistock.

Dahrendorf, R. (1979). *Life chances*. Chicago: University of Chicago Press.

Dean, K. (1989). Self-care components of lifestyles: The importance of gender, attitudes and the social situation. *Social Science and Medicine, 29*, 137-152.

Denzin, N. K. (1991). *Images of postmodern society*. London: Sage.

d'Houtaud, A., & Field, M. G. (1984). The image of health: Variations in perception by social class. *Sociology of Health and Illness, 6*, 30-59.

DuBos, R. (1959). *Mirage of health*. New York: Harper & Row.

Featherstone, M. (1987). Lifestyle and consumer culture. *Theory, Culture and Society, 4*, 55-70.

Featherstone, M. (1991). *Consumer culture and postmodernism*. London: Sage.

Frisby, D. (1985). *Fragments of modernity*. Oxford, England: Polity Press.

Gallagher, E. B. (1988). Modernization and medical care. *Sociological Perspectives, 31*, 59-87.

Giddens, A. (1991). *Modernity and self-identity*. Stanford, CA: Stanford University Press.

Glassner, B. (1989). Fitness and the postmodern self. *Journal of Health and Social Behavior, 30*, 180-191.

Green, H. (1986). *Fit for America: Health, fitness, sport, and American society*. New York: Pantheon.

Greenacre, M., & Blasius, J. (1994). *Correspondence analysis in the social sciences*. London: Academic Press.

Harris, D. M., & Guten, S. (1979). Health-protective behavior: An exploratory study. *Journal of Health and Social Behavior, 20*, 17-29.

Herzlich, C., & Pierret, J. (1987). *Illness and self in society*. Baltimore: Johns Hopkins University Press.

Hradil, S. (1987). *Sozialstrukturanalyse in einer fortgeschrittenen Gesellschaft*. Leverkusen, Germany: Leske + Budrich.

Jenkins, R. (1992). *Pierre Bourdieu*. London: Routledge.

Kotarba, J. A., & Bentley, P. (1988). Workplace wellness participation and the becoming of self. *Social Science and Medicine, 26*, 551-558.

Kronenfeld, J. J., Jackson, K. L., Davis, K. W., & Blair, S. N. (1988). Changing health practices: The experience from a worksite health promotion project. *Social Science and Medicine, 26*, 515-524.

Lüschen, G., Cockerham, W. C., & Kunz, G. (1987). Deutsche und amerikanische Gesundheitskultur—oder what they say when they sneeze. *Mensch Medizin Gesellschaft, 12*, 59-69.

Lüschen, G., Cockerham, W. C., & Kunz, G. (1989). *Health and illness in America and Germany*. Munich: Oldenbourg.

Lüschen, G., Cockerham, W. C., van der Zee, J., Stevens, F., Diederuicks, J., Ferrando, M., d'Houtaud, A., Peters, R., Abel, T., & Niemann, S. (1995). *Health systems in the European Union: Diversity, convergence, and integration*. Munich: Oldenbourg.

Münch, R. (1988). *Understanding modernity*. London: Routledge.

Münch, R. (1994). *Sociological theory: Vol. 3*. Chicago: Nelson-Hall.

Otten, M. W., Teutsch, S. M., Williamson, D. F., & Marks, J. S. (1990). The effect of known risk factors on the excess mortality of black adults in the United States. *Journal of the American Medical Association, 268*, 845-850.

Ransford, H. E. (1986). Race, heart disease worry, and health protective behavior. *Social Science and Medicine, 12*, 1355-1362.

Reid, I. (1989). *Social class differences in Britain* (3rd ed.). Glasgow, UK: Fontana Press.

Ross, C. E., & Bird, C. E. (1994). Sex stratification and health lifestyle: Consequences for men's and women's perceived health. *Journal of Health and Social Behavior, 35*, 161-178.

Scheuch, E. K. (1989). Recent social changes and their consequences for the health care system in the Federal Republic of Germany. In G. Lüschen, W. Cockerham, & G. Kunz (Eds.), *Health and illness in America and Germany* (pp. 147-166). Munich: Oldenbourg.

Shilling, C. (1993). *The body and social theory*. London: Sage.

Smart, B. (1992). *Modern conditions, postmodern controversies*. London: Routledge.

Smart, B. (1993). *Postmodernity*. London: Routledge.

Turner, B. S. (1988). *Status*. Milton Keynes, UK: Open University Press.

Turner, B. S. (1992). *Regulating bodies*. London: Routledge.

Wacquant, J. D. (1992). Toward a social praxeology: The structure and logic of Bourdieu's sociology. In P. Bourdieu & L. Wacquant (Eds.), *An invitation to reflexive sociology* (pp. 1-61). Chicago: University of Chicago Press.

Weber, M. (1978). *Economy and society* (2 vols.; G. Roth & C. Wittch, Eds.). Berkeley: University of California Press.

13

Social Attachments, Group Structures, and Health Behavior

Reed Geertsen

The connection between group ties and personal well-being was first demonstrated by Durkheim's (1897/1951) classic study of suicide. A century of research has expanded his integration hypothesis to include other forms of mortality and broader measures of social integration. Numerous studies have shown that the socially isolated are less healthy and more likely to die (Cohen & Syme, 1985). For example, early prospective studies of mortality, such as the Alameda County Study (Berkman & Syme, 1979) and the Tecumseh Community Health Study (House, Robbins, & Metzner, 1982), reported higher mortality for those with fewer social ties at several levels of social involvement. More recent cross-community comparisons confirm the broad-based mortality risks of social isolation (Seeman et al., 1993). In reviewing the evidence, House, Landis, and Umberson (1988, p. 543) concluded that "the evidence regarding social relationships and health increasingly approximates the evidence in the

1964 Surgeon General's report that established cigarette smoking as a cause or risk factor for mortality and morbidity from a range of diseases."

Although the evidence on mortality is impressive, the precise contributions of social variables to health outcomes are ambiguous (Bloom, 1990). Several questions need further clarification. Of special interest in this chapter are four questions that relate to health behavior, particularly medical orientations and use of medical services. The first question concerns different types of group ties: How do household ties, informal ties with relatives and friends, and religious ties influence health behaviors? The second question concerns parochial group structures and individual orientations toward medicine: Are strong in-group ties correlated with distinctive medical orientations and medical behaviors? The third question deals with the sociocultural context of group-related health behaviors: Are group ties and health behaviors influenced by the cultural background of the socially connected individuals? The fourth and final question concerns lay consultations with group members in situations of possible illness: How does advice on medical issues influence the process of seeking medical help?

Reed Geertsen • Department of Sociology, Utah State University, Logan, Utah 84322-0730.

Handbook of Health Behavior Research I: Personal and Social Determinants, edited by David S. Gochman. Plenum Press, New York, 1997.

This chapter examines the role of social attachments and group structures in health behavior. It includes an assessment of some common strategies employed in measuring group ties. Special attention is paid to the influence of different types of social contacts in the decision to seek medical help. The chapter concludes with a discussion of some key issues in group structures research.

GROUP TIES AND HEALTH BEHAVIOR

Durkheim's (1897/1951) approach to the study of social integration and its consequences paved the way for modern research on group structures and health behavior. He believed that frequent social contacts promoted social integration by reducing tendencies toward self-centeredness and egoism. The price of social integration was a loss of freedom; the payoff, however, was emotional support and a sense of belonging. His research on social ties examined the association between marital status and suicide. Married persons, particularly those with children, were considered to be more highly integrated in society and thus less likely to commit suicide. His research confirmed this hypothesis. Most people have attachments at other levels of social interaction as well, including social ties with relatives and friends and memberships in various types of organizations. Research on health behavior has searched for connections at all three levels of social involvement. The first part of this chapter examines some of the research on mortality and health behavior with respect to household ties, relatives and friends, and organizational participation.

Household Ties

The household is a significant social group in the lives of many individuals. In fact, it has been argued elsewhere that a close-knit family household is the most significant group influence on health behavior (Geertsen, 1988). Frequent and recurrent interactions take place in the family setting. Meal preparation, child feeding, child care, sanitary practices, waste disposal, home remedies, self-care, accommodations to illness, and spending on health services are all centered in this unit of social organization. Research on mother–child interactions shows how older children, especially boys, develop a "stiff upper lip, business as usual approach to illness" as part of their sick role socialization (Campbell, 1978). Health professionals have urged a renewed emphasis on the household as a producer of health (e.g., Berman, Kendall, & Bhattacharyya, 1994).

Measures of household ties typically include marital status, household size, age and gender of household members, and working status of adults, especially mothers. Additional measures are sometimes used to measure household cohesion, patterns of expected and actual support, and household conflict. All of these factors have been linked with health behavior in some way through research. Studies using health diaries documented the diversity of health maintenance and self-care practices utilized in the home (Punamaki & Aschan, 1994). These findings showed the wide variety of behaviors that are defined by household members as being part of health maintenance. In addition, other studies showed that everyday health behaviors such as physical exercise are easier to sustain when other household members support the behaviors through encouragement or mutual participation (Treiber et al., 1991), as are exercise regimens prescribed by medical professionals (Dishman, 1982).

Husband–wife households tend to engage in better health behaviors. For example, Broman's (1993) research showed that married persons are less likely to be smokers and heavy drinkers. Even when these known risk factors are controlled, however, marital status continues to predict mortality. Some research shows that its importance relative to other types of social ties varies by age. One study (Seeman, Kaplan, Knudsen, Cohen, & Guralnik, 1987) extended the original 9-year mortality risks in the well-known Alameda County Study to 17-year mortality risks.

The findings indicated that marital status has a greater impact on those under 60 years of age at baseline, whereas frequency of contact with friends and relatives has a greater impact on older persons. Findings from the Massachusetts Women's Health Study supported and amplified these findings (Avis, Brambilla, Vass, & McKinlay, 1991). Older women who lose a spouse do not report more physical symptoms compared with pre-widowhood baselines; however, widows do make more frequent visits to doctors and use more prescribed medications. Other research described in the next few paragraphs has documented the importance of household support for persons under 60.

The connection between adult mortality and health service use is unclear. Frequent users do not necessarily have higher mortality. For example, women make more frequent use of medical services, and yet they live longer than men. Nevertheless, in comparisons of the married and unmarried, health service use and mortality tend to vary in the same direction; i.e., the unmarried have higher mortality and make more frequent use of health services. Ingham and Miller (1983, 1986) conducted extensive research on the connection between marital status and medical utilization. Their studies were based on 1416 adults enrolled in a health center. Persons who used the facility during the year were matched with controls of the same age and sex who were enrolled but had not recently used the facility. The research included adjustments for symptom severity and explored possible interactions with the gender of respondents. Widowed, separated, and divorced women were found to be the highest users regardless of the severity of symptoms. Gender differences occur in other research on the medical visits of married persons. Chien and Schneiderman (1975) compared the medical behaviors of married couples. They found that married women made far more visits to doctors than their spouses. This finding held for nearly all types of visits, including well-care and somatic illness.

Health care utilization also varies by symptom attribution and marital status. Ingham and Miller (1986) found that most symptoms are attributed to internal physical factors, and of the unmarried who did so, 92% were frequent utilizers. On the other hand, only 78% of the married who did so were frequent users. Symptoms attributed to psychological factors revealed even sharper contrasts. Among the unmarried who attributed symptoms to psychological factors, 68% were frequent users compared to only 44% of the married respondents with similar attributions. These findings were summarized by Ingham and Miller (1986, p. 56) as follows:

> People who attribute their symptoms to an internal physical cause, or at least in part to psychological factors, are more likely to consult their doctors if they are unmarried, widowed, divorced or separated than if they are married or in a stable relationship with a cohabitee. Those who have no close intimate relationship with someone to whom they can turn for support and advice in the event of psychological problems are most likely to seek such support in a confidential relationship with their doctors.

Household demands influence a mother's perception of the possibility of illness. Geertsen and Gray (1970) examined more than 800 families with at least one child under 6 years of age. Mothers with more children tended to ignore the seriousness of symptoms with respect to the need to seek medical help. Preschool children are particularly demanding, and their presence in households further accentuated the tendency to downplay symptoms. In households with four or more children, mothers with more than one preschool child were 2.2 times less likely to seek medical help than other mothers. This study also looked at familism, or the importance of family and relatives in the life of the individual. The Bardis (1959) familism scale was used by Geertsen and Gray to measure the perceived sense of obligation among family members to provide assistance in time of need and to place family concerns ahead of personal interests. Mothers with low familism scores were 2.1 times less likely to seek medical help than mothers with high scores. In fact, mothers with low familism who had four or more children were 2.67 times less likely to seek medical help in response to symptoms of possible illness.

These findings are important for two reasons. First, there is evidence in other research that household members engage in similar health behaviors. Second, there is evidence that the influence of mothers on children's utilization behavior is especially pronounced. Schor, Starfield, Stidley, and Hankin (1987) followed 693 families for 6 years who were enrolled in a prepaid health plan. They found medical utilization rates for different family members to be highly correlated. In fact, family membership explained approximately 30% of the variance in individual use of medical services. Although both parents had an influence, the utilization rates of mothers were 2–3 times more powerful in predicting children's utilization than the utilization rates of fathers. Similar findings were reported by Riley et al. (1993), who found mothers' utilization patterns to be "powerful predictors" of child pediatric visits. The findings of Horwitz, Morgenstern, and Berkman (1985) added further support to this circle of influence. They found that children in larger households made less frequent use of pediatric services.

Household demands are often complicated by work responsibilities outside the home. The result is added stress and less frequent medical visits for children. In ethnographic accounts of their health, women claim a stress connection between heavy family responsibilities and challenging outside employment (Walters, 1993). Working women with higher family responsibilities have an increased risk for heart disease, and the relationship appears to be linear. As the number of children in the household increases, so does the mother's risk for heart disease (Haynes & Feinleib, 1980). The consequence of additional heavy demands is less frequent health care for children, particularly in low-income populations. Alexander and Markowitz (1986) followed users of an innercity hospital clinic for 6 months. Women who worked outside the home had greater daily stress and better social supports; nevertheless, their children had fewer pediatric visits than children of housewives.

There is some indication that more cohesive families make less frequent use of maternity and pediatric services. Researchers examined the prenatal care utilization of 185 low-income, inner city patients in Seattle. Those who sought the least care had stronger ties in the immediate family and closer ties with nearby relatives (St. Clair, Smeriglio, Alexander, & Celentano, 1989). Other researchers tabulated the health maintenance organization (HMO) pediatric visits of 450 children over a 2-year period. Interviews with mothers were used to assess family functioning and conflict. Children from families experiencing conflict were found to have a higher volume of care (Riley et al., 1993).

The foregoing research documents the influence of household ties on health behavior. Having fewer adult ties predicts mortality. More demanding ties such as being married or having many children predicts lower use of health services. This outcome is conditioned by the age, gender, socioeconomic status, and perceived social support of persons sharing the same living quarters. The household influence on health behavior is no doubt shaped by the fact that common residence facilitates daily interaction. The added effect of social support shows, however, that household ties represent only part of the overall social connections of individuals. Other social ties connect the household to broader circles of social influence outside the home, and these ties too have been found to predict health behavior.

Relatives and Friends

Relatives and friends are frequently lumped together in research on group structures and health behavior. Questions about these contacts typically fall into two main categories. One group of questions deals with the structure of social involvement such as number of friends and relatives, frequency of contacts, intimacy and duration of relationships, and geographic proximity of social partners (O'Reilly, 1988). Another group deals with perceptions of social support such as material assistance and emotional encouragement (Winemiller, Mitchell, Sutliff, & Cline, 1993).

Different levels of specificity are also reflected in the strategies used to collect information on social contacts. The most common strategy asks for combined estimates about social interaction with relatives and friends. The Duke Social Support Index makes frequent use of questions such as, "Are you satisfied with how often you see your friends and relatives?" The index also asks for estimates on matters such as how many times per week respondents talk with friends or relatives on the telephone (Koenig et al., 1993). This strategy obscures potential differences, if any, between relatives and friends. Another strategy gets around this problem by asking for specific information on persons listed by name as close friends or relatives. Salloway and Dillon (1973) used this method to assess the separate effects of friends and relatives on medical behavior. The main problem with this strategy is that many more questions are required for measuring these differences. This is probably why most researchers have opted to use simpler though less definitive measures of this dimension of group structure.

A precedent for lumping relatives and friends together in a measurement scale was set in the Alameda County mortality study. Separate questions were asked about the number of close associates in both categories; however, the investigators had to combine these two questions with a third question on frequency of monthly contacts to see a pronounced effect on mortality (Berkman & Syme, 1979). It is easy to see how separate measures might give biased estimates of social isolation outside the household. By way of illustration, let us say that one person has no close friends and five close relatives, while another has five close friends and no close relatives. Both have the same number of close ties (5), but each could be tabulated quite differently (0 or 5) if one type of relationship is used without the other. In this instance, some sort of combined measure

would give the most reasonable indication of overall social involvement, and yet the individual with exclusive close ties with relatives might have stronger in-group ties.

Research on social involvement with relatives and friends reveals mixed outcomes with respect to medical care utilization. Like household ties, these outcomes vary according to the age, gender, and socioeconomic characteristics of the respondents. One set of studies shows more frequent use of medical services for those who have greater social involvement. A study of the utilization behavior of 500 children in a prepaid group practice at Yale University examined several dimensions of social contact (Horwitz et al., 1985). Network size was measured by asking mothers how many close friends and relatives they had. They were also asked how far away different network members lived. Both network size and geographic proximity were positively correlated with acute care utilization over a 12-month period. The positive effect of social contacts on utilization was explained primarily by the number of friends a mother saw monthly, rather than by contacts with relatives. The investigators attributed part of this positive correlation to the high levels of education and promedical health beliefs of social network members.

The network measures used in the Yale study were derived from earlier research by Salloway and Dillon (1973). Their population was taken from a racially and ethnically mixed suburb of Boston with a 40% black population. They measured frequency of contact with friends and relatives (including telephone calls) and expected support in the form of grocery shopping, house cleaning, and lending money. Family networks were analyzed separately from friendship networks. These investigators hypothesized that family networks were more likely to be closed and close-knit with many interlocking ties, and would thus provide many alternatives to seeking outside help. Conversely, friendship networks were more likely to be open, with less mutual contact and sharing of ideas, and thus less likely to keep the individual from seeking outside help.

Though not conclusive, the findings showed that friend and family networks might operate in opposite ways in terms of delay in the use of health services (friends occasioning less delay, family more delay).

Some segments of the elderly population reveal positive correlations between social involvement and medical use. Wan (1987) found more physician visits among those reporting the availability of a social interaction network in a study of the elderly who were functionally disabled but not institutionalized. He also found that the availability of material support was associated with less frequent doctor visits for those reporting the poorest health. Arling's (1985) research on older people found that high social support was associated with more frequent medical visits among those with *severe* functional impairments.

Another set of studies associates higher medical utilization with weak social support from relatives and friends. In one study (Blake, 1991), low social supports were correlated with increased bed days and more follow-up visits with physicians among older adults with chronic lung disease. The medical outcomes were measured prospectively by mailed questionnaires over a 6-month period. Demographic characteristics failed to account for the low support effect on physician visits. Counte and Glandon (1991) conducted a multiyear panel study of two groups of older persons who were HMO members and fee-for-service clients. They found more frequent health service utilization among older persons with low social supports, but only in situations of high life stress.

Pilisuk, Boylan, and Acredolo (1987) found more frequent clinic visits in a middle-aged HMO population with less support from friends and family. The low utilizers were also found to have less positive orientations toward their social networks. Broadhead, Gehlbach, DeGruy, and Kaplan (1989) looked at the volume of continued use among patients who were established medical utilizers. Their study population consisted of 343 adults using a family medicine center at Duke University. Follow-up visits were not associated with frequency of contact with friends and relatives, but were influenced by social supports. Social support measures included multiple-item scales measuring confidant support (chances to talk and seek advice) and affective support (people who care and provide help). Low social supports were found to predict up to 1.6 extra visits per year to the doctor's office (i.e., 5.2 visits vs. 3.6 visits). Patients with weak social supports also made visits of longer than average duration and spent more money for medical care.

Collectively, the studies show correlations between health service use and social involvement with relatives and friends. The direction of this influence varies, however, by type of visit and population group investigated. In HMOs and family practice groups, follow-up visits are more prevalent among patients who lack social support. In highly educated populations, acute care visits for children are more frequent when mothers have greater social contacts. These contrasting findings, as well as the findings on older persons, imply that the connection between social contacts and medical utilization is mediated by other factors. Social contacts may be more influential for younger persons, while social supports may have greater importance for the elderly. The impact of types of support may also vary by gender and age. A pediatric study (Horwitz et al., 1985) indicates that contact with friends and relatives may work at cross-purposes in more ethnically diverse populations. Race and ethnicity are further complicated by religious background. Membership in church groups and voluntary associations constitutes a third level of social involvement extending beyond households ties, relatives, and friends.

Religious and Social Participation

Durkheim's (1897/1951) study of suicide included a religious dimension in social integration. He believed that religious norms reduced social alienation and helped attach individuals to society by providing direction and purpose. The

Protestant emphasis on individualism was thought to provide less normative direction than the Catholic or Jewish emphasis on group ritual. His research went on to identify systematic differences in suicide rates for Protestants, Catholics, and Jews. Though some of his conclusions have been challenged by other research, the connection between religious participation and mortality has been confirmed (Breault & Barkey, 1982; Stark, 1978).

The indices used to measure religious and social participation are typically less precise than those used to assess contact with relatives and friends. Social participation in clubs and voluntary associations is variously measured by summing the number of memberships and offices held in different organizations. Religion is usually included in medical studies as a control variable, so fairly broad categories are used. For example, it is often categorized as Protestant, Catholic, Jewish, and Other. Broad categories such as "Protestant" are used because more precise distinctions yield subsample sizes that are too small for meaningful analysis. In some studies, respondents are asked to specify a religious preference without indicating current levels of activity. In others, frequency of attendance is used to measure religious participation.

Reviews of the literature on religion and health show that frequency of religious attendance is positively associated with better health (Levin, 1994; Levin & Schiller, 1987). Membership in a church or temple was correlated with lower mortality in the Alameda County Study (Berkman & Syme, 1979). Comparisons of religious groups show lower mortality in denominations with stricter behavioral norms. For example, Mormons, Seventh-Day Adventists, Orthodox Jews, and the clergy of all faiths have less cardiovascular disease, less uterine and cervical cancer, better general health, and less overall cause-specific mortality. Higher levels of religiosity (religious attendance and church membership) are also associated with lower blood pressure (Levin & Vanderpool, 1989).

Religious participation has been investi-gated in many areas of health care utilization. The most consistent findings were reported by those who identified with the Jewish religion. Jews had more physician visits than any other religious group (Solon, 1966; Wan & Soifer, 1974) and the highest rates for dental utilization (Wan & Yates, 1975). In other research, Jews were more likely than Catholics to participate in breast cancer screening (Fink, Shapiro, & Lewison, 1968) and to travel long distances for hospital care (Bashshur, Shananon, & Metzner, 1971). Research on frequent religious attenders across different religious groups showed greater variation. The most conclusive finding related to older persons. The highly religious elderly made more frequent visits to doctors (Wan & Soifer, 1974). Research on other age groups was less conclusive. Among women of child-bearing age, postpartum family planning services were used more by infrequent religious attenders (Collver, Ten Have, & Speare, 1967). On the other hand, highly religious mothers had higher utilization rates for acute pediatric care (Horwitz et al., 1985). Other research suggests that religious activity may have an indirect effect on health service through other health-related variables. For example, Schiller and Levin (1988) reported more frequent physician visits for more active religious participants in a diverse religious population in Appalachia; however, most of the effect was attributed to predisposing and need variables.

Utilization patterns for Protestants and Catholics are inconsistent and often vary by type of medical problem (Greenlick, Hurtado, Pope, Saward, & Yoshioka, 1968). Utilization patterns also vary by race. For example, among frequent attenders, Catholics had lower prenatal care use than Protestants (Collver et al., 1967). On the other hand, Protestant African-Americans were less likely than Catholics to use family planning services prior to having a baby (Notzon, 1977); however, they were more likely to use these services than Catholics after delivery (Collver et al., 1967). Part of the problem is undoubtedly due to imprecise measurement. A wide variety of diverse religious groups are identified as Protestant. Many studies on health care are forced to use this broad label due to the limited response categories used in most surveys. Other studies that attempt to use more precise distinctions in Protestant denominations suffer from small sample size. For example, Schiller and Levin (1988) compared physician visits for seven different religious denominations in Appalachia. Visits were broken down into six categories ranging from less than once a year (0) to more than once a month (5). Considerable variation was reported, but the differences lacked statistical significance because five of the eight religious groups had too few subjects (13, 13, 19, 27, and 31). Those reporting no religion had a mean score of only 0.69 compared to a mean score of 3.34 for Pentecostals.

Utilization studies on other forms of social participation such as club memberships and participation in voluntary associations are often difficult to interpret, because of the practice of adding organizational memberships to other social ties to form composite measures of network size. There is some evidence, however, that social participation is less important in health behavior than religious participation. For example, Broadhead et al. (1989) examined organizational memberships independent of other types of social ties. No association was found between participation in voluntary associations and frequency of health service use among recent users of an outpatient clinic. Nevertheless, belonging to organizations has been linked with lower mortality risks for women (Berkman & Syme, 1979), less frequent smoking and drinking, and greater use of seat belts (Broman, 1993).

Research on religious membership points to the potential importance of group culture in health behavior. The consistently high use of medical services by members of the Jewish faith underscores this possibility. Overlooked in most studies, however, is the potential diversity of other cultural groups subsumed under global labels such as "Catholic" and "Protestant." Cultural distinctions among Jews may also hide potentially important internal variations. According to Levin, religion has received inadequate treatment in medical research. In most health studies, "one or more religious indicators have made a serendipitous 'guest appearance' alongside of scores of other psychosocial measures" (Levin, 1994, p. 1475). The potential importance of group culture in the relationship between social ties and health behavior is examined in the next section.

PAROCHIAL STRUCTURES AND MEDICAL ORIENTATIONS

Social ties at the three different levels of social interaction sometimes interlock to form strong in-group structures. In these situations, group members tend to have much closer ties with a more limited or exclusive set of long-time associates. At the other extreme are individuals with abundant and varied group ties of shorter duration and weaker intensity. Several typologies in the sociological literature have tried to capture this distinction in group structure (McKinney, 1966). These typologies typically represent polar extremes on a continuum of personal to impersonal relations. For example, the terms *gemeinschaft* versus *gesellschaft*, *folk* versus *urban*, *primary* versus *secondary*, and *mechanical* versus *organic* solidarity reflect this contrast. The first term in each pair refers to a group structure characterized by close and personal relationships with strong sentiments and mutual support; the second term refers to opposite group structures, in which relationships are distant and impersonal with weak sentiments and limited or no support.

Suchman (1965) was the first to apply this distinction in group structure to health behavior. He used the terms *parochial* and *cosmopolitan* to represent the polar opposites on his continuum of group structure. Parochial or in-group tendencies were assessed at family, friend, and community levels of social interaction. In his view, parochial family structures were characterized by authority and tradition. Family authority measured deference to an authority figure in the household and respect for old-time customs.

Friendship solidarity measured close, interlocking friendships of long duration. Parochial community ties were defined as ethnic exclusivity. To measure this parochialism, he asked questions about the tendency to limit interactions to persons of similar background.

Parochial Structures in New York City

Suchman hypothesized that group structures influence attitudes, which in turn shape health-related behaviors. An examination of 1883 adults in the Washington Heights section of New York City showed significant positive correlations among the three measures of social group organization. Persons who tended to limit community ties to persons of their same ethnicity also tended to report higher friendship solidarity and higher family authority, and vice versa. From this finding, he concluded that the three variables could be combined to form a single index ranging from "parochial" to "cosmopolitan" group structures.

Individual medical orientations were measured through questions designed to tap how people thought (knowledge of disease), felt (skepticism of medical care), and behaved (dependency during illness) with respect to illness and medical care. Persons with low knowledge of disease were found to be more skeptical toward medical care and to have a higher dependency in illness. Consequently, these three variables were combined to form an index called "scientific" versus "popular" health orientation, with "popular" representing low knowledge, high skepticism, and high dependency. Health behavior was limited to health status and usual source of care. Usual source of care was assessed as the respondent's first point of contact with the health care system and dichotomized as either private (e.g., private physician) or public (e.g., outpatient clinics). Suchman assumed that persons with parochial group ties would tend to use a private physician rather than impersonal outpatient facilities as the point of first contact in those instances in which medical visits were made.

Suchman's most important finding was the apparent strong connection between group structures and medical orientations. For example, high ethnic exclusivity was found to be associated with significantly lower knowledge about disease, higher skepticism of medical care, and higher dependency in illness. Suchman's (1964) analysis of ethnic subgroups in the Washington Heights population supported this finding. For example, Puerto Ricans reporting more cosmopolitan group structures tended to be more scientific in their health orientations than Puerto Ricans reporting parochial group structures. Similar findings were obtained for other racial and ethnic groups. From this study, he concluded that parochial structures tend to produce nonscientific medical orientations regardless of the cultural background of respondents.

Parochial Structures in Salt Lake City

A full-scale replication of the Suchman study using another population was not completed until ten years later (Geertsen, Klauber, Rindflesh, Kane, & Gray, 1975). Support of rather than opposition to modern medicine on the part of parochial group structures appeared to be a strong possibility in the predominantly Mormon population of Salt Lake City, Utah. Mormons are admonished to abstain from tobacco and hard liquor and to follow good health practices. Church-operated hospitals using modern medical technology were once widespread in Utah. Continued contacts with relatives and strong family ties are facilitated through family reunions and genealogy records. Frequent associations with like-minded church members are promoted through various church programs and organizations such as neighborhood "wards" (O'Dea, 1964).

The Salt Lake City data revealed significant discrepancies in how Suchman's variables were related in the two populations. Family authority was found to coincide with friendship solidarity, but not with ethnic exclusivity. For medical orientations, individuals who scored low on knowledge of disease were not found to be more skeptical of medical care or to have a higher dependency in illness. Further differences were uncovered in the associations between social group structures and medical orientations. Whereas Suchman found that high family authority and strong friendship solidarity were related to low knowledge of disease, just the opposite was found in the Salt Lake City study. Likewise, family authority and friendship solidarity were found to be associated with low rather than high skepticism.

One significant shortcoming in Suchman's research was the limited measurement of medical behavior. Although usual sources of care (defined as private or public at time of first contact) and health status were examined, no data were collected on the frequency of use of medical services (Suchman, 1965). This data gap created a problem because his hypothesized connections of the social group and medical orientation variables with source of care proved to be inconsistent and were probably influenced more by socioeconomic status than by the study variables. The Utah study examined the actual utilization of health services instead of just the source of care. Only two of the six variables—family authority and knowledge of disease—were found to be associated with utilization, regardless of the socioeconomic status of respondents. Friendship solidarity was found to be associated with utilization, but only among respondents of lower socioeconomic status.

A Sociocultural Explanation

Suchman (1964, 1965) chose Washington Heights because of its racial and ethnic diversity. In addition to white Protestant (9%) and white Catholic (20%), the sample included African-Americans (25%), Jews (27%), Irish-born Catholics (10%), and Puerto Ricans (9%). The diversity of the population was considered to be useful in testing the consistency of the group structure hypothesis across different cultural groups. The experience of recent immigration, however, may have transcended some of the assumed cultural

differences. In Suchman's ethnically diverse sample, more than one third of the white ethnics were foreign-born, and many of the African-Americans were recent immigrants from the South (Lendt, 1960). Research on assimilation reveals a general distrust of the dominant society and its institutions among recent immigrants from contrasting cultural backgrounds. Strong ingroup tendencies have also been observed as ways of easing the adjustment to unfamiliar surroundings as members find security through familiar customs and social support (Gordon, 1964).

The comparative findings from the two studies suggested a link between group structures and health behaviors different from that given by Suchman (Geertsen, 1988; Geertsen et al., 1975). In-group structures were redefined as intervening variables in the connection between cultural beliefs and health behaviors. The sociocultural explanation argues that cultural beliefs are reinforced by in-group ties when all members of the social network know and interact with each other and share the same cultural background. Furthermore, the comparative absence of intercultural or socially diverse ties protects members of the network from alternative responses. In other words, individuals with close and exclusive group ties respond to a medical problem by (1) seeking professional medical care when doing so is consistent with cultural beliefs and practices or (2) not seeking professional medical care when cultural beliefs and practices emphasize skepticism and distrust. In the second situation, the individual is more likely to seek alternative means for treating medical problems, such as self-care, folk medicine, or alternative healing.

GROUP CULTURE AND HEALTH BEHAVIOR

Is skepticism of medical care a natural reaction to the culture shock associated with recent immigration? If it is, participation in parochial group structures would reinforce this distrust until the cultural barriers that separate strong in-groups from larger society subside through processes of acculturation and assimilation. Is there any evidence of medical skepticism and institutional distrust among recent immigrants in other research? What does research on other cultural groups show about medical skepticism and health service use as members become more familiar with medical institutions and practices?

New Immigrants and Medical Resistance

The utilization behaviors of new immigrants with a variety of different racial/ethnic backgrounds are reported in the literature. A consistent pattern of longer delay and infrequent use emerges from these studies. Weitzman and Berry (1992) collected data on 387 immigrant females working as home attendees in New York City; they also gathered utilization data on 355 of their minor children. Although the attendees were covered by insurance, they made even less frequent use of medical services than other poor Americans without insurance. On the other hand, the immigrant women and children were more likely to report poor or fair health than working but poor nonimmigrant women and children. In fact, the rates of annual visits for women and children were about half the rates reported for poor adults and poor children in national samples. Zambrana, Ell, Dorrington, Wachsman, and Hodge (1994) studied Latina immigrant mothers who used emergency pediatric services. They found "a clear pattern of delayed care for acute problems in the children, a high number of reported barriers to pediatric care, and high mental distress reported by mothers."

Garret, Zyzanski, and Alemagno's (1990) research on Puerto Ricans showed how adaptation to the dominant culture can reverse the negative effect of recent immigration on health service use. Ramakrishna and Weiss (1992) believed that cultural barriers to using American medicine are pronounced for some immigrant groups. India

has a pluralistic medical system and uses Ayurvedic humoral concepts of health and illness. As a result, even those familiar with Western medicine before leaving India have difficulty adjusting to American medicine and consider it to be one option among many for several types of illness. Another study (Gilman, Justice, Saepharn, & Charles, 1992) showed how Laotian refugees attempt to integrate American medical services with their cultural beliefs and practices. Tung (1980) pointed to superstitions and traditional beliefs as common barriers to utilization for other Indochinese refugees. Refugees present a special challenge to health services research because medical screening is required for entry into this country. The result is frequent use during the first year, followed by a systematic decline in visits for subsequent years. For example, in Strand and Jones's (1983) research on Indochinese refugees, only 38.3% of respondents had a low volume of physician use during their first year in this country. In contrast, 75% had a low volume of use 6 years after entry.

May (1992) has done the most complete research on the group structures of an immigrant group. She examined patterns of help seeking for children among Middle Eastern immigrants who had been in America an average of 10 years. What emerged was a pattern of limited health care use (May, 1992, p. 910):

> Most parents handled a non-serious situation themselves or consulted a lay source. Some parents made telephone calls to family in the Middle East for consultation about child care. Others relied on nearby relatives or a friend because a mother or other relative in the Middle East was less available. It was stated that Middle-Eastern immigrant families are available to each other for help, relying on shared traditional values about family and other relationships. Some parents expressed feelings misunderstood by USA health providers when parents went to them for help.

The variety of social group measures used indicate a strong tendency toward parochial group structures—smaller, high-density social circles with considerable ethnic exclusivity. For nearly two thirds of the sample, all network relationships were with co-ethnics (ethnic exclusivity). Network densities were extremely high (0.87), indicating that nearly all relationships were with individuals who knew each other (friendship solidarity). Average number of network ties (7.62) was approximately half that reported for nonimmigrant populations (12.39) using identical measures. The majority of these ties were with relatives rather than friends. Compared with nonimmigrant populations, weaker social supports were found because of geographic fragmentation in network structures. Some 26% of network members resided outside the United States, whereas 62% lived in close physical proximity (May, 1992).

Hispanics and Modern Medicine

Four decades of research on Hispanics provides some evidence of a recent acculturation effect in the attitudes and utilization of health services. Early portrayals of Hispanic culture (e.g., Saunders, 1954) emphasized negative orientations toward modern medical care. Folk beliefs emphasizing magic and herbs, "nonscientific" healers such as *curanderos* and *medicas* with alternative treatments, and various rituals and attitudes of fatalism and skepticism were cited as obvious hindrances to modern medical care. Nall and Speilberg (1967) found evidence of social interference with modern medicine among rural Hispanics. For example, poor participation in treatment regimens for tuberculosis was associated with family factors such as being married and having relatives in the home and with other factors such as seeking advice from associates. On the other hand, Hispanics characterized as being socially alienated were the most likely to accept treatment. All of the 53 subjects (a small sample size) were mostly unskilled residents of a small rural community in Texas. Others writing at about the same time reaffirmed the importance of the extended family in the delay or "last resort" orientation of Hispanics toward Anglo medicine (Madsen, 1964; Rubel, 1966).

A decade later, Farge (1978) replicated Such-

man's measures among Hispanics in the Houston area. Positive correlations were found for all three social group variables. Parochial group ties, however, were associated with more rather than less accurate knowledge of disease and low rather than high skepticism of medical care. No information on health services utilization was reported in this study, but other research (Hoppe & Heller, 1975; Quesada & Heller, 1977) during the 1970s reported better access to care in Hispanic families with strong family ties. In addition, data from general population surveys reported adjusted utilization rates for Hispanics that were similar to those of other population groups. One study (Andersen, Lewis, Riachello, Aday, & Chiu, 1981), using 1976 national survey data for the Southwest, found lower use of physician services among Hispanics before making statistical adjustments for need and socioeconomic status. After adjustments, the differences nearly disappeared. The adjusted figures showed that 73% of the Hispanics saw a physician during the previous year, compared with 76% of the total United States population. According to the authors, unadjusted differences in utilization were explained by younger age (need), lower income (socioeconomic status), and lower insurance coverage, rather than by negative cultural orientations. A three-generation study in San Antonio, Texas, conducted in 1985 further supported the view that Hispanics do not underutilize physician services. Although the oldest generation reported the fewest Anglo friends, they had the most doctor visits (6.2) during the year (Markides, Levin, & Ray, 1985).

African-Americans and Medical Utilization

Utilization information on African-Americans shows trends similar to those observed for Hispanics. Early studies found lower rates of utilization and more negative attitudes toward physicians among African-Americans in the 1960s and early 1970s (Dutton, 1978; Hines, 1972). Other research in the 1970s reported active networks of informal ties in lower-class urban neighborhoods (Martineau, 1977) and active kinship networks in middle-income urban and suburban neighborhoods (McAdoo, 1978). African-American females were found to have especially strong friendship and kinship networks (Feagin, 1970). These studies imply a possible connection between strong in-group ties and poor utilization similar to Suchman's findings in the 1960s in New York City.

Sharp, Ross, and Cockerham's (1983) study of African-Americans in 1980 was one of the first to document a change in attitudes. Their analysis of survey data for Illinois revealed an absence of skepticism toward the medical profession and a strong awareness of symptom seriousness. In their words (Sharp et al., 1983, p. 260):

> We find a comparative lack of skepticism among Blacks and the less educated about visiting the doctor. In fact, the reverse seems true; these groups held attitudes and evaluated symptoms in such a way that would predispose them to use physician services when ill. These data support our original hypothesis that attitudes and beliefs among the less privileged no longer serve as barriers to utilization.

Wan's (1982) research supported this position among elderly African-Americans. In his research, they were found to have a higher number of physician visits than other elderly Americans. Wolinsky's (1982) findings on health care utilization in a rural Southern county revealed no differences between African-Americans and whites after controlling for the predisposing, enabling, and need characteristics often used in health service research. He did find significant differences, however, in the specific effects of these characteristics, thus suggesting a possible cultural influence in the response of African-Americans to the use of physicians, hospitals, and dentists.

A decade after these studies, a national study of contact with friends and relatives showed gender differences in the utilization behavior of elderly African-Americans (Nelson, 1993). Males with more frequent contact with relatives had more physician visits, while those who had more frequent contact with friends had fewer physi-

cian visits. The opposite was true for African-American females. Frequent contact with friends resulted in more physician visits than frequent contact with relatives. Unfortunately, the measures of contact with friends and relatives do not provide information on the parochial structure of these relationships.

Berkanovic and Telesky (1985) examined social network variations for African-Americans, Hispanic-Americans, and Anglo-Americans. They discovered significant network interactions with ethnicity. For example, network advice was more influential in the decision to seek care among Anglos and Hispanics than among African-Americans, while having a regular source of care was much more important in this decision for African-Americans than for Anglos and Hispanics. In addition, general health orientations were influential in the decision of African-Americans to seek medical care, but not in the decision of Anglos or Hispanics to do so. These and other differences emphasize the potential importance of cultural differences. According to Berkanovic and Telesky (1985, p. 1025):

> The present analysis indicates that ethnicity plays a role in determining responses to illnesses through its interaction with networks and cognitive orientations. Thus, Black-Americans and Mexican-Americans, the two distinguishable ethnic groups in this analysis, differ both from each other and from the Whites with respect to the variables that predict the reporting of illnesses, disability and the decision to seek medical care.

Other research on the social ties of African-Americans has examined overall network size, but the findings are inconsistent. Some later research (Gaudin & Davis, 1985; Hogan, Hao, & Parish, 1990) claimed larger kin networks among African-Americans than among Anglo-Americans. Another study using national data (Cross, 1990), however, showed larger kin networks among ethnic white mothers than among nonwhite mothers. A study of African-American parents with chronically ill children found smaller-sized networks with less geographic dispersion and higher perceived supports from network members for

African-Americans than for Anglo-Americans (H. A. Williams, 1993). None of these findings addressed the influence of in-group ties on the use of medical services.

LAY CONSULTATIONS AND ADVICE ON MEDICAL ISSUES

Group ties represent potentially important sources of information about appropriate medical behavior. One of the oldest theoretical traditions in sociology, symbolic interactionism, characterizes human action as a constructed process in which taking the role of others plays an important part. According to this theory, individuals respond to situations by seeking cues from others as to the appropriateness of various courses of action. Social interactions provide an important context for defining situations and constructing courses of action (Blumer, 1969; Turner, 1991, pp. 392–394). Research on social contacts and advice on medical matters provides a clearer picture of the social dynamics involved in the interpretation of and reaction to symptoms of possible illness.

Lay Referral Systems

Freidson (1960) saw social interactions as playing an important role in situations of illness. These social contacts constituted what he called a "lay referral system" that could significantly influence the individual's response to medical symptoms. In his words (Freidson, 1960, p. 377):

> Indeed, the whole process of seeking help involves a network of potential consultants, from the intimate and informal confines of the nuclear family through successively more select, distant, and authoritative laymen, until the "professional" is reached. This network of consultants, which is part of the structure of the local lay community and which imposes form on the seeking of help, might be called the "lay referral structure." Taken together with the cultural understandings involved in the process, we may speak of it as the "lay referral system."

Supporting research shows that the perceived urgency of seeking medical care is influenced by the social role of the person contacted. For example, Calnan (1983) studied the contributions of more formal contacts in the consultation process for injuries and illness episodes. Police, bystanders, and neighbors were found to be more likely to suggest seeking medical attention than other consultants. Those who gave advice to seek help were influenced to do so by the legal and social pressures associated with the broader network context of their positions. Other research shows that the use of medical advice varies by gender and age. Meininger (1986) investigated the self-treatments and lay consultations among white, married individuals. Pronounced differences were found between men and women in the use of lay consultants. Furstenberg and Davis (1984) found discussions about health to be everyday occurrences in the lives of most older people. Their case study method described how new information is acquired and health actions are reinforced on a near-daily basis. Some subjects reported active interventions from lay consultants in matters related to health.

McKinlay (1973) examined the relationship between lay consultations and medical utilization among lower working-class families in Aberdeen, Scotland. Respondents were asked whom they consulted on problems such as sickness, pregnancy, and finances. Women who underutilized maternity services sought advice from a wider variety of readily available friends and relatives, especially mothers, as alternatives to outside help. Delay in seeking care was also most common among those with strong, undifferentiated network ties among relatives and friends.

Timing of Advice

The study of social groups and medical advice may be biased by the potential unreliability of respondent recall. One way to overcome this limitation is to recontact participants at short intervals during the course of the study. For example, in a study conducted in Los Angeles (Berkanovic, Telesky, & Reeder, 1981), 1210 individuals were re-interviewed every 6 weeks over a 12-month period. Some 769 reported a health problem during the year. At the beginning of the study, general information was collected on group ties, including frequency of contact, consultation with others on health matters, and social support in various situations of need. During the re-interviews, more specific information was obtained on the actual use of social contacts when symptoms were experienced. Over 40% of the variance in seeking medical care was explained by the perceived seriousness of symptoms, the perceived efficacy of care, and specific network advice to see a doctor. In contrast, respondents who reported frequent general contact and consultation with network members at the beginning of the study were somewhat less likely to see a doctor than those with less frequent contact and consultation. Thus, the two different forms of data collection gave contradictory views of how social networks influenced the seeking of medical help. Perhaps more frequent social contact exposed network members to a wider range of alternative actions besides the seeking of professional medical help. In any case, more appears to be involved than the overall frequency of contact with network members.

Another study by Berkanovic and Telesky (1982) showed how network influences may vary when advice is congruent or incongruent with personal beliefs about the seriousness of symptoms. Persons who considered symptoms to be serious were much more likely to see a doctor (85.6%) if network members also advised this action than if no such advice was received (65.2%). When symptoms were not considered to be serious, those who received network advice to see a doctor were much more likely to visit the doctor (49.3%) than were those who received no such advice (13.4%). Of special interest is Berkanovic and Telesky's (1982) finding that "when the network advises seeking care but beliefs do not support this behavior, fewer individuals actually

seek care than in the other incongruent condition" (p. 1026). The "other incongruent condition" consisted of no network advice to seek care when beliefs supported care. In instances in which network advice contradicted what the individual personally believed, general network characteristics (contact, consulting, support) were found to have a positive influence on the seeking of medical help. This finding points to the possible contingent nature of network influences. In this case, structural network factors worked against the seeking of help except in cases in which informational conflicts developed in the immediate situation.

RESEARCH ISSUES

Group Structures

A social isolation bias is inevitable in population studies with low participation rates. The socially isolated are harder to find and tend to resist participation in studies when they are contacted. Persons with weak social ties are more likely to be lost in longitudinal studies with periodic recontacts (Berkman, 1986). Equally problematic is the full representation of strong ingroups in immigrant cultures. Individuals with very strong ties in parochial groups are likely to resist answering questions in population surveys. The disproportionate absence of the socially isolated and the strongly connected is especially problematic in studies of social attachments. These potential problems underscore the need for extra efforts to obtain high participation rates in group structures research.

Another difficulty in group structures research is the interpretation of abundant social ties. Do such ties mean higher social integration? Some studies have interpreted social attachment to mean a larger number of social ties. On the other hand, strong in-group ties may coincide with smaller circles of social involvement, as indicated in May's (1992) research on immigrants.

This possibility may explain why some studies attribute greater importance to social support than to network size. Smaller in-group networks, however, probably provide more emotional than material support (Granovetter, 1983). Emotional support is more likely in close relationships among persons who have known each other for many years. According to Suchman, friendship solidarity or close friendship ties of long duration are indicative of parochial or in-group ties. This view suggests that large network size implies a different type of social involvement and support.

The group structures tradition in sociology emphasizes intersecting patterns of group affiliations. According to Simmel (1955), most individuals participate in multiple social circles. With advances in transportation and communication, people are less confined to particular localities. As a result, their in-group contacts in one circle of associations are less likely to coincide with other circles of associations. Suchman's parochial groups are exceptions to this tendency toward diversity in social ties.

Blau's macrostructural theory of social integration (Blau, 1977; Blau & Schwartz, 1984) expands on Simmel's view of group structures. In Blau's theory, diverse social ties are a natural by-product of increasing heterogeneity and social diversity in modern society. The erosion of interlocking in-group ties weakens the influence of cultural values and social norms. According to Blau and Schwartz (1984, p. 1):

> Simmel's imaginative analysis of intersecting circles draws attention to their significance for various aspects of contemporary culture—the diverse human personalities, the individualized situations of people, the lesser domination by social norms and pressures, the potentiality for subjectivity and departure from conformity, and the greater individual freedom.

Thus, social diversity means increased freedom. Blau attributes part of this freedom to the offsetting influences of countersocial forces. With diverse friendship ties, social pressures or advice in one relationship may be offset by counterpressures or different advice in another relationship. Abundant social ties give increased exposure to diverse perspectives and cross-cutting influences. Granovetter (1983) sees a number of advantages to casual acquaintances and broadly based friendship ties because social contacts connect people to resources and increase their options.

My own research suggests that strong in-group ties are likely to be fostered in subcultural groups that are trying to maintain particular cultural values and norms. These parochial group structures tend to reaffirm cultural tendencies in behavior. On the other hand, cross-cutting social circles and diverse social ties tend to broaden individual perspectives and weaken subcultural influences on behavior. More research is needed on the group structures of different religious, racial/ethnic, and immigrant group cultures.

Sociocultural Contexts

Freidson (1960) saw an important cultural element in the lay referral system. He believed that all referral systems had two critical dimensions, the first of which was the culture of the client and its similarity with that of the medical profession. In his view (Freidson, 1960, p. 377):

> Considerations of culture have relevance to the diagnosis and prescriptions that are meaningful to the client and to the kinds of consultants considered authoritative. Consideration of the extensiveness of the lay referral structure has relevance to the channeling and reinforcement of lay culture and to the flowing-in of "outside" communications.

The research on religious cultures and immigrant cultures cited earlier underscores Freidson's emphasis on the cultural context of medical help seeking.

Responses to questions on social attachments and supports, however, are conditioned by cultural meanings. Misinterpretations of questions can give highly distorted views of social contacts. Jacobson (1986) described a woman in his research who said she had "no contact with the family, only on holidays," in response to a question about contacts with family. The woman interpreted the question to mean gatherings in which the entire family got together. In a follow-up interview the same woman indicated that she took care of a retarded sister who lived across the street. Since the sister lived with her father and a brother, she saw the three of them every day. She also had another sister whom she called at least once a week. This lady was initially mislabeled as a social isolate. Comparisons across cultural groups require careful attention to cultural misinterpretations of questions.

Other measurement problems are apparent in the assessments commonly used to represent group culture. Most studies have attributed certain cultural orientations to particular ethnic and religious groups. Recent studies showing new attitudes and cultural outlooks among Hispanics and African-Americans question the validity of such global indicators. The problem is particularly troublesome in large cross-sectional studies in which persons are treated as being culturally similar due to ethnicity or race, without adequate empirical verification. This concern is reflected in a review of the literature on how race and ethnicity have been employed in health services research (D. R. Williams, 1994). Past studies are criticized for using race to represent assumed social and cultural factors. D. R. Williams (1994, p. 261) states:

> Researchers and practitioners must give more careful attention to the conceptualization and measurement of race. An understanding of racial/ethnic differences in patterns of health service utilization will require efforts to catalog and quantify the specific social and cultural factors that are differentially distributed by racial and ethnic status.

The use of religion in the study of health behavior reveals further complications. The Protestant label glosses over considerable religious and cultural diversity. Congregationalists, Mormons, and Pentecostals are radically different cultural groups, yet the Protestant label applies to them all. The Catholic label is also too broad because it includes multiple ethnic groups besides Anglo-Americans; respondents of Hispanic, Italian, and Irish descent typically belong to the Catholic faith. What is clear from this analysis of group structures is that many of the measures typically used in health behavior research hide potentially important subcultural differences.

Data Collection Strategies

One of the persistent problems in health behavior research is the issue of population sampling versus convenience sampling. Several studies examined in this chapter used population groups who were either enrolled in prepaid or family practice clinics or had visited a particular clinic during a specified period of time. These studies may reflect variations only among particular types of utilizers in the larger population. The extreme nonutilizers of health care services are excluded from prepaid practice groups. To the extent that the socially isolated tend to avoid memberships in these types of health organizations, the findings from these studies may underestimate the importance of social ties in health care use.

Part of the inconsistency in the findings emerging from group structures research and its relationship with health behavior may be attributed to the diverse outcome measures employed. Utilization has been defined and measured in terms of source of care, total number of visits, acute episode visits, delay in seeking care, and participation in specific treatment programs. Some studies have ignored utilization completely and looked only at attitudes. Group influences may be stronger for some health behaviors than for others, but any differences are hard to untangle due to wide variations in study samples and measurements used. The separation of psychiatric disorders from other types of medical problems in most utilization studies reduces some of the potential confusion in health behavior research. Distinctions between other types of problems, however, such as acute episodes versus chronic conditions and undiagnosed concerns versus well-care practices, may be necessary to specify more clearly the relationships between group structures and health behavior.

Retrospective surveys inevitably have a problem with recall bias. Social contacts and medical visits are typically underreported. Shorter recall periods result in more accurate medical information, but do not give a very broad picture of past utilization patterns. Some longitudinal studies address both issues by using periodic re-interviews with shorter recall. Others studies eliminate this bias by measuring health service use from clinic records of persons enrolled in prepaid medical programs. More troublesome is the finding that people often underreport or overlook taken-for-granted relationships in which daily contact is customary. Their doing so gives a distorted view of social attachments (Berkman, 1985, pp. 256–257).

Health care diaries avoid recall bias by having respondents make daily entries about their health behavior. This approach indicates that social contacts are more important in the day-to-day response to medical symptoms than survey studies typically indicate. Health diaries show that the majority of everyday symptoms and illness experiences are handled through self-care and lay consultations. Daily accounts of symptoms show that the most frequent complaints are respiratory and musculoskeletal in nature. The most frequent reactions to both are drugs, followed by lay consultations, activity restrictions, and, last, seeking professional care (Verbrugge & Ascione, 1987). In other studies, fewer than one third of the illness episodes result in the use of professional medical care (Hannay, 1980; Pill, 1988, p. 140). In one study (Punamaki & Aschan, 1994), respondents were asked to record daily what was done to care for their health or the health of those close to them. Some 49.6% of the respondents reported some form of lay care during the 2 weeks that diaries were kept, whereas only 10.1% reported the use of official health care.

Health diaries offer some advantages and disadvantages in health behavior research. One advantage is the symptom-specific information that is available. Another advantage is a substantial reduction in recall bias. The diaries also provide a clearer picture of how people arrive at definitions of illness. Most important, however, is the rich detail on the everyday context of health and illness. The greatest problem in using medical diaries is the difficulty of getting people to record daily information for any extended period of time. Relatively low completion rates (55%) compared to those in most health surveys (80–95%) are not uncommon in diary studies (Punamaki & Aschan, 1994). This difference brings back the issue of underrepresenting the socially isolated in studies with low participation rates.

SUMMARY AND CONCLUSIONS

Social attachments and group affiliations influence health behaviors, but the precise nature of this influence varies by age, gender, race, socioeconomic status, and perception of social support. The research reviewed at three separate levels of social attachment—household ties, relatives and friends, and religious and social participation—confirms this view. Some studies have taken a broader view of group structures and have examined the influences of interconnecting group ties on health behavior. At one time, strong and interlocking in-group structures were thought to have a negative influence on health beliefs and the seeking of medical help. Suchman's research in New York City in the 1960s reflects this position. A more recent sociocultural hypothesis suggests that interlocking group ties tend to reinforce cultural beliefs when network members know and interact with each other and share the same cultural background. According to this view, strong group ties may oppose or support the seeking of medical help depending on the shared sociocultural experiences of social network members. Research on new immigrants tends to support a group structures link between cultural beliefs and health behavior. Other research on Hispanics and African-Americans provides some evidence of change in the relationship between group ties and health behavior as the earlier cultural distrust of medical institutions has been eroded by broadened participation and acculturation.

Improved research designs are needed to help us better understand the role of group structures in health behavior. Longitudinal research on lay consultations shows how the timing of advice on medical matters can make a significant difference in the decision to seek medical help if network members are consulted during actual episodes of possible illness. On the other hand, more general network measures conceal this influence. Studies of group structure also require greater effort to find the socially isolated who are typically missed in social surveys. More cautious interpretations of abundant social ties and group culture are needed. The assumed connection between abundant social ties and social integration is dubious and requires further investigation. Likewise, more precise measures of the sociocultural beliefs attributed to racial/ethnic and religious groups should be used. Finally, the potential problem of underreporting in social surveys requires more careful scrutiny due to the apparent recall bias uncovered in more recent studies using health care diaries.

REFERENCES

Alexander, C. S., & Markowitz, R. (1986). Maternal employment and use of pediatric clinic services. *Medical Care, 24*, 134–147.

Andersen, R., Lewis, S. Z., Giachello, A. L., Aday, L. A., & Chiu, G. (1981). Access to medical care among the Hispanic population of the southwestern United States. *Journal of Health and Social Behavior, 22*, 78–89.

Arling, G. (1985). Interaction effects in a multivariate model of physician visits by older people. *Medical Care, 23*, 361–371.

Avis, N. E., Brambilla, D. J., Vass, K., & McKinlay, J. B. (1991). The effect of widowhood on health: A prospective analysis from the Massachusetts Women's Health Study. *Social Science and Medicine, 33*, 1063–1070.

Bardis, P. D. (1959). A familism scale. *Marriage and Family Living, 21*, 340–341.

Bashshur, R. L., Shananon, G. W., & Metzner, C. A. (1971). Some ecological differentials in the use of medical services. *Health Services Research, 6*, 61–75.

Berkanovic, E., & Telesky, C. (1982). Social networks, beliefs, and the decision to seek medical care: An analysis of congruent and incongruent patterns. *Medical Care, 20*, 1018–1026.

Berkanovic, E., & Telesky, C. (1985). Mexican-American, black-American and white-American differences in reporting illnesses, disability and physician visits for illness. *Social Science and Medicine, 20*, 567–577.

Berkanovic, E., Telesky, C., & Reeder, S. (1981). Structural and social psychological factors in the decision to seek medical care for symptoms. *Medical Care, 19*, 693–709.

Berkman, L. F. (1985). The relationship of social networks and social support to morbidity and mortality. In S. Cohen & S. L. Syme (Eds.), *Social support and health* (pp. 241–262). New York: Academic Press.

Berkman, L. F. (1986). Social networks, support, and health: Taking the next step forward. *Journal of Epidemiology, 123*, 559–562.

Berkman, L. F., & Syme, S. L. (1979). Social networks, host resistance and mortality: A nine year follow-up study of Alameda County residents. *American Journal of Epidemiology, 109*, 186–204.

Berman, P., Kendall, C., & Bhattacharyya, K. (1994). The household production of health: Integrating social science perspectives on micro-level health determinants. *Social Science and Medicine, 38*, 205–215.

Blake, R. L., Jr. (1991). Social stressors, social supports, and self-esteem as predictors of morbidity in adults with chronic lung disease. *Family Practice Research Journal, 11*, 65–74.

Blau, P. M. (1977). *Inequality and heterogeneity: A primitive theory of social structure*. New York: Free Press.

Blau, P. M., & Schwartz, J. E. (1984). *Crosscutting social circles*. New York: Academic Press.

Bloom, J. R. (1990). The relationship of social support and health. *Social Science and Medicine, 30*, 635–637.

Blumer, H. (1969). *Symbolic interactionism: Perspective and method*. Englewood Cliffs, NJ: Prentice-Hall.

Breault, K. D., & Barkey, K. (1982). A comparative analysis of Durkheim's theory of egoistic suicide. *Sociological Quarterly, 23*, 321–331.

Broadhead, W. E., Gehlbach, S. H., DeGruy, F. V., & Kaplan, B. H. (1989). Functional versus structural support and health care utilization in a family medicine outpatient clinic. *Medical Care, 27*, 221–233.

Broman, C. L. (1993). Social relationships and health-related behavior. *Journal of Behavioral Medicine, 16*, 335–350.

Calnan, M. (1983). Social networks and patterns of help-seeking behavior. *Social Science and Medicine, 17*, 25–28.

Campbell, J. D. (1978). The child in the sick role: Contributions of age, sex, parental status, and parental values. *Journal of Health and Social Behavior, 19*, 35–51.

Chien, A., & Schneiderman, L. J. (1975). A comparison of health care utilization by husbands and wives. *Journal of Community Health, 1*, 118–126.

Cohen, A. S., & Syme, L. (1985). *Social support and health*. New York: Academic Press.

Collver, A., Ten Have, R., & Speare, M. C. (1967). Factors

influencing the use of maternal health services. *Social Science and Medicine, 1*, 293-308.

Counte, M. A., & Glandon, G. L. (1991). A panel study of life stress, social support, and the health services utilization of older people. *Medical Care, 29*, 348-361.

Cross, W. (1990). Race and ethnicity: Effects on social networks. In M. Cochran, M. Larner, D. Riley, L. Gunnarsson, & C. R. Henderson, Jr. (Eds.), *Extended families: The social networks of parents and their children* (pp. 67-85). Cambridge, England: Cambridge University Press.

Dishman, R. K. (1982). Compliance/adherence in health-related exercise. *Health Psychology, 1*, 237-267.

Durkheim, E. (1897/1951). *Suicide: A study in sociology.* (Translated by J. A. Spaulding and G. Simpson; edited by G. Simpson.) Glencoe, IL: Free Press.

Dutton, D. B. (1978). Explaining the low use of health services by the poor: Costs, attitudes, or delivery systems. *American Sociological Review, 43*, 348-368.

Farge, E. J. (1978). Medical orientation among a Mexican-American population: An old and a new model reviewed. *Social Science and Medicine, 12*, 277-282.

Feagin, J. (1970). A note on the friendship ties of black urbanites. *Social Forces, 49*, 303-308.

Fink, R., Shapiro, S., & Lewison, J. (1968). The reluctant participant in breast cancer screening programs. *Public Health Reports, 83*, 479-490.

Freidson, E. (1960). Client control of medical practice. *American Journal of Sociology, 65*, 374-382.

Furstenberg, A. L., & Davis, L. J. (1984). Lay consultations of older people. *Social Science and Medicine, 18*, 827-837.

Garrett, R. E., Zyzanski, S. J., & Alemagno, S. A. (1990). Immigration, health status, and physician visits in a Puerto Rican community. *Family Medicine, 22*, 14-19.

Gaudin, J., & Davis, K. (1985). Social networks of black and white rural families: A research report. *Journal of Marriage and the Family, 47*, 1015-1021.

Geertsen, R. (1988). Social group characteristics and health behavior. In D. S. Gochman (Ed.) *Health behavior: Emerging research perspectives* (pp. 131-148). New York: Plenum Press.

Geertsen, R., & Gray, R. M. (1970). Familistic orientations and inclination toward adopting the sick role. *Journal of Marriage and the Family, 32*, 638-646.

Geertsen, R., Klauber, M. R., Rindflesh, M., Kane, R. L., & Gray, R. (1975). A re-examination of Suchman's views on social factors in health care utilization. *Journal of Health and Social Behavior, 16*, 226-237.

Gilman, S. C., Justice, J., Saepharn, K., & Charles, G. (1992). Use of traditional and modern health services by Laotian refugees. *Western Journal of Medicine, 157*, 310-315.

Gordon, M. M. (1964). *Assimilation in American life.* London: Oxford University Press.

Granovetter, M. (1983). The strength of weak ties: A network theory revisited. In R. Collins (Ed.), *Sociological theory* (pp. 201-233). San Francisco: Jossey-Bass.

Greenlick, M. R., Hurtado, A. V., Pope, C. R., Saward, E. W., & Yoshioka, S. S. (1968). Determinants of medical care utilization. *Health Services Research, 3*, 296-315.

Hannay, D. R. (1980). The "iceberg" of illness and "trivial" consultations. *Journal of the Royal College of General Practitioners, 30*, 551-554.

Haynes, S. G., & Feinleib, M. (1980). Women, work and coronary heart disease: Prospective findings from the Framingham Heart Study. *American Journal of Public Health, 70*, 133-141.

Hines, R. (1972). The health status of black Americans: Changing perspectives. In E. Jaco (Ed.), *Patients, physicians and illness* (pp. 40-50). New York: Free Press.

Hogan, D., Hao, L., & Parish, W. (1990). Race, kin networks, and assistance to mother-headed families. *Social Forces, 68*, 797-812.

Hoppe, S. K., & Heller, P. L. (1975). Alienation, familism, and the utilization of health services by Mexican Americans. *Journal of Health and Social Behavior, 16*, 304-314.

Horwitz, S. M., Morgenstern, H., & Berkman, L. F. (1985). The impact of social stressors and social networks on pediatric medical care use. *Medical Care, 23*, 946-959.

House, J. S., Landis, K. R., & Umberson, D. (1988). Social relationships and health. *Science, 241*, 540-545.

House, J. S., Robbins, C., & Metzner, H. L. (1982). The association of social relationships and activities with mortality: Perspective evidence from the Tecumseh community health study. *American Journal of Epidemiology, 116*, 123-140.

Ingham, J. G., & Miller, P. (1983). Self-referral: Social and demographic determinants of consulting behavior. *Journal of Psychosomatic Research, 27*, 233-242.

Ingham, J. G., & Miller, P. (1986). Self-referral to primary care: Symptoms and social factors. *Journal of Psychosomatic Research, 30*, 49-56.

Jacobson, D. E. (1986). Types and timing of social support. *Journal of Health and Social Behavior, 27*, 250-264.

Koenig, H. G., Westlund, R. E., George, L. K., Hughes, D. C., Blazer, D. G., & Hybels, C. (1993). Abbreviating the Duke Social Support Index for use in chronically ill elderly individuals. *Psychosomatics, 34*, 61-69.

Lendt, L. A. (1960). *A social history of Washington Heights, New York City.* New York: Columbia-Washington Heights Community Mental Health Project.

Levin, J. S. (1994). Religion and health: Is there an association, is it valid, and is it causal. *Social Science and Medicine, 38*, 1475-1482.

Levin, J. S., & Schiller, P. L. (1987). Is there a religious factor in health? *Journal of Religion and Health, 26*, 9-36.

Levin, J. S., & Vanderpool, H. Y. (1989). Is religion therapeutically significant for hypertension? *Social Science and Medicine, 29*, 69-78.

Madsen, W. (1964). *Mexican Americans of south Texas.* Chicago: Holt, Rinehart & Winston.

Markides, K. S., Levin, J. S., & Ray, L. A. (1985). Determinants of physician utilization among Mexican Americans: A three generation study. *Medical Care, 23*, 236-246.

Martineau, W. (1977). Informal social ties among urban black Americans. *Journal of Black Studies, 8*, 83-104.

May, K. M. (1992). Middle-Eastern immigrant parents' social networks and help-seeking for child health care. *Journal of Advanced Nursing, 17*, 905-912.

McAdoo, H. (1978). Factors related to stability in upwardly mobile black families. *Journal of Marriage and the Family, 40*, 761-776.

McKinlay, J. B. (1973). Social networks, lay consultation and help-seeking behavior. *Social Forces, 51*, 275-292.

McKinney, J. C. (1966). *Constructive typology and social theory.* New York: Appleton-Century-Crofts.

Meininger, J. C. (1986). Sex differences in factors associated with use of medical care and alternative illness behaviors. *Social Science and Medicine, 22*, 285-292.

Nall, F. C., & Speilberg, J. (1967). Social and cultural factors in the responses of Mexican-Americans to medical treatment. *Journal of Health and Social Behavior, 8*, 299-308.

Nelson, M. A. (1993). Race, gender, and the effect of social supports on the use of health services by elderly individuals. *International Journal of Aging and Human Development, 37*, 227-246.

Notzon, R. (1977). Utilization of family planning services by currently married women 15-44 years of age, United States, 1973. *Vital Health Statistics, 23*(1), 1-36.

O'Dea, T. F. (1964). *The Mormons.* Chicago: University of Chicago Press.

O'Reilly, P. (1988). Methodological issues in social support and social network research. *Social Science and Medicine, 26*, 863-873.

Pilisuk, M., Boylan, R., & Acredolo C. (1987). Social support, life stress and subsequent medical care utilization. *Health Psychology, 6*, 273-288.

Pill, R. (1988). Health beliefs and behavior in the home. In R. Anderson, J. K. Davies, I. Kickbusch, D. V. McQueen, & J. Turner (Eds.), *Health behaviour: Research and health promotion* (pp. 140-153). Oxford, England: Oxford University Press.

Punamaki, R., & Aschan, H. (1994). Self-care and mastery among primary health care patients. *Social Science and Medicine, 39*, 733-741.

Quesada, G. M., & Heller, P. L.(1977). Sociocultural barriers to medical care among Mexican Americans in Texas. *Medical Care, 15*(Supplement), 93-101.

Ramakrishna, J., & Weiss, M. G. (1992). Health, illness, and immigration: East Indians in the United States. *Western Journal of Medicine, 157*, 265-270.

Riley, A. W., Finney, J. W., Mellits, E. D., Starfield, B., Kidwell, S., Quaskey, S., Cataldo, M. F., Filipp, L., & Shematek, J. P. (1993). Determinants of children's health care use: An investigation of psychosocial factors. *Medical Care, 31*, 767-783.

Rubel, A. J. (1966). *Across the tracks: Mexican Americans in a Texas city.* Austin: University of Texas Press.

Salloway, J. C., & Dillon, P. B. (1973). A comparison of family networks and friend networks in health care utilization. *Journal of Comparative Family Studies, 4*(Special Issue), 131-142.

Saunders, L. (1954). *Cultural difference and medical care.* New York: Russell Sage Foundation.

Schiller, P. L., & Levin, J. S. (1988). Is there a religious factor in health care utilization? A review. *Social Science and Medicine, 27*, 1369-1379.

Schor, E., Starfield, B., Stidley, C., & Hankin, J. (1987). Family health: Utilization and effects of family membership. *Medical Care, 25*, 616-626.

Seeman, T. E., Berkman, L. F., Kohout, F., Lacroix, A., Glynn, R., & Blazer, D. (1993). Intercommunity variations in the association between social ties and mortality in the elderly: A comparative analysis of three communities. *Annals of Epidemiology, 3*, 325-335.

Seeman, T. E., Kaplan, G. A., Knudsen, L., Cohen, R., & Guralnik, J. (1987). Social network ties and mortality among the elderly in the Alameda County Study. *American Journal of Epidemiology, 126*, 714-723.

Sharp, K., Ross, C. E., & Cockerham, W. C. (1983). Symptoms, beliefs, and the use of physician services among the disadvantaged. *Journal of Health and Social Behavior, 24*, 255-263.

Simmel, G. (1955). *Conflict and the web of group affiliations.* (Translated and edited by K. H. Wolff & R. Bendix.) New York: Free Press.

Solon, J. A. (1966). Patterns of medical care: Sociological variations among a hospital's outpatients. *American Journal of Public Health, 56*, 884-894.

St. Clair, P. A., Smeriglio, V. L., Alexander, C. S., & Celentano, D. D. (1989). Social network structure and prenatal care utilization. *Medical Care, 27*, 823-832.

Stark, S. (1978). Suicide: A comparative analysis. *Social Forces, 57*, 644-653.

Strand, P. J., & Jones, W., Jr. (1983). Health service utilization by Indochinese refugees. *Medical Care, 21*, 1089-1098.

Suchman, E. A. (1964). Sociomedical variations among ethnic groups. *American Journal of Sociology, 70*, 319-331.

Suchman, E. A. (1965). Social patterns of illness and medical care. *Journal of Health and Human Behavior, 6*, 2-16.

Treiber, F. A., Baranowski, T., Braden, D. S., Strong, W. B., Levy, M., & Knox, W. (1991). Social support for exercise: Relationship to physical activity in young adults. *Preventive Medicine, 20*, 737-750.

Tung, T. M. (1980). The Indochinese refugees as patients. *Journal of Refugee Resettlement, 1*, 53.

Turner, J. H. (1991). *The structure of sociological theory.* Belmont, CA: Wadsworth.

Verbrugge, L. M., & Ascione, F. J. (1987). Exploring the iceberg: Common symptoms and how people care for them. *Medical Care, 25*, 539-569.

Walters, V. (1993). Stress, anxiety and depression: Women's

accounts of their health problems. *Social Science and Medicine, 36,* 393–402.

Wan, T. T. (1982). Use of health services by the elderly in low-income communities. *Millbank Memorial Fund Quarterly/Health and Society, 60,* 82–107.

Wan, T. T. (1987). Functionally disabled elderly: Health status, social support and use of health services. *Research on Aging, 9,* 61–78.

Wan, T. T., & Soifer, S. J. (1974). Determinants of physician utilization: A causal analysis. *Journal of Health and Social Behavior, 15,* 100–108.

Wan, T. T., & Yates, A. S. (1975). Prediction of dental services utilization: A multivariate approach. *Inquiry, 12,* 143–146.

Weitzman, B. C., & Berry, C. A. (1992). Health status and health care utilization among New York City home attendants: An illustration of the needs of working poor, immigrant women. *Women and Health, 19,* 87–105.

Williams, D. R. (1994). The concept of race in health services research: 1966–1990. *Health Services Research, 29,* 261–274.

Williams, H. A. (1993). A comparison of social support and social networks of black parents and white parents with chronically ill children. *Social Science and Medicine, 37,* 1509–1520.

Winemiller, D. R., Mitchell, M. E., Sutliff, J., & Cline, D. J. (1993). Measurement strategies in social support: A descriptive review of the literature. *Journal of Clinical Psychology, 49,* 638–648.

Wolinsky, F. D. (1982). Racial differences in illness behavior. *Journal of Community Health, 8,* 87–101.

Zambrana, R. E., Ell, K., Dorrington, C., Wachsman, L., & Hodge, D. (1994). *Health and Social Work, 19,* 93–102.

14

Sick Role Concepts and Health Behavior

Alexander Segall

INTRODUCTION

Parsons's sick role concept (e.g., Parsons, 1951) and the identity of the field of medical sociology are closely interrelated and over the past four decades have undergone a similar process of historical transformation. This chapter will begin by summarizing the basic dimensions of Parsons's sick role model and the type of early empirical research stimulated by this conceptual framework. The discussion will then shift to the major limitations of the sick role concept and comment briefly on past efforts to reformulate and extend the Parsonian model. The parallel between the declining influence of Parsons's sick role concept and the changing research focus in the sociological analysis of health and illness behavior will be highlighted.

In view of the ongoing struggles to transform medical sociology into health sociology, and to shift the primary research focus of the

Alexander Segall • Department of Sociology, University of Manitoba, Winnipeg, Manitoba R3T 2N2, Canada.

Handbook of Health Behavior Research I: Personal and Social Determinants, edited by David S. Gochman. Plenum Press, New York, 1997.

field from patient illness behavior to the study of population health behavior, it is important to attempt to reconceptualize the dimensions of the sick role and situate it in the social context of lay health beliefs and behavior. The concluding section of the chapter will discuss the relevance of a redefined sick role concept for the study of health behavior and the type of research initiatives required to advance our understanding of this new sick role as a potential social determinant of health behavior.

Emergence of the Sick Role Construct: The Era of Influence

Due to the widespread nature of illness, it is not surprising that many past studies attempted to identify and describe the social position of the sick person in society. This unique social position includes a set of expectations regarding the behavior of both the sick person and those with whom the sick person interacts (e.g., family members and health professionals). It has been recognized for many years that the sick person occupies a special social position with an associated behavioral pattern and set of reciprocal role relationships. Not until Parsons (1951) theoretically formulated the behavioral dimensions of this status, however, did the sick role emerge as a central concept in the sociological analysis of illness behavior. In fact, the development of the sick role concept has been described as "a major turning point in the history of medical sociology" (Turner, 1992, p. 136).

Sick Role Behavioral Expectations

The specific features of the role of the sick person were outlined by Parsons in terms of two major rights and two major duties. Briefly, the occupant of the sick role is exempt from responsibility for the incapacity, as it is beyond the sick person's control (Right 1). Definition of the condition as an illness also exempts the sick person from usual well roles and task obligations (Right 2). Parsons acknowledged that the sick person's exemption from these obligations would vary in terms of degree (partial versus complete) and duration (temporary versus permanent), depending upon the nature and severity of the illness.

In addition, these rights or exemptions depend, in part, upon how well the sick person fulfills the obligations associated with this social role. For example, the occupant of the sick role is expected to recognize that to be ill is inherently undesirable, and the sick person therefore has an obligation to try to get well (Duty 1). According to Parsons, the sick person also has an obligation to seek technically competent help and to cooperate in the process of trying to get well (Duty 2). In Parsons's model, the sick role requires the incumbent to seek a specific type of help, i.e., the services of a physician. Thus, sick role occupancy is perceived by others as legitimate only if the sick person clearly demonstrates a desire to get well by seeking medical care and complying with the physician's recommended treatment regimen.

The Parsonian Paradigm and the Identity of Medical Sociology

Parsons's sick role model inspired an extensive body of empirical research beginning in the late 1950s and continuing throughout the 1960s and thus played a major part in defining the identity of medical sociology. During this period, the sick role concept was accepted widely (and often uncritically) and guided the research of many investigators in the emerging field of medical sociology. This versatile conceptual framework was applied to the study not only of typical illness episodes, but also of conditions as diverse as pregnancy (Rosengren, 1962) and alcoholism (Roman & Trice, 1968), as well as the aging process (Lipman & Sterne, 1969).

A number of insightful reviews of this research literature are available (e.g., Gerhardt, 1987; Levine & Kozloff, 1978). Without going into detail at this time, this discussion must point out that Parsons's sick role concept was of fundamental importance to the development of this field of inquiry. In fact, in the early 1960s, researchers extolled the virtues of the sick role as a unifying theme for integrating diverse research efforts and shaping the character of medical sociology (Goldstein & Dommermuth, 1961). Consequently, for a number of years, research guided by the Parsonian paradigm focused primarily on aspects of illness behavior and pathways to medical care (i.e., the process of becoming a patient and the dynamics of the patient–physician interaction).

Parsons conceptualized sickness in large part as a form of deviant behavior and raised concerns about the potential for secondary gains to be derived from claims to the sick role that might not actually be legitimate. For example, an individual might feign illness as a means of gaining role exemptions and avoiding work or family responsibilities or both. According to Wolinsky (1988), the sick role may be used as a coping device, as an avoidance mechanism, or as a justification for failure. In all three cases, the efforts by the individual to deal with the social pressures of role and task performance by seeking sick role legitimation may in fact violate the presumed normative expectation of the undesirability of being sick. Wolinsky cautioned that increasing levels of stress in contemporary society may result in more prevalent claims to the privileges and temporary exemptions associated with the sick role.

Consequently, the Parsonian paradigm tied the duties of the sick person (i.e., an obligation to get well) to the power of the physician to regulate entry into the sick role. Parsons presented the physician as a prototype professional and an important agent of social control. While the illness experience might begin with individuals' seeking information and advice about their symptoms from family and friends and engaging in self-treatment of their symptomatic conditions, it is ultimately the physician who possesses the knowledge and expertise to define illness and legitimate claims to the sick role. In the words of Wolinsky (1988, p. 182): "Although provisional validation from the lay referral system permits the sick role to be adopted on a temporary basis, the ill individual does not become a bona fide occupant of the sick role until patient status has been legitimated by the physician."

As a result of this perspective, research influenced by Parsons's model typically operationally defined and measured willingness to adopt the sick role in terms of the individual's tendency or inclination to use the services of a physician (e.g., Mechanic & Volkart, 1961; Phillips, 1965). Thus, at this early stage in its development, medical sociology accepted the legitimate authority of the medical profession and the preeminence of physician-centered healing and devoted a great deal of research attention to the social control issues inherent in Parsons's sick role concept.

LIMITATIONS OF THE SICK ROLE CONCEPT: A DECADE OF CRITICAL COMMENTARY

"The Parsonian model has proven to be remarkably controversial as well as provocative" (Arluke, 1988, p. 172). Despite the obvious importance of Parsons's contribution to the development of medical sociology, and the fact that the sick role has been described as perhaps the single most important concept in the sociological analysis of health and illness behavior, this concept also stimulated a great deal of critical commentary throughout the 1970s and early 1980s (e.g., see Arluke, Kennedy & Kessler, 1979; Honig-Parnass, 1981; McCormack, 1981; Segall, 1976a). Wolinsky (1988, p. 181) contended, however, that "nearly all subsequent theoretical or conceptual frameworks in sociological approaches to health behavior have emerged as the result of attempts to refute or to extend the sick-role concept."

Major Criticisms of Parsons's Sick Role Concept

Many aspects of the Parsonian paradigm have been subjected to careful scrutiny. Parsons's sick role model has been criticized because it applies only to temporary, acute physical illness episodes and not to chronic illness. It has been convincingly argued that the sick role does not provide a relevant explanatory framework for understanding the behavior of individuals who experience long-term or permanent conditions such as chronic illness and disability (e.g., Arluke, 1988; Kassebaum & Baumann, 1965; Segall, 1976a).

Furthermore, the model not only is limited to selected physical conditions, but also does not pertain to psychosocial conditions (e.g., mental and emotional health problems). For example, Blackwell (1967) explored expectations about entering the sick role for physical and psychiatric conditions and reported that in the case of physical illness, the social norms are relatively clear (i.e., the individual should consult a physician as soon as possible). When, however, the health problem "has both physical and psychological connotations, and when the question of extent of personal responsibility for both causing and coping with the dysfunction is introduced, the appropriateness of applying the norms relating to the sick role becomes uncertain" (Blackwell, 1967, p. 93). In other words, it appears that the relevance of sick role behavioral expectations decreases as the social and psychological aspects of the illness condition increase.

In addition, Parsons's sick role model has been characterized as "medicocentric," since it places the physician at the center of the health care system (Gallagher, 1976). The type of patient activity acknowledged by the Parsonian model is extremely restricted and essentially entails being submissive and compliant. The physician is presented as controlling and dominating this asymmetrical relationship, while the patient is portrayed as a passive object, as opposed to an active, reflexive subject participating in an interactional process. Certainly the patient (even one who is experiencing an acute physical illness) possesses a greater degree of autonomy than is recognized by this model.

Thus, in formulating the sick role concept, Parsons paid little attention to the possible variations that may occur in the nature of the patient–physician relationship and the attendant differences in role expectations and performance. Honig-Parnass (1981) empirically investigated the extent to which lay sick role conceptions correspond to the behavioral dimensions outlined in the Parsonian model. More specifically, this study focused on lay expectations regarding the relative degrees to which sick persons with acute versus chronic physical illnesses would be dependent on formal professional medical treatment and on the care and support of informal members of their social networks. The findings did not support Parsons's assumption that medical professionals typically play a dominant part both in caring for sick persons and in shaping their sick role expectations. In fact, the study identified two distinct sets of behavioral expectations corresponding to the sick role for acute versus chronic illness conditions; furthermore, in the case of the chronically ill, a more crucial caregiving role was assigned to lay significant others. Thus, Honig-Parnass (1981, p. 616) concluded that "the professionalist bias of Parsons' model becomes particularly noticeable in the case of chronic illness."

It is important to note that the "professionalist bias" inherent in the sick role model not only attributed a central position to the physician and medical care, but also diverted attention from the fact that lay persons are not simply consumers of professional medical services, but are actually active primary health care providers. In other words, Parsons's conceptual framework overestimated the therapeutic impact of the physician and medical care and at the same time underestimated the importance of the caregiving functions performed by members of the informal social network. As a result, research attention was long diverted from a systematic exploration of the nature and extent of lay self-health management practices.

Finally, Parsons's sick role model has also been criticized because this conceptual model failed to consider adequately the potential influence of factors such as culture, class, and gender on the behavioral pattern expected of the sick person. According to Arluke (1988, p. 175), "the Parsonian model is based on an ideal type of American middle-class family, and is therefore culture-bound and class-bound." The patterned behavioral expectations associated with the rights and duties of the sick role are far from universal. In fact, on the basis of cross-cultural comparisons, Butler (1970) argued unequivocally that the behavior expected of the sick person (as described by Parsons) cannot be viewed as the role prescription for all types of illness in diverse sociocultural contexts.

Butler (1970) raised a number of questions that still need to be addressed, including, "What importance is attached in different cultures to the various components of the sick role, and what variations exist in the normative definitions of them?" (p. 243). The available research evidence, though limited, indicates that the behavioral expectations associated with sick role performance are indeed shaped by sociocultural factors such as ethnic group membership and religious affiliation (Segall, 1976b, 1988). In addition, there is evidence that perceived legitimacy to adopt the sick role is also affected by social class standing (e.g., Petroni, 1969). The inherent emphasis in Parsons's conceptual model on individual responsibility and the desirability of good health clearly reflects dominant middle-class values. Finally, it should be noted that potential gender differences in sick role behavior have essentially been overlooked.

Although Parsons's critics acknowledge that the sick role may apply to acute and episodic physical illnesses, serious questions have been raised even for such cases about the validity of the normative basis of the behavioral expectations embodied in Parsons's sick role concept. Most surveys of lay conceptions of the rights and duties of the sick person have failed to provide empirical support for the behavioral dimensions outlined in Parsons's sick role model (e.g., Arluke et al., 1979; Berkanovic, 1972; Segall, 1976b; Twaddle, 1969). Overall, these limitations suggest that Parsons's model does not provide an adequate conceptual framework for analyzing the behavioral expectations and role performance of the sick person.

Reformulating and Extending the Parsonian Model

In 1975, Parsons revisited the sick role and attempted to respond to some of his critics, dismissing many of the criticisms outlined in the preceding section as misrepresentations resulting from incorrect understandings of the original model. For example, Parsons denied that the sick role was confined to cases of acute illness and omitted chronic illness. In addition, he argued that it is quite incorrect to assume that the asymmetrical structure of the patient–physician relationship implies that the role of the patient is purely passive. At the same time, however, he attempted to justify the dominance of the physician inherent in the sick role model by arguing that "... there must be a built-in institutionalized superiority of the professional roles, grounded in responsibility, competence, and occupational concern," for therapeutic agents to function effectively (Parsons, 1975, p. 271). Basically, then, Parsons's views on the sick role and the role of the physician remained unchanged.

In the mid-1970s, a number of other authors attempted to combine their critical reviews of the sick role with an effort to revise and extend the Parsonian paradigm (e.g., Gallagher, 1976; Gerhardt, 1979). For example, Gallagher (1976) was critical of the extreme emphasis in medical sociology on the conception of illness as deviance and the physician as an agent of social control and recommended Parsons's alternative formulation of illness as impaired adaptive capacity. According to Gallagher (1976, p. 208), "... the lines of theoretical extension necessitated by shortcomings in the deviance conception can be supplied from a full analysis of illness as a problem in adaptation...."

Gerhardt (1979) also argued that the Parsonian paradigm includes two models of illness: a structural model focusing on illness as incapacity for role performance and a psychodynamic model focusing on illness as motivated deviance. According to Gerhardt, most criticism of Parsons's sick role has been based on an incomplete and often confused understanding of the full paradigm: "In fact, contemporary medical sociology seems to have adopted a view of the Parsonian paradigm which is truncated and leaves out important aspects" (Gerhardt, 1979, p. 230).

RECONCEPTUALIZING AN ALTERNATIVE SICK ROLE: FROM SICKNESS TO HEALTH BEHAVIOR

Although it is possible to debate the distinctiveness of these two illness models, it is quite evident that Parsons's sick role concept occupied a position of central importance in the development of the field of medical sociology. In the process of reflecting on some of the major changes that had occurred in medical sociology since the 1950s, Levine (1987, pp. 2–3) commented that "we owe much to Talcott Parsons for his classic analysis of the sick role several decades ago in which the concept of sickness was wrested from the biological sphere and raised to the social level." The Parsonian paradigm forcefully emphasized the importance of understanding the social aspects of ill health (sickness), as well as the psychological (illness) and biological (disease) components. Today, health is generally understood as a multidimensional phenomenon consisting of physical, psychological, and social dimensions.

While Parsons's sick role concept was described some years ago as "the most important single theoretical contribution to medical sociology to date" (Cockerham, 1983, p. 1516), it currently receives very little research attention. The declining influence of structural–functionalism as a dominant theoretical paradigm and ongoing ideological struggles to redefine medical sociology as health sociology are both reflected in the ensuing dramatic decrease in the number of studies devoted to an exploration of traditional sick role behavioral expectations and performance. Past efforts to revise and extend the Parsonian paradigm failed to revitalize the sick role concept. Consequently, it seems that the sick role concept is now "… in need of a major theoretical overhaul" (Wolinsky, 1988, p. 190), if this construct is to become relevant to the study of health behavior and a future component in the conceptual framework of the emerging field of health sociology.

Transformation of Medical Sociology into Health Sociology

In a historical analysis of institutional trends in medical sociology, Bloom (1986) traced the sociological analysis of health and illness behavior from its roots in public health to the emergence of social medicine and the eventual recognition (around 1950) of medical sociology as an area of academic specialization. Turner (1992) described the history of social medicine as complex and changing. He contended, however, that social medicine provided an important historical precursor to the development of social and behavioral medical sciences. In turn, a growing emphasis on the social and political functions of the physician's role provided the intellectual origins of medical sociology.

Medical sociology was defined by Bloom (1986, p. 265) as a "… specialized field of learning that applies the concepts and methods of sociology to the systematic study of medicine as a social institution, the fabric of the health system, and the problems of health and illness." After offering this definition, Bloom then summarized the internal tensions that characterize this specialized field of inquiry as applied versus basic research, and the "insider–outsider" perspective. In doing so, he inadvertently perpetuated Straus's (1957) outdated, false dichotomy between sociology in medicine and the more critical sociology of medicine.

At an early stage in the history of medical sociology, Straus suggested that the field could be divided into two patterns of research. Sociology in medicine (the insider view) was described as the application of sociological concepts and research methods with the intention of clarifying questions defined by the medical profession. In contrast, the research focus of sociology of medicine (the outsider view) concentrated on medical practitioners, their institutions and organizations, and their relationships with others (e.g., patients), in an effort to clarify sociological questions. Over the intervening years, this distinction has had an enduring impact on the dual focus of medical sociology on applied and basic research issues (e.g., Mechanic, 1990; Twaddle, 1982).

It is important to recognize that in either case, the underlying assumption is that sociological inquiry should focus primarily on the nature of medical practice and the process of transforming diverse populations into compliant patients. In other words, sociological imaginations have for many years been constrained (either directly or indirectly) by the priorities established by organized medicine. For example, Gold (1977) carefully documented the nature of medical domination of the subject matter of medical sociology. A review of research articles published in the *Journal of Health and Social Behavior* between 1960 and 1976 revealed that the majority focused on patient populations and investigated issues such as access to medical care, and utilization behavior. On the basis of this analysis, Gold (1977, p. 166) contended that "the medical sociologist who incorporates medical values into her or his research may become a deliberate or unwitting agent of social control." This perspective was reinforced by Gill and Twaddle's (1977) argument that the research emphasis in this field on physician-treated disease, patient compliance, and the benefits of medicine indicates that medical sociology has been coopted by medical interests.

It is time for the sociological analysis of health and illness behavior to rid itself of the persistent medical dominance that has characterized the discipline and return to the intellectual roots that gave rise to this field of inquiry. In other words, the proper focus of the sociology of health and health care should be population health issues, the social meaning and management of health and illness, and the socio-political dynamics of the health care sector. To a great extent, medical sociology has restricted its research focus to the study of patient illness behavior, access to medical care, and the role of organized medicine. This approach not only ties sociological analysis to the profession of medicine, but also tends to equate medicine with health care. Transforming the field into health sociology will entail a shift in conceptual and methodological emphasis to population health behavior and consequently broader research horizons.

In the early 1980s, Twaddle characterized health sociology as an emerging paradigm and argued that in the process of trying to transform itself, "sociology is divorcing from the medical perspective and medicocentric perspective to one that takes medicine as one element associated with the health of both individuals and populations ..." (Twaddle, 1982, p. 349). Divorce is sometimes a lengthy and difficult process. For the past decade, the debate regarding the past, present, and future of medical sociology has continued and has attracted the attention of a number of scholars who have made distinguished contributions to this field.

In fact, over the decade beginning in the mid-1980s, a number of recipients of the Leo G. Reeder Award for Distinguished Scholarship in Medical Sociology have commented on the changing nature of the sociological analysis of health and illness behavior and the political struggle to transform the field from medical sociology into health sociology (Elinson, 1985; Levine, 1987; Zola, 1991). Elinson (1985) addressed the decline and possible demise of the field of medical sociology and staunchly defended the future of traditional sociomedical research. Levine (1987) focused his comments on the evolution, rather than the end, of medical sociology and contended that the intellectual terrain of this field has changed over the years. He restricted his analysis, however, to the ways in which medical sociology has expanded its relationship with medicine.

Finally, Zola (1991) also concentrated his comments on the profession of medicine and medical dominance, but presented a rather different perspective. Zola advocated incorporating the notions of power and patriarchy in future analyses of the patient–physician relationship. Furthermore, he concluded his discussion by calling for a shift in the focus of sociological analysis of health and illness behavior from patients to people! This shift is necessary, Zola (1991, p. 10) argued, because "the great majority of the people we study and write about neither think of themselves as 'patients' nor are they necessarily functioning in that role when we are studying them." This illuminating statement clearly signals a need to reconceptualize a nonmedicalized sick role to guide the investigation of everyday health and illness behavior.

The New Sick Role Concept and Lay Health Beliefs and Behavior

In the Parsonian paradigm, the occupant of the sick role is, by definition, a potential patient of the professional medical care system. For many years, due to the pervasive influence of Parsons's analytical framework, "we were locked firmly into a view of ourselves as patients in the sick role" (Zola, 1991, p. 3). It is both theoretically and practically possible, however, to enter and exit the sick role without seeking the assistance of a physician and formally becoming a patient. In fact, the majority of everyday illness episodes are self-managed and are never brought to the attention of a health care professional.

It is therefore necessary to separate the sick role from the patient role and to respond finally to Honig-Parnass's (1981, p. 622) call for a "redimensionalization of the sick role concept." Doing so will require a reconceptualization of the behavioral pattern associated with the status of the sick person in contemporary society. In addition, there must be an improved specification of the type of behavior appropriate for both the sick person and a range of potential care providers, as well as further clarification of the conditions under which the sick role may be legitimately assumed.

It is clear that Parsons's sick role is not a unitary concept that applies equally well to all people who experience illness. At the empirical level, the behavioral dimensions included in Parsons's model vary extensively and do not necessarily constitute a patterned role (Arluke et al., 1979; Berkanovic, 1972; Segall, 1976b; Twaddle, 1969). It could be argued that this lack of unidimensionality stems from the fact that Parsons's model embodies aspects of both the informal sick role and the formal patient role.

Furthermore, a close examination reveals that the rights and duties described by Parsons are not reciprocal in nature. The rights of the person experiencing illness (i.e., exemption from responsibility for the condition and from usual well roles) translate into duties for members of the sick person's informal social network. In contrast, the duties of the person experiencing illness (i.e., the obligation to get well and to seek technically competent help) translate into rights for physicians and formal health care providers. Parsons failed, however, "... to describe in matching clarity and detail the corresponding structure of exemptions and obligations" that characterize the physician's role (Gerhardt, 1987, p. 115). As a result, the rights and duties of the sick role and the physician role are not complementary.

It is time to distinguish conceptually between being sick and being a patient. Redefining the behavioral expectations associated with the social position of the sick person involves situating the sick role completely within the context of lay health beliefs and behavior. A reconceptualized sick role must reflect the fact that laypersons routinely self-evaluate and self-treat many of their health problems as a part of daily living (Dean, 1981; Segall & Goldstein, 1989). To illustrate, Segall and Goldstein (1989) found that the interpretation and evaluation of the meaning of various physical conditions (self-diagnosis) and the decision to engage in some form of self-treatment are symptom-specific. While the majority of participants in a cross-sectional population health survey would see a physician without delay if they experienced an unexplained loss of weight or shortness of breath, they would routinely self-treat symptomatic conditions such as stomach upset, bowel irregularity, and difficulty sleeping at night. In fact, self-care appears to be the predominant mode of treatment for many daily symptoms.

Furthermore, everyday self-care behaviors include health maintenance activities, as well as the management of symptomatic conditions. An alternative sick role concept must recognize that laypersons are not only consumers of professional medical care, but also primary providers and active participants in the health care process. Physician contact and the use of professional medical services may be understood as an aspect of self-management of health, but must be reinterpreted as patient role behavior rather than sick role behavior.

An alternative (nonmedicalized) sick role would include a reciprocal set of expectations regarding the behavior of the person who is experiencing illness and the members of the sick person's informal social network who serve as lay care providers. While it must be acknowledged that these behavioral expectations reflect their historical antecedents to some extent, they differ significantly from the Parsonian model of the patient–physician role relationship. A redimensionalized sick role concept would consist of the following rights: the right to make decisions about health-related behavior (Right 1), the right to be exempt from performing usual well roles (Right 2), and the right to become dependent on lay others for care and social support (Right 3).

The right to make health-related decisions includes a range of potential lay initiatives regarding health-protective behaviors and illness-management strategies (such as lifestyle choices and the selection of appropriate self-care practices). The right of the occupant of the sick role to abdicate well roles means that the sick person must have the opportunity to stop performing certain daily activities while not feeling well and be able to depend on others (informal and formal caregivers) for assistance.

In an alternative sick role, the rights of the role occupant continue to be partially dependent upon how well the individual fulfills the associated obligations (as is the case in all patterned roles). Now, however, the reciprocal behavioral expectations relate more directly to the actual participants involved in this role relationship. For example, in order for the sick person to relinquish usual well roles and become dependent on others, members of the individual's social network must be prepared to take on added responsibilities and to function as caregivers. Informal social support may take the form of instrumental, emotional, or informational assistance. In practical terms, provision of this support may mean performing additional specific social roles and task obligations and helping the sick person cope psychologically with the illness experience. Discussing health problems with members of the informal social network may enable the occupant of the sick role to acquire the type of information required to make sense of the sickness, to evaluate alternative sources of help and forms of treatment, and consequently to make appropriate health-related decisions.

A redimensionalized sick role concept would also consist of the following duties: the duty to maintain health and overcome illness (Duty 1), the duty to engage in routine self–health manage-ment (Duty 2), and the duty to make use of a range of health care resources (Duty 3). While the Parsonian model was limited to a duty to try to get well (by seeking medical assistance), the new sick role includes lay responsibility to maintain good health, along with an obligation to overcome ill health.

Self-health management encompasses lay activities undertaken to promote health, to prevent illness, and to detect and treat illness when it occurs. These activities involve a range of behaviors such as health maintenance activities (e.g., exercise and dietary practices), illness prevention (e.g., immunization), symptom evaluation, self-treatment (e.g., medication practices), and the use of a variety of health resources (e.g., informal social network members, health care practitioners including medical care services). In each case, the critical factor is that these behaviors are undertaken as a result of a self-determined decision-making process.

Thus, the rights of the alternative sick role are partially dependent upon the individual's willingness to engage actively in self–health management. By situating the sick role in the context of lay health beliefs and behavior, this nonprofessional reconceptualization of the rights and duties associated with the sick role should more accurately reflect the everyday health and illness experiences of the individual and more fully recognize the pervasive nature of self-care. In fact, according to Dean (1981, p. 673), "self-care in its various forms, preventive, curative and rehabilitative,... is the basic health behavior in all societies past and present."

Finally, the issue of legitimating claims to this alternative sick role must also be addressed. As previously discussed, Parsons considered the physician to be the source of authoritative validation for entry into the sick (patient) role. As a result of Parsons's early influence, legitimation was operationalized in many studies in terms of a specific form of medical intervention. For example, physician sick role legitimation typically takes the form of prescribed medication, hospitalization, or written communication (i.e., a medical certificate), often required to be eligible for formal sick leave benefits (Wolinsky, 1988; Wolinsky & Wolinsky, 1981).

In reality, health care professionals sanction claims to the patient role. Obviously, to be a patient means by definition that the sick person has been accepted by a physician (or other health professionals) for medical treatment. While the occupant of the patient role must be willing to utilize professional health care services, doing so is not a prerequisite for adopting the sick role. The occupant of the sick role depends essentially on self-health management and the care and support of members of his or her informal social network. Nevertheless, even though self-care is typically described as the basic or primary level of care in all societies, "lay care continues to be viewed as residual and supplemental to professional care in spite of the well documented fact that professional care is the supplemental form of health care" (Dean, 1986, p. 275). In fact, the vast majority of health problems are handled by lay care—a form of care that existed prior to the professionalization of medical care.

It is important to repeat that it is possible to enter and exit the sick role without being treated by a physician. It must therefore be recognized that in the reconceptualized sick role, it is members of the individual's informal social network who legitimate claims to this role by their willingness to become active caregivers and to provide assistance. Indicators of informal sick role legitimation might include restricted activity days (i.e., the number of days on which a person cuts down on his or her usual activity level due to a health problem) and bed days (i.e., the number of days spent in bed due to a health problem). These sick role exemptions depend upon the willingness of family members, friends, and other lay caregivers to fulfill their reciprocal role responsibilities.

Thus, the reconceptualized sick role fully acknowledges that the rights of the sick person translate into duties for lay others. For example, family members and friends may be expected to help with child or elder care duties or various household tasks when an individual is sick. In addition, if the sick person is in the paid labor force and the illness results in an absence from work, coworkers may be expected to take on additional duties. It is this type of informal social support that enables the sick person to exercise the rights of the sick role (i.e., to relinquish the usual well role and engage in dependent behavior). In summary, the behavioral expectations associated with the reconceptualized sick role are clearly embedded in the web of informal, reciprocal role relationships that comprise the sick person's everyday social world.

IS THERE A FUTURE FOR SICK ROLE RESEARCH?

Parsons's model of the sick (patient) role assigned to the physician and the utilization of professional health care services a position of central importance and thus stimulated a large body of empirical research that focused upon issues such as the role of the physician, the dynamics of the patient–physician relationship, and patient compliance. The Parsonian paradigm, and the ensuing research in medical sociology, have been criticized for failing "to account for preventive health care, or health maintenance, as an element of normative lay conduct …" (Gallagher, 1976, p. 209). It has been well documented that research guided by this conceptual model concentrated on illness behavior and professional healing within the confines of the Parsonian sick (patient) role and essentially diverted attention away from the study of lay health beliefs and behavior.

It must be recognized, however, that Parsons (1951) also acknowledged the fundamental importance of the notion of health in his overall analytical framework. In fact, Parsons characterized health as a basic individual and societal value and in his own terminology described health as a functional prerequisite of the social system. Gerhardt (1987, p. 118) argued that "Parsons' strong endorsement of health as a most important concern in a democratic social structure ... has often been overlooked by medical sociology."

The sick role construct and health behavior should not be viewed as mutually exclusive. By redimensionalizing the expectations of this role and recognizing that the behavior of the sick person typically takes place within the context of the family and informal social networks, it may be possible to build a conceptual bridge between the sick role concept and health behavior. The alternative sick role model outlined in this chapter incorporates behavior undertaken both to overcome ill health and to protect good health. Thus, the sick role may now be understood as a patterned role consisting of positive behavioral dimensions intended to protect and restore health, and not as a negatively achieved illness-based role as depicted by Parsons.

Studies designed to measure willingness to adopt this new sick role must focus upon whether the individual is ready to be relieved of usual well role responsibilities and become dependent upon lay caregivers. There is some evidence that research on sick role expectations is beginning to reflect this shift in emphasis and to explore factors such as the extent of dependency granted to those who are experiencing ill health and the type of support provided by nonprofessional significant others (e.g., Honig-Parnass, 1983; Segall, 1988). Future research on role release and dependency must develop more comprehensive measures of these behavioral expectations and the linkage between occupying the sick role and engaging in self-care health behavior.

If the sick role is to be understood as a social determinant of health behavior, sick role behavior must be removed from the physician's office and the hospital (and the confusion with the patient role) and situated within the social context of family, friends, informal caregiving networks, and the broader sociocultural environment. This revitalized sick role concept has the potential to become a central research focus in the developing field of health sociology. A number of years ago, Twaddle (1982, p. 95) asserted

that "examination of the future health care agenda makes it abundantly clear that if we didn't have a sociology of health we would now have to invent one."

The sociology of health perspective has actually been developing gradually over the past several decades. In fact, it is a logical extension of the pioneering work done in medical sociology. According to Twaddle (1982), the ongoing struggles to transform medical sociology into health sociology involve a fundamental paradigm shift from the study of individual disease, illness, and sickness to the study of population health and well-being. Furthermore, this shift includes a changing conception of key healing roles and the organizational settings in which care is provided to include lay healers and informal settings.

Despite these changes, this field of inquiry continues to be officially designated as medical sociology, "instead of using what would really be a more appropriate and accurate designation ... the Sociology of Health" (Levine, 1987, p. 2). Health sociology offers a more intellectually autonomous and more relevant framework for understanding population health issues and the environmental factors that contribute to health problems. It has been suggested that the future agenda of health sociology might include research issues such as unmet health care needs, social change and the health professions, social networks, personal health practices and health status (Elinson, 1985), quality of life (Elinson, 1985; Levine, 1987), and a greater understanding of the gendered aspects of health and health care (Zola, 1991).

Furthermore, an analysis of the relationship between the reconceptualized sick role and health behavior may also find a place on the agenda of health sociology. The redefined rights and duties of the nonmedicalized sick role highlight central research concerns in the sociological analysis of health behavior, i.e., freedom of choice (the right to make health-related decisions) and personal effectiveness in dealing with health problems (the duty to engage in self-health management). Renewed interest in an alternative conception of the sick role may provide a means of integrating ongoing research activities in health sociology, gaining a greater understanding of the nature of lay health beliefs and behavior, and consequently enhancing the social organization of community-based health care.

REFERENCES

Arluke, A. (1988). The sick role concept. In D. S. Gochman (Ed.), *Health behavior: Emerging research perspectives* (pp. 169–180). New York: Plenum Press.

Arluke, A., Kennedy, L., & Kessler, R. (1979). Reexamining the sick role concept: An empirical assessment. *Journal of Health and Social Behavior, 20,* 30–36.

Berkanovic, E. (1972). Lay conceptions of the sick role. *Social Forces, 51,* 53–64.

Blackwell, B. L. (1967). Upper middle class adult expectations about entering the sick role for physical and psychiatric dysfunctions. *Journal of Health and Social Behavior, 8,* 83–95.

Bloom, S. W. (1986). Institutional trends in medical sociology. *Journal of Health and Social Behavior, 27,* 265–276.

Butler, J. R. (1970). Illness and the sick role: An evaluation in three communities. *British Journal of Sociology, 21,* 241–261.

Cockerham, W. C. (1983). The state of medical sociology in the United States, Great Britain, West Germany and Austria: Applied vs. pure theory. *Social Science and Medicine, 20,* 1513–1527.

Dean, K. (1981). Self-care responses to illness: A selected review. *Social Science and Medicine, 15A,* 673–687.

Dean, K. (1986). Lay care in illness. *Social Science and Medicine, 22,* 275–284.

Elinson, J. (1985). The end of medicine and the end of medical sociology? *Journal of Health and Social Behavior, 26,* 268–275.

Gallagher, E. B. (1976). Lines of reconstruction and extension in the Parsonian sociology of illness. *Social Science and Medicine, 10,* 207–218.

Gerhardt, U. (1979). The Parsonian paradigm and the identity of medical sociology. *Sociological Review, 27,* 229–251.

Gerhardt, U. (1987). Parsons, role theory, and health interaction. In G. Scambler (Ed.), *Sociological theory and medical sociology* (110–133). London: Tavistock.

Gill, D., & Twaddle, A. (1977). Medical sociology: What's in a name? *International Social Science Journal, 29,* 369–385.

Gold, M. (1977). A crisis of identity: The case of medical sociology. *Journal of Health and Social Behavior, 18,* 160–168.

Goldstein, B., & Dommermuth, P. (1961). The sick role cycle: An approach to medical sociology. *Sociology and Social Research, 46,* 36–47.

Honig-Parnass, T. (1981). Lay concepts of the sick-role: An examination of the professionalist bias in Parsons' model. *Social Science and Medicine, 15A,* 615–623.

Honig-Parnass, T. (1983). The relative impact of status and health variables upon sick-role expectations. *Medical Care, 21,* 208–224.

Kassebaum, G. G., & Baumann, B. O. (1965). Dimensions of the sick role in chronic illness. *Journal of Health and Human Behavior, 6,* 16–27.

Levine, S. (1987). The changing terrains in medical sociology: Emergent concern with quality of life. *Journal of Health and Social Behavior, 28,* 1–6.

Levine, S., & Kozloff, M. A. (1978). The sick role: Assessment and overview. *Annual Review of Sociology, 4,* 317–343.

Lipman, A., & Sterne, R. S. (1969). Aging in the United States: Ascription of a terminal sick role. *Sociology and Social Research, 53,* 194–203.

McCormack, T. (1981). The new criticism and the sick role. *Canadian Review of Sociology and Anthropology, 18,* 30–47.

Mechanic, D. (1990). The role of sociology in health affairs. *Health Affairs, 9,* 85–97.

Mechanic, D., & Volkart, E. H. (1961). Stress, illness behavior and the sick role. *American Sociological Review, 26,* 51–58.

Parsons, T. (1951). *The social system.* New York: Free Press.

Parsons, T. (1975). The sick role and the role of the physician reconsidered. *Milbank Memorial Fund Quarterly, 53,* 257–278.

Petroni, F. A. (1969). Social class, family size and the sick role. *Journal of Marriage and the Family, 31,* 728–735.

Phillips, D. L. (1965). Self-reliance and the inclination to adopt the sick role. *Social Forces, 43,* 555–563.

Roman, P. M., & Trice, H. M. (1968). The sick role, labelling theory, and the deviant drinker. *International Journal of Social Psychiatry, 14,* 245–251.

Rosengren, W. R. (1962). The sick role during pregnancy: A note on research in progress. *Journal of Health and Human Behavior, 3,* 213–218.

Segall, A. (1976a). The sick role concept: Understanding illness behavior. *Journal of Health and Social Behavior, 17,* 163–170.

Segall, A. (1976b). Sociocultural variation in sick role behavioural expectations. *Social Science and Medicine, 10,* 47–51.

Segall, A. (1988). Cultural factors in sick role expectations. In D. S. Gochman (Ed.), *Health behavior: Emerging research perspectives* (pp. 249–260). New York: Plenum Press.

Segall, A., & Goldstein, J. (1989). Exploring the correlates of self-provided health care behaviour. *Social Science and Medicine, 29,* 153–161.

Straus, R. (1957). The nature and status of medical sociology. *American Sociological Review, 22,* 200–204.

Turner, B. S. (1992). *Regulating bodies: Essays in medical sociology.* London: Routledge.

Twaddle, A. C. (1969). Health decisions and sick role variations: An exploration. *Journal of Health and Social Behavior, 10,* 105–114.

Twaddle, A. C. (1982). From medical sociology to the sociology of health: Some changing concerns in the sociological study of sickness and treatment. In T. Bottomore, M. Sokolowska, & S. Nowak (Eds.), *Sociology: The state of the art* (pp. 323–358). Beverly Hills, CA: Sage.

Wolinsky, F. D. (1988). Sick role legitimation. In D. S. Goch-

man (Ed.), *Health behavior: Emerging research perspectives* (pp. 181–192). New York: Plenum Press.

Wolinsky, F. D., & Wolinsky, S. R. (1981). Expecting sick-role legitimation and getting it. *Journal of Health and Social Behavior, 22,* 229–242.

Zola, I. K. (1991). Bringing our bodies and ourselves back in: Reflections on a past, present and future "medical sociology." *Journal of Health and Social Behavior, 32,* 1–16.

15

Changing Gender Roles and Gender Differences in Health Behavior

Ingrid Waldron

INTRODUCTION

This chapter describes patterns and trends in gender differences in health behavior. In addition, this chapter analyzes the causes of gender differences in health behavior, with a major focus on the contributions of gender roles to gender differences in health behavior. Health behavior is defined broadly to include behaviors that influence health or are generally believed to influence health. Gender roles are defined broadly to include the social roles, behaviors, attitudes, and psychological characteristics that are more common, more expected, and more accepted for one sex or the other.

One hypothesis proposes that gender differences in health behavior are due primarily to two complementary aspects of gender roles, namely, males' greater risk taking and females' greater health concerns. Specifically, this hypothesis proposes that males are socialized to be brave and

bold and take risks, whereas females are socialized to be more cautious and more concerned with protecting health; consequently, males engage in more risky behavior, while females engage in more preventive and protective behavior, as well as more treatment seeking and self-care for illness (Nathanson, 1977; Veevers & Gee, 1986). Several lines of evidence support this hypothesis. Some types of risk taking are more often encouraged in boys and discouraged in girls (Rosen & Peterson, 1990). Also, survey evidence indicates that women worry more about health and place somewhat greater value on preserving health (Nathanson, 1977; Waldron, 1988; Weissfeld, Kirscht, & Brock, 1990). Finally, gender differences in many types of health behavior conform to the predicted pattern of more risky behavior for males and more preventive and health care behavior for females (Nathanson, 1977). Thus, several types of evidence suggest that gender differences in general attitudes toward risk-taking and health may contribute to gender differences in many types of health behavior.

Other authors have argued that gender differences in health behavior are influenced by multiple social and biological influences, including varied aspects of gender roles (del Boca,

Ingrid Waldron • Department of Biology, University of Pennsylvania, Philadelphia, Pennsylvania 19104-6018.

Handbook of Health Behavior Research I: Personal and Social Determinants, edited by David S. Gochman. Plenum Press, New York, 1997.

1994; Hayes & Ross, 1987; Waldron, 1983, 1988, 1991a). For example, the female gender role includes an emphasis on appearance, and females' greater concern with appearance, in combination with the contemporary slender beauty ideal, has influenced gender differences in dieting, exercise, and several other health behaviors. Other aspects of gender roles, such as women's greater parental responsibilities and males' greater assertiveness and rebelliousness, also appear to contribute to gender differences in specific types of health behavior. In addition, biological factors contribute to gender differences in some types of health behavior. As a result of these diverse psychosocial and biological influences, gender differences in health behavior do not show a consistent male excess for risky behaviors or a consistent female excess for health-promoting behaviors (Waldron, 1988). For example, males have higher rates than females for one major type of health-promoting behavior, vigorous exercise (Piani & Schoenborn, 1993).

Additional hypotheses have been proposed concerning trends in gender differences in health behavior. The "convergence hypothesis" proposes that as male and female roles have become more similar, gender differences in health behavior have decreased and may even be eliminated (Perkins, 1992; Veevers & Gee, 1986). A more specific version of the convergence hypothesis focuses on the effects of decreasing gender differences in employment. In the United States in 1960, 84% of men, but only 38% of women, were in the labor force. This gender difference decreased steadily over the next three decades, and by 1992, 76% of men and 58% of women were in the labor force (U.S. Bureau of the Census, 1993). It has been hypothesized that the decreasing gender difference in employment has resulted in decreasing gender differences in income and social influences, which have contributed to decreasing gender differences in health behavior (Waldron, 1991a).

An alternative point of view predicts more varied trends in gender differences in health behavior. Many different causes influence trends in

health behavior, and some of these causes may contribute to increasing, rather than decreasing, gender differences in health behavior. This argument is supported by evidence that in the United States during the 1980s, some types of health behavior showed decreasing gender differences, but other types of health behavior showed increasing gender differences (Waldron, 1995).

As a basis for evaluating these hypotheses, this chapter describes gender differences and trends in gender differences for several major types of health behavior and reviews evidence concerning the causes of gender differences in these health behaviors. Cigarette smoking and alcohol consumption are discussed in depth; accident-related behavior, exercise, dieting, eating disorders, and physician visits are discussed more briefly. The descriptions of gender differences and trends in gender differences for these behaviors are based primarily on data for national samples in the United States from the 1960s through the early 1990s. Data for other Western countries and for non-Western societies are briefly summarized, and limited data are presented for earlier time periods. Evidence concerning the relationships of health behaviors to other characteristics has been drawn primarily from studies in the contemporary United States and other Western countries, with limited evidence from non-Western countries, as noted.

Methodological Cautions

Gender differences may be assessed as a sex difference (male minus female rates) or a sex ratio (the ratio of male to female rates). These two measures may show opposite trends under certain circumstances. For example, if male and female rates for a health behavior decrease from 80% and 20%, respectively, to 50% and 10%, respectively, then the sex difference decreases from 60% to 40%, while the sex ratio increases from 4 to 5. In this chapter, the terms *sex difference* and *sex ratio* refer to the specific measures defined above, while the term *gender differences* is used to encompass both measures.

An additional caution concerns the distinction between risky and protective behavior, which is not as clear-cut as it may appear. For example, the health effects of dieting are controversial and uncertain at present (French & Jeffery, 1994). Also, a behavior may have beneficial effects on health when practiced in moderation, but harmful effects on health when practiced to excess (e.g., vigorous physical exercise [evidence for younger women] or alcohol consumption [evidence for older adults] [Poikolainen, 1995; Putukian, 1994]). Thus, this chapter discusses health behaviors that affect health or are generally believed to affect health, but the health consequences of some of these behaviors are complex or controversial or both. In addition, the motivations that influence these health behaviors frequently have little or nothing to do with their health effects.

SMOKING

Gender Differences in Tobacco Use, Smoking Initiation, and Smoking Cessation

In the early 20th century in the United States, tobacco use was much more common for males than for females; males had much higher rates of smokeless tobacco use and pipe, cigar, and cigarette smoking (Waldron, 1991a). During the mid-20th century, cigarette smoking became the primary form of tobacco use, and gender differences in cigarette smoking decreased substantially for all age groups (Figure 1) (Waldron, 1991a). By the early 1990s, gender differences in the prevalence of cigarette smoking were quite small, with sex ratios between 1.1 and 1.3 for various adult age groups and between 1.0 and 1.1 for teenagers (calculated from data in National Center for Health Statistics, 1980–1994; U.S. Department of Health and Human Services, 1994a). Other aspects of tobacco use continue to show substantial gender differences (Grunberg, Winders, & Wewers, 1991; Johnston, O'Malley, &

Bachman, 1994; Piani & Schoenborn, 1993; Schoenborn & Boyd, 1989; U.S. Department of Health and Human Services, 1994a; Waldron, 1991a). Males are much more likely than females to smoke pipes or cigars or to use smokeless tobacco. Among cigarette smokers, males smoke more cigarettes per day, on average.

In other Western countries, patterns of gender differences have been generally similar to those observed in the United States, although in some Western countries, current gender differences in cigarette smoking are larger and the timing of trends has varied in different countries (Grunberg et al., 1991; Waldron, 1991a). In most non-Western societies, more men than women are smokers or use tobacco in some form, but in some groups and time periods, there has been little or no gender difference in smoking or tobacco use (Grunberg et al., 1991; Waldron et al., 1988).

This discussion will focus on the causes of the changing gender differences in the prevalence of cigarette smoking, primarily in Western countries. Space limitations preclude discussion of the causes of gender differences in other forms of tobacco use (Grunberg et al., 1991; Waldron, 1991a).

One major reason why gender differences in the prevalence of cigarette smoking have decreased is that gender differences in smoking initiation rates have decreased. For example, in the United States in the early 20th century, males had much higher rates of smoking initiation than females, but during the mid-20th century, females' smoking initiation rates increased and gender differences decreased (Waldron, 1991a). In the 1960s and 1970s, smoking initiation rates decreased more for males than for females, and, by the late 1970s and 1980s, smoking initiation rates were generally higher for females than for males (Johnston et al., 1994; Lee, Gilpin, & Pierce, 1993; U.S. Department of Health and Human Services, 1994a). By the early 1990s, however, it appeared that these trends had been reversed and males had slightly higher smoking initiation rates than females. In summary, United

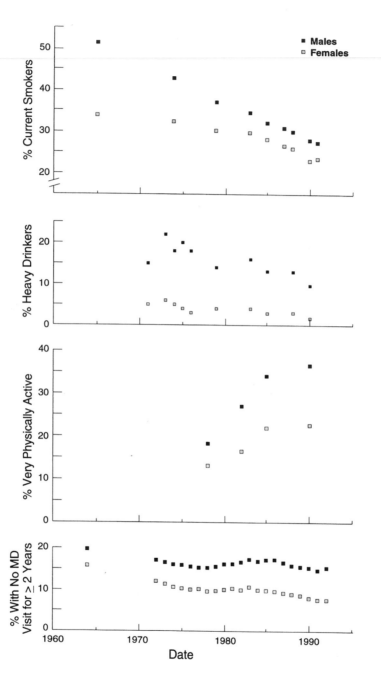

Figure 1. Trends in smoking, drinking, exercise, and physician visits in the United States: 1960–1992. The prevalence of current cigarette smoking is age-adjusted for adults (18 and over). Heavy drinkers consume an average of 1.00 or more ounces of absolute alcohol (ethanol) per day; rates of heavy drinking are given for adults (18 and over). Very physically active individuals expend an average of 3 or more kcal/kg per day in vigorous leisure-time activity; data are for adults (18 and over). No MD visit for ≥ 2 years is defined as no contact with a physician in person or by phone for 2 years or more previous to the survey; data are age-adjusted (all age groups included). For several of these data series, there have been minor changes in methods during the time period considered. All data are for national samples (National Center for Health Statistics, 1980–1994; Piani & Schoenborn, 1993; Schoenborn, 1988; Stephens, 1987; White et al., 1987).

States data indicate that gender differences in smoking initiation decreased during the mid-20th century, and gender differences in smoking initiation were small and inconsistent from the late 1970s through at least the early 1990s.

Among smokers in the United States, men have been more likely than women to quit smoking cigarettes, and this has been another reason for the decreasing gender differences in the prevalence of cigarette smoking (Waldron, 1991a). This gender difference in quit rates began during the late 1950s and was large during the 1960s. During the late 1970s and 1980s, it appears, men had slightly higher quit rates than women; national data indicate little or no gender difference in rates of serious quit attempts, but, among smokers who made a serious attempt to quit, women were somewhat more likely to experience late relapse (Hatziandreu et al., 1990; Mc-Whorter, Boyd, & Mattson, 1990; Waldron, 1991a). It should be noted that, at least during the earlier decades, much of the gender difference in rates of quitting cigarette smoking was accounted for by men who switched from cigarettes to cigars (Jarvis, 1984). For teenagers, quit rates have been higher for males in some time periods, but higher for females in other time periods (U.S. Department of Health and Human Services, 1994a). In summary, gender differences in quit rates have varied in the United States, but, since the mid-1950s, men have generally had higher rates of quitting cigarette smoking than women, especially during the late 1950s and 1960s. Data for other Western countries generally show similar patterns, although women have had higher quit rates than men in a few countries in certain time periods (Waldron, 1991a). In non-Western countries, women have often had higher quit rates than men (Waldron et al., 1988).

Effects of Gender Differences in Risk Taking and Health Concerns

Evidence for adolescents suggests that a general tendency to risk taking is associated with increased likelihood of smoking initiation (U.S. Department of Health and Human Services, 1994a). Since this type of propensity for risk taking is greater for males, it would tend to contribute to greater smoking initiation by males (Waldron, Lye, & Brandon, 1991).

With respect to concerns about the health-damaging effects of smoking, current evidence does not support the hypothesis that these health concerns lead females to reduce smoking more than males. Surveys have found small and inconsistent gender differences in knowledge of and concern about the health-damaging effects of smoking (Piani & Schoenborn, 1993; Schoenborn & Boyd, 1989; Waldron, 1991a; Waldron et al., 1988). Behavioral data also do not support the hypothesis that health concerns have resulted in greater reductions in smoking for females (Waldron, 1991a). For example, males' smoking appears to have decreased as much as or more than females' smoking in response to publicity about the health-damaging effects of smoking during the 1950s, 1960s, and early 1970s (Lee et al., 1993; Waldron, 1991a). One reason males may have responded more to antismoking campaigns during this early period is that both the research evidence and personal familiarity with the health-damaging effects of smoking related primarily to men, since smoking-related disease was still relatively uncommon for women.

Gender differences in smoking have also been influenced by two more specific health-related concerns, that is, concerns about the effects of smoking during pregnancy and concerns about the effects of smoking on physical fitness. Women smokers who become pregnant have relatively high quit rates, and, despite significant relapse during the first year after birth, it appears that roughly 10% of smokers who become pregnant may become long-term quitters (Kruse, Le Fevre, & Zweig, 1986; Waldron, 1991a). In the United States, about 10% of women who have quit smoking give pregnancy as their reason for quitting (Schoenborn & Boyd, 1989).

In contrast, males are more likely than females to mention concerns about the effects of smoking on physical fitness or athletic ability as a reason not to smoke (Waldron, 1991a). Males are more involved in athletics, and athletes are less likely to begin smoking and may be more likely to quit (Pedersen, Poulin, Lefcoe, Donald, & Hill,

1992; U.S. Department of Health and Human Services, 1994a; Waldron et al., 1991). Thus, concerns about the effects of smoking on physical fitness tend to lead to greater reductions in smoking for males.

In summary, limited evidence suggests that males' greater propensity for risk taking tends to increase smoking initiation for males. Concerns about the health-damaging effects of smoking, however, have had mixed effects on gender differences in smoking. Pregnancy-related concerns have increased quit rates for women; concerns about the effects of smoking on physical fitness and the early publicity concerning the health-damaging effects of smoking appear to have reduced smoking more for males.

Other Effects of Gender Roles

Traditional gender roles have often included substantial restrictions on women's behavior, and these restrictions have often included proscriptions against women's smoking. In non-Western societies, many women are deterred from smoking by widespread social disapproval of women's smoking and social attitudes that often label women who smoke as unfeminine or promiscuous (Waldron et al., 1988). Similarly, in Western countries in the early and mid-20th century, strong social disapproval of women's smoking was a major reason for women's lower rates of smoking (Waldron, 1991a). Even as late as the mid-1960s, it appears, social disapproval of girls' and women's smoking and social encouragement of boys' and men's smoking accounted for a major portion of the gender difference in smoking. By the 1980s, social attitudes toward girls' smoking were still somewhat more negative than social attitudes toward boys' smoking, but the difference was relatively small (U.S. Department of Health and Human Services, 1994a; Waldron, 1995). Thus, decreasing differences in social attitudes toward women's and men's smoking have been a major cause of decreasing gender differences in smoking. These trends in attitudes toward smoking were part of a general trend toward

decreasing restrictions on women's behavior and increasing acceptance of gender equality. Increases in women's employment probably contributed to these general trends. Thus, historical trends in women's employment probably contributed indirectly to decreasing gender differences in smoking (Waldron, 1991a).

A more direct relationship between women's employment and smoking has also been hypothesized. Specifically, this hypothesis proposes that employed women are more likely to be smokers because employed women have more money to buy cigarettes and because smoking may be stimulated by work stresses or the social environment on the job. This hypothesis receives indirect support from evidence that limited financial resources have contributed to women's lower rates of smoking in some non-Western societies and in the mid-20th-century United States (Waldron, 1991a; Waldron et al., 1988). Also, United States data suggest that, in the early to mid-20th century, employed women were more likely than homemakers to be smokers. It is unclear, however, whether employed women were more likely to smoke because employment increased smoking or because in the early 20th century, unconventional women were more likely to take up both employment and smoking. By the 1980s, there appears to have been little or no association between women's employment status and smoking (Ebi-Kryston, Higgins, & Keller, 1990; Waldron, 1991a).

Another hypothesis proposes that a woman is more likely to smoke if she has nontraditional attitudes toward women's roles and gender equality. In the United States in the 1920s, college women often explicitly asserted their right to smoke as part of their equal rights with men. Recent evidence, however, provides only limited and inconsistent support for this hypothesis; data for the 1970s and 1980s indicate an association between nontraditional gender role attitudes and smoking in one study of adult women, but not in other studies of young adult women or teenage girls (Waldron, 1991a).

In summary, in Western countries in the

early 20th century, restrictive attitudes toward women's behavior included strong social disapproval of women's smoking. In this context, few women smoked, and it appears that the women who did smoke may have had nontraditional gender role attitudes and a greater likelihood of being employed, another type of nontraditional behavior for women. In contrast, in the contemporary era of much less restrictive attitudes toward women's behavior, more women smoke and there is little or no association between women's smoking and employment or gender role attitudes.

Thus, general social trends toward fewer restrictions on women's behavior have contributed to increasing acceptance of women's smoking and decreasing gender differences in smoking. These trends have been reinforced by the increasingly aggressive efforts of tobacco companies to market cigarettes to women. Beginning in the late 1920s and extending through the 1980s, it appears that increased cigarette advertising oriented toward women has contributed to increased smoking adoption by women and decreased gender differences in smoking (Pierce, Lee, & Gilpin, 1994; U.S. Department of Health and Human Services, 1994a; Waldron, 1991a).

Traditional gender roles have had a variety of additional effects on gender differences in smoking (Waldron, 1991a; Waldron et al., 1991). For example, military service has traditionally been expected and even required of males, and, for much of the 20th century, military service fostered smoking, so males' higher rates of military service contributed to their higher rates of smoking. Rebelliousness and rejection of adult authority have been more expected and accepted for males, and males' greater rebelliousness tends to increase male rates of smoking adoption. Conversely, females' greater religiosity tends to reduce their rates of smoking.

One other aspect of gender roles, the emphasis on females' appearance, combined with the very slender contemporary beauty ideal, appears to increase smoking among females. Smokers generally weigh less than nonsmokers, and people who quit smoking tend to gain weight, at least

temporarily (Chen, Horne, & Dosman, 1993). As would be expected, more females than males report weight control as a motivation for smoking, and among smokers, more females than males express concern that quitting would result in weight gain (Lando, Hellerstedt, Pirie, & McGovern, 1991; U.S. Department of Health and Human Services, 1994a; Waldron, 1991a).

In addition, it appears that females may more often use smoking to cope with stress, although the evidence for this gender difference has been inconsistent (Waldron, 1991a). Another observation suggests that emotional or psychological factors may tend to increase smoking more for females than for males; females are more likely than males to be depressed, and depression decreases the likelihood of smoking cessation and may also increase the likelihood of smoking initiation (Anda et al., 1990).

Effects of Sex Differences in Biology

Males may metabolize nicotine more rapidly than females and may require higher nicotine intake to achieve similar plasma nicotine levels, which may be one reason males smoke more cigarettes per day than females (Grunberg et al., 1991). Another postulated effect of sex differences in nicotine metabolism is that among first-time smokers, females may be more likely to feel sick; this effect may have contributed to females' lower rates of smoking adoption. However, evidence for this hypothesis is inconsistent, and it appears that this effect has probably made only a minor contribution to gender differences in smoking adoption (Waldron, 1991a). Similarly, it has been proposed that females experience more withdrawal symptoms and consequently are less likely to quit smoking; again, however, available evidence is inconsistent, and it appears that this effect has not been a major cause of gender differences in smoking cessation (Waldron, 1991a).

A final biological hypothesis proposes that higher testosterone levels may increase smoking initiation rates, possibly via effects of testosterone on psychological characteristics that may contribute to smoking initiation (Bauman, Foshee, & Haley, 1992; Waldron, 1991a). However, studies of the relationships between testosterone levels and smoking have yielded inconsistent results, and any relationship between testosterone and smoking could be due to effects of smoking on testosterone levels, rather than vice versa. Thus, the possible effects of sex hormones on smoking remain unknown at present.

Summary

The prevalence of smoking has been much higher for men than for women, both in Western countries in the first half of the 20th century and in many contemporary non-Western societies. A major cause of this gender difference in smoking has been social disapproval of women's smoking and social acceptance of men's smoking. Social disapproval of women's smoking appears to have been one component of generally greater restrictions on women's behavior. In the United States and other Western countries, as women's roles changed and restrictions on women's behavior decreased during the 20th century, there was less social disapproval of women's smoking, and gender differences in smoking decreased substantially.

Other factors appear to have contributed to males' higher rates of smoking adoption, including males' greater risk taking and rebelliousness, males' greater participation in the military, and males' lesser involvement with religion. Health-related concerns have had mixed effects on gender differences in smoking.

In the contemporary United States, gender differences in the prevalence of cigarette smoking are relatively small, but there are gender differences in the motivations that influence cigarette smoking. For example, females' smoking is motivated more by weight concerns and reduced by pregnancy-related health concerns. In contrast, rebelliousness and risk taking may contribute more to males' smoking initiation, and males' greater interest in athletics and physical fitness tends to reduce their smoking.

ALCOHOL CONSUMPTION

Gender Differences in Drinking

In the United States and other Western countries, males drink more than females (see Figure 1) (Johnston et al., 1994; Rossow & Rise, 1994; United States Department of Health and Human Services, 1994b; Waldron, 1988; Zemp & Ackermann-Liebrich, 1988). Males are much more likely than females to be daily drinkers or heavy drinkers. Conversely, more females than males are abstainers, although this gender difference is small among teenagers in the United States. This section discusses trends and causes of these gender differences in frequency and quantity of alcohol consumption; it does not discuss gender differences in problem drinking, alcohol dependence, or alcoholism (del Boca, 1994; U.S. Department of Health and Human Services, 1994b).

Historical data for the United States suggest that gender differences in drinking decreased during the mid-20th century (Whitehead & Ferrence, 1976). Since the 1970s, however, gender differences in drinking have shown inconsistent trends (Waldron, 1988, 1995). In this recent period, inconsistent trends have been observed for gender differences in the proportion who abstained from drinking and for gender differences in the proportion who were heavy drinkers (data from National Center for Health Statistics, 1980–1994). For example, from the mid-1970s to the late 1980s, as rates of heavy drinking decreased for both men and women, sex differences decreased, but sex ratios tended to increase (Figure 1). This same pattern of decreasing sex differences and increasing sex ratios was observed within each adult age group (data for 1985–1990 from Piani & Schoenborn, 1993; Schoenborn, 1988). The trend toward increasing sex ratios for heavy drinking may seem somewhat surprising, but the validity of this trend is supported by the observation that sex ratios for alcohol-related mortality also increased during the 1980s (Waldron, 1995). Trend data for teenagers show more evidence of decreasing gender differences in alcohol consumption; for high school seniors between 1975 and 1993, sex differences decreased for several measures of alcohol use and sex ratios also decreased slightly (Johnston et al., 1994). In summary, United States data for the 1970s through the early 1990s indicate that gender differences in drinking have decreased for teenagers, but gender differences in drinking have shown variable trends for adults.

Data for non-Western societies indicate that in many groups, men drink more than women, although in many other groups, there has been little or no gender difference in drinking (Fuller, Edwards, Sermsri, & Vorakitphokatorn, 1993; Waldron, 1988; Westermeyer, 1988).

Effects of Gender Differences in Risk Taking and Health Concerns

Several lines of evidence suggest that gender differences in risk taking and health concerns may make a modest contribution to gender differences in alcohol consumption. Males report more motivation to engage in physically dangerous activities and a greater general predisposition to risk taking, and these types of predisposition to risk taking appear to be associated with greater alcohol consumption (Cherpitel, 1993; Kraft & Rise, 1994).

Females rate alcohol use as more risky than do males (Beck & Summons, 1987; Spigner, Hawkins, & Loren, 1993; Waldron, 1988). To some extent, this difference may reflect females' concerns with nonhealth risks, such as possible sexual misadventures or social disapproval; these concerns may contribute to gender differences in drinking styles, with females more likely to avoid intoxication and blackouts (Fillmore, 1987; Johnston et al., 1994; C. A. Robbins & Martin, 1993). In addition, females appear to be somewhat more aware of the health risks of heavy drinking or drinking and driving, and males may believe more in the health benefits of moderate drinking (Beck & Summons, 1987; Piani & Schoenborn, 1993; Svenson, Jarvis, & Campbell, 1994; Waldron, 1988).

Pregnancy provides an additional health-related motivation for reduced drinking by women. Among women who drink, many abstain or reduce their alcohol intake during pregnancy out of concern for the health of the baby, and to some extent this reduced alcohol consumption is maintained during the first year after delivery (Fried, Barnes, & Drake, 1985; Kruse et al., 1986). The continued reduction in alcohol intake may be motivated primarily by concerns that heavy alcohol consumption interferes with maternal responsibilities for child care, as discussed below.

Other Effects of Gender Roles

One major cause of gender differences in drinking has been social disapproval of heavy drinking by women, together with greater social acceptance of men's drinking (Waldron, 1988). Even as recently as the 1980s in the United States, there continued to be substantial social disapproval of frequent or heavy drinking by females, whereas there was more social acceptance and even encouragement of males' drinking (Lemle & Mishkind, 1989; U.S. Department of Health and Human Services, 1994b; Waldron, 1995).

Social disapproval of heavy drinking by women appears to be linked to concerns that heavy drinking may interfere with a woman's responsibilities for child care and may leave a woman vulnerable to seduction or rape (Klee & Ames, 1987; U.S. Department of Health and Human Services, 1994b; Waldron, 1988). For example, a study of blue-collar couples with children found that many of the women explicitly stated that they had given up heavy drinking in order to be able to care for their children, whereas many men continued to drink as a component of male socializing and friendship (Klee & Ames, 1987). In other studies, both women and men have reported that drinking reduces sexual inhibition and has sometimes resulted in unintended sexual activities (Klassen & Wilsnack, 1986; Perkins, 1992; Plant & Plant, 1992). Although both sexes report sexual disinhibition, this effect carries greater risk of negative consequences for women, because of women's risk of pregnancy and because of greater social disapproval of sexual promiscuity for women. Thus, it appears that traditional roles and expectations for women, namely, responsibility for child care and restrictions on sexual behavior, contribute to stronger social disapproval of heavy drinking by women.

In contrast, there has been greater social acceptance and even encouragement of men's drinking, and in many cultures, drunkenness has been more acceptable for men (Gefou-Madianou, 1992; Waldron, 1988). In many traditional non-Western societies, men's roles appear to have been more compatible with occasional heavy drinking or drunkenness, since the demands of men's roles appear to have been more episodic or intermittent, compared to the more constant demands of women's roles (Waldron, 1988; Westermeyer, 1988). Evidence for Western countries indicates additional reasons why drinking has been more socially acceptable for males. Drinking is associated with characteristics such as toughness, rebelliousness, and aggressiveness, which are often considered desirable for males, and drinking has been considered a sign of masculinity (Chassin, Tetzloff, & Hershey, 1985; Lemle & Mishkind, 1989). In addition, in many groups, drinking is an important component of male socializing (Gefou-Madianou, 1992; Klee & Ames, 1987). The divergent social attitudes toward men's and women's drinking have been a major cause of gender differences in drinking.

Additional evidence indicates that boys' greater rebelliousness and involvement in antisocial behavior contribute to their greater alcohol consumption (Chassin et al., 1985; Waldron, 1988). Conversely, girls' and women's drinking may be reduced by their greater involvement with religion, since strong religious commitment is generally associated with lower alcohol consumption (Waldron, 1988).

Since traditional gender roles have contributed to gender differences in drinking, it has been predicted that gender differences in drinking would be larger for individuals who have more traditional gender role attitudes. This pre-

diction has been confirmed by evidence for contemporary teenagers (Huselid & Cooper, 1992; Lye & Waldron, 1996). As expected, among males, more traditional gender role attitudes were associated with heavier drinking. Among females, gender role attitudes and alcohol consumption were not related (in analyses that included controls for relevant confounding variables [Lye & Waldron, 1996]). These findings suggest that trends toward less traditional gender role attitudes may have contributed to decreases in teenage boys' alcohol consumption, and this may be one reason that gender differences in teenage alcohol consumption have decreased somewhat in recent decades (Johnston et al., 1994). Comparable trends have not been observed for adults.

It has also been hypothesized that employment contributes to increased drinking, since employment provides income, time away from the family context, and in some cases social encouragement for drinking. Data for the 1970s and 1980s provide limited support for this hypothesis. Some studies have found that full-time homemakers are more likely to be abstainers and employed women drink more, but other studies have found no significant relationship or inconsistent relationships between women's employment and drinking (Darrow, Russell, Cooper, Mudar, & Frone, 1992; Ebi-Kryston et al., 1990; Parker & Harford, 1992; Waldron, 1988; Wilsnack & Wilsnack, 1992). A related hypothesis proposes that recent increases in women's employment have resulted in increased drinking by women and decreased gender differences in drinking. However, the available evidence does not support this hypothesis. It appears that from 1970 to 1990, as women's employment increased, there was a decrease in women's heavy drinking and mixed trends in gender differences in drinking (Figure 1) (National Center for Health Statistics, 1980–1994; Waldron, 1988). In summary, the available evidence suggests that women's employment has not had a major effect on women's drinking or on gender differences in drinking.

Another hypothesis suggests that the contemporary slender beauty ideal for women may motivate some women to reduce alcohol consumption as part of a general effort to reduce caloric intake. Surprisingly, research evidence indicates that greater alcohol consumption is not related to greater obesity or weight gain (Liu, Serdula, Williamson, Mokdad, & Byers, 1994; Poikolainen, 1995). Nevertheless, the belief that drinking increases the risk of obesity may contribute to gender differences in drinking. No evidence was found to test this hypothesis.

It has also been proposed that men more often use alcohol to cope with stress, whereas women more often use other stress-coping techniques, such as psychotropic medications, prayer, or talking with friends and relatives. However, research evidence indicates inconsistent sex differences in the use of alcohol to cope with stress (Cooper, Russell, Skinner, Frone, & Mudar, 1992; del Boca, 1994; Waldron, 1988).

Effects of Sex Differences in Biology

After consumption of a given quantity of alcohol, women have higher blood alcohol levels than men (Blume, 1994). One reason is that women weigh less than men, and a higher proportion of women's body weight is fat, so a given quantity of alcohol is diluted in a smaller volume of body water in the average woman. This sex difference in biology appears to contribute significantly to the sex difference in amount of alcohol consumed. In the United States, average daily alcohol consumption is about 3.1 times higher for men than for women, but the amount of alcohol consumed per volume of body water is only about 2.1 times higher for men than for women (calculated from data in Dawson & Archer, 1992).

It appears that another biological sex difference also contributes to lower blood alcohol levels in men for equivalent alcohol intake. Current evidence indicates that more alcohol is metabolized by stomach enzymes in men, so less alcohol enters the blood (Frezza et al., 1990). The magnitude of this effect is uncertain at present. However, several observations indicate that males' alcohol intake is greater than females', even after correcting for all aspects of biological sex differences in alcohol metabolism. First, males report substantially higher frequencies of having been intoxicated or having blacked out, both among teenagers and adults (Fillmore, 1987; Johnston et al., 1994; C. A. Robbins & Martin, 1993). Second, among adults, men are substantially more likely than women to drink every day or nearly every day, whereas women are more likely to abstain from alcohol consumption completely or to consume alcohol infrequently (Dawson & Archer, 1992; Fillmore, 1987; Rossow & Rise, 1994; U.S. Department of Health and Human Services, 1994b; Zemp & Ackermann-Liebrich, 1988).

It has also been proposed that genetic factors may have different effects on male and female drinking. However, studies of genetic influences on the amount and frequency of alcohol consumption in general population samples have found that genetic influences are important for both men and women, with no clear evidence for a sex difference in the genetic contribution (Clifford, Fulker, Gurling, & Murray, 1981; Jardine & Martin, 1984; U.S. Department of Health and Human Services, 1994b).

Summary

Males drink more than females in Western countries and in many non-Western societies. In the contemporary United States, there are substantial gender differences in drinking, particularly heavy drinking, and trends in gender differences in drinking have been inconsistent during the 1970s and 1980s. Gender differences in amount of alcohol consumed result in part from biological factors, including sex differences in body size, body composition, and alcohol metabolism. It appears, however, that males drink more than females, even after taking these biological differences into account. One major cause of gender differences in drinking is greater social acceptance of men's drinking and social disapproval of heavy drinking by women. These social attitudes are related to the perceived compatibility of drinking with traditional masculine characteristics and the perceived incompatibility of heavy drinking with women's traditional responsibility for child care and sexual restraint. It appears that gender differences in alcohol consumption are also due in part to males' generally greater risk-taking and rebelliousness and women's greater concern about the risks of drinking, e.g., during pregnancy. Thus, multiple biological and social factors contribute to gender differences in drinking.

OTHER HEALTH BEHAVIORS

Accident-Related Behavior

Males have had higher accident mortality than females in almost all contemporary and historical data for Western and non-Western countries (Waldron, 1988, in press). In the United States, males have higher accident rates than females for both fatal and non-fatal accidents, for almost all types of accidents, and for almost all age groups (National Center for Health Statistics, 1969–1994, Veevers & Gee, 1986; Waldron, 1988, 1995). These gender differences in accident rates result from gender differences in many different types of accident-related behavior, including driving habits, employment, and recreation.

Male drivers have higher rates of fatal motor vehicle accidents than female drivers because males both drive more and have more fatal accidents per mile driven (Figure 2) (Evans, 1991; U.S. Department of Transportation, 1993, 1994). Males have more fatal accidents per mile driven because they drive faster, more often violate traffic regulations and take risks in driving, and are more likely to drive with high blood alcohol levels (Evans, 1991; Svenson et al., 1994; Veevers & Gee, 1986; Waldron, 1988, 1995).

Trends in gender differences have varied for different types of behavior related to motor vehicle accidents. United States data from the late 1960s through the early 1990s indicate a general tendency to decreasing gender differences for the proportion who were licensed drivers, miles driven per adult, and rates of fatal accidents per billion miles driven, although there have been some inconsistencies in these trends (Figure 2) (data from U.S. Department of Transportation, 1993, 1994; Waldron, 1995). In contrast, gender differences in seat belt use have increased. Before the 1980s, there was little or no gender difference in seat belt use, but by the late 1980s, more women than men used seat belts (Figure 2) (Waldron, 1983, 1995). One possible reason why women's seat belt use increased more than men's is that women may have been more likely to comply with the mandatory seat belt use laws that were enacted during the mid- and late 1980s. However, the available evidence provides only very weak support for this interpretation (Escobedo et al., 1991; Wagenaar & Wiviott, 1986). Another possible interpretation is that women may have responded more than men to public health campaigns encouraging seat belt use.

Data for the United States indicate that work-related accidents also contribute significantly to men's higher accident rates (National Center for Health Statistics, 1969–1994; Waldron, 1991b). Men have higher rates of fatal and nonfatal work accidents because more men are employed and employed men are more likely than employed women to have physically hazardous jobs. Men drive more as part of their jobs, and employment-related driving contributes substantially to men's greater miles driven and consequent greater exposure to motor vehicle accident risk (data from U.S. Department of Transportation, 1993, 1994). Trend data for the United States indicate that gender differences in nonfatal work accidents decreased during the 1980s, due to decreases in males' rates of nonfatal work accidents (data from National Center for Health Statistics, 1969–1994).

Other behaviors that contribute to gender differences in accident risk include recreational activity and gun use. Males more often take risks in swimming and boating and more often use guns; consequently, males have much higher

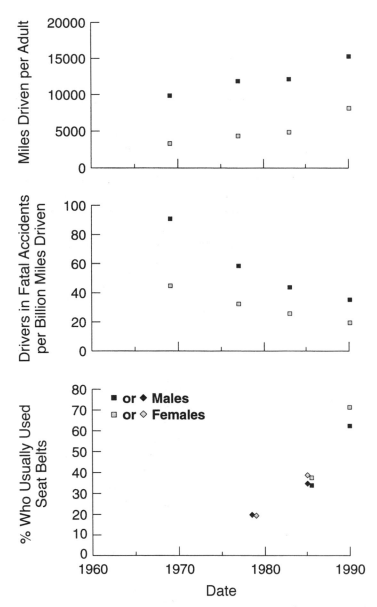

Figure 2. Trends in motor vehicle accident–related behavior in the United States: 1960–1990. Miles driven per adult and rates of fatal accidents are for adults (16 and over); for accident rates, there was a change in methods between 1983 and 1990 (calculated from data in National Safety Council, 1972, 1985, 1991; U.S. Department of Transportation, 1993, 1994). Seat belt use data are the proportion who "usually" used seat belts for adults aged 20–64 (for 1979 and 1985) or the proportion who used seat belts "all or most of the time when riding in a car" for adults aged 18 and over (for 1985 and 1990) (National Center for Health Statistics, 1988; Piani & Schoenborn, 1993; Schoenborn, 1988). All data are based on national samples.

rates of drownings and fatal gun accidents (Rosen & Peterson, 1990; Veevers & Gee, 1986; Waldron, 1988). Limited evidence suggests that gender differences in these types of accident-related behavior have not decreased recently; indeed, data for young adults in the U.S. indicate that during the 1980s, there were slight increases in sex mortality ratios for drownings and for fatal gun accidents (Waldron, 1995).

One important reason for boys' higher accident rates is that boys engage in more risky play than girls (Rosen & Peterson, 1990; Waldron, 1983, in press). Parents appear to discourage risk taking more in girls, so gender differences in socialization appear to contribute to gender differences in risk taking. Biological effects may also contribute to gender differences in accident risk; effects of male sex hormones may contribute to males' higher levels of physical activity, which in turn contribute to males' higher accident risk (Berenbaum & Snyder, 1995; Waldron, 1988, in press).

The evidence reviewed suggests that males have a greater predisposition to physical risk taking, and that their risk taking is a major cause of their higher accident rates. Some additional evidence supports this interpretation (Cherpitel, 1993; Plant & Plant, 1992; Rosen & Peterson, 1990; Veevers & Gee, 1986). However, unexpected findings from a study of a national sample of United States adults indicate the need for more systematic evidence concerning the proposed association between a general predisposition to risk taking and higher accident rates for males. This study found that the risk of serious accidents was not related to measures of risk taking and impulsivity, thrill seeking, or risk perception, once controls for alcohol consumption and gender were introduced (Cherpitel, 1993). For teenagers and adults, it appears that gender differences in amount of alcohol consumed and gender differences in responses to drinking may be important causes of gender differences in accident risk (Cherpitel, 1993; Waldron, 1983).

In summary, males' higher accident rates have been due to a variety of behaviors that have been more socially accepted or expected of males, including taking risks physically in driving and recreation, working at physically hazardous jobs, use of guns, and heavy drinking. Gender differences in accident-related behavior appear to be due in part to differential socialization of males and females, and may also be due in part to hormonal effects. United States data indicate mixed trends in gender differences in accident-related behavior in recent decades. The male excess has decreased for driving and for nonfatal work accidents, but not for drownings or for gun accidents, and there has been a growing female advantage in seat belt use. One interpretation of the observed trends is that women have increasingly adopted behaviors that can contribute to the well-being of families in the modern world, including driving, employment, and seat belt use. In contrast, women have not adopted the high-risk behaviors that contribute to drownings and gun accidents.

Exercise

In the United States, more women are sedentary and more men engage in vigorous physical exercise both in their leisure time and in their main daily activity (see Figure 1) (Piani & Schoenborn, 1993; Schoenborn, 1988; Stephens, 1987). The male excess in leisure-time exercise has been observed in some other Western countries, but has not been found in surveys in some Scandinavian countries (e.g., Rossow & Rise, 1994; Zemp & Ackermann-Liebrich, 1988).

In the United States during the 1970s and 1980s, leisure-time exercise increased for both men and women, and trends in gender differences varied depending on the time period and measure considered. During the 1970s, the proportion who were sedentary decreased, and the magnitude of sex differences in this measure decreased, while sex ratios showed inconsistent trends (data from Stephens, 1987). During the 1980s, the proportion who were very physically active in leisure time increased, and sex differences and sex ratios increased (Figure 1). These contrasting trends were observed within specific adult age groups, as well as for all adult age groups combined. Gender differences in the amount of exercise involved in a person's main daily activity appear to have changed very little from 1985 to 1990 (data from Piani & Schoenborn, 1993; Schoenborn, 1988). Thus, gender differences in exercise have decreased, increased, or stayed the same depending on the specific time period and measure considered. These variable trends contrast with the steady decrease in gender differences in employment during the same time period, which suggests that the employment trends have not substantially influenced the trends in gender differences in exercise. This conclusion is compatible with survey evidence that indicates no consistent relationship between women's employment status and exercise levels (Piani & Schoenborn, 1993; Schoenborn, 1988).

Gender differences are observed not only for the amount of exercise, but also for the type of exercise and the motivation for exercising. Men's participation substantially exceeds women's participation for team sports, while women are more likely to engage in noncompetitive activities such as walking and calisthenics (Piani & Schoenborn, 1993; Schoenborn, 1988; Stephens, 1987; White, Powell, Hogelin, Gentry, & Forman, 1987). One reason for these differences appears to be that competition is a more important motivation for men's participation in vigorous physical activity (Finkenberg, DiNucci, McCune, & McCune, 1994). Women's participation in vigorous exercise appears to be motivated more by concerns about weight control and appearance (Finkenberg et al., 1994; McDonald & Thompson, 1992). For example, in a 1985 national sample of United States adults, 25% of women versus 15% of men reported that they exercised in order to lose weight (data from Stephenson, Levy, Sass, & McGarvey, 1987). No gender differences have been found in the reported importance of health or fitness as motivators for exercise (data for physically active college students) (Finkenberg et al., 1994; McDonald & Thompson, 1992).

Gender differences in exercise appear to be due in part to differential socialization of males and females. Boys are encouraged more than girls to be physically active (Rosen & Peterson, 1990). Males are also expected and encouraged more than females to participate in competitive sports and physically demanding jobs. Biological influences may also play a role. Prenatal exposure to testosterone may predispose males to high-energy physical activity, although the evidence for this effect is inconsistent and subject to methodological problems (Berenbaum & Snyder, 1995; Waldron, 1988, in press). Thus, the available evidence suggests that gender differences in exercise may be due to the combined effects of hormonal and social influences.

Dieting and Eating Disorders

Dieting and Other Weight Loss Behaviors. In the United States and other Western countries, females are substantially more likely than males to judge themselves overweight, to wish to lose weight, and to diet in order to lose weight (French & Jeffery, 1994; Whitaker et al., 1989; Zemp & Ackermann-Liebrich, 1988). For example, national data for the United States indicate that women's rates of dieting were roughly twice as high as men's from the 1950s through the 1980s. In 1956 and 1966, approximately 14% of women compared to 7% of men reported that they were on a diet (Dwyer & Mayer, 1970). In 1985, 36% of women compared to 19% of men reported trying to lose weight by eating less (data from Stephenson et al., 1987).

Evidence for the United States indicates that females also engage in other types of weight loss behavior more often than males. For example, more females than males report that they use diet pills, induce vomiting, or use laxatives to reduce weight (French & Jeffery, 1994; Johnston et al., 1994; Warheit, Langer, Zimmerman, & Biafora, 1993; Whitaker et al., 1989).

Females' higher rates of dieting and other weight loss behaviors are to a large extent the result of the greater social pressures on girls and women to be slender, reflecting the greater emphasis on appearance for females, in combination with the very slender contemporary beauty ideal (Hayes & Ross, 1987; Hsu, 1989; Waldron, 1988). Males place greater emphasis than females on appearance as a very major determinant of a potential partner's desirability, and being overweight results in greater social disadvantages for females (Feingold, 1994; Harris, Walters, & Waschull, 1991; Hsu, 1989; Waldron, 1988). The emphasis on a slender beauty ideal and dieting for women is reinforced by media images and articles on dieting (Dolan & Gitzinger, 1994).

Informal observation suggests that appearance-related motivations contribute much more than health-related motivations to gender differences in dieting, and this conclusion is supported by several research findings. Indirect evidence is provided by United States survey data that show that gender differences in "trying to lose weight" are larger for younger adults, for whom appearance motivations may be more important; conversely, gender differences in "trying to lose weight" are smaller for older adults, for whom health motivations may be more important (data from Stephenson et al., 1987). More direct evidence is provided by a survey of high school students that found that, among students who were dieting, girls were substantially more likely than boys to give reasons related to appearance, both sexes were equally likely to give health-related reasons, and boys were more likely to give reasons related to athletics (Whitaker et al., 1989). In summary, there are strong social pressures on females to be slender, and these social pressures appear to be the primary reason for females' higher rates of dieting and weight loss behaviors.

Eating Disorders. Females have much higher rates than males for the eating disorders anorexia nervosa and bulimia nervosa (evidence for the United States and the United Kingdom in Hsu, 1989). Females' higher rates of eating disorders are due in large part to social pressures on females to be slender and to harmful effects of

dieting (French & Jeffery, 1994; Hsu, 1989; Waldron, 1988).

One type of bulimic behavior, binging, has not shown consistent gender differences (Drewnowski, Hopkins, & Kessler, 1988; Warheit et al., 1993; Whitaker et al., 1989). The inconsistent gender differences in binging are probably the result of two opposing influences. On the one hand, greater social pressures on females to eat small amounts and to be slender may tend to reduce their risk of binging (Rolls, Federoff, & Guthrie, 1991). On the other hand, dieting tends to increase the risk of binging, so females' more frequent dieting probably increases their risk of binging (French & Jeffery, 1994; Waldron, 1988).

Gender differences in eating disorders may also be influenced by gender differences in relevant psychological characteristics. It appears that anxious, constricted, and conforming children have a higher risk of developing an eating disorder (Vitousek & Manke, 1994). Conversely, the risk of eating disorders and bulimic behaviors may be reduced by "masculinity" (assessed as assertiveness and independence) and associated higher self-esteem (Klingenspor, 1994; Lancelot & Kaslow, 1994). Thus, females' higher risk of developing an eating disorder may be due in part to their higher anxiety and lower assertiveness and self-esteem (Feingold, 1994). Although psychological "masculinity" may be protective, no consistent relationship has been found between bulimic behavior or eating disorders and "femininity" (assessed as being oriented to others, with more affective expressiveness) or women's gender role attitudes or nontraditional aspirations (Dolan & Gitzinger, 1994; Klingenspor, 1994; Lancelot & Kaslow, 1994; Morgan, Affleck, & Solloway, 1990; Rost, Neuhaus, & Florin, 1982).

Biological factors may also contribute to females' higher rates of eating disorders. The conflict between the inherent tendency of female bodies to accumulate fat during puberty and the contemporary slender beauty ideal may increase teenage girls' risk of developing eating disorders (Waldron, 1988). There may also be sex differences in brain chemistry that may contribute to girls' and women's higher risk of eating disorders (Cowen, Anderson, & Fairburn, 1992).

In summary, females' higher rates of dieting, weight loss behaviors, and eating disorders are due in large part to greater social pressures on females to be slender. In addition, gender differences in psychological and biological characteristics may contribute to females' greater vulnerability to eating disorders.

Physician Visits

In the United States and other Western countries, women have higher rates of physician visits than men (Gijsbers van Wijk, van Vliet, Kolk, & Evenaerd, 1991; Waldron, 1983). In the United States, more males than females have had no contact with a physician within the previous 2 years, and this gender difference increased from the mid-1960s through the early 1990s (see Figure 1). Women's higher rates of physician visits are part of a general pattern of gender differences in health care behavior; women also visit dentists more often, use more prescribed and nonprescribed medicines, and more often take a day of bed rest or restricted activity because of illness or injury (Gijsbers van Wijk et al., 1991; National Center for Health Statistics, 1969–1994; Waldron, 1983).

Although women visit physicians more than men in Western countries, this gender difference is not observed for children in the United States (National Center for Health Statistics, 1969–1994; Waldron, 1983). Also, for adults in non-Western countries, gender differences in physician visits have varied, with higher rates for women in some regions and time periods, but higher rates for men in other regions and time periods (Fuller et al., 1993; Waldron, 1983).

Gender Differences in Need and Motivation for Medical Care. In Western countries, one major reason for women's higher rates of physician visits is that women have much higher rates of reproduction-related visits (Gijsbers van Wijk et al., 1991; Waldron, 1983, 1988). Among

young and middle-aged adults, it appears that reproduction-related visits account for about one third to two thirds of the gender difference in physician visits. Similarly, for young and middle-aged adults in Bangkok, Thailand, it appears that pregnancy and menstrual problems make a substantial contribution to women's higher rates of physician visits (Fuller et al., 1993). However, in some non-Western countries, women have had limited access to obstetric and gynecological care, and women have had lower rates of physician visits than men, even during peak reproductive ages (Waldron, 1983, 1988). Thus, the contribution of inherent sex differences in reproductive biology to gender differences in physician visits varies substantially depending on cultural and socioeconomic conditions.

Additional evidence for Western countries indicates that women report more symptoms and health problems than men, and women's higher rates of symptoms and health problems appear to be another important reason for women's higher rates of physician visits (Verbrugge, 1985; Waldron, 1983; Zemp & Ackermann-Liebrich, 1988). Gender differences in self-reported symptoms and health problems may be due to sex differences in actual physical problems, possible sex differences in sensory sensitivity, and possible gender differences in the psychological predisposition to identify and report a given sensation as a symptom or health problem.

To test for possible gender differences in reporting, studies have compared self-report with more objective measures of health problems. Some of these studies suggest a greater female propensity to report health problems, but others suggest a greater male propensity to report health problems, and others find no evidence for a gender difference in reporting (MacIntyre, 1993; Stenberg & Wall, 1995; Waldron, 1983). A related line of research, using controlled pain stimuli in laboratory settings, indicates that, relative to men, women tend to have a lower threshold for reporting pain and women tend to report a given pain stimulus as more unpleasant (Feine, Bushnell, Miron, & Duncan, 1991; Otto &

Dougher, 1985). Limited evidence suggests that these gender differences in pain reporting may be due in part to sex differences in sensory processes. Additional evidence suggests that psychological gender differences, such as women's greater anxiety or men's greater "masculinity" (assertiveness and instrumentality), may contribute to gender differences in reports of pain, symptoms, and health problems (Annandale & Hunt, 1990; Feingold, 1994; Otto & Dougher, 1985; A. S. Robbins, Spence, & Clark, 1991). Taken together, the available evidence suggests that both physiological and psychological gender differences contribute to women's higher rates of self-reported symptoms and health problems, which in turn contribute to women's higher rates of physician visits.

Women may also be somewhat more predisposed than men to visit a physician for a given level of symptoms or health problems, and women may make more preventive visits than men, although evidence concerning these possible gender differences has been inconsistent in different studies (Verbrugge, 1985; Waldron, 1983; Zemp & Ackermann-Liebrich, 1988). Interestingly, men seek medical care as promptly or more promptly than women for symptoms of many types of serious illness, including myocardial infarctions and various types of cancer (Dracup et al., 1995; Waldron, 1983). This observation suggests that gender differences in the likelihood of physician visits may occur primarily for conditions that are not life-threatening. Women may be more prone to seek medical help for these less serious conditions for several reasons. Women appear to be less willing to ignore or tolerate pain, may be generally more willing to seek help and care taking, and appear to have greater concern about health and more confidence in the benefits of medical care (Nathanson, 1977; Otto & Dougher, 1985; Waldron, 1983, 1988; Weissfeld et al., 1990).

Women report more psychological distress, and greater psychological distress may contribute to women's higher rates of physician visits for somatic symptoms, since psychological distress increases the occurrence and perception of so-matic symptoms and the likelihood of seeking treatment for somatic symptoms (Fuller et al., 1993). In addition, women have more physician visits for explicit psychological symptoms. Women also have higher rates of physician visits for weight gain, reflecting women's greater concern with weight control (based on United States data in Waldron, 1983).

Gender Differences in Access to Medical Care. In addition to gender differences in need and motivation for medical care, there may be gender differences in access to medical care. In the United States, young women are somewhat more likely than young men to have health insurance (Salem, 1995). However, for ages 35 and older in the United States and for most Western countries there is little or no gender difference in health insurance coverage (National Center for Health Statistics, 1987; Salem, 1995). In some non-Western societies, males have greater access to scarce resources such as medical care due to males' higher status and the perception that males are more valuable (Waldron, 1983, 1988). Also, restrictions on women's travel and norms concerning modesty for women limit women's access to medical care in some non-Western societies. Thus, gender differences in access to medical care contribute to gender differences in physician visits in some circumstances.

Another hypothesis proposes that, because more men than women are employed, men have more "fixed role" obligations, and the inflexible time demands of these fixed role obligations may make it difficult for men to arrange time for a physician visit. This hypothesis receives little support from the available evidence for Western countries (Lutz, 1989; Waldron, 1983, 1988). One study found evidence that gender differences in employment may make a modest contribution to gender differences in physician visits. However, other studies have not found consistent relationships between women's employment status and the propensity to seek preventive health care or visit a physician when ill. Also, men are no more likely than women to report inconvenience in arranging time for physician visits. It appears that there may be a balance between men's greater role obligations due to employment and women's greater role obligations due to responsibility for care of family and home, so differences in role obligations may not contribute substantially to gender differences in physician visits. The conclusion that gender differences in employment status are not a major determinant of gender differences in physician contacts is congruent with the observation that gender differences in physician contacts have not decreased as gender differences in employment rates have decreased in recent decades (Figure 1) (data from National Center for Health Statistics, 1969–1994).

In summary, women visit physicians more often than men in Western countries and in some non-Western countries. Women's more complex and demanding reproductive functions are one major reason for their higher rates of physician visits. Despite this biological contribution to women's physician visits, men have had higher rates of physician visits than women in some non-Western countries, apparently due to greater access to medical care for men. In Western countries, women's higher rates of physician visits may be due to additional factors, which may include women's higher rates of perceived symptoms and health problems and possibly a greater propensity of women to visit a doctor for preventive purposes or for conditions that are not life-threatening. Underlying factors may include gender differences in attitudes toward pain and health care and in psychological distress. Thus, a variety of sociocultural and biological factors contributes to gender differences in physician visits.

CONCLUSIONS

This section presents general conclusions based on the preceding analyses of gender differences in various types of health behavior. These conclusions apply primarily to the United States and other Western countries in the period since about 1960, with limited discussion of non-Western countries or earlier periods, as noted.

Risk Taking and Health Concerns

As discussed in the Introduction, previous authors have hypothesized that gender differences in risk taking and health concerns are major causes of gender differences in health behavior. The evidence reviewed provides partial support for this hypothesis. Physical risk taking is more common and more accepted and encouraged for males. For example, males take more risks in driving, swimming, and children's play. Males' greater propensity for risk taking may also contribute to their higher rates of heavy drinking; heavy drinking in turn contributes to males' increased risk taking. A general propensity to risk taking may also be associated with increased likelihood of smoking initiation; however, there is currently little gender difference in smoking initiation in the United States.

Gender differences in explicit health concerns appear to make only a limited contribution to gender differences in health behavior. It appears that women are somewhat more concerned than men about health, and this greater concern may contribute to women's higher rates of physician visits. Females may be more aware of the health risks of heavy drinking, and this greater awareness may contribute to gender differences in heavy drinking. However, concerns about the health-damaging effects of smoking appear to have reduced cigarette smoking at least as much for men as for women. Also, it appears that health-related motivations make little or no contribution to gender differences in dieting and exercise.

These observations suggest that gender differences in risk taking and health concerns make a significant contribution to gender differences in some types of health behavior, but have little effect on gender differences in other types of health behavior. This conclusion is supported by the observation that some types of health behavior show the predicted pattern of greater male risk taking or greater female health-promoting behavior, but other types of health behavior do not show this pattern. In the contemporary United States, males take more health risks in driving, recreation, employment in hazardous jobs, and heavy drinking, but females take more health risks in excessive weight loss behaviors and eating disorders. More males smoke cigarettes, but the male excess in smoking has decreased as the health risks of smoking have become more widely known. With respect to health-promoting behavior, women use seat belts more, but men exercise more. Women are more likely to visit doctors, but are not more prompt in seeking medical attention for many types of major life-threatening illness. Taken together, the evidence reviewed indicates that males have a greater propensity for physical risk taking, but gender differences in many types of health behavior are influenced relatively little by gender differences in risk taking and health concerns and more by other causal factors.

Other Effects of Gender Roles

Gender differences in health behavior are influenced by several additional characteristics of male and female roles. For example, females' greater concern with appearance, in combination with the contemporary slender beauty ideal, is a major contributor to females' higher rates of dieting, other weight loss behaviors, and eating disorders. Females' concern with weight control also tends to increase their rates of physical exercise and smoking, which reduces gender differences in these behaviors.

Males are encouraged more to be physically active and competitive, and this contributes to males' higher rates of vigorous exercise and accidents. Males' greater rebelliousness and lesser involvement with religion tend to increase their rates of smoking adoption and drinking. Males' greater assertiveness and lesser anxiety appear to reduce their risk of eating disorders. Thus, gender roles include a variety of psychological characteristics and attitudes that are more common,

more expected, and more accepted for one sex or the other, and these characteristics in turn contribute to gender differences in various types of health behavior.

In addition, some health behaviors can be seen as part of male or female gender roles, since these health behaviors are much more common and socially acceptable for one sex than for the other. For example, dieting can be considered part of the female gender role for teenage girls and young women in some social groups, and competitive sports, heavy drinking, and/or gun use can be considered part of the male gender role in some social groups. Clearly, these health behaviors are related to other aspects of male and female gender roles. For example, heavy drinking is associated with toughness and other aspects of masculinity, and this is one reason why heavy drinking is more socially acceptable for males. Conversely, heavy drinking is less socially acceptable for females, in part because heavy drinking is seen as incompatible with important aspects of female roles, including women's primary responsibility for child care and sexual restraint. In summary, a gender role can be seen as a group of interrelated behaviors, attitudes, and psychological characteristics that includes some types of health behavior and also includes multiple psychological characteristics and attitudes that influence many types of health behavior.

One additional aspect of gender roles appears to be particularly important in some non-Western societies. In many traditional societies, men have greater power and access to scarce resources, and greater restrictions are placed on women's behavior. These aspects of traditional societies appear to be important reasons for women's lower rates of smoking or physician visits, or both, in various non-Western societies. This type of effect seems less important in contemporary Western societies, probably because there is less scarcity of resources and greater equality between the sexes. Although women's employment tends to increase their financial resources and power, there is little relationship between women's employment status and health behavior in contemporary Western countries. Specifically, no consistent differences have been found between employed women and full-time homemakers in smoking, exercise, or physician visits, although some evidence suggests that employed women drink more than full-time homemakers.

Multiple Psychosocial and Biological Influences

It is clear that gender differences in health behavior are influenced by multiple aspects of gender roles. In addition, social influences such as advertising and public health campaigns may affect gender differences in health behavior. Biological factors also contribute to gender differences in health behavior. For example, women's more complex and demanding reproductive functions are a major cause of their higher rates of physician visits. Females' smaller lean body mass appears to be one reason for the lower quantity of alcohol consumed by females. Greater exposure to prenatal testosterone may predispose males to greater physical activity, which contributes to males' higher rates of vigorous exercise and accidents. In summary, multiple psychosocial and biological factors influence gender differences in health behavior.

It should also be noted that, even when males and females engage in similar health behavior, they may have different motivations. For example, females' smoking appears to be motivated more by concerns about weight control, whereas males' smoking adoption may be motivated more by risk taking and rebelliousness. Women's smoking is reduced by pregnancy-related health concerns, while males' smoking is reduced more by concerns about the effects of smoking on physical fitness. Similarly, there appear to be sex differences in the motivations for exercise. Weight control appears to be a more important motivation for exercise for females, whereas enjoyment of competitive sports appears to be a more important motivation for exercise for males.

Trends

As discussed in the Introduction, it has been hypothesized that gender differences in health behavior have decreased as male and female roles have become more similar in recent decades. This hypothesis is not supported by data for the United States from the 1960s through the early 1990s, which have shown inconsistent trends in gender differences in health behavior. Gender differences generally decreased for the proportion who smoked cigarettes, mileage driven, and drivers' risk of fatal accidents per mile driven. However, gender differences in seat belt use increased during the 1980s, as did gender differences in the proportion who saw a doctor infrequently. For heavy drinking and exercise, trends in gender differences varied, depending on the measure and/or time period considered. Thus, gender differences decreased for some types of health behavior, but not for others.

A closely related hypothesis proposes that decreasing gender differences in employment have resulted in decreasing gender differences in health behavior. This hypothesis is also not supported since women's employment status appears to have relatively little effect on their health behavior, and there has not been a consistent trend toward decreasing gender differences in health behavior, despite substantial decreases in gender differences in employment. Thus, in recent decades, trends in employment have had little or no direct effect on trends in gender differences in health behavior. However, historical evidence suggests that changing gender differences in employment may have had significant indirect effects on gender differences in some types of health behavior, particularly if the time frame is extended back to the early and mid-20th century. During this period, it appears, the trend toward increasing employment of women contributed to a general decrease in restrictions on women's behavior, including decreased social disapproval of women's smoking, and this trend in attitudes was a major cause of the decrease in gender differences in smoking.

This chapter has not systematically analyzed the causes of the varied recent trends in gender differences in health behavior, but a partial interpretation can be suggested. It appears that these varied trends have been influenced by the differing compatibility of various types of health behavior with fundamental aspects of female gender roles. For example, heavy drinking appears to be incompatible with important aspects of female gender roles, and this appears to contribute to the continuing large gender differences in heavy drinking. In contrast, females use smoking more for weight control, reflecting females' greater concern with appearance, and this has contributed to the decrease in gender differences in smoking. Similarly, women have adopted behaviors such as driving and employment, which help women to meet traditional family care responsibilities in the modern world; consequently, gender differences in driving and employment have decreased, which has contributed to decreasing gender differences for some types of accidents. However, it appears that women have not adopted the high-risk behaviors that contribute to drownings and gun accidents. These observations suggest that fundamental aspects of traditional gender roles continue to influence changing gender differences in health behavior, contributing to more rapid change for some types of health behavior and more resistance to change for other types of health behavior.

QUESTIONS FOR FUTURE RESEARCH

In future research, it will be of interest to explore additional questions and hypotheses concerning the possible causes of trends in gender differences in health behavior. What changes have there been in the socialization of males and females, and how have these changes affected gender differences in characteristics such as the propensity to physical risk taking, rebelliousness, or assertiveness? Have any changes in socialization or psychological characteristics had an effect on gender differences in health behavior? Have social trends, such as increased divorce rates, increases in female-headed households, or changing parental roles, influenced trends in gender differences in health behavior? Have there been differential effects on male and female health behavior due to public health campaigns, due to relevant laws, such as laws requiring seat belt use, or due to advertising for products such as cigarettes or alcoholic beverages? In future research, it will also be important to assess patterns and trends in gender differences for other types of health behavior and for various age groups, ethnic groups, and social classes in the United States and in other countries. Clearly, many questions remain to be answered concerning the patterns and causes of changing gender differences in health behavior.

Finally, although this chapter has focused on gender differences in health behavior, it is important to note that there are many similarities in the patterns and causes of male and female health behavior. For example, in recent decades, many types of health behavior have shown similar trends for males and females. Both males and females have increased their rates of exercise, seat belt use, and mileage driven. Similarly, both males and females have had decreasing rates of smoking and heavy drinking and decreasing risk of fatal accidents per mile driven. These observations indicate that, to a large extent, recent trends in male and female health behavior have been influenced by similar causal factors. In conclusion, gender roles and sex differences in biology contribute to significant gender differences in many types of health behavior, but there are also many shared influences on male and female health behavior.

ACKNOWLEDGMENTS. I am grateful to Sarah Cookinham, Jessie Eyer, Katie Eyer, Mahan Ghaznavi, Leigh Ann Simmons, and Paulette Staum for their help in preparing this chapter.

REFERENCES

Anda, R. F., Williamson, D. F., Escobedo, L. G., Mast, E. E., Giovino, G. A., & Remington, P. L. (1990). Depression and the dynamics of smoking. *Journal of the American Medical Association, 264,* 1541-1545.

Annandale, E., & Hunt, K. (1990). Masculinity, femininity and sex: An exploration of their relative contribution to explaining gender differences in health. *Sociology of Health and Illness, 12,* 24-46.

Bauman, K. E., Foshee, V. A., & Haley, N. J. (1992). The interaction of sociological and biological factors in adolescent cigarette smoking. *Addictive Behaviors, 17,* 459-467.

Beck, K. H. & Summons, T. G. (1987). Adolescent gender differences in alcohol beliefs and behaviors. *Journal of Alcohol and Drug Education, 33,* 31-44.

Berenbaum, S. A., & Snyder, E. (1995). Early hormonal influences on childhood sex-typed activity and playmate preferences: Implications for the development of sexual orientation. *Developmental Psychology, 31,* 31-42.

Blume, S. B. (1994). Gender differences in alcohol related disorders. *Harvard Review of Pyschiatry, 2,* 7-13.

Chassin, L., Tetzloff, C., & Hershey, M. (1985). Self-image and social-image factors in adolescent alcohol use. *Journal of Studies on Alcohol, 46,* 39-47.

Chen, Y., Horne, S. L., & Dosman, J. A. (1993). The influence of smoking cessation on body weight may be temporary. *American Journal of Public Health, 83,* 1330-1332.

Cherpitel, C. J. (1993). Alcohol, injury, and risk-taking behavior: Data from a national sample. *Alcoholism: Clinical and Experimental Research, 17,* 762-766.

Clifford, C. A., Fulker D. W., Gurling, H. M. D., & Murray, R. M. (1981). Preliminary findings from a twin study of alcohol use. *Progress in Clinical and Biological Research, 69,* 47-52.

Cooper, M. L., Russell, M., Skinner, J. B., Frone, M. R., & Mudar, P. (1992). Stress and alcohol use: Moderating effects of gender, coping and alcoholic tendencies. *Journal of Abnormal Psychology, 101,* 139-152.

Cowen, P. J., Anderson, I. M., & Fairburn, C. G., (1992). Neurochemical effects of dieting: Relevance to changes in eating and affective disorders. In G. H. Anderson & S. H. Kennedy (Eds.), *The biology of feast and famine* (pp. 269-284). San Diego, CA: Academic Press.

Darrow, S. L., Russell, M., Cooper, M. L., Mudar, P., & Frone, M. R. (1992). Sociodemographic correlates of alcohol consumption among African-American and white women. *Women and Health, 18,* 35-51.

Dawson, D. A., & Archer, L. (1992). Gender differences in alcohol consumption: Effects of measurement. *British Journal of Addiction, 87,* 119-123.

del Boca, F. K. (1994). Sex, gender and alcoholic typologies. *Annals of the New York Academy of Sciences, 708,* 34-48.

Dolan, B., & Gitzinger, I. (Eds.). (1994). *Why women? Gender issues and eating disorders.* London: Athlone Press.

Dracup, K., Moser, D. K., Eisenberg, M., Meischke, H., Alonzo, A. A., & Braslow, A. (1995). Causes of delay in seeking treatment for heart attack symptoms. *Social Science and Medicine, 40,* 379-392.

Drewnowski, A., Hopkins, S. A., & Kessler, R. C. (1988). The prevalence of bulimia nervosa in the US college student population. *American Journal of Public Health, 78,* 1322-1325.

Dwyer, J. T., & Mayer, J. (1970). Potential dieters: Who are they? *Journal of the American Dietetic Association, 56,* 510-514.

Ebi-Kryston, K. L., Higgins, M. W., & Keller, J. B. (1990). Health and other characteristics of employed women and homemakers in Tecumseh, 1959-1978. *Women and Health, 16*(2), 5-21.

Escobedo, L. G., Chorba, T. L., Remington, P. L., Anda, R. F., Sanderson, L., & Zaidi, A. A. (1991). State laws and the use of car safety seat belts. *New England Journal of Medicine, 325,* 1586-1587.

Evans, L. (1991). *Traffic safety and the driver.* New York: Van Nostrand Reinhold.

Feine, J. S., Bushnell, M. C., Miron, D., & Duncan, G. H. (1991). Sex differences in the perception of noxious heat stimuli. *Pain, 44,* 255-262.

Feingold, A. (1994). Gender differences in personality: A meta-analysis. *Psychological Bulletin, 116,* 429-456.

Fillmore, K. M. (1987). Women's drinking across the adult life course as compared to men's. *British Journal of Addiction, 82,* 801-811.

Finkenberg, M. E., DiNucci, J. M., McCune, S. L., & McCune, E. D. (1994). Analysis of course type, gender, and personal incentives to exercise. *Perceptual and Motor Skills, 78,* 155-159.

French, S. A., & Jeffery, R. W. (1994). Consequences of dieting to lose weight: Effects on physical and mental health. *Health Psychology, 13,* 195-212.

Frezza, M., di Padova, C., Pozzato, G., Terpin, M., Baraona, E., & Lieber, C. S. (1990). High blood alcohol levels in women—The role of decreased gastric alcohol dehydrogenase activity and first-pass metabolism. *New England Journal of Medicine, 322,* 95-99.

Fried, P. A., Barnes, M. V., & Drake, E. R. (1985). Soft drug use after pregnancy compared to use before and during pregnancy. *American Journal of Obstetrics and Gynecology, 151,* 787-792.

Fuller, T. D., Edwards, J. N., Sermsri, S., & Vorakitphokatorn, S. (1993). Gender and health: Some Asian evidence. *Journal of Health and Social Behavior, 34,* 252-271.

Gefou-Madianou, D. (Ed.). (1992). *Alcohol, gender and culture.* London: Routledge.

Gijsbers van Wijk, C. M. T., van Vliet, K. P., Kolk, A. M., & Everaerd, W. T. A. M. (1991). Symptom sensitivity and sex differences in physical morbidity: A review of health surveys in the United States and the Netherlands. *Women and Health, 17,* 91-124.

Grunberg, N. E., Winders, S. E., & Wewers, M. E. (1991). Gender difference in tobacco use. *Health Psychology, 10,* 143-153.

Harris, M. B., Walters, L. C., & Waschull, S. (1991). Gender and ethnic differences in obesity-related behaviors and attitudes in college sample. *Journal of Applied Social Psychology*, *21*, 1545–1566.

Hatziandreu, E. J., Pierce, J. P., Lefkopoulou, M., Fiore, M. C., Mills, S. L., Novotny, T. E., Giovino, G. A., & Davis, R. M. (1990). Quitting smoking in the United States in 1986. *Journal of the National Cancer Institute, 82*, 1402–1406.

Hayes, D., & Ross, C. E. (1987). Concern with appearance, health beliefs, and eating habits. *Journal of Health and Social Behavior, 28*, 120–130.

Hsu, L. K. G. (1989). The gender gap in eating disorders: Why are the eating disorders more common among women? *Clinical Psychology Review, 9*, 393–407.

Huselid, R. F., & Cooper, M. L. (1992). Gender roles as mediators of sex differences in adolescent alcohol use and abuse. *Journal of Health and Social Behavior, 33*, 348–362.

Jardine, R., & Martin, N. G. (1984). Causes of variation in drinking habits in a large twin sample. *Acta Geneticae Medicae et Gemellologiae (Roma), 33*, 435–450.

Jarvis, M. (1984). Gender and smoking: Do women really find it harder to give up? *British Journal of Addiction, 79*, 383–387.

Johnston, L. D., O'Malley, P. M., & Bachman, J. G. (1994). *National survey results on drug use from the Monitoring the Future Study, 1975–1993: Vols. 1 & 2.* Rockville, MD: National Institute on Drug Abuse.

Klassen, A. D., & Wilsnack, S. C. (1986). Sexual experience and drinking among women in a U.S. national survey. *Archives of Sexual Behavior, 15*, 363–391.

Klee, L., & Ames, G. (1987). Reevaluating risk factors for women's drinking. *American Journal of Preventive Medicine, 3*, 31–41.

Klingenspor, B. (1994). Gender identity and bulimic eating behavior. *Sex Roles, 31*, 407–431.

Kraft, P., & Rise, J. (1994). The relationship between sensation seeking and smoking, alcohol consumption and sexual behavior among Norwegian adolescents. *Health Education Research, 9*, 193–200.

Kruse, J., Le Fevre, M., & Zweig, S. (1986). Changes in smoking and alcohol consumption during pregnancy: A population-based study in a rural area. *Obstetrics and Gynecology, 67*, 627–632.

Lancelot, C., & Kaslow, N. J. (1994). Sex role orientation and disordered eating in women: A review. *Clinical Psychology Review, 14*, 139–157.

Lando, H. A., Hellerstedt, W. L., Pirie, P. L., & McGovern, P. G. (1991). Survey of smoking patterns, attitudes, and interest in quitting. *American Journal of Preventive Medicine, 7*, 18–23.

Lee, L., Gilpin, E. A., & Pierce, J. P. (1993). Changes in the patterns of initiation of cigarette smoking in the United States: 1950, 1965 and 1980. *Cancer Epidemiology, Biomarkers and Prevention, 2*, 593–597.

Lemle, R., & Mishkind, M. E. (1989). Alcohol and masculinity. *Journal of Substance Abuse Treatment, 6*, 213–222.

Liu, S., Serdula, M. K., Williamson, D. F., Mokdad, A. H., &

Byers, T. (1994). A prospective study of alcohol intake and change in body weight among US adults. *American Journal of Epidemiology, 140*, 912–920.

Lutz, M. E. (1989). Women, work and preventive health care: An exploratory study of the efficacy of HMO membership. *Women and Health, 15*, 21–33.

Lye, D. N., & Waldron, I. (1996). *Relationships of substance use to attitudes toward gender roles, family, and cohabitation.* Manuscript submitted for publication.

Macintyre, S. (1993). Gender differences in the perceptions of common cold symptoms. *Social Science and Medicine, 36*, 15–20.

McDonald, K., & Thompson, J. R. (1992). Eating disturbance, body image dissatisfaction, and reasons for exercising: Gender differences and correlation findings. *International Journal of Eating Disorders, 11*, 289–292.

McWhorter, W. P., Boyd, G. M., & Mattson, M. E. (1990). Predictors of quitting smoking: The NHANES I followup experience. *Journal of Clinical Epidemiology, 43*, 1399–1405.

Morgan, C. S., Affleck, M., & Solloway, O. (1990). Gender role attitudes, religiosity, and food behavior: Dieting and bulimia in college women. *Social Science Quarterly, 71*, 142–151.

Nathanson, C. A. (1977). Sex roles as variables in preventive health behavior. *Journal of Community Health, 3*, 142–155.

National Center for Health Statistics. (1969–1994). Current estimates from the Health Interview Survey: United States, 1967–1992. *Vital and Health Statistics*, Series 10.

National Center for Health Statistics. (1980–1994). *Health, United States, 1979–1993.* Hyattsville, MD: U.S. Public Health Service.

National Center for Health Statistics. (1987). Health coverage by age, sex, race, and family income: United States, 1986. *Advance Data from Vital and Health Statistics, 139*, 1–8.

National Center for Health Statistics. (1988). Adult health practices in the United States and Canada. *Vital and Health Statistics*, Series 5, No. 3.

National Safety Council. (1972). *Accident facts 1972.* Chicago: National Safety Council.

National Safety Council. (1985). *Accident facts 1985.* Chicago: National Safety Council.

National Safety Council. (1991). *Accident facts 1991.* Chicago: National Safety Council.

Otto, M. W., & Dougher, M. J. (1985). Sex differences and personality factors in responsivity to pain. *Perceptual and Motor Skills, 61*, 383–390.

Parker, D. A., & Harford, T. C. (1992). Gender-role attitudes, job competition and alcohol consumption among women and men. *Alcoholism: Clinical and Experimental Research, 16*, 159–165.

Pederson, L. L., Poulin, M., Lefcoe, N. M., Donald, A. W., & Hill, J. S. (1992). Does cigarette smoking affect the fitness of young adults? *Journal of Sports Medicine and Physical Fitness, 32*, 96–105.

Perkins, H. W. (1992). Gender patterns in consequences of collegiate alcohol abuse: A 10-year study of trends in an undergraduate population. *Journal of Studies on Alcohol*, *53*, 458–462.

Piani, A., & Schoenborn, C. (1993). Health promotion and disease prevention, United States, 1990. *Vital and Health Statistics*, Series 10, No. 185.

Pierce, J. P., Lee, L., & Gilpin, E. A. (1994). Smoking initiation by adolescent girls, 1944 through 1988: An association with targeted advertising. *Journal of the American Medical Association*, *271*, 608–611.

Plant, M., & Plant, M. (1992). *Risk-takers: Alcohol, drugs, sex and youth*. New York: Tavistock/Routledge.

Poikolainen, K. (1995). Alcohol and mortality: A review. *Journal of Clinical Epidemiology*, *48*, 455–465.

Putukian, M. (1994) The female triad: Eating disorders, amenorrhea and osteoporosis. *Medical Clinics of North America*, *78*, 345–356.

Robbins, A. S., Spence, J. T., & Clark, H. (1991). Psychological determinants of health and performance: The tangled web of desirable and undesirable characteristics. *Journal of Personality and Social Psychology*, *61*, 755–765.

Robbins, C. A., & Martin, S. S. (1993). Gender, styles of deviance, and drinking problems. *Journal of Health and Social Behavior*, *34*, 302–321.

Rolls, B. J., Fedoroff, I. C., & Guthrie, J. F. (1991). Gender differences in eating behavior and body weight regulation. *Health Psychology*, *10*, 133–142.

Rosen, B. N., & Peterson, L. (1990). Gender differences in children's outdoor play injuries: A review and an integration. *Clinical Psychology Review*, *10*, 187–205.

Rossow, I., & Rise, J. (1994). Concordance of parental and adolescent health behaviors. *Social Science and Medicine*, *38*, 1299–1305.

Rost, W., Neuhaus, M., & Florin, I. (1982). Bulimia nervosa: Sex role attitude, sex role behavior, and sex role related locus of control in bulimarexic women. *Journal of Psychosomatic Research*, *26*, 403–408.

Salem, N. (1995). Health insurance coverage and receipt of preventive health services—United States, 1993. *Morbidity and Mortality Weekly Report*, *44*, 219–224.

Schoenborn, C. A. (1988). Health promotion and disease prevention: United States, 1985. *Vital and Health Statistics*, Series 10, No. 163.

Schoenborn, C. A., & Boyd, G. M. (1989). Smoking and other tobacco use: United States, 1987. *Vital and Health Statistics*, Series 10, No. 169.

Spigner, C., Hawkins, W., & Loren, W. (1993). Gender differences in perception of risk associated with alcohol and drug use among college students. *Women and Health*, *20*, 87–97.

Stenberg, B., & Wall, S. (1995). Why do women report "sick building symptoms" more often than men?. *Social Science and Medicine*, *40*, 491–502.

Stephens, T. (1987). Secular trends in adult physical activity: Exercise boom or bust? *Research Quarterly for Exercise and Sport*, *58*, 94–105.

Stephenson, M. G., Levy, A. S., Sass, N. L., & McGarvey, W. E. (1987). 1985 NHIS findings: Nutrition knowledge and baseline data for the weight-loss objectives. *Public Health Reports*, *102*, 61–67.

Svenson, L. W., Jarvis, G. K., & Campbell, R. L. (1994). Gender and age differences in the drinking behaviors of university students. *Psychological Reports*, *75*, 395–402.

U.S. Bureau of the Census. (1993). *Statistical Abstract of the United States: 1993*. Washington DC: U.S. Government Printing Office.

U.S. Department of Health and Human Services. (1994a). *Preventing tobacco use among young people—A report of the Surgeon General*. Office on Smoking and Health, Public Health Service, USDHHS. Washington DC: U.S. Government Printing Office.

U.S. Department of Health and Human Services. (1994b). *Alcohol and health*. Washington DC: U.S. Government Printing Office.

U.S. Department of Transportation. (1993). *Nationwide personal transportation survey: 1990 NPTS databook: Vol. I*. Washington, DC: Federal Highway Administration.

U.S. Department of Transportation. (1994). *Nationwide personal transportation survey: 1990 NPTS databook: Vol. II*. Washington, DC: Federal Highway Administration.

Veevers, J. E., & Gee, E. M. (1986). Playing it safe: Accident mortality and gender roles. *Sociological Focus*, *19*, 349–360.

Verbrugge, L. M. (1985). Triggers of symptoms and health care. *Social Science and Medicine*, *20*, 855–876.

Vitousek, K., & Manke, F. (1994). Personality variables and disorders in anorexia nervosa and bulimia nervosa. *Journal of Abnormal Psychology*, *103*, 137–147.

Wagenaar, A. C., & Wiviott, M. B. T. (1986). Effects of mandating seatbelt use: A series of surveys on compliance in Michigan. *Public Health Reports*, *101*, 505–513.

Waldron, I. (1983). Sex differences in illness incidence, prognosis and mortality: Issues and evidence. *Social Science and Medicine*, *17*, 1107–1123.

Waldron, I. (1988). Gender and health-related behavior. In D. S. Gochman (Ed.), *Health behavior: Emerging research perspectives*. (pp. 193–208). New York: Plenum Press.

Waldron, I. (1991a). Patterns and causes of gender differences in smoking. *Social Science and Medicine*, *32*, 989–1005.

Waldron, I. (1991b). Effects of labor force participation on sex differences in mortality and morbidity. *In* M. Frankenhaeuser, U. Lundberg, & M. Chesney (Eds.), *Women, work, and health: Stress and opportunities* (pp. 17–38). New York: Plenum Press.

Waldron, I. (1995). Contributions of changing gender differences in behavior and social roles to changing gender differences in mortality. In D. Sabo & D. Gordon (Eds.), *Men's health and illness: Gender, power and the body* (pp. 22–45). Thousand Oaks, CA: Sage.

Waldron, I. (in press). Sex differences in infant and early child mortality—Major causes of death and possible biological causes. In *Sex differentials in infant and child mortality*. New York: United Nations.

Waldron, I., Bratelli. G., Carriker, L., Sung, W.-C., Vogeli, C., & Waldman, E. (1988). Gender differences in tobacco use in Africa, Asia, the Pacific and Latin America. *Social Science and Medicine, 27*, 1269-1275.

Waldron, I., Lye, D. & Brandon, A. (1991). Gender differences in teenage smoking. *Women and Health, 17*, 65-90.

Warheit, G. J., Langer, L. M., Zimmerman, R. S., & Biafora, F. A. (1993). Prevalence of bulimic behaviors and bulimia among a sample of the general population. *American Journal of Epidemiology, 137*, 569-576.

Weissfeld, J. L., Kirscht, J. P., & Brock, B. M. (1990). Health beliefs in a population: The Michigan blood pressure survey. *Health Education Ouarterly, 17*, 141-155.

Westermeyer, J. (1988). Sex differences in drug and alcohol use among ethnic groups in Laos, 1965-1975. *American Journal of Drug and Alcohol Abuse, 14*, 443-461.

Whitaker, A., Davies, M., Shaffer, D., Johnson, J., Abrams, S., Walsh, B. T., & Kalikow, K. (1989). The struggle to be thin: A survey of anorexic and bulimic symptoms in a non-referred adolescent population. *Psychological Medicine, 19*, 143-163.

White, C. C., Powell, K. E., Hogelin, G. C., Gentry, E. M., & Forman, M. (1987). The Behavioral Risk Factor Surveys: The descriptive epidemiology of exercise. *American Journal of Preventive Medicine, 3*, 304-310.

Whitehead, P. C., & Ferrence, R. G. (1976). Women and children last. In M. Greenblatt & M. Schuckit (Eds.), *Alcoholism problems in women and children* (pp. 165-191). New York: Grune and Stratton.

Wilsnack, R. W., & Wilsnack, S. C. (1992). Women, work, and alcohol: Failures of simple theories. *Alcoholism: Clinical and Experimental Research, 16*, 172-179.

Zemp, E., & Ackermann-Liebrich, U. (1988). Geschlechtsunterschiede in Gesundheit und Gesundheitsverhalten. *Sozial- und Präventivmedizin, 33*, 186-192.

V

INSTITUTIONAL AND CULTURAL DETERMINANTS

Institutions and the communities of which they are parts have been only minimally investigated as determinants of health behavior, especially in comparison with the number of studies relating to other social entities or social systems. Although health behavior is presumed to be affected by characteristics of non-health-related institutions and of the communities in which the behavior takes place, relatively few studies of such relationships have been reported. (The impact on health behavior of health care institutions such as physicians' offices, hospitals, and professional groupings, is covered systematically in Volume II.) In contrast, culture, which institutions and communities reflect and of which they are integral parts, has been far more widely studied as a determinant of health behavior, particularly by medical anthropologists.

INSTITUTIONAL DETERMINANTS

The term *institutional determinants* refers to factors associated with organizations (or bureaucracies, in the original meaning of the term), namely, those social units that are deliberately planned in order to accomplish certain goals (e.g., Etzioni, 1964). Schools, for example, have the potential for being enabling factors in areas such as dental health. They can offer space for the provision of dental services such as fluoride programs, encourage daily "brush-ins," provide dental screenings, limit the availability of sweets, and make only noncariogenic food options available (Silversin & Coombs, 1981). Although there is a rich literature on school-based health education and health promotion programs (see Chapter 8 by Glanz & Oldenburg and Chapter 14 by Kelder, Lytle, & Edmundson in Volume IV), there is little research linking schools as social and physical environments with health behaviors (in all likelihood reflecting the absence of such enabling features within institutions).

Workplaces also have great potential for determining health behaviors. There is a slowly emerging literature linking workplace characteristics to health behaviors, particularly to risk behaviors. The evidence concerning relationships between workplace characteristics and smoking and alcohol and other drug use remains inconclusive. Some studies (e.g., Mensch & Kandel, 1989) reveal no specific concentration of drug and alcohol users in particular industries and find that job conditions such as complexity and control over work do not consistently contribute much to alcohol and drug use, although there may be some negative linkage between some job characteristics, such as intellectual demands, and smoking. Cole, Berger, and Garrity (1988), on the other hand, showed how organizational environments were related to workplace safety behaviors.

329

In Chapter 16, Eakin examines the way workplace characteristics are related to health behaviors within a political and economic context. In Volume II, Chapter 20, of this *Handbook*, Cohen and Colligan look at workplace characteristics in relation to acceptance of safety behaviors. In Volume IV, Chapter 17 of this *Handbook*, Cole systematically examines the use of narrative representations in workplace safety programs.

COMMUNITY DETERMINANTS

Communities include large numbers of institutions, such as schools, businesses and workplaces, governments and judicial organizations, markets, recreational facilities, and places of worship. Communities also include topographic and geographic features such as parklands, rivers, hills, and woodlands. Although there are an increasing number of community-focused health promotion programs (see Volume IV, Chapter 15, of this *Handbook*, by Schooler & Flora), there are few nonintervention studies linking community characteristics to health behaviors. The results of the few extant studies are inconsistent. A large-scale study of 396 locations in the United Kingdom revealed a minimal community or locational impact on risk behaviors (Duncan, Jones, & Moon, 1993). At the same time, in a study of 15 United States communities, mostly in California, appreciable community variability was observed for smoking, alcohol use, consumption of dietary fat, and use of seat belts (Diehr et al., 1993). These equivocal data suggest the need for further study and for more refined conceptualizations of community and community-level variables.

CULTURAL DETERMINANTS

The selection of materials on the cultural determinants of health behavior as these materials are presented here, reflects the "pattern theory" of culture (e.g., Singer, 1968), which views culture as consisting of explicit or implicit patterns of expected and endorsed behavior, acquired and transmitted by symbols, and constituting the distinctive achievements of human groups. Such patterns include norms; standards for behavior; ideologies; justifications and rationalizations of selected ways of behaving; artifacts; and traditional ideas.

Unfortunately, much research that has been labeled or indexed as cultural or sociocultural is simply demographic. There is, however, a rather small corpus of research that deals with culture in terms more congruent with the broader, "pattern" definition. Moreover, culture permeates other levels of determinants of health behavior. Cultural values, norms, and expectations shape individual belief systems, lifestyles, family interactions, role systems, social organizations, and institutions. The cultural pattern predominant within the United States emphasizes values of optimal health, democracy, individualism, achievement, cleanliness, time, and automation in relation to health behavior and health care (e.g., Leininger, 1990).

To the degree that there are identifiably different pattern systems within a larger system, often associated with different ethnic backgrounds, religions, race, and other demographic characteristics, these smaller systems can be thought of as distinctive subcultures. It is often through observations of subcultural differences that the impact of culture is itself appreciated. The term *cultural*, however, can be understood to embrace subcultural effects.

Saunders (1954) was among the earliest researchers to show how cultural factors impinge on a variety of health-related behaviors. The importance of cultural influences on perspectives of health, illness, and disease is discussed by Gochman (Chapter 1) and Fabrega (Chapter 2). The totality of a culture's beliefs and behaviors related to health, and its sanctioning and organization of healing practices, are referred to as a *health culture*. Other cultural influences can be observed in beliefs that underlie utilization of services and in responses to pain and to signs and symptoms of illness.

Health Culture

A "health culture" has meaning and integrity for its members. Health cultures, moreover, do not exist in isolation from one another. Within the United States, there is ongoing acculturation between the health culture of the larger society and of the ethnic and other subcultural groupings of which it is constructed. Moreover, the bidirectionality of "acculturation" has often been overlooked; elements of pre-Columbian, indigenous health culture, particularly beliefs about herbs and disease prevention, traveled back to Europe and became incorporated in the Eurocentric health culture (Berlinguer, 1992).

Durie's (1985) elaboration of the Maori conception of health leads to an awareness that health pervades the totality of Maori culture. For the Maori, health involves spiritual, mental (psychic), somatic (physical), and family dimensions. The spiritual dimension includes not only religious beliefs, but also beliefs about humans and their needs to be linked spiritually with their environment. The mental dimension embraces styles of thinking that go beyond Western linearity and analysis, and emphasizes holistic and synthetic thought. The somatic dimension extends beyond the traditional Western concern for the body to include concern for ritualized behaviors relating to a variety of bodily functions, particularly to the preparation and eating of food. The family dimension provides the Maori with much of their sense of identity and rootedness. Within the somatic dimension, they have a highly polarized view of activities that involve food preparation and cleanliness, and they maintain beliefs and behaviors that keep these two functions separated. Accordingly, they will perceive a highly sanitized hospital setting with a hidden bedpan or urinal close to the eating tray as *un*-hygienic and hazardous. Moreover, in being so

different from a strictly personal view, such as that found in Western societies, the Maori conception embraces and assigns high priority to community concerns such as pollution of streams and to children's health.

Fabrega and Hunter's (1977, 1978) investigation of the *Ladino* population in a community in Mexico revealed a consistency—or a pattern—in beliefs about how personality and emotional factors contribute to both susceptibility and severity of certain diseases (Fabrega & Hunter, 1978). In other words, a "lay theory" of disease was maintained by members of this culture. Furthermore, there was consistency in the way this population perceived specific diseases to have effects on daily behavior (Fabrega & Hunter, 1977).

A. Kleinman and Sung (1979), in their analysis of the success of "indigenous healers," provided insight into how healing itself must be considered as a part of the entire social system and must be seen as a way of not only controlling the sickness but also providing meaning to the individual's experience of the sickness. Eisenberg and Kleinman (1981), paradoxically, warn against the reverse ethnocentrism involved in "the celebration of the wisdom of *the* folk healer as part of the myth of a Golden Age.... Healing ceremonies can be efficacious, but hardly substitute for anti-biotics or surgery ..." (p. 10).

Young's (1981) decision-tree analysis of nonuse of physicians in a rural Mexican community moved beyond the more typical study of demographic characteristics to relate nonuse to a broader context of cultural beliefs related to the effectiveness of alternative, traditional healers. Young pointed out that the cultural tradition itself is less important than the belief in the effectiveness of a particular curer—for a specific condition. Related to such findings are the observations of Martin, Martinez, Leon, Richardson, and Acosta (1985), who noted the distribution of reports of folk illnesses, e.g., *susto* (trauma, fright), and found that those physicians who reported receiving more such reports were more sensitive in "psychosocial orientations" and were closer to Hispano-Mexican culture.

Hagey's (1984) narrative of the way in which urban Canadian Ojibway Indians view diabetes provided evidence that the illness is viewed as a metaphor in terms of a total cultural phenomenon: It represents concerns about stress, balance, and imbalance and is "personified" in cultural legends about Windigo, a mythological gluttonous figure who represents the Ojibway conception of lack of morality, namely, excess, or lack of balance or harmony.

Another way of viewing "health culture" is provided by Frankle and Heussenstamm's (1974) observations of youth culture and food zealotry, involving vegetarianism, natural and organically grown foods, and Zen macrobiotic diets. Ostrowska's (1983) integration of data related to patient characteristics, perceptions of availability of care, confidence in medical institutions, availability of care alternatives, and other factors, and how these factors were related to responses to illness, formed the basis for her delineation of contemporary Polish health culture. Among her findings was the association between lack of confidence in medical institutions and medical care and delay in seeking such care and resort to self-care.

Weidman (1988) synthesized and amplified the discussion of "health culture" in an extensive analysis of cultural differences in health and medical beliefs and culture-bound syndromes. She identified the important concepts of *emic* (phenomenological, or insider) and *etic* ("objective," or outsider) approaches and the "transcultural perspective" and discussed their implications for health professionals and health institutions.

Health Beliefs and Health Services Utilization

Concepts of cultural patterning were implicit in Suchman's (1965/1972) research on social organization and use of health services, which is discussed in Chapter 13. Farge (1978), for example, was unable to replicate the signifi-

cant linkages between all three of the Suchman medical orientation variables, but did observe a relationship between skepticism of medical care and dependency in illness. Moreover, the few observed linkages between social group and medical orientation variables related to ethnic exclusivity only, and were opposite in direction to Suchman's findings; e.g., high ethnic exclusivity was related to *greater* knowledge of health and disease. Farge argued for the development of a model of Chicano health care, based on Geertsen's model (e.g., Geertsen, Klauber, Rindflesh, Kane, & Gray, 1975), that would include the positive effects on medical orientation of maintaining Mexican cultural traditions in the home and of self-determination.

Berkanovic and Reeder's (1974) review of the literature suggested that cultural factors may selectively determine the psychological cost of using certain services, misfitting expectations and priorities of professionals and consumers, and differences in vulnerability to the "ego assault" of interventions and treatments. These cultural differences were believed to be more important than income in determining utilization of health services.

Berkanovic and Telesky (1985) found that while Mexican-Americans, black Americans, and white Americans do not show differences in reporting of illnesses, days in bed or of restricted activity due to illness, or frequency of seeking medical attention for illnesses, the factors that lead to seeking medical care are different among blacks than among whites and Mexicans. These observations suggest cultural and ethnic variability in the decision processes that underlie utilization.

More recent research on the Mexican-American community (Guendelman & Abrams, 1995) revealed that despite lower socioeconomic status, first-generation Mexican-American women have more healthful nutritional intake than second-generation or white non-Hispanic women. The second-generation women have begun to show acculturation to the larger community. Although these behaviors might be presumed to reflect belief differences, such differences were not examined in the study.

Hoppe and Heller's (1975) study of the Mexican-American cultural value of familism showed that it was not necessarily a barrier to use of scientific medical services, but rather served as a support for coping mechanisms. Moreover, familism was positively related to the timing of prenatal care, although not to use of curative services. More recent research has shown familism to have a positive impact on acceptance of mammography use among Mexican-American women; those women who were "least acculturated"—who were least removed from traditional Mexican values—were the ones most likely to have had a mammogram (Suarez, 1994).

Welch, Comer, and Steinman (1973) explored the effect of cultural beliefs about doctors and health care, social characteristics, and financial factors among Mexican-Americans. Their data suggested that assumptions about the impact of cultural factors on attitudes and use of health care should be questioned. Involvement with Mexican-American culture did not appear to explain as much as did social status and economic factors.

While recently arrived immigrants are less likely to have contact with health providers than are other population groups, when other variables are controlled, data show that after 10 years of residence in the United States, their profiles of health care utilization resemble those of the native-born population (LeClere, Jensen, & Biddlecom, 1994).

Cassel (1957) reported on the way in which cultural beliefs about foods may hinder acceptance of new, improved dietary patterns. For example, although milk had historically been an important part of the diet of the Zulu and other Bantu-speaking peoples of Africa, attempts to restore their milk consumption to healthful levels were impaired by their cultural beliefs about menstruating women coming in contact with milk herds and about drinking milk only from the herd of a kinship group. Other cultural beliefs impeded the introduction of green vegetables

and new grains. Jenny's (1975) observations about cultural conceptions of beauty, which often lead people into painful and traumatic scarification processes, have implications about the acceptability and use of orthodontic services, above and beyond considerations of health and occlusion.

The Appalachian subculture, which is markedly similar to the mainstream North American culture in terms of race, religion, ancestry, and language, differs appreciably in terms of beliefs about health, illness, and treatment (e.g., Hansen & Resick, 1990). Ethnographic evidence, framed by the health belief model, showed that illness was accepted as a cultural norm and that there was appreciable denial of illness coupled with beliefs in fatalism (Hansen & Resick, 1990).

Davis (1984) reported consistent anecdotal evidence that Newfoundland women exhibit a culturally patterned complaint of "nerves." For these women, nerves may mean any number of stresses or complaints. They can elicit concern from others and—with proper etiquette—can be choreographed by a woman to manipulate her friends and family into assuring that she seek care. Davis additionally points out that physicians who are unaware of the meaning of "nerves" will not understand the woman's complaint and will not respond to it appropriately.

Too often, culture and race are used interchangeably in an inappropriate way. Scott's (1974) research carefully avoided the all too prevalent confounding of race, ethnicity, and culture. Her examination of five distinct black ethnic groups all living in close proximity—Bahamian, Cuban, Haitian, Puerto Rican, and southern United States blacks—revealed that they maintained culturally distinct beliefs about health, illness, and health care and used a variety of available health systems, both traditional and "scientific." P. H. Kleinman and Lukoff's (1978) research demonstrated cultural differences in frequency and type of drug use among West Indian blacks, American blacks, and American whites, as well as different sources of influences on drug use.

Strauss's (1976) research, while it confounded economic and class factors with racial identity, nonetheless pointed out differences in perceptions between blacks and whites in the area of dental services. Blacks anticipate to a higher degree than whites that a tooth will be extracted and show more concern for the value of maintaining dental health.

Oller (1984) observed that within Judaism, anything that promotes health is advocated. Moreover, there is no endorsement of risk-taking behavior. Oller also notes that there is an over-concern with pain and symptoms, together with an accepted use of the physician as a way of dealing with stress.

Patrick, Sittampalam, Somerville, Carter, and Bergner (1985) demonstrated a general agreement between British and American respondents in the values attached to aspects of health status, particularly where severe dysfunction was involved. There were some disagreements in areas where dysfunction was minimal.

Uyanga (1983) observed marked differences in conceptions of illness and health, as well as use of health services, between rural and migrant-urban Nigerians. For example, the rural residents were more likely than the migrant-urban residents to attribute illness to anger of the gods or to witchcraft and to use traditional healers who share personal relationships and symbol systems with them. Among the migrant-urban residents, however, when modern hospital treatment fails, traditional healers are sought.

In Chapter 17, Dressler and Oth examine culture and cultural differences in health behaviors within a framework of information exchange and social interaction. Patterns of information exchange are shown to define health and illness and to affect decision making about treatment.

Responses to Pain and to Signs and Symptoms

Zborowski's (1952) seminal analysis of ethnic differences in interpretation of and response to pain in Americans of Jewish, Italian, Irish, and "Yankee" backgrounds was a landmark study in generating research that increased understanding of cultural determinants of health behavior. Greenblum's (1974) study took a critical look at ethnic differences, reexamining Zborowski's conclusions about responses to pain as well as Suchman's (1965/1972) conclusions on the relationship between ethnicity, social status and social integration, and acculturation, and reported that ethnic differences in health behaviors diminish with increasing acculturation and upward social mobility.

Koopman, Eisenthal, and Stoeckle (1984) found that while older Italian-American women were more likely to report pain than older Anglo-American women, this ethnic difference was not observable among younger women or among men. The effects of acculturation are apparently mediated by age and gender. Guttmacher and Ellinson's (1971) observations of how diverse ethnic and religious groups differentially attribute mental illness to personal behaviors that depart from group patterns or subcultural norms shed additional light on the effect of cultural factors in tolerating deviance through medicalizing it.

Medical Pluralism

Durkin-Longley (1984) pointed out that medical pluralism, defined as the "coexistence in one society of divergent medical traditions" (p. 867), is more the norm than the exception in complex societies and that there are regularities in the way the different medical practices are used. Such medical pluralism reflects the cultural pluralism within many such societies. She notes two basic patterns of use: multiple therapeutic use, referring to use of more than one therapeutic system during a single illness, and illness-specific use, referring to use of specific therapies for the treatment of specific disorders. Her analysis of use of healers in Nepal revealed that while patients' reports of why they sought treatment substantiate illness-specific use, their actual behavior was consistent with multiple therapeutic use. Moreover, there was no consensus among respondents about which types of illnesses required which specific therapies. She did observe, however, that patients used multiple therapies to deal with different aspects of chronic conditions, i.e., one healer for medication and another to build strength or to deal with stresses.

REFERENCES

Berkanovic, E., & Reeder, L. G. (1974). Can money buy the appropriate use of services? Some notes on the meaning of utilization data. *Journal of Health and Social Behavior*, *15*, 93-99.

Berkanovic, E., & Telesky. C. (1985). Mexican-American, black-American and white-American differences in reporting illnesses, disability and physician visits for illnesses. *Social Science and Medicine*, *20*, 567-577.

Berlinguer, G. (1992). The interchange of disease and health between the Old and New Worlds. *American Journal of Public Health*, *82*, 1407-1413.

Cassel, J. (1957) Social and cultural implications of food and food habits. *American Journal of Public Health*, *47*, 732-740.

Cole, H. P., Berger, P. K., & Garrity, T. F. (1988). Analogues between medical and industrial safety research on compliance behavior. In D. S. Gochman (Ed.), *Health behavior: Emerging research perspectives* (pp. 337-353). New York: Plenum Press.

Davis, D. L. (1984). Medical misinformation: Communication between outport Newfoundland women and their physicians. *Social Science and Medicine*, *18*, 273-278.

Diehr, P., Koepsell, T., Cheadle, A., Psaty, B. M., Wagner, E., & Curry, S. (1993). Do communities differ in health behaviors? *Journal of Clinical Epidemiology*, *46*, 1141-1149.

Duncan, C., Jones, K., & Moon, G. (1993). Do places matter? A multi-level analysis of regional variations in health-related behaviour in Britain. *Social Science and Medicine*, *37*, 725-733.

Durie, M. H. (1985). A Maori perspective of health. *Social Science and Medicine*, *20*, 483-486.

Durkin-Longley, M. (1984). Multiple therapeutic use in urban Nepal. *Social Science and Medicine*, *19*, 867-872.

Eisenberg, L., & Kleinman, A. (Eds.). (1981). *The relevance of social science for medicine*. Dordrecht, Holland: Reidel.

Etzioni. A. (1964). *Modern organizations*. Englewood Cliffs, NJ: Prentice-Hall.

Fabrega, H., Jr., & Hunter, J. E. (1977). The effects of disease on behavior: Analysis of *Ladino* medical beliefs. *Ethos*, *5*(2), 119-137.

Fabrega, H., Jr., & Hunter, J. E. (1978). Judgements about disease: A case study involving *Ladinos* of Chiapas. *Social Science and Medicine*, *12*, 1-10.

Farge, E. J. (1978). Medical orientation among a Mexican-American population: An old and a new model reviewed. *Social Science and Medicine*, *12*, 277-282.

Frankle, R. T., & Heussenstamm, F. K. (1974). Food zealotry and youth: New dilemmas for professionals. *American Journal of Public Health*, *64*, 11-18.

Geertsen, R., Klauber, M. R., Rindflesh, M., Kane, R. L., & Gray, R. (1975). A re-examination of Suchman's views on social factors in health care utilization. *Journal of Health and Social Behavior*, *16*, 226-237.

Greenblum, J. (1974). Medical and health orientations of American Jews: A case of diminishing distinctiveness. *Social Science and Medicine*, *8*, 127-134.

Guendelman, S., & Abrams, B. (1995). Dietary intake among Mexican-American women: Generational differences and a comparison with white non-Hispanic women. *American Journal of Public Health*, *85*, 20-25.

Guttmacher, S., & Elinson, J. (1971). Ethno-religious variation in perceptions of illness: The use of illness as an explanation for deviant behavior. *Social Science and Medicine*, *5*, 117-125.

Hagey, R. (1984). The phenomenon, the explanations and the responses: Metaphors surrounding diabetes in urban Canadian Indians. *Social Science and Medicine*, *18*, 265-272.

Hansen, M. M., & Resick, L. K. (1990). Health beliefs, health care, and rural Appalachian subcultures from an ethnographic perspective. *Family and Community Health*, *13*(1), 1-10.

Hoppe, S. K., & Heller, P. L. (1975). Alienation, familism and the utilization of health services by Mexican Americans. *Journal of Health and Social Behavior*, *16*, 304-314.

Jenny, J. (1975). A social perspective on need and demand for orthodontic treatment. *International Dental Journal*, *25*, 248-256.

Kleinman, A., & Sung, L. H. (1979). Why do indigenous practitioners successfully heal? *Social Science and Medicine*, *13B*, 7-26.

Kleinman, P. H., & Lukoff, I. F. (1978). Ethnic differences in factors related to drug use. *Journal of Health and Social Behavior*, *19*, 190-199.

Koopman, C., Eisenthal, S., & Stoeckle, J. D. (1984). Ethnicity in the reported pain, emotional distress and requests of medical outpatients. *Social Science and Medicine*, *18*, 487-490.

LeClere, F. B., Jensen, L., & Biddlecom, A. E. (1994). Health care utilization, family context, and adaption among immigrants to the United States. *Journal of Health and Social Behavior*, *35*, 370-384.

Leininger, M. (1990). The significance of cultural concepts in nursing. *Journal of Transcultural Nursing*, *2*(1), 52-59.

Martin, H. W., Martinez, C., Leon, R. L., Richardson, C., & Acosta, V. R. (1985). Folk illnesses reported to physicians in the lower Rio Grande Valley. *Ethnology*, *24*, 229-236.

Mensch, B. S., & Kandel, D. B. (1988). Do job conditions influence the use of drugs? *Journal of Health and Social Behavior*, *29*, 169-184.

Oller, D. T. (1984). Jewish genetic diseases and Jewish illness behavior: A review of selected socio-cultural literature. *Jewish Social Studies, 46,* 177–187.

Ostrowska, A. (1983). Elements of the health culture of Polish society. *Social Science and Medicine, 17,* 631–636.

Patrick, D. L., Sittampalam, Y., Somerville, S. M., Carter, W. B., & Bergner, M. (1985). A cross-cultural comparison of health status values. *American Journal of Public Health, 75,* 1402–1407.

Saunders, L. (1954). *Cultural difference and medical care: The case of the Spanish-speaking people of the Southwest.* New York: Russell Sage Foundation.

Scott, C. S. (1974). Health and healing practices among five ethnic groups in Miami, Florida. *Public Health Reports, 89,* 524–532.

Silversin, J. B., & Coombs, J. A. (1981). Institutions and oral health behavior. *Journal of Behavioral Medicine, 4,* 297–320.

Singer, M. (1968). Culture: The concept of culture. In D. L. Sills (Ed.), *International encyclopedia of the social sciences: Vol. 3* (pp. 527–543). New York: Macmillan & The Free Press.

Strauss, R. P. (1976). Sociocultural influences upon preventive health behavior and attitudes toward dentistry. *American Journal of Public Health, 66,* 375–377.

Suarez, L. (1994). Pap smear and mammogram screening in Mexican-American women: The effects of acculturation. *American Journal of Public Health, 84,* 742–764.

Suchman, E. A. (1965/1972). Stages of illness and medical care. In E. G. Jaco (Ed.), *Patients, physicians and illness: A sourcebook in behavioral science and health* (2nd ed.). New York: Free Press. [Reprinted from *Journal of Health and Human Behavior,* 1965, *6,* 114–128.]

Uyanga, J. (1983). Rural–urban migration and sickness/health care behaviour: A study of eastern Nigeria. *Social Science and Medicine, 17,* 579–583.

Weidman, H. H. (1988). A transcultural perspective on health behavior. In D. S. Gochman (Ed.), *Health behavior: Emerging research perspectives* (pp. 261–280). New York: Plenum Press.

Welch, S., Comer, J., & Steinman, M. (1973). Some social and attitudinal correlates of health care among Mexican-Americans. *Journal of Health and Social Behavior, 14,* 205–213.

Young, J. C. (1981). Non-use of physicians: Methodological approaches, policy implications, and the utility of decision models. *Social Science and Medicine, 15B,* 499–507.

Zborowski, M. (1952). Cultural components in responses to pain. *Journal of Social Issues, 8*(4), 16–30.

16

Work-Related Determinants of Health Behavior

Joan M. Eakin

Among the external influences that shape us, the work we do is probably the most powerful one in adult life.

—Frankenhaeuser (1991, p. 49)

Work is of core significance to human experience generally (Erikson & Vallas, 1990), and has been a major focus of inquiry in the social sciences. This chapter explores what is known about the impact of work specifically on behavior related to health. In what way does one's occupation and the physical and social circumstances in which one works affect perceptions, attitudes, beliefs, and actions regarding health?

First, the concepts of "work" and "health behavior" used in this chapter are outlined. The literature linking work and health behavior is then described and discussed. Finally, findings from two empirical studies of health and safety behavior in small workplaces are used to illus-

Joan M. Eakin • Department of Behavioural Science, Faculty of Medicine, University of Toronto, Toronto, Ontario M5S 1A8, Canada.

Handbook of Health Behavior Research I: Personal and Social Determinants, edited by David S. Gochman. Plenum Press, New York, 1997.

trate and make concrete the major points raised in the review.

DEFINITIONS AND CONCEPTS

Figure 1 presents a conceptual schema for considering the impact of work on health behavior. This framework is not intended as a comprehensive classification or explanatory map, but as a heuristic device for demonstrating different conceptual levels and dimensions of work, and the regions of health behavior for which they may have consequence.

Health Behavior

In this chapter, behavior is defined broadly to include cognitions (attitudes, conceptions, beliefs) and actions. Health behavior refers to individual cognitions and actions that are related to the improvement, maintenance, and restoration of health. Notably, the definition includes behavior that is *emic* (behavior that individuals consciously direct toward or recognize as related to their own health) and *etic* (behavior that external observers believe is related to health, regard-

Work

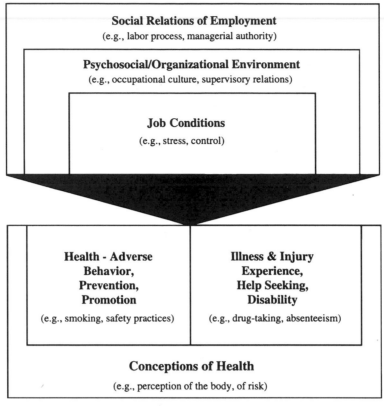

Figure 1. Dimensions of work and health behavior.

less of the awareness or motivation of the behaver). This distinction is captured in Kickbusch's (1988) differentiation between "health-directed" and "health-related" behavior (Kickbusch, 1988). With the breadth of current definitions of health (e.g., physical, mental, and social well-being, not just the absence of disease or disability [World Health Organization, 1946]) and its determinants (e.g., the "social determinants of health" framework [Ottawa Charter for Health Promotion, 1986]), almost all human behavior might qualify as health behavior. On the other hand, to limit the discussion to deliberate health-directed behavior would be to ignore behavior that is known to affect health adversely but that may not be motivated by health considerations (e.g., smoking).

This chapter does not try to resolve this particular conceptual problem, but considers health behavior to mean behavior that is believed, by either the behaver or the observer, to affect health.

Figure 1 conveys three facets of health behavior. First are conceptions, attitudes, and beliefs regarding health in general, including definitions and representations of health and perceptions of the body. Second is behavior related to prevention and promotion, including the perception of risk. Health-adverse activities, such as risk taking, are also included here. The third facet of health behavior concerns illness, injury, and disability, including perception of and responses to symptoms and disorder, help seeking, the experience of illness and injury, recovery, and rehabilitation.

These groups of health behaviors, of course, overlap conceptually; they are separated here only to demonstrate the range of health behaviors on which work can have influence.

Work

The concept of work has most commonly referred to paid employment, although more recently the notion has been extended to include unpaid labor such as child care and domestic activities. This chapter addresses work only as paid employment.

Work is a general conceptual domain comprised of many interrelated dimensions. Figure 1 includes levels of analysis ranging from relatively concrete job conditions to the psychosocial and organizational environment to the social relations of employment in the society more generally. The most tangible level is that of the job: its material nature, the physical and psychological demands of the task or product, the technology, the immediate arrangement of the work process. At a more abstract level is the organizational dimension of work: its occupational structure, division of labor, managerial hierarchy, supervisory practices, reward system, organizational culture, and unionization. Broader still are the social relations of production, including employment relations and the labor process. Both the concrete and the organizational aspects of work are shaped by these more general relations of employment.

Given these very broad notions of health behavior and work, the next step is to identify how the various aspects of work might influence the various forms of health behavior.

IMPACT OF WORK ON HEALTH BEHAVIOR

We have every reason in the world to think, for example, that taking drugs and drinking too much and sinking into a kind of numbed depression are correlated with alienating work conditions.
—Erikson and Vallas (1990, p. 32)

Despite these authors' confident "every rea-son," assembling and assessing what is known about work as a determinant of health behavior is a challenging undertaking. There is no clearly defined research or scholarly field focused on the relationship between work and behavior related to health. Although there is much literature on the behavioral implications of work, occupations, and organizations, it is scattered across many disciplines, such as sociology, organizational behavior, labor studies, and industrial psychology. Further, while some of the behavior studied could be considered health behavior as the terms are defined here, the analytical problem is rarely framed in these generic terms. In addition to making relevant literature hard to locate (e.g., health behavior is not used as a key word), disciplinary isolation and conceptual variation inhibit collective development of the topic.

On the other hand, however, knowledge of the impact of work on health behavior can often be extracted from literature that does not identify the research problem in such terms. For example, L. Jackson, Highcrest, and Coates's (1992) study of sex practices among street prostitutes was not conceptualized in terms of work, but it reveals several aspects of sex trade work that affect risk-taking behavior (e.g., condom use was influenced by the ambiguity and unpredictability of work in certain locales, such as in cars). Mining such relevant literature broadens our perspective on the topic (but finding it can be serendipitous).

Although there is much literature on the determinants of health behavior, occupational and workplace determinants are rarely addressed (Mullen, 1992). Epidemiological literature shows that certain health behaviors (e.g., drinking) are more or less prevalent in particular occupations (Olkinuora, 1984; Shore & Peiri, 1992). Although this research is suggestive, it seldom illuminates what the work-related determinants might be. In other instances, particular occupational groups are selected for study of health behaviors, but selection of an employee sample appears to be primarily for methodological reasons (access to an adult population, control for sociodemographic variables), and the influence of work or occupation on the behaviors under investigation is not explored per se. Furthermore, in many instances, occupational variations in health behaviors cannot be straightforwardly attributed to the nature of the work because occupation is so confounded with gender and class (Casswell & Gordon, 1984; Ganster & Schaubroeck, 1991).

Even literature focused directly on behavior that occurs in the workplace makes surprisingly little reference to the work-relatedness of the behaviors being examined. For example, in the fields of workplace health promotion and occupational health and safety, studies of health behavior emphasize personal determinants rather than the nature of the work environment (Daykin, 1990). An example of this is Lebovits' study of smoking behavior among asbestos workers, in which explanation was sought in personal employee attributes, with no reference to the potential contributory role of working conditions (Lebovits & Strain, 1990).

The literature that explicitly links work and health behavior often tends to treat the latter as the independent rather than the dependent variable. That is, health behavior is viewed as the determinant of work-related outcomes rather than vice versa. An example is the extensive research on the implications of employee alcohol and drug use for work productivity and performance (e.g., Manning, Keeler, Newhouse, Sloss & Wasserman, 1991; Rice, Kelman, Miller, & Dunmeyer, 1990).

In sum, the occupational and workplace determinants of health behavior have not been widely explored, and it is necessary to piece together fragments of relevant knowledge from widely diverse literatures. Examples of the literature will be provided here to illustrate the nature and range of relationships suggested in Figure 1. The review will start with concrete job conditions and then proceed to consider more abstract organizational and structural aspects of work. Within each level, examples will include the various forms of health-related behavior.

Job Conditions

A variety of job characteristics or features of the work task have been found to influence health-related behavior. Two themes are particularly common in the literature: job stress and job control.

Job stress is widely understood to be an important determinant of physical and mental health (Frankenhaeuser, Lundberg, & Chesney, 1991; Quick, Murphy, & Hurrell, 1992). It is the subject of an extensive and rapidly growing field of research that cuts across many disciplines and professions (Ganster & Schaubroeck, 1991). Although the emphasis has been on its implications for health status, job stress has also been linked to various health-related behaviors. For example, inability to stop smoking was associated with higher levels of occupational stress (Kalimo, 1987), heavy smoking was more frequent among workers in high-strain jobs (Green & Johnson, 1990), and participation in a worksite exercise program was more likely among employees who were experiencing job stress (Davis, Jackson, Kronenfeld, & Blair, 1987).

In such research, the interest in job stress lies primarily in its consequences rather than in its causes. Elsewhere, however, job stress and health behavior are linked with particular working conditions. For example, Caplan, Cobb, French, Harrison, and Pinneau (1975) compared the job characteristics of assembly-line and continuous-process workers and found that smoking was more prevalent among those whose abilities were being underused and who were in monotonous and repetitive jobs. In Johansson, Johnson, and Hall's (1991) survey of Swedish men and women, smoking and sedentary behavior were associated with certain job characteristics (psychological demands, physical load, hazardous exposures, monotony, shiftwork and piecework) and with work resources (personal freedom, learning opportunities, control over the work process, extent of social interaction). Although the findings were generally in the expected direction (job demands associated with unhealthy behavior and job resources with healthy behavior), patterns of association were different for smoking and sedentary behavior, as well as for men and women. In this and other work, job stress is assumed (although not always explicitly) to be the mechanism whereby working conditions are linked to health-related behavior.

The nature of the job has also been associated with behavior related to illness, injury, and use of health care services. Individuals in jobs characterized by monotonous, repetitive tasks, interpersonal conflict, high production demands, and low levels of autonomy have been found to have higher rates of sick leave (Frankenhaeuser & Johansson, 1986; Karasek, Gardell, & Lindell, 1987), to take more tranquilizers and sleeping pills (Billette & Piche, 1987; Karasek et al., 1987), to make greater use of the company dispensary (Caplan et al., 1975), to underreport minor injuries incurred on the job (Wrench & Lee, 1982), and to be more susceptible to "sick building syndrome" (Boxer, 1990) and to workplace health problems considered by some to be "mass psychogenic illness" (Colligan & Murphy, 1979).

Although these studies include a range of different indicators of job conditions, a cluster of indicators—primarily monotony, low skill, and low autonomy—appear repeatedly and are most consistently found to have health-related outcomes. The notion of *job control* captures many of these characteristics and has become a core concept in the field of occupational health (Sauter, Hurrell, & Cooper, 1989). Job control refers to the nature and amount of discretion workers have over their jobs, including their ability to influence the volume, speed, and terms of their work. Job control is the conceptual centerpiece of the influential "control–demand" model of workplace health (Karasek & Theorell, 1990). This model proposes that employee health status is compromised in work situations marked by low control over work (low autonomy regarding task activities), high psychological demands (high expectations, time constraints), and low social support from coworkers and supervisors. Most of the research conducted in this tradition has focused on health status outcomes of job control, with limited exploration of how health behavior may mediate the relationship between job control and mortality and morbidity.

Smoking, alcohol use, and exercise have been the main behaviors linked to low job con-trol, probably because of their association with coronary heart disease, the health status outcome widely used in this research. For example, there is evidence that employees in positions with low decision latitude (i.e., little control over the work process) are more passive in their non-working lives than those with more discretion over their work (Gardell, 1982). Individuals in low-control jobs are more likely to smoke (Marmot & Theorell, 1991; Karasek et al., 1987), less likely to engage in health practices such as exercising (Allison & Coburn, 1985), and less likely to participate in community activities (Meissner, 1971).

Evidence of the consequences of work for nonwork health behavior is not consistent. Abel, Cockerham, Lueschen, and Kunz's (1989) study of the "spillover effect" (as the impact of work on nonwork behavior is often called) found that measures of self-direction in American men were not associated with smoking, dietary practices, exercise, or seeking medical checkups. High control over work was not related to preventive health behavior (Coburn & Pope, 1974). Contradictory findings regarding spillover effects of control over work may stem from the possibility, as Abel et al. (1989) suggested, that certain health behaviors have become normative and cross class and occupational boundaries. Alternatively, class may be more important than occupation as a determinant of health behavior (Casswell & Gordon, 1984; Johansson et al., 1991). It is also possible that inconsistent findings may arise from differing conceptualizations of control. Aronsson (1989) noted that the concept can refer to control over or control within a situation or to such varied notions as predictability, participation, or influence over outcomes.

Less research has been devoted to linking job control and explicitly occupational health behavior, such as workers' self-protective behavior at work (e.g., compliance with safety regulations) or efforts to address occupational health problems (e.g., exercising legal rights, health activism). James (1987) found that workers' perceptions of danger, acceptance of risks, and informal coping strategies (e.g., "spelling" or helping out coworkers) varied by job task and by the degree of autonomy workers had over their work. S. Jackson (1989) found that workers with greater job control tended to use problem-solving, proactive strategies for dealing with occupational stress, rather than emotion-focused, reactive strategies.

The pathways between various working conditions, occupational stress, and various behavioral outcomes are frequently conceived in terms of coping; i.e., health-related behaviors are seen as coping strategies for dealing with stressful working conditions (e.g., S. Jackson, 1989; James, 1987; Mullen, 1992). Mullen's qualitative study of health behavior among Glaswegian men is an example. One way in which workers responded to the stresses and strains of their jobs, particularly boredom and time constraints, was through "compensatory coping," such as drinking and smoking. The author called these health behaviors "self-contradictory" because they were used to limit the negative health effects of occupation, but were themselves health-damaging. Kristensen (1991) noted a similar contradiction in a study of sickness absence among Danish slaughterhouse workers. Absence appeared to be an individual coping strategy for dealing with job strain, but the author suggested that this behavior can serve to sustain health-damaging working conditions insofar as it does not address the sources of job strain.

In sum, job conditions—particularly job control—are seen to influence levels of occupational stress, which in turn have been linked to a range of health behaviors, particularly smoking and drinking and sickness absence. These health behaviors are frequently conceived as coping with job stress, although coping is generally viewed as a function of individual style not necessarily related to the work environment.

Psychosocial and Organizational Environment

In addition to the more tangible conditions of work, health-related behavior is associated with the psychosocial and organizational environment, the organizational and group process dimensions of work. Two aspects of this environment are illustrated here: occupational culture and supervisory relations.

Individual health-related behavior is frequently observed to reflect occupational culture, or group norms and practices. There is considerable evidence, for example, of a "drinking culture" in various occupations. Applebaum's (1981) anthropological study of working life in the construction industry suggested how drinking was core to coworker solidarity and was even part of the process of securing work assignments. Ames and James (1987) also found that the social organization of work and the evolution of a drinking culture were associated with a high level of alcohol use among blue-collar workers, particularly those with family difficulties outside of work. Attitudes and practices regarding diet, smoking, and exercise have also been associated with occupational culture (Mullen, 1992). Group norms were also invoked by Green and Johnson (1990) to account for smoking cessation behavior among chemical workers, particularly the unexpected finding that a higher level of coworker social support was associated with a lower likelihood of smoking cessation among older workers.

Work group culture has also been linked to occupational health behavior. It is argued that group life and social support in work subcultures shape the discourse of health, including how workers define situations of threat and danger and how they formulate strategies for coping and change (Johnson, 1989; Nelkin & Brown, 1984). In his field study of hospital workers' perceptions of radiation hazards on the job, Rayner (1986) identified four organizational cultures or "contexts," each with its own rationality concerning risk. For example, staff in a "competitive–individualist" context (e.g., medical specialists) tended to view the risk of radiogenic harm as a legitimate risk to be accepted in return for the autonomy and financial and status rewards of specialist practice, and drew their confidence from a sense of personal control. This behavior contrasted with that of staff working in a "bureaucratic" context (e.g., administrators, technicians), whose confidence was derived from the routinization of risk and careful adherence to established procedures. Trust in management and confidence in institutional procedures varied among the groups, reflecting their different positions in the hierarchy and experience of team membership.

Like location in the organizational hierarchy, work group dynamics have also been related to health behavior. Haas's (1977) study of risk taking among high-rise steel construction workers found that safety-related practices were influenced by strong group norms. For example, denial of fear functioned to preserve group solidarity and foster mutual self-protection among the workers. Similar cultural norms regarding risk taking were observed in Duclos' (1987) study of "group consensus" on risk and denial strategies among chemical workers and Brewer's (1990) exploration of vocabularies of danger and risk in the police force. The influence of occupational culture on health behavior is also evident in the applied literature (although it is often not labeled in this way). For example, Zohar's (1980) study of a training program for increasing the use of ear protectors on the job suggested that initial behavior change was sustained by "group norms."

Another theme in the work organization literature is the influence on health behavior of supervisory relations in the workplace. An absence of supervision, for example, has been associated with problem drinking (Trice & Roman, 1972) and with occupational self-protective practices (Dwyer, 1981). Conversely, too much supervision in the form of pressure to produce and performance monitoring has been observed to legitimate and encourage hazardous work practices (Nichols, 1975) and, as seen earlier, to affect health through reducing workers' control over the work process.

Perceived support from one's boss or supervisor has been associated with a variety of other health-related behaviors. Use of sleeping pills and tranquilizers was greater among women managers reporting unsupportive bosses than among those who felt supported (Greenglass, 1985). Participation in a worksite health promotion program was more likely among employees reporting supervisory supportiveness (Sloan & Gruman, 1988). Absenteeism and use of medical services for children's illnesses among single working mothers was related to their assessment of their bosses' flexibility and empathy (Semchuk & Eakin, 1989).

Relations with coworkers may also influence employee health behavior. Dodier's (1985) study of a mostly white-collar French workplace viewed the taking of sick leave as a response to processes of "moral evaluation" from coworkers and supervisors. Sickness claims were legitimated on the basis of implicit, nonmedical assessments related to the sick person's age, occupation, past behavior, and the "microculture" at the workplace. Rules of conduct concerning sickness absence were tied to social control mechanisms in the workplace and functioned to sustain key social relationships at work. Bellaby's (1990) analysis of sickness absence in an English pottery factory drew out the gender, age, and class relations that underlie coworkers' and managers' evaluation of sick role behavior. Ambiguities in these relations, power associated with work discipline, and worker resistance are "reproduced in the negotiation of genuine sickness" (Bellaby, 1990, p. 47).

In sum, work organization—exemplified here in terms of supervisory relations and occupational group culture—has implications for health and illness behavior. Notions of legitimacy and group solidarity are key in many analyses.

Social Relations of Employment

The term *social relations of employment* refers to the ideologies, assumptions, and structural forces that, explicitly or otherwise, underlie systems of production and the labor process. The two previously discussed dimensions of work—job conditions and psychosocial and organizational environment—produce and are produced by these broader relations of work. Literature that formulates the work–health behavior relationship in terms of the more general social relations of employment is considered here.

Health behavior can be viewed as a cultural phenomenon embedded in practical everyday experience and the broader social and political context (Crawford, 1984; Douglas & Wildavsky, 1982). From this perspective, health behavior is constituted in daily work experience and in the social relations of employment. The relation between work and the body, for example, has been conceived in this way. Boltanski (1976) and others (e.g., Surault, 1979) noted the links between manual labor and body perception and management. Boltanski wrote of a "somatic culture" among lower-class French workers that is associated with the physical nature of their work and that fosters a restricted awareness of the body and of its capacities. In their study of images of health among French workers, d'Houtaud and Field (1984) proposed that those who do manual work tend to perceive their health only in terms of their labor and are "alienated" from their own health.

Pierret (1988) suggested that workers' conceptions of health and illness were related to their position in the system of production and their "representational frameworks" for handling the relations between themselves and society. In her research, workers' understanding of and response to health issues were related to their working conditions and power in the workplace. Workers with unskilled and insecure jobs saw sickness as unpredictable and largely unpreventable; consequently, their interest in health was primarily framed in terms of access to health services rather than prevention.

The relationship between work and health has also been approached from the perspective of labor process theory. In this research, the effort has been to identify how behaviors are related to the central themes of labor–capital conflict, the commodification of labor, and the structures of control and compliance in the

workplace (Dwyer, 1991; James, 1987; Quinlan, 1988). As Quinlan (1988, p. 195) wrote:

> [Workplace stressors are dealt with in] a fragmented or taxonomic fashion which belies a broad understanding of power structure and dominant value systems within the workplace and industry.

An assertion of this literature is that the market capitalist mode of production sets the fundamental context in which health-related behavior can be understood. Workers sell their labor and are expected to accept management's prerogative to control this labor. Although they have become important objects of labor negotiation, health issues remain fundamentally subordinate to the need for corporate profit. Consideration of the health of workers is often in direct contradiction to capital accumulation.

In such a context, health claims are necessarily problematic—a key point in understanding health behavior in the workplace. The issue of legitimacy is, of course, central to illness behavior more generally (Gerhardt, 1989; Parsons, 1975), but is magnified in the context of employment, where work discipline, productivity, and rights to compensation are at issue.

The problem of legitimacy and suspicion of malingering in work-related illness behavior is illustrated in Reid, Ewan, and Lowy's (1991) study of the experience of help-seeking among women with the controversial occupational disorder repetitive strain injury. The skepticism of coworkers, employers, and medical personnel regarding the validity of these women's disorder appeared to produce illness behavior (e.g., demonstrating the existence of their pain and inability to work) that, the authors proposed, contributed to their suffering and inhibited recovery. In a study of the experience of occupational back injury, Tarasuk and Eakin (1994) suggested that rehabilitation and return to work may be impeded by workers' perception that their supervisors doubted the validity of their suffering and need for time off work.

The social relations of employment also

shape perception and management of risk. Nelkin and Brown's (1984) interviews with workers employed in hazardous occupations pointed to the way in which workers' perspectives on risk are framed by the terms and conditions of the employment relationship. Workers made trade-offs between their health and their jobs, particularly in relation to issues of financial incentives, job security, and career advancement.

Sickness and injury absenteeism have also been related to the social relations of employment. In a study of sickness absences in a Finnish metal factory, Virtanen (1994) found that absences and use of health services were sharply reduced during a time of threatened layoffs. The author took an "interactionalist" perspective on health behavior, viewing sickness absences as intersubjectively and situationally construed social activity.

Sickness absenteeism is also viewed in terms of the social relations of production in the literature that construes illness and injury absenteeism as "restrictive labor practices" (James, 1987) or as a mode of industrial conflict (e.g., as an alternative to strikes) (Quinlan, 1988). This literature takes the clear position that occupational health behavior is best understood, not as an individualized psychological response, but as a function of the power structure in the workplace and of dominant value systems regarding employment and managerial prerogative.

Summary

In sum, despite the lack of a clearly defined field of research, there is considerable literature that speaks to the impact of work on health behavior. Although differentiated for purposes of this chapter, the various levels of work are nested within each other, and certain concepts are relevant to more than one level. Job control, for example, can refer to characteristics of specific work tasks or procedures, or to much more abstract features of the work, such as predictability, or participation in corporate decision making.

Occupational culture is a feature of workplace organization, but it reproduces the broader power relations of work.

The range of health behaviors linked to work is narrow, with much attention being devoted to lifestyle health behaviors, coping, and sickness absenteeism. Less is known about how work affects occupational health behaviors, especially behaviors related to workplace change or collective action. Many aspects of work have been associated with health behavior, although the literature focuses more on job conditions and the psychosocial and organizational environment than on the structural and ideological features of work. Job stress, job control, group norms and occupational culture, supervisory relations, and the nature of power and authority vested in the employment relationship have been linked in various ways with workers' perception of risk, self-protective practices, and illness behavior.

ETIOLOGICAL, POLITICAL, AND GENDER ISSUES

Several issues cross-cut the various aspects of work and types of health behavior addressed in the literature: the issue of where the source of the behavior is located (etiological stance), the issue of ideological position (political stance), and the issue of gender.

Etiological Stance

A primary distinction between the different levels of work illustrated in this chapter is etiological perspective. How far "upstream," to use McKinlay's (1994) classic analogy, are the determinants of behavior to be located? In the immediate physical working environment? In the way work is organized and behavior controlled? In the broader societal power relations and ideology that govern employment?

The particular case of repetitive strain injury (RSI) provides a useful contemporary illustration of the different etiological stances that can be taken on the work–health behavior relationship. RSI generally refers to ailments characterized by progressively debilitating pain in the arms and upper body. Its incidence has risen dramatically in the last decade among both blue- and white-collar workers, particularly among women (Ireland, 1992). RSI is marked by clinical uncertainty, an absence of physiological markers, and controversy over its cause, treatment, and prognosis (Ireland, 1992).

It is widely agreed that RSI involves musculoskeletal disorder related to overuse through repetitive movements. Some researchers accept the organic reality of the problem, account for it in terms of the physical demands of work, and seek ergonomic solutions (e.g., more appropriate design of tools and work spaces) (McDermott, 1986). Others, while not denying that physical demands may be the immediate cause of the disorder, prefer to account for the problem in terms of the forces that produce the specific working conditions: specialization, mechanization, and productivity-centered management practices driven by changing technology and the capitalist labor process (Williams, 1985). Other researchers perceive RSI as a more complex behavioral phenomenon that arises from social, psychological, and organizational dislocation. RSI is seen as a condition that arises from and is aggravated by work environments marked by conflictful labor relations, alienation, lack of power, a gendered division of labor, and access to compensation (Bammer & Martin, 1992; Deves & Spillane, 1989). Symptom experience and help-seeking behavior are influenced by the suspicion of fraud and illegitimacy bred of the inherent conflict of corporate/capital and worker interests (Reid & Reynolds, 1990). RSI-related behavior—from preventive activity to recovery—becomes an expression of and metaphor for current strains in the social relations of production.

The etiological stance of the literature is on the whole relatively downstream, in the eddies of occupational culture and organizational stress. Recognition of the structural and ideological dimensions of health-related behavior occurs more frequently in the literature of the 1990s, reflecting increased sociological input into occupational health and perhaps a post-industrial concern with institutional "embedded" power.

Political Stance

The literature on work and health behavior can also be differentiated by political stance, particularly its labor–management orientation and its assumptions about the nature and significance of work and health.

Much of the relevant literature reveals a managerialist perspective—as is evident, for example, in the type of health behavior that is selected for research. Behaviors that have import for the achievement of organizational goals are the ones that tend to be investigated. The extensiveness of the literature on employee drinking, drug use, and sickness and injury absenteeism perhaps reflects this managerial orientation, as does the prevalence of "victim-blaming" conceptualizations of work-related health behavior, such as accident proneness, carelessness, ignorance, machismo, and malingering (Quinlan, 1988).

A managerialist stance is also suggested by the discourse itself. For example, the same employee behavior is labeled "counterproductivity" in one study (Jones & Boye, 1992) and "resistance" in another (Jermier, Knights, & Nord, 1994). The former is framed from the point of view of organizational management, the latter more from the employees' perspective. The notion of absenteeism, to take another example, has the employment relationship as its point of reference, rather than the significance of the behavior for the employee.

The concepts of management support and organizational climate are frequently used variables for explaining health-related behavior. A supportive environment fostered by management is viewed as a positive force that encourages health-promoting practices among employees (Lovato & Green, 1990). From a different political stance, however, a supportive environment can be seen as a manipulative extension of corporate managerial control into the nonwork lives of employees (Conrad & Walsh, 1992).

A generalized mangerialist posture toward health behavior may account for the relative emphasis on downstream explanations of health behavior. Labor-oriented studies are likely to emphasize working conditions and structural forces (e.g., piecework, time pressures) as determinants of health behavior, while management-oriented research is more likely to focus on individual attributes and traits (e.g., lack of knowledge, coping ability). It is also possible that a managerialist posture toward health behavior contributes more generally to the relative scarcity of research on work as a determinant of health behavior.

Gender Issues

Work-related health behavior is widely noted to vary by sex. It remains unclear, however, whether and how this behavior reflects different working conditions or gendered responses to similar working conditions.

There is evidence that men and women do different jobs. They are highly segregated into different occupations (Armstrong & Armstrong, 1993; Heaney, 1993) and have different kinds and amounts of control over their work (Hall, 1991). Much less recognized is that even within the same job categories or occupations, women have different responsibilities and tasks (Messing, Dumais, & Romito, 1993; Statham, 1993) and shoulder different unpaid workloads (Frankenhaeuser, 1991). As Hall (1991, p. 98) put it, women and men "inhabit relatively distinct occupational universes." Failure to examine differences in the work and work environment of men and women may lead researchers to inappropriately attribute sex differences to gender-related health behavior.

There is also evidence to suggest that women experience work differently than do men and that this difference has corresponding implications for their work-related health behavior. For example, women and men have been found to appraise occupational risks and hazards differently. Daykin (1990) suggested that women do not identify with prevailing "masculinized" conceptions of workplace hazards and do not always recognize, or define as occupational, such work hazards as violence and sexual harassment. This viewpoint may reflect the fact that women are socialized into an occupational health discourse that has been derived from studies that do not include women or examine women's jobs (Messing, 1993–1994). It has been noted, for example, that women differ from men in their response to lack of control and monotony (Johansson et al., 1991) and to occupational stress (Statham, 1993). This difference may reflect the fact that the conceptualization and operationalization of job control may not capture the way women understand the term or the specific contingencies of women's occupational circumstances (Heaney, 1993).

Gender differences in health behavior may also stem from different role expectations of men and women. Bellaby (1990) found substantial differences between men and women in a factory setting in terms of their response to pain and to stress at work. When asked about the "bad" aspects of work, men mentioned supervisors "getting on their backs" (i.e., autonomy), while women thought first of the work environment, often the health and safety aspect (i.e., working conditions). Men sought to exert mental control over their bodies in order to sustain performance at work and offer more resistance to the harmful invasion of their bodies by the work environment; women sought instead to fend off the dangers of their hostile physical surroundings. Gender was central in the negotiation of whether or not and under what terms sickness and absence were considered acceptable in the work-group. Domestic obligations, for example, were a compelling legitimator of work absence for women, but not for men.

A curious sexist undertone seems to characterize some of the research on gender issues in work-related health behavior. For example, there is some suggestion that there is a confluence of the absence of organic pathology, the suspicion of "psychosocial origins," and the acknowledgment of gender issues. For example, the fact that disorders such as RSI, sick building syndrome, and stress are more prevalent among women (Hedge, Erikson, & Rubin, 1992; Steinberg & Wall, 1995) has spawned diagnoses of hysterical contagion and somaticization. It is interesting that when there is no measurable pathology and women are the primary sufferers, symptoms are likely to be deemed "behavioral" or psychosomatic. When determined as a "behavioral" issue, problems tend to be viewed as personal (individual sensitivity, coping style), rather than social (arising from gendered social relations in the workplace).

Summary

In sum, in terms of etiological and political stance, the literature tends to be concerned primarily with the social–psychological and organizational determinants of health behavior. The underexploration of the broader sociological forces that impinge on such behavior may be associated in part with a certain mangerialist bias in the research process. The literature raises a number of gender issues, including the suggestion that women's health behavior is not affected by work in the same way as is men's. Pursuit of this question will require disentangling gendered differences in health behavior from the gendered division of labor.

The links between work and health behavior have been treated thus far on a general level. To provide some specific and concrete illustration of these links, the last part of the chapter considers selected findings from the author's research on health behavior in small workplaces.

HEALTH BEHAVIOR IN SMALL BUSINESSES

Two ethnographic studies of health and working life in small businesses offer empirical examples of how responses to workplace health problems and issues are affected by work at the job, organization, and labor process levels.

Background and Methods

About one third of the Canadian labor force works in businesses with fewer than 50 employees (Thompson, 1995). The small-business sector consists predominantly of industrial and service enterprises, including retail trade, construction and repair, restaurants, dry cleaners, printing, manufacturing, social service agencies, and the like. Compared to larger enterprises, small businesses are likely to have, on average, employees with lower levels of skill and education, lower pay, higher rates of part-time work, limited benefits, multifunction job categories, and low rates of unionization (Armstrong, 1991). The failure rate of new businesses is very high, and financial marginality and instability are major problems for many enterprises. Small firms are more likely to include family members, immigrants, young entry-level workers, and women (Curran & Stallworth, 1979; Messite & Welch, 1987). Particularly in the smallest enterprises (fewer than 20 employees), there are few if any supervisory- or management-level employees other than the owner. Thus, many owners fulfill all managerial functions themselves, including pitching in when necessary on the shop floor, and employees often do a little bit of everything.

In terms of health and safety, small businesses have higher rates of injury and ill health (MacKinnon, 1987; Rutsohn, Schoolfield, & McLeod, 1981; Thomas, 1991), are disproportionately engaged in certain high-hazard industries (MacKinnon, 1987), and have numerous health and safety problems (A.R.A. Consultants, 1987; Spiegel & Yassi, 1989; Tuskes & Key, 1988). Yet small businesses are widely considered hard to reach in terms of prevention and change.

To understand the context of such health problems, a series of studies were undertaken by the author. Findings from two of these studies are drawn upon in this discussion, one focusing on the owners and managers of small enterprises (*N* = 53 [Eakin, 1992]), the other on employees (*N* = 39 [Eakin, unpublished]). The data consist of transcripts from in-depth ethnographic interviews with individuals working in many different types of small-business settings. The interviews explored the nature of working life (e.g., physical and organizational environment, the labor process, relations with coworkers and employers/ employees) and health and safety experiences, perceptions, and practices (perception of risk, prevention activities, occupational illness/injury experience). Both studies attempted to understand and explain occupational health behavior in relation to its organizational and interactional context. The data presented here are representative of the data sets upon which the analysis was based and are in the form of verbatim excerpts from the transcripts (in which the emphases are the author's).

Small-Business Owners: "Leaving It Up to the Workers"

Owners understood the concept of workplace health primarily in terms of the personal behavior of their employees (e.g., carelessness, wearing self-protective equipment). As an electrical contractor noted, "... the worker is one of the biggest unsafe things you have." Owners tended to take the working conditions as given and to perceive employee behavior as the locus of intervention. For example, one owner observed that calcium chloride is "rough on the hands," but identified the "problem" as one of workers not liking to wear gloves.

In terms of their perceived roles and responsibilities regarding the health-related behavior of employees, owners could be placed on a continuum from "coming down hard on" to "leaving it up to" the workers. Two thirds of the owners in this sample were clustered in the latter end of the continuum, sounding something like this owner of a heating and ventilation business:

> We provide them with a mask and then *it's their option*. If they use it, they use it; if they don't, they don't.

This stance was usually accompanied by expressed reluctance to intervene forcefully in the health behavior of their employees:

> You always make sure there's a set [of goggles] hanging right by the grinder, so if they don't use them, you know, *I'm not going to go around slapping them.* (Ted, auto repair)

Owners often appeared to perceive health and safety intervention by management to be inappropriately paternalistic, insisting: "You can't baby-sit them [workers]," "You can't welfare them," "You can't mother them."

The owners' health-related behavior in general, and the "leave it up to the workers" posture in particular, were embedded in the three levels of work identified earlier: practical everyday workplace contingencies, organizational culture, and the social relations of work.

At the concrete job level, the "leave it up to the workers" stance was linked to the challenges of managing a small business. First, in a context in which economic survival is paramount and owners are confronted with a plethora of demands on their time and energies, health-related matters were clearly of low priority. As Joe, a machine shop owner, put it:

> ... [health and safety] is a very minor thing, very minor. Compared to problems of getting business, and collecting money, and dealing with bankers, and things like that. Oh yes, *it's way down the line.*

A "leaving it up to the workers" perspective was easily sustained in a context in which owners were struggling, often through 14-hour days, to address problems they perceived to be more critical to the welfare of the business. Even when owners did perceive health to be a significant concern (the conditions for this concern being also related to workplace contingencies but not discussed here), other practical constraints contributed to the "leave it up to the workers" perspective. For example, in many small enterprises, employees are scattered over multiple job sites belonging to the client. Supervision and other prevention measures were considered impossible because, as one owner put it, "I can't be everywhere at once."

Factors at the cultural and social organizational levels also influenced the owners' posture toward health and safety. One example is the norm of independence that appeared to pervade many small businesses. When asked what they liked about being the owner of a small business, over half of the informants referred foremost to the issue of personal autonomy, using such phrases as "being your own boss." Owners acknowledged the same need or desire for independence in their employees. For example, subcontracted workers were noted to perform better because they "work for themselves." The "good" employee was seen as someone who could work "without being told what to do." Employees, particularly tradespersons, were often seen to require a "free hand."

Although the "leave it up to the workers" stance was embedded in broader normative beliefs about autonomy in the workplace, it was also prompted by the owners' perceived lack of control over employees. Some owners spoke of this deficit in terms of employee "type":

> Take welders — my God, there is no way you can tell a welder what to do! They're a special breed. (Reg, auto repair)

Others felt reluctant to exert authority over employees because of their dependence on them. As Jake, the owner of a floor-laying company, pointed out:

> It's hard to find real conscientious craftsmen. And if you do, you treasure them ... *you bust your butt trying to keep the good ones.*

This dependence has consequences for the owners' authority, as is suggested by Garth, the owner of a pest control company, who was not willing to make his employees wear masks despite known toxicity of the chemicals because:

> Once a guy's around for a while, they start doing their own thing, and *you can't tell them what to do,* that's for sure ... *you're not about to let him go* because he

knows what he's doing, and he's built his customer relationships.

For some owners, this lack of control stemmed in part from what many called their "one of the boys" relationship with their employees:

> I work with them [employees] *as if I'm not the boss here,* I just work with them. I never wanted to sit here with my white shirt and tie on.... I just get into a pair of blue jeans and work with them. (Bob, plastic tube manufacturing)

As "one of the boys," however, an owner appeared at times to compromise his or her authority over employees.

> The relations we [co-owners] have with the guys, it's basically as a friend, but *I find it hard myself to really come down and say,* "*No* I don't want it done this way." (Kate, auto repair)

Being hard on employees over health and safety (and other) matters appeared to be additionally difficult for owners who had themselves come up through the ranks and had experienced first-hand the inconvenience or discomfort associated with self-protective devices and practices. Ray, himself a former auto body mechanic, said:

> I sympathize with these guys ... it's a dirty, hard, thankless job.... I have a lot of trouble being hard on anybody who has been in the trade for a long time.

The owners' health-related behavior was influenced not only by practical job contingencies and cultural norms regarding authority and control, but also by more abstract social relations of employment. One example of this ambiguity is the relationship between the "leave it up to the workers" stance and the owners' understanding of the nature of their responsibility for workplace health. In contrast to some who perceived health and safety as a legal and bureaucratic function of office (a normal function of business management), many owners appeared to perceive the management of health and safety in personal terms. When intervening in the health behavior of employees, they saw themselves as acting not as business managers but as individual persons.

Intervention was thus seen as carrying certain "moral" imputations (in Goffman's sense) about the owners' values and motivations. For example, one owner said that he is called a "worry-wart" for raising health issues; others believed that they would be considered "health freaks" and "goody-goodys" if they insisted on certain safety practices.

The personalization of health and safety intervention may have been linked in many cases to owners' close identification with and great emotional investment in their companies. Many appeared to perceive their businesses as an extension of themselves. Such personal identification with the business sometimes appeared to make it difficult for owners to acknowledge work-related health issues. If the work is harmful, then the owners themselves must be harmful. Such personalization was evident in the words of the owner who declared "I sure ain't out to poison anybody" while describing the chemical hazards in his workplace, and in the defensive assertion "I care for my guys" from an employer who perceived government inspectors to be "knights" who "charge in to save the workers."

The findings from the owner study presented here illustrate how health behavior (in this case the owners' posture toward the management of health and safety in the workplace) is related to the nature of work and social relations in small businesses (in this case the owners' authority relations with employees).

Small-Business Employees: "But What Can You Do?"

Like the owners, the employees' health-related attitudes and practices are also embedded in the everyday context of work in small-business settings. Because they occupy a different structural position in the workplace, however, workers have perceptions of risk and actions regarding the management of health and safety problems that are distinctly different from those of their employers.

Several patterns of employee responses are evident in the data, including variations on Hirshman's (1971) notions of "exit" (a market mechanism) and "voice" (a change mechanism). In this case, exit behavior involves quitting the job, while voice involves protest and participation in change. Other types of responses are found in the data, including "accommodation" (e.g., adapting, accepting, enduring) and "resistance" (e.g., absenteeism, sabotage, retaliation).

Which responses are made is contingent to a large extent upon the work environment itself. A look at accommodation behavior provides an illustration. Accommodation includes a variety of behaviors, such as acceptance ("That's just the kind of work it is"), self-protection ("I take my breaks outside"), resignation ("... it wasn't good for me but I did it anyway"), and compensation ("We go out for a drink after the shift"). The central question in this analysis is not so much *how* workers accommodate as *why* they accommodate. The case of Ahpo, a cashier in a corner convenience store, provides an example of how accommodative responses to workplace health and safety hazards are influenced by the constraints of the immediate job and the social and organizational character of work.

Ahpo is a 32-year-old Asian woman who has lived in Canada for eight years. During the day, she is training to become qualified as a teacher, so she supports herself by an evening job in a family-run convenience store. The store employs two managers (the owner's son and daughter-in-law) and two employees, a cashier (Ahpo) and a stockman. Ahpo works the evening shift and weekends with the stockman. Ahpo's major health concern at work is having to stand for most of the seven hours of her shift. She finds this very tiring, and her back and legs hurt. She is dismayed by her varicose veins, which she attributes to having to stand, noting with distress that they are "nothing good to a woman." Ahpo notes other health-related concerns, such as the fact that she works even when she is sick, has no time for any health-promoting activities such as exercise, has no break for a meal, and is constantly distressed by the family conflicts in which the members of the family that owns the store try to get her to take sides. Despite her concerns, Ahpo has neither tried to find another job (exit) nor spoken out about her discomfort (voice). Instead, she appears to take an accommodative stance toward health and safety. She rejects the possibility that she could use a stool at the cash register or eat in front of customers. She sometimes tries to alleviate discomfort by exercising surreptitiously at the cashier's station ("If nobody come in ... I actually myself sit down and, you know, up and down ... I disco in place"), but otherwise suffers silently.

Ahpo's health-related behavior—specifically that she does not try to assert her health needs at work—is produced, at least in part, by the work environment. At the level of the immediate job situation, Ahpo feels unable to change her situation because she cannot leave the till unattended and there is only the stockman to take over temporarily. She says that she never takes sick leave because she knows it would be difficult for the managers to replace her: "Even I have sick I go to work. I don't make some other people have trouble, you know." Being sick or raising health concerns would cause "trouble" for her employer (and ultimately for her as well) and so is avoided. Ahpo has only one coworker with whom to share her concerns, and he, she notes, does not "understand" her discomfort from standing and thinks her job is an "easier woman's job." She says that she will not sit down because the owner might think she is "lazy" and not working. She herself appears to share the normative expectation in a business setting that the customers' needs are paramount. Thus, sitting would be "rude" to the customers and would not be good for business. Ahpo does not speak to the manager about her discomfort, in part because they have little actual opportunity to talk; he works the day shift and leaves when she arrives in late afternoon.

Ahpo's health-related behavior is influenced by other less concrete aspects of her work situation. A significant feature of the small-business sector is family involvement. Companies are of-

ten co-owned by family members, and relatives are employed in the business or do unpaid work such as accounting or helping out at busy times. The juxtaposition of family and employment relations has implications for the distribution of authority and control in the workplace, for worker solidarity, and ultimately for health and safety behavior. Ahpo's boss is a friend of her brother (who owns another small business). The boss' wife helps him manage the store. Ahpo is friendly with a sister-in-law of the manager. The presence of this family web in the workplace appears to inhibit Ahpo from addressing workplace issues and her health concerns. She fears that any action on her part might harm her brother's reputation or spawn unpleasant rumors in the family and the community.

In addition to control from such family relations, Ahpo is subject to control by employment relations. Her boss had once rejected a suggestion she made about the layout of the store, telling her, "This is not your store," and implying that she was usurping his authority as "boss."

Family and employment roles sometimes conflict. Ahpo reported instances in which fulfilling her duties as an employee violated family norms (e.g., angering her boss by telling a family member where he was). For Ahpo, the strain of combining work and family roles prompts her to be "deeply thinking if it's better to quit the job or not" and ultimately deters her from leaving and from raising any issues at all.

Ahpo's unwillingness to make claims for her own health and safety also reflects the ideological ambivalence of many employees in small-business settings. For a variety of reasons that cannot be explored here (e.g., visibility of corporate issues, mobility between supervisory and line positions, aspirations of many small-business employees to own their own businesses), many employees have no clear "we–they" identity vis-à-vis worker–management relations. One implication of this situation is that employees may deny their own claims to a safe workplace. For example, many employees in this study mentioned health needs, but did not pursue them because "the company cannot afford it." Ahpo's family connection to the management made it very difficult for her to assert her legal rights as an employee. To do so would be to highlight the inherent conflict of interest between labor and capital and would run counter to normative practices in the workplace.

A final set of reasons for Ahpo's health behavior stems from broad structural aspects of work. Ahpo is part of the growing "contingent" labor market that includes part-time work and other impermanent and flexible working arrangements such as contract work, home work, and moonlighting. Workers in such jobs generally lack the power to influence the terms and nature of their work. Ahpo can do little to alter the working conditions that affect her health, yet she cannot leave because she needs the income to support herself, the store is near her home, and her hours fit in with her school schedule. As with many others in this study, Ahpo trades her health for other considerations.

In sum, Ahpo's health-related behavior (specifically her reluctance to assert her health needs in the workplace) is influenced by the context in which she works—the characteristics of her day-to-day job circumstances, the social organization of the business, and normative expectations and assumptions about her incongruent roles as employee and as family/community member.

CONCLUSION

Although both the employer and the employee study echo the concepts and relationships noted in the literature, they have a somewhat different take on the topic. These studies take a contextual perspective on the topic, revealing how health behavior is a contingent product of, and has a reciprocal influence on, the material, social, and ideological context in which it is embedded. Taking this perspective means, first, approaching the notion of health behavior, not as a discrete, predetermined phenomenon, but as an emergent property of more general work-related behavior. Health behavior is inseparable from

work behavior. The analytical point is reflected empirically in the oft-noted observation in the literature that workers often see occupational injury and risk as "just part of the job."

Second, and partly flowing from the preceding point, the concept of health behavior encompasses a much more diverse set of behaviors than is generally evident in the literature. Thus, the health behavior of a bar waitress includes not only her drinking behavior or sickness absences, but also her strategic use of her "regulars" to protect herself against violent customers, as well as other attitudes and behaviors that are intrinsic to her daily work experience.

Third, meaning and standpoint are viewed as central to understanding health-related behavior. Employees and employers have different perspectives on health because they occupy different social statuses within the workplace. To explain health-related behavior, it is necessary to take account of the meanings that individuals attribute to health and health-related action within their particular work settings.

Research and Methodological Issues

Suggestions for future research emerge from the literature reviewed in this chapter and observations from the small-business studies. It is proposed that health behavior cannot sensibly be understood separate from the setting and circumstances in which it occurs. Since work plays such a significant part in people's lives, it warrants more attention than it has received from researchers interested in the determinants of health behavior. The theoretical development of the topic has been limited by the use of preconceived, observer-centered notions of health behavior. More effort should be made to identify forms of health behavior that are woven into the fabric of people's daily work lives. Consideration of a broader range of behaviors may enhance our capacity to identify new properties of the concept and to generate fresh theoretical possibilities.

Also needed is empirical research on the less

visible ideological and organizational structures of work that appear to have consequence for health-related behavior. Although the literature makes broad-brush assertions about the relationship between health behavior and such structures, there is little empirical demonstration of this relationship or of its actual manifestation at the level of individual behavior and experience.

REFERENCES

A.R.A. Consultants. (1987). *A report to the Occupational Health and Safety Education Authority: Volume One. Needs Assessment Survey.* Toronto, Ontario: A.R.A. Consultants.

Abel, T., Cockerham, W. C., Lueschen, G., & Kunz, G. (1989). Health lifestyles and self-direction in employment among American men: A test of the spillover effect. *Social Science and Medicine, 28*(12), 1269-1274.

Allison, K., & Coburn, D. (1985). Explaining low levels of exercise amongst blue collar workers. *Canadian Association of Health, Physical Education and Recreation Journal, 5*(7), 34-37.

Ames, G., & James, C. (1987). Heavy and problem drinking in an American blue-collar population: Implications for prevention. *Social Science and Medicine, 25*(8), 949-960.

Applebaum, H. (1981). *Royal blue: The culture of construction workers.* New York: Rinehart & Winston.

Armstrong, P. (1991). *"Under 10s": Small establishments in the private sector.* Ontario Ministry of Labour.

Armstrong, P., & Armstrong, H. (1993). *The double ghetto.* Toronto: McClelland & Stewart.

Aronsson, G. (1989). Dimensions of control as related to work organization, stress and health. *International Journal of Health Services, 19*(3), 459-468.

Bammer, G., & Martin, B. (1992). Socio-political aspects of work-related musculoskeletal disorders. In M. Haglnig & A. Kilbom (Eds.), *International scientific conference on prevention of work-related musculoskeletal disorders* (pp. 34-36). Stockholm: Premus.

Bellaby, P. (1990). What is genuine sickness? The relationship between work-discipline and the sick role in a pottery factory. *Sociology of Health and Illness, 12*(1), 47-68.

Billette, A., & Piche, J. (1987). Health problems of data entry clerks and related job stressors. *Journal of Occupational Medicine, 29*(12), 942-948.

Boltanski, L. (1976). Die soziale Verwendung des Körper. In D. Kamper & V. Rittner (Eds.), *Zur Geschichte des Körpers* (pp. 138-183). Munich: Hanser.

Boxer, P. (1990). Indoor air quality: A psychosocial perspective. *Journal of Occupational Medicine, 32*(5), 425-428.

Brewer, J. D. (1990). Talking about danger: The RUC and the paramilitary threat. *Sociology, 24*(4), 657-674.

Caplan, R. D., Cobb, S., French, J. R. P., Harrison, R. V., & Pinneau, S. R. (1975). *Job demands and worker health.* Washington, DC: U.S. Government Printing Office.

Casswell, S., & Gordon, A. (1984). Drinking and occupational status in New Zealand men. *Journal of Studies on Alcohol, 45*(2), 144-148.

Coburn, D., & Pope, C. (1974). Socioeconomic status and preventive health behavior. *Journal of Health and Social Behavior, 15*, 67-77.

Colligan, M. J., & Murphy, L. R. (1979). Mass psychogenic illness in organizations: An overview. *Journal of Occupational Psychology, 52*(2), 77-90.

Conrad, P., & Walsh, D. C. (1992). The new corporate health ethic: Lifestyle and the social control of work. *International Journal of Health Services, 22*(1), 89-111.

Crawford, R. (1984). A cultural account of "health": Control, release, and the social body. In J. McKinaly (Ed.), *Issues in the political economy of health care* (pp. 60-103). New York: Tavistock.

Curran, J., & Stanworth, J. (1979). Self-selection and the small firm worker—A critique and an alternative view. *Sociology, 13*(3), 427-444.

d'Houtaud, A., & Field, M. (1984). The image of health: Variations in perception by social class in a French population. *Sociology of Health and Illness, 16*(1), 30-60.

Davis, K., Jackson, K. L., Kronenfeld, J. J., & Blair, S. N. (1987). Determinants of participation in worksite health promotion activities. *Health Education Quarterly, 14*(2), 195-205.

Daykin, N. (1990). Health and work in the 1990's: Towards a new perspective. In P. Abbott & G. Payne (Ed.), *New directions in the sociology of health* (pp. 153-164). London: Falmer Press.

Deves, L., & Spillane, R. (1989). Occupational health, stress, and work organization in Australia. *International Journal of Health Services, 19*(2), 351-363.

Dodier, N. (1985). Social uses of illness at the workplace: Sick leave and moral evaluation. *Social Science and Medicine, 20*(2), 123-128.

Douglas, M., & Wildavsky, A. (1982). *Risk and culture.* Berkeley: University of California Press.

Duclos, D. (1987). La construction sociale du risque: Le cas des ouvriers de la chimie face aux dangers industriels. *Revue Française de Sociologie, 28*(1), 17-42.

Dwyer, T. (1981). The production of industrial accidents: A sociological approach. *Australian and New Zealand Journal of Sociology, 17*(2[July]), 59-65.

Dwyer, T. (1991). *Life and death at work: Industrial accidents as a case of socially produced error.* New York: Plenum Press.

Eakin, J. (1992). Leaving it up to the workers: Sociological perspective on the management of health and safety in small workplaces. *International Journal of Health Services, 22*, 689-704.

Eakin, J. (unpublished). The social production of health in small workplaces. University of Toronto.

Erikson, K., & Vallas, S. P. (Eds.). (1990). *The nature of work: Sociological perspectives*. New Haven, CT: Yale University Press.

Frankenhaeuser, M. (1991). A biopsychosocial approach to work life issues. In J. Johnson & G. Johansson (Eds.), *The psychosocial work environment: Work organization, democratization and health* (pp. 49–60). Amityville, NY: Baywood.

Frankenhaeuser, M., & Johansson, G. (1986). Stress at work: Psychobiological and psychosocial aspects. *International Review of Applied Psychology, 35*, 287–299.

Frankenhaeuser, M., Lundberg, U., & Chesney, M. (Eds.). (1991). *Women, work, and health: Stress and opportunities*. New York: Plenum Press.

Ganster, D. C. (1989). Worker control and well-being: A review of research in the workplace. In S. L. Sauter, J. J. Hurell, & C. L. Cooper (Ed.), *Job control and worker health* (pp. 3–23). London: Wiley.

Ganster, D., & Schaubroeck, J. (1991). Work stress and employee health. *Journal of Management, 17*(22), 235–271.

Gardell, B. (1982). Autonomy and participation in work. *Human Relations, 30*(6), 515–533.

Gerhardt, U. (1989). *Ideas about illness: An intellectual and political history of medical sociology*. New York: New York University Press.

Green, K. L., & Johnson, J. V. (1990). The effect of psychological work organization on patterns of cigarette smoking among male chemical plant employees. *American Journal of Public Health, 80*(11), 1368–1371.

Greenglass, E. R. (1985). Psychological implications of sex bias in the workplace. *Academic Psychology Bulletin, 7*, 227–240.

Haas, J. (1977). Learning real feelings: A study of high steel ironworkers' reactions to fear and danger. *Sociology of Work and Occupations, 4*, 147–170.

Hall, E. (1991). Gender, work control, and stress: A theoretical discussion and an empirical test. In J. Johnson & G. Johansson (Eds.), *The psychosocial work environment: Work organization, democratization and health* (pp. 89–108). Amityville, NY: Baywood.

Heaney, C. A. (1993). Perceived control and employed men and women. In B. C. Long & S. E. Kahn (Eds.), *Women, work and coping* (pp. 193–215). Montreal & Kingston: McGill-Queen's University Press.

Hedge, A., Erickson, W. A., & Rubin, G. (1992). Effects of personal and occupational factors on sick building syndrome reports in air-conditioned offices. In J. C. Quick, L. R. Murphy, & J. J. Hurrell (Eds.), *Stress and well-being at work* (pp. 286–298). Washington, DC: American Psychological Association.

Hirshman, A. (1971). *Exit, voice and loyalty*. Cambridge, MA: Harvard University Press.

Ireland, D. (1992). The Australian experience with cumulative trauma disorders. In L. C Millender, D. Lewis, & B. Simmons (Eds.), *Occupational disorders of the upper extremity* (pp. 79–88). New York: Churchill Livingstone.

Jackson, L., Highcrest, A., & Coates, R. (1992). Varied potential risks of HIV infection among prostitutes. *Social Science and Medicine, 35*(3), 281–286.

Jackson, S. (1989). Does job control control job stress? In S. L. Sauter, J. J. Hurrell, Jr., & C. L. Cooper (Ed.), *Job control and worker health* (pp. 25–53). London: Wiley.

James, C. (1987). Occupational injury: Accidental or a reflection of conflict between capital and labour? *Australian and New Zealand Journal of Sociology, 23*(1), 47–64.

Jermier, J., Knights, D., & Nord, W. (Eds.). (1994). *Resistance and power in organizations*. New York: Routledge.

Johansson, G., Johnson, J., & Hall, E. (1991). Smoking and sedentary behavior as related to work organization. *Social Science and Medicine, 32*(7), 837–846.

Johnson, J. V. (1989). Collective control: Strategies for survival in the workplace. *International Journal of Health Services, 19*(3), 469–480.

Jones, J., & Boye, M. (1992). Job stress and employee counterproductivity. In J. Quick, L. Murphy, & J. Hurrell (Eds.), *Stress and well-being at work* (pp. 239–251). Washington, DC: Americal Psychological Association.

Kalimo, R. (1987). Psychosocial factors and workers' health: An overview. In R. Kalimo, M. A. El-Batawi, & C. L. Cooper (Eds.), *Psychosocial factors at work and their relation to health*. Geneva: World Health Organization.

Karasek, R., Gardell, B., & Lindell, J. (1987). Work and nonwork correlates of illness and behaviour in male and female Swedish white collar workers. *Journal of Occupational Behaviour, 8*(3), 187–207.

Karasek, R., & Theorell, T. (1990). *Healthy work: Stress, productivity, and the reconstruction of working life*. New York: Basic Books.

Kickbusch, I. (1988). New perspectives for research in health behaviour. In R. Anderson, J. K. Davis, I. Kickbusch, D. V. McQueen, & J. Turner (Eds.), *Health behaviour research and health promotion* (pp. 237–243). New York: Oxford University Press.

Kristensen, T. (1991). Sickness absence and work strain among Danish slaughterhouse workers: An analysis of absence from work regarded as coping behaviour. *Social Science and Medicine, 32*(1), 15–27.

Lebovits, A., & Strain, J. (1990). The asbestos worker who smokes: Adding insult to injury. *Health Psychology, 9*(4), 405–417.

Lovato, C. Y., & Green, L. W. (1990). Maintaining employee participation in workplace health promotion programs. *Health Education Quarterly, 17*(1), 73–88.

MacKinnon, B. (1987). *Work-related injuries and illnesses: Small employers 1977–1985*. Research and Statistics Section, Research Branch, Occupational Health and Safety Division, Alberta Community and Occupational Health.

Manning, W. G., Keeler, E. V., Newhouse, J. P., Sloss, E. M., &

Wasserman, J. (1991). *The costs of poor health habits*. Cambridge MA: Harvard University Press.

Marmot, M., & Theorell, T. (1991). Social class and cardiovascular disease: The contribution of work. In J. Johnson & G. Johansson (Eds.), *The psychosocial work environment: Work organization, democratization and health* (pp. 21–48). Amityville, NY: Baywood.

McDermott, F. (1986). Repetition strain injury: A review of current understanding. *Medical Journal of Australia, 144*, 196–200.

McKinlay, J. (1994). A case for refocussing upstream: The political economy of illness. In P. Conrad & R. Kern (Eds.), *Sociology of health and illness: Critical perspectives* (pp. 509–523). New York: St. Martin's Press.

Meissner, M. (1971). The long arm of the job: A study of work and leisure. *Industrial Relations, 10*(3), 239–260.

Messing, K. (1993–1994). Women's occupational health and androcentric science. *Canadian Women's Studies, 14*(3), 11–16.

Messing, K. (1994). Can safety risks of blue-collar jobs be compared by gender? *Safety Science, 18*, 95–112.

Messing, K., Dumais, L., & Romito, P. (1993). Prostitutes and chimney sweeps both have problems: Towards full integration of both sexes in the study of occupational health. *Social Science and Medicine, 36*(1), 47–55.

Messite, J., & Welch, L. S. (1987). An overview: Occupational health and women workers. *Women and Work, 2*:21–43.

Mullen, K. (1992). A question of balance: Health behaviour and work context among male Glaswegians. *Sociology of Health and Illness, 14*(1), 73–97.

Nelkin, D., & Brown, M. S. (1984). *Workers at risk*. Chicago: University of Chicago Press.

Nichols, T. (1975). The sociology of accidents and the social production of industrial injury. In G. Esland, G. Salaman, & M. Speakman (Eds.), *People and work* (pp. 217–229). Edinburgh: Homers McDougall.

Olkinuora, M. (1984). Alcoholism and occupation. *Scandinavian Journal of Work Environment and Health, 10*(6), 511–515.

Ottawa Charter for Health Promotion. (1986). *Health Promotion, 1*(4), iii–iv.

Parsons, T. (1975). The sick role and role of the physician reconsidered. *Milbank Memorial Fund Quarterly, 53* (Summer), 257–278.

Pierret, J. (1988). What social groups think they can do about health. In R. Anderson, J. Davies, I. Kickbusch, D. McQueen, & J. Turner (Eds.), *Health behaviour research and health promotion* (pp. 45–52). New York: Oxford University Press.

Quick, J. C., Murphy, L. R., & Hurrell, J. J. (Eds.). (1992). *Stress and well-being at work*. Washington, DC: American Psychological Association.

Quinlan, M. (1988). Psychological and sociological approaches to the study of occupational illness: A critical review. *Australian and New Zealand Journal of Sociology, 24*(2), 189–207.

Rayner, S. (1986). Management of radiation hazards in hospitals: Plural rationalities in a single institution. *Social Studies of Science, 16*, 573–591.

Reid, J., Ewan, C., & Lowy, E. (1991). Pilgrimage of pain: The illness experiences of women with repetitive strain injury and the search for credibility. *Social Science and Medicine, 32*(5), 601–612.

Reid, J., & Reynolds, L. (1990). Requiem for RSI: The explanation and control of an occupational epidemic. *Medical Anthropology Quarterly, 9*, 162–190.

Rice, D. P., Kelman, S., Miller, L. S., & Dunmeyer, S. (1990). *The economic costs of alcohol and drug abuse and mental illness*. Report submitted to the office of Financing and Coverage Policy of the Alcohol and Drug Abuse and Mental Health Administration, U.S. Department of Health and Human Services, San Francisco California. San Francisco: Institute for Health and Aging, University of California.

Rutsohn, P., Schoolfield, M., & McLeod, M. (1981). Comprehensive occupational health: Is it beyond the reach of small businesses? *Journal of Small Business Management*, April, 52–60.

Sauter, S. L., Hurrell, J., & Cooper, C. (Eds.). (1989). *Job control and worker health*. New York: Wiley.

Semchuk, K., & Eakin, J. (1989). Children's health and illness behaviour: The single working mother's perspective. *Canadian Journal of Public Health, 80*(September/October), 346–350.

Shore, E., & Pieri, S. (1992). Drinking behaviors of women in four occupational groups. *Women and Health, 19*(4), 55–64.

Sloan, R. P., & Gruman, J. C. (1988). Participation in workplace health promotion programs: The contribution of health and organizational factors. *Health Education Quarterly, 15*(3), 269–288.

Spiegel, J., & Yassi, A. (1989). Community health centre-based occupational health services for the small workplace: An Ontario study of employer acceptability. *Canadian Journal of Public Health, 80*(5), 355–358.

Statham, A. (1993). Examining gender in organizational relationships and technological change. In B. Long & S. Kahn (Eds.), *Women, work, and coping* (pp. 111–130). Montreal & Kingston: McGill-Queen's University Press.

Steinberg, B., & Wall, S. (1995). Why do women report "sick building symptoms" more often than men? *Social Science and Medicine, 40*(4), 491–502.

Surault, J. (1979). *L'inegalite devant la mort: Analyse, socio-economique de ses determinants*. Paris: Economica.

Tarasuk, V., & Eakin, J. (1994). The problem of legitimacy in the experience of work-related back injury. *Qualitative Health Research, 5*(2), 204–221.

Thomas, P. (1991). Safety in smaller manufacturing establishments. *Employment Gazette*, January, 20–24.

Thompson, P. (1995). Small business and job creation in Canada 1992. Canadian Federation of Independent Business, Toronto, Ontario, Canada.

Trice, H., & Roman, P. (1972). Spirits and demons at work: Alcohol and other drugs on the job. Ithaca, NY: New York State School of Industrial and Labor Relations, Cornell University.

Tuskes, P. M., & Key, M. M. (1988). Potential hazards in small business—A gap in OSHA protection. *Applied Industrial Hygiene, 3*(2), 55-57.

Virtanen, P. (1994). "An epidemic of good health" at the workplace. *Sociology of Health and Illness, 16*(3), 394-401.

Williams, T. (1985). Visual display technology, worker disablement, and work organization. *Human Relations, 38*(11), 1065-1084.

World Health Organization: (1946) Constitution of the World Health Organization. *Official Record of the World Health Organization, 20*, 100.

Wrench, J., & Lee, G. (1982). Piecework and industrial accidents: Two contemporary case studies. *Sociology, 16*(4), 512-525.

Zohar, D. (1980). Promoting increased use of ear protectors through information feedback. *Human Factors, 22*, 69-79.

17

Cultural Determinants of Health Behavior

William W. Dressler and Kathryn S. Oths

INTRODUCTION

In the behavioral sciences in medicine, discussions of health behaviors have often had a very specific and focused aim. For example, with respect to adherence to prescribed drug regimens, the goal has been to identify those factors that interfere with or otherwise compromise an individual's success in following a recommended regimen. Once those factors have been identified, steps can then be taken to modify characteristics of the regimen, or to try to alter the patient's beliefs and values, in order to increase adherence to and the effectiveness of the prescribed treatment.

There are two characteristics of such an approach that can, in the long run, limit its effectiveness in understanding health behaviors. First, such an approach breaks down and isolates discrete behaviors, such as adherence, from behav-

iors, such as symptom recognition and definition, that logically must be part of a larger process and that must share empirical determinants. Second, much of the research on health behaviors conducted within the United States assumes the dominance of Western biomedicine; i.e., there is an assumption that biomedicine is simply "true" and that research ought to be devoted to understanding how the behaviors of individual patients can be made to conform better to the requirements of biomedical regimens.

These are limiting characteristics of much, although of course not all, research on health behaviors. The approach to discussing health behaviors in this chapter will be different. In the first place, the use of biomedical treatment and the behaviors associated with it are just one dimension, albeit a very large dimension, of the general issue of health behavior. Any model that purports to account for health behaviors must be capable of dealing equally with the decision to seek treatment from and adhere to the advice of an internist in Cleveland and a *curandero* in Chicago.

In the second place, discrete health behaviors must be seen in the context of an ongoing process of the definition of states of health and

William W. Dressler and Kathryn S. Oths • Department of Anthropology, University of Alabama, Tuscaloosa, Alabama 35487-0210.

Handbook of Health Behavior Research I: Personal and Social Determinants, edited by David S. Gochman. Plenum Press, New York, 1997.

sickness, a process that is not initiated upon the receipt of a biomedical diagnosis, but rather forms a part of daily life. Every time a person decides, for example, that a headache is the result of a lack of sleep and only needs an over-the-counter analgesic or, conversely, that it is a sign of an impending brain tumor and needs an MRI scan, that person is engaging in health behaviors that need to be understood as part of a single process.

The approach adopted in this chapter demands a refined social and cultural perspective. Not surprisingly, given the emphasis on biomedicine, with its individualistic biases, health behaviors are often examined narrowly in terms of individual motives and attributions; that aim, after all, is to arrive at a definition of the problem that can be resolved within the confines of the doctor–patient relationship, or at least within the confines of the health care facility. Where social and cultural factors are brought into the explanatory framework, these factors are often defined in such a way that they are hopelessly confounded with other characteristics of groups and individuals, such as ethnicity or social class or national origin. It will be argued instead that culture, viewed as a set of interlocking cognitive schemata that literally constructs much of what people do on a daily basis, is fundamental to understanding health behaviors. Culture often directly influences health behaviors; just as frequently, however, culture plays a moderating role, modifying the effects of other influences on behaviors in the natural history of disease and illness.

This chapter will discuss the importance of the role of cultural factors in understanding health behaviors. It will first examine contemporary culture theory as a background to research on culture and health behaviors. Next, a model for understanding the natural history of health and illness will be discussed, focusing on the direct and indirect impact of culture in the various stages of the process. From the standpoint of this conceptual framework, the chapter will then examine some of the classic and contemporary studies of health behavior, including methodological issues involved in this research. Finally, the chapter will conclude with a discussion of the theoretical and practical implications of this model.

CULTURE THEORY

Anthropologists have struggled for decades with the concept that is the defining feature of their discipline. There has been a trend in culture theory away from a perspective that views culture in terms of discrete traits or behaviors and toward a perspective that emphasizes information processing and systems of meaning (Keesing, 1994). Throughout the first half of the 20th century, culture theorists placed a much greater emphasis on discrete culture "traits," which could be anything from a particular technology to a particular ideology. Whether cultural processes were seen to operate in terms of historical diffusion or in terms of the variety of functionalist theories, an emphasis was placed on these traits that were, fundamentally, behaviorally defined (Bohannon & Glazer, 1973).

Since the early 1950s, however, more emphasis has been placed on culture as information. That is, for a refined understanding of the culture of a particular social group, it is less important, for example, to catalogue their ritual implements used in curing ceremonies than it is to examine the storage and transmission of the information required to produce those implements. Similarly, it is more important to understand the storage and transmission of the information (or rules, or recipes, or strategies) used to guide mate selection, or child rearing, or sacred devotion, than it is to simply describe the observed behaviors that result from that information.

Implicit in this approach to thinking about culture are two fundamental assumptions. First, this information is *learned* by the individuals who make up a society. Second, this information is *socially transmitted*, and hence socially patterned.

361

The increasing emphasis on culture as information has led anthropologists to pay greater attention to human beings as creatures capable of creating and manipulating symbols. Culture has thus come to be viewed as a system of symbols or abstract elements that are learned and socially patterned, that in turn can be manipulated and altered, and that underlie all forms of behavior. As D'Andrade (1984) describes it, culture comprises a system of meanings with four fundamental properties. First, culture is *constitutive*, in that cultural propositions define, for example, what it is, or what it is not, to be married, or to be a sibling, or to engage in any of the myriad of mundane tasks that make up a life. Second, culture is *representational*, in the sense that what goes with what (e.g., parenting accompanies marriage in traditional American culture) is stored in a set of propositions by which we all are acculturated. Third, culture is *directive*, defining the normative expectations for behavior and social interaction. Fourth, culture is *evocative*, in the sense that sets of emotions are organized in such a way as to be consistent with the directive functions of meaning. It is the sharing of cultural meaning systems that helps make sense of human behavior in mundane social interaction. Because people share knowledge of how things are done, they can make meaningful distinctions and know what things to attend to and what things to ignore.

D'Andrade (1984) provides a brief, simple, and elegant example of the pervasive influence of cultural meaning systems in our lives. He describes an experiment in artificial intelligence in which a computer was programmed to understand the grammar of the English language and was provided with an extensive lexicon. It could then "understand" simple stories about, for example, a man going into a restaurant and ordering something from the menu. When the machine was questioned about what the man had to eat, however, it was stumped. It did not understand that "ordering something from the menu" and "eating" were in any way connected. While it could readily understand and respond to questions phrased solely in terms of the language used in the tale, it could not make sense of questions with answers that depended heavily upon the wealth of cultural knowledge that constitutes the whole enterprise known as "eating out." (Anyone who has coped for the first time with getting into an English pub for a meal and then out may sympathize with the computer.)

This mundane example helps to explicate the more literary descriptions spun by contemporary culture theorists such as Geertz (1973), who describes human beings as suspended in webs of significance of their own making. It also clarifies the foundations of a contemporary perspective on culture referred to as a "constructivist" perspective (Gaines, 1992). Both of these notions emphasize that individual behaviors are shaped to a great extent by implicit systems of meaning and that it is in many respects more important to understand the meaning of some event or circumstance to the individual in accounting for that individual's behavior than it is to understand some "objective" quality of the event or circumstance. Indeed, the emphasis on culture as meaning has led some to embrace a radical cultural determinism that, carried to its logical extreme, would essentially preclude the scientific comparison of societies. A complete examination of these issues is beyond the scope of this chapter; the interested reader is referred to Spiro (1986) for a critique.

The approach adopted in this chapter, while it embraces the perspective of cultural meaning systems as defined by D'Andrade (1984), stops short of the more radical notions of cultural determinism. It certainly argues that there are cultural influences that permeate all of human thought and behavior. Like Burkett (1991), the authors reject the "onion" metaphor for understanding human behavior. In this metaphor, human behavior can be considered as an onion, in that successive layers, such as "culture" and then "ethnic group" and then "social class," can be peeled away to reveal the more fundamental (and usually perceptual–motivational) determinants of behavior. A more satisfying perspective is to think of determinants of human behavior as being described by a set of nested systems, as in the multilayered framework of the biopsychosocial model (Engel, 1977), but incorporating culture-as-meaning as a kind of suspension medium that links those systems in novel ways, much as cells cultured in different media will grow and develop in different ways. The web of significance or meaning in which each of us is suspended will indeed profoundly influence our behaviors, including health behaviors, but this influence does not preclude the influences of other kinds of social and psychological factors. Rather, cultural meaning systems are likely to modify social and psychological processes associated with health behaviors.

The final consideration to be noted in contemporary thinking about the concept of culture involves the notion that culture is socially patterned. Traditionally, this social patterning was assumed to refer to the shared nature of culture, which seems so obvious that it hardly needs stating. Without shared meanings regarding the most mundane matters (remember the restaurant example), one could not make it through an average day. What is probably incorrect, however, is what Pelto and Pelto (1975) referred to as a *cultural uniformist* assumption, meaning that everyone within a single social group shares a complete set of the same knowledge. Clearly, especially in a complex society (but most likely also in so-called "traditional" societies), there are vast amounts of information—culture—that individuals do not share. Yet this differential does not necessarily impede social interaction. Obviously, part of this nonsharing comes about because some knowledge is specialized and some individuals (e.g., physicians) are specialists. The division of labor in society, and especially in a highly differentiated society, allows for some to be given the responsibility of learning specialized knowledge. This provision is merely efficient.

There is accumulating evidence, however, that even mundane knowledge is not shared throughout a society with the kind of consistency that a conventional concept of culture presumes (Boster, 1987). Rather, some individuals simply know more about their own culture than do others. Also, some features of culture are more salient for some members of a group than they are for other members. It is not so much that individuals do not know the same things as it is that the same things are not of equal importance for everyone. These two dimensions of what is termed *intracultural diversity* might be referred to as *differential fluency* and *differential salience*; these dimensions in turn are patterned, especially in relation to social interaction.

This perspective on culture demands a much greater sensitivity to the social relational contexts within which cultural meaning systems guide behaviors and interactions or, in short, those contexts within which culture is or is not shared (Dressler, 1989). Put differently, the study of culture cannot be divorced from the study of the specific settings of social interaction in which cultural meaning systems come constantly into play.

In sum, for a refined understanding of cultural influences on health behaviors, the concept of culture will be used here to refer to learned systems of meaning that are socially patterned. These systems of meaning make mundane social interaction possible. Cultural knowledge and the salience of that knowledge are not shared equally throughout a society, but rather are distributed systematically in relation to patterns of social interaction.

CULTURE AND HEALTH BEHAVIOR: A MODEL

The model used here as a point of departure in examining culture and health behaviors is a modification of what Chrisman (1977) introduced as a model of the "health seeking process," which itself drew heavily upon the classic works of Parsons (1951), Suchman (1965), and Kasl and Cobb (1966). In the words of Chrisman (1977, p. 351): "The health seeking model is an attempt to conceptualize people's experiences with sickness *holistically* as *natural histories of illness* ...” (emphasis in the original). Given this emphasis on natural history, sickness is viewed explicitly in a temporal framework. The following five stages structure this model: symptom definition, illness-related shifts in role behavior, lay consultation and referral, treatment actions, and adherence. Chrisman emphasized in his original presentation that any given episode of sickness will not necessarily pass through all five stages, nor are these stages necessarily sequential in all episodes. Rather, these stages of health behavior describe the range of possible actions taken by any individual in attempting to define a state of dysfunction and to return to a state of health.

There has remained, however, a tendency to view this entire process as one that moves in a linear fashion and is guided by individual information processing and decision making. This emphasis is probably inappropriate. Rather, the model needs to be conceptualized as a nonrecursive process in which sickness becomes not simply a property of individuals, but a property of a social context (A. Young, 1982). Of course, since the work of McKinlay (1981), at least, the influence of other persons on decisions about sickness has been recognized in the sense of social network members and their influences on treatment choice and other factors. But even this formulation of the issue defines the sickness episode as something happening *to* an individual, with social network influences serving as another set of causal factors impinging on that individual.

This chapter adopts a perspective in which episodes of health problems are viewed as embedded in a social context involving the exchange of information regarding health. A. Young (1982) has perhaps argued most clearly for this contextualized view of human health and disease. To correct the individualistic view of disease or illness, he suggests specifically the study of what he terms *sickness*, or the contextualized definition of dysfunction. The definition of sickness is a process by which signs and symptoms are given socially recognizable meanings (i.e.,

they are converted into socially significant events). Every culture, including the dominant culture of Western society through biomedicine, follows prescribed rules for this translation process, a process of considerable import for the study of health behaviors.

The perspective of this work is more along the lines of Janzen’s (1978) work in Africa or of Pescosolido’s (1992) theoretical contribution. The emphasis is on the exchange of cultural information in social interaction to define health and sickness. Janzen was critical of the decision-making models of treatment choice, arguing instead that the sickness episode was embedded in a social group process from the beginning of symptom definition through the evaluation of treatment outcome. Pescosolido applies similar reasoning to help seeking in the United States, going so far as to offer the provocative argument that the individual may be an inappropriate unit of analysis for studying health behaviors. Here it is important to note that examining health behaviors as embedded in a social context is fundamentally important for understanding cultural influences in the process. As noted, in any society (and especially in any complex society), there is going to be intracultural diversity. This diversity is organized by social context, in that cultural knowledge is going to be more highly shared within a network or group among whose members there is regular, face-to-face social interaction (Holland, 1987; Swartz, 1991). Attempting to understand cultural influences on individual behavior, without simultaneously taking into account the social substrate in which information is shared or exchanged, would be ineffective.

One further modification that must be introduced into this model, recognized by Chrisman (1977, p. 352) but not incorporated explicitly into the model, is the distinction between disease and illness (Kleinman, Eisenberg, & Good, 1978). Typically, especially in common language use, but even in professional discourse in biomedicine, the terms *illness* and *disease* are used completely interchangeably. Kleinman et al. (1978) suggested that the concepts should be distinguished. Disease is defined as a malfunctioning of biological structures and functions. Illness is defined as the individual experience of disvalued states of being and functioning. Put differently, disease is the measurable deviation of an organic system from some independently defined optimum, while illness is the human experience of suffering or distress.

Clearly, disease and illness need not overlap. Essential hypertension is the classic case of the presence of disease in the absence of illness. The state of chronically elevated arterial blood pressure is well understood as a precursor of coronary artery disease and stroke, yet it is virtually without symptoms and entirely out of the conscious awareness of the individual. Until a diagnosis is made, there literally is no illness. By the same token, it is estimated that as many as 40% of all patients seek out medical care for presenting complaints for which there are no clear and unambiguous labels (Kleinman et al., 1978). In other words, the patient suffers an illness for which the disease is problematic. Also, of course, there are the classic presentations described by the term *somatization* or *hypochondriasis*, in which there is illness with no indication of disease. Disease and illness are therefore useful tools for describing deviations from some preferred or optimal level of functioning, but they need not overlap.

The distinction between disease and illness should not be confused with the presence or absence of symptoms. For example, it is somewhat of a truism in the literature on "patient compliance" that individuals will adhere more assiduously to a drug regimen when it provides symptomatic relief. But the disease–illness distinction strikes closer to issues of meaning. Returning to the example of hypertension, for some persons the knowledge of a borderline high blood pressure reading can very quickly transform blood pressure from an unacknowledged physiological parameter into a grave illness problem. Such a transformation may be accompanied by careful and frequent monitoring of blood pressure, a reduction of salt in the diet,

and an increase in physical activity. For other persons, this same knowledge leads to no such behavior changes. It is therefore the *meaning* of knowledge that is at issue, not the equivalent lack of symptoms in both cases.

It is necessary to expand the model of health behavior used here to recognize that individuals acting within the natural history of a sickness episode may be behaving relative to issues raised either as illness problems or as disease problems or, of course, as both. Heuristically, it may be useful to conceive of illness and disease problems as separate tracks of a single episode of sickness, although in many instances illness and disease problems will not be independent.

The chapter next examines the literature on cultural influences in this health-seeking process.

PROBLEM DEFINITION

Although Chrisman (1977) originally used the term *symptom definition*, the term *problem definition* is preferable, since, as argued above, the process may or may not begin with a symptom. Rather, this health-seeking process could begin with an elevated blood pressure reading on an automated sphygmomanometer in a shopping mall, or with the reading of an article in the popular press on the danger of dietary tropical oils. Or, as argued in the classic literature on health beliefs, the health-seeking process may be put in motion by the experience of some persistent deviation from a self-defined (and socially defined) optimal functioning, a deviation that carries a substantial threat to the affected individual. In whatever way it begins, in conventional terms of the process, some health issue becomes salient for the individual.

In each example cited, however, there is a substantial foundation of cultural knowledge that enables the individual to interpret the information meaningfully, whether it is an experienced symptom or some other kind of information. Certainly social–psychological issues, such as the degree of threat associated with the symptom or information, or the individual's self-perceived susceptibility, are important, but these issues define the personal or idiosyncratic meaning of the symptom or information. Serving as background to these individual interpretations is the cultural information that defines meaning—cultural information that is embedded in a social relational context.

An interesting example of this process is provided in a study of a small-scale society, a religious cult (Kliger, 1994). Female members of this cult, located in New York and San Francisco, expressed, in somatic terms, symptoms of distress arising from a forced separation from their families and communities. These symptoms included such clear physical outcomes as rapid and excessive weight gain and amenorrhea, because the concept of "mental illness," or even "psychological distress," was not tolerated in the belief system of the social group. The specific sociocultural expression of distress was rigorously shaped by group consensus regarding the appropriate manifestation of illness.

As another example, take common symptoms of fatigue, listlessness, loss of interest in everyday activities, and a sense of helplessness. On one hand, these symptoms can be interpreted very straightforwardly in a biomedical framework (although even within the biomedical framework they are liable to a variety of interpretations). They could be interpreted as consistent with depression, chronic fatigue syndrome, or even poor nutrition (Ware & Kleinman, 1992). On the other hand, these symptoms could be interpreted as a manifestation of *susto*, a so-called "folk" illness of the Hispanic community sometimes translated as "magical fright" (Rubel, 1964; Rubel, O'Nell, & Ardon, 1984). In *susto*, the affected individual experiences some very concrete event, such as a narrow escape from being struck by a car. The fright associated with this experience can sometimes be sufficiently intense to separate the soul from the body and give rise to the symptoms described above.

It does not appear that these symptoms can be experienced neutrally; rather, affected individuals, or more often immediate social network members, actively interpret the occurrence of symptoms. Kleinman (Kleinman, 1980; Kleinman et al., 1978) introduced the construct of *explanatory model* precisely to account for this process. An explanatory model (EM) is a cognitive model of health processes, based on both cultural knowledge and idiosyncratic experience, that is used to guide interpretation and action regarding states of health. Kleinman distinguishes EMs from general health beliefs through the EMs' specificity and utility in interpreting discrete episodes of illness. The EM is structured along five basic dimensions: etiology, timing of the onset of symptoms, pathophysiology, course of sickness, and treatment (Kleinman, 1980, p. 105). For example, with respect to *susto*, the etiology of the illness involves the occurrence of the frightening experience. The pathophysiology is the displacement of the soul from the body, and in some ethnographic accounts of the illness, it is compounded by poor nutrition (resulting from the lassitude). The course of the illness is downhill; without treatment, it will only get worse and may lead to death. Treatment involves undertaking the appropriate ritual activity to reunite the soul with the body. The important point here is that the EM provides the afflicted individual and the individual's social network with a ready framework within which the fundamental existential state of sickness can be understood.

The EM has been found to be useful in understanding a variety of health problems, one of the more interesting examples of which is the aforementioned essential hypertension. Blumhagen (1980, 1982) examined EMs within a Veteran's Administration hospital medicine outpatient clinic for hypertension. Among the findings of his research, which included EM interviews with over 100 patients, was that in commonsense understandings of the disease, there were actually two separate illness states. One, "hyper-tension," consisted of a state of excitation of the whole being. This sort of generalized state of arousal was in turn prodromal to the more serious condition, "high blood pressure." "Hypertension" was under the influence mainly of social and psychological factors, while high blood pressure could also be influenced by overweight, family history, and sodium intake.

This group consensus EM for essential hypertension could be viewed as an imperfect approximation of a biomedical understanding of the disease state, which it probably is, but that conclusion would be premature. In the first place, it is striking that a consensus, or sharing, of beliefs about this disease would be found. In the second place, it is likely that this shared knowledge was generated out of social interaction. It is likely that EMs are shared, compared, and even contested, as individuals in interaction work out the business of understanding health and disease. Kleinman (1980) argues that the EM can be defined at various levels of social abstraction, including a "popular culture EM," as well as EMs at the level of the family and the profession (e.g., physician EMs). The EM was developed in part as a way of understanding the interaction and negotiation taking place between physician and patient, but it is important to recognize the social relational process out of which emerges a group consensus EM that is independent of the formal health care delivery system.

NEGOTIATING SICKNESS AND SHIFTS IN ROLE BEHAVIOR

The second stage in Chrisman's (1977) model—illness-related shifts in role behavior—refers to changes in social role behaviors associated with sickness. The classic view of this shift is the concept of the sick role, first articulated by Parsons (1951, pp. 436–437). The sick role involves changes in role behavior such that the individual is exempted from typical obligations for the performance of social roles and is expected to engage in appropriate behaviors required to regain a state of health, including seeking and cooperating with technically competent providers (Chrisman, 1977, p. 356). The label used by Chrisman is again altered here, to empha-

size that the process is one in which cultural models guide and are modified in the process of social interaction.

The way in which the sick role has typically been conceptualized could almost be viewed as the liminal process associated with certain rites of passage: The individual's role remains ambiguous up to the point at which an appropriate and acceptable labeling of the episode of sickness is made; after that point, the sick role can be adopted and accepted by the social group. While the process is no doubt played out in this way in many instances, what is missing from this formulation is the extent to which sickness is the result of negotiation, or the exchange of information. A part of this negotiation takes place in interaction with a health care provider (of whatever sort), in which ambiguous symptoms are presented in a clinical encounter and diagnosis acceptable (to both parties) is worked out in the visit. Mishler (1981a) discussed this point in some detail with respect to biomedical diagnosis. That is, despite the seemingly "objective" nature of the diagnosis of disease, the relatively low reliability of clinical diagnoses makes it apparent that other factors are at work in the definition of disease. Even in seemingly straightforward diagnoses such as diabetes or menopause, there is ample room, in many clinical presentations, for social and cultural influences operating on both patient and provider to affect the ultimate label applied (Kirmayer, 1994; Lock, 1985).

Certainly, however, a part of this process of the negotiation of symptoms takes place within the primary social network of the individual, a process in which symptoms are evaluated by network members and EMs are compared and contrasted until the definition of the current episode is worked out. It is in this sense that illness becomes a contested category, one that can be employed strategically in social interaction. The family unit is a system within which sickness episodes are both generated and their meanings negotiated (Fisher, Terry, & Ransom, 1990). Much of the research on family and health has been conducted using the stress model as a framework, emphasizing how stresses within the family generate health problems. Neglected in the study of family and health, however, is a detailed examination of how signs and symptoms are interpreted and come to be defined as salient episodes in need of intervention. One example to follow is that provided by Crandon-Malamud (1991) in her study of sickness in the context of a village in Bolivia. She found that, within families, the labeling of illness symptoms was contested because of the way in which the illness label could reflect on the status and prestige of the family. In case studies, family members were observed to advocate for one or another label because of the way in which that label might reflect ethnic or class identity.

Epidemiological research also suggests that such processes take place. Dressler (1994) examined family health in relation to social status in a general population sample from England and Wales. He was specifically interested in examining how social status incongruence might be associated with reported sickness in this sample. Reasoning that status incongruence and other social stresses might place whole families at risk, as opposed to individuals within families, he chose the family as the unit of analysis. In addition to status incongruence, he examined job stressors experienced by employed persons in the household, as well as a variety of sociodemographic variables (e.g., economic dependency ratio, socioeconomic status) and health habits (e.g., alcohol use, tobacco use). Net of household size and age of the household head, family job stressors and status incongruence were found to be the best predictors of household morbidity (defined as the number of persons in the household reported to be chronically sick). Even more intriguing, however, was the finding that these same variables were the best predictors of the number of children in the household reported to be chronically sick.

One possible interpretation of these findings, of course, would be that stress and psychosomatic processes lead directly to the occurrence of disease in members of families in which

that stress is endemic. By the same token, however, the specific measurement of chronic health problems depended upon the reporting of long-term illness that interfered with satisfactory functioning. Dressler (1994) argued that it is equally likely that the designation of particular family members as sick resulted from a process of negotiation within families, one in which the mundane symptoms of one family member became the focus of the frustrations and distress experienced within the social unit as a whole. Nor do these processes of direct causation and illness negotiation need not be mutually exclusive.

Mishler (1981b) discussed the literature on family interaction patterns and mental illness from a similar perspective. That is, he criticized this literature on the grounds that most of the research was done after a family member had already been biomedically diagnosed as, for example, schizophrenic. He argued that, instead, more research needs to be devoted to the study of family interaction patterns prior to the diagnosis of disorder in one of its members, to better understand how stresses within the family interact with behavior patterns and symptoms of particular family members, the end result being the identification of those members as sick. Such research needs to be devoted to the negotiation and construction of mundane illness episodes, as well as to dramatic diagnoses such as schizophrenia.

LAY CONSULTATION AND REFERRAL

In traditional linear models of health behavior, it was at the stage of "lay consultation," in which the ill individual would seek the advice of others, that social factors would become prominent. After individual decisions about the definition of symptoms had been made, and shifts in social role behavior had become either manifest or contested, individuals were seen as turning to their social networks for advice in terms of further refining the tentative diagnosis they had adopted and seeking information regarding referral to an appropriate practitioner (McKinlay, 1981). One can conclude, following especially the argument of Pescosolido (1992), that the entire process is more deeply embedded in a social interaction and the exchange of cultural information than previous decision-based models suggested. Rather, the shared knowledge and information that is culture underlies the recognition and definition of symptoms. The definition of states of health and sickness takes place largely in terms of the social relational processes by which this information is stored, transmitted, and exchanged.

It is still useful, however, to separate out a distinct stage at which the illness episode comes to encompass a wider range of social network members; at least, incorporating this distinct stage can help highlight the cultural and ethnic diversity in social organization that will influence an individual's choice of whom to turn to for assistance in help seeking. It is likely that the process of problem definition, and the contention over changing role definitions occur within the most intimate of social relationships: the primary kinship links of the family. As Swartz's (1991) comparative research on family culture clearly shows, the sharing of culture, including beliefs about health and the treatment of sickness, is greater within families than within social statuses that cut across families. Once these issues have been worked out, however, the resources of the family, especially with respect to information, are often too limited to serve as a guide to action. The notion that the illness episode comes to encompass a wider network of relationships at this point is therefore a useful one. Social network members, including extended kin, friends, neighbors, coworkers, and members of voluntary associations such as churches, can serve as important sources of information regarding appropriate courses of action in response to a particular problem.

Numerous large-scale, longitudinal epidemiological studies of social networks and health have appeared, Berkman and Syme's (1979) work being among the first. While their aim was to examine the association of social networks and overall mortality, they also showed that having more network ties was associated with engaging in more positive health habits, as well as an increased likelihood of visiting health professionals for preventive care. Ethnographically, work such as Stack's (1974) research in a low-income African-American community demonstrates the importance of extensive social networks in help seeking of all kinds.

The intersection of culture, social organization, and ethnicity is prominent in an examination of social networks. Numerous studies of ethnicity in the United States have demonstrated the importance of networks of extended kin in the adaptation of minority groups to American society, including Mexican-Americans (Keefe, Padilla, & Carlos, 1979), Samoans (Janes, 1990), and Asian-Americans (Lin, Ensel, Simeone, & Kuo, 1979). Additionally, the importance of extended kin networks in the adjustment of African-Americans to years of economic marginality and social inequality has been demonstrated (Dressler, 1991). The importance of extended kin networks in ethnic groups in the United States becomes clear when the nature of social support groups is examined cross-culturally (Dressler, 1994a). Many ethnic groups in the United States have migrated here from peasant economic systems in which systems of extended kinship are essential in controlling land and labor, both for subsistence cultivation and for marketing. Even within the United States, social organization within the African-American community has its roots in agrarian economic adaptations of the rural South in the 19th century. Not surprisingly, in migration to and adaptation to novel situations in urban contexts, there is a heavy reliance, at least initially, on these same networks of extended kin with respect to the sharing of material resources, emotional support, and, especially, information. This information sharing includes the cultural dimensions of health and disease. In contrast, in middle-class European-American communities, there is a much greater emphasis placed on "voluntarism" in the formation of support systems; that is, support systems outside the nuclear family household consist largely of relationships formed through voluntary interaction (i.e., "friends"), as opposed to relationships with kin.

Beyond this broad generalization about the importance of kin versus nonkin relationships, the process by which salient support networks are formed becomes a function of the specific ethnohistory of the group under consideration. For example, in Mexico and Central America, the system of *compadrazgo* (which can be given the unwieldy translation "godparenthood") looms large in the formation of support networks. Selecting and enlisting individuals as *comadres* and *compadres* for one's children at critical junctures (e.g., baptism, first communion, marriage) has functioned in traditional villages in Mexico as a way of forging social network ties across barriers of social inequality. It also is important with respect to political organization. Furthermore, it has been shown that those individuals, especially men, who perceive greater levels of support from *compadres* also enjoy better health status, as measured by arterial blood pressure (Dressler, 1994a). The system of *compadrazgo* has arrived with Hispanic migrants in United States urban communities as a part of social organization and, as such, may be of considerable importance in defining the social network within which states of sickness are defined and treatment decisions are made.

Culturally distinct groups in the United States exhibit a variety of patterns with respect to the nature of social networks and support systems. Janes (1980) described support systems for Samoans in detail, and the Samoan case is instructive because of the large and highly structured nature of their kin groups. In general terms, in Samoan social organization, there are formal leaders of large kin groups who can demand from all members of the kin group contributions of material resources that are in turn invested and redistributed to carry out family business; these contributions can sometimes reach proportions that place considerable strain on individual nuclear family households that make up the larger kin

groups. Counterbalancing the demands that such leaders can legitimately make are what are referred to as "core networks," largely composed of adult siblings who maintain affectively close relationships throughout life. The point here is that extended kin groups can incorporate both considerable support and considerable demand for individual members of those groups, and a refined understanding of the nature of social networks within any one group requires an understanding of the ethnohistory of that group. One observation that can be made about specific patterns of social organization within culturally distinct groups is that, in general, these patterns of social relationships enable such groups to adapt to the conditions of economic marginality that ethnic minorities in the United States must often face.

It is also important to recognize, however, that there is considerable diversity within ethnic groups in the United States. This diversity can be structured along a generational dimension, as well as along dimensions of social class. The result of this intraethnic differentiation is that the patterns of social support within particular segments of an ethnic group may correspond more closely to a basic middle-class pattern of social support than to a modal pattern described in cultural uniformist terms (Dressler, 1991).

There are thus likely to be two ideal types when it comes to the help seeking associated with social networks. On one hand, there are segments of an ethnic group for whom social support networks are effective precisely because they enable the members of that group to exist separately from the majority society and its institutions. On the other hand, other segments of the ethnic group are characterized by networks that are effective in the mastery of the barriers and obstacles that typically are faced by ethnic minorities. With respect to health behaviors, it seems likely that in the first instance, these social network referral systems help to support the existence of alternatives to the majority health care system, such as *espiritismo* and *santeria* in the Puerto Rican community (Garrison, 1977), various forms of herbalists in the Samoan community (Janes, 1990), and complicated patterns of alternative self-care in the African-American community (Snow, 1993). In the second instance, these social network referral systems are more likely to be ones that enable the members of the ethnic minority to cope effectively with the arcane intricacies of bureaucratic systems of health care, especially the complicated mix of programs designed to assist those who have been historically denied access to the professional health care system. Understanding cultural influences on health behaviors requires a sensitivity to these kinds of differences in social organization.

TREATMENT CHOICE

Much of the early research in medical anthropology was devoted to studies of treatment choice. In the decades following World War II, anthropologists began examining non-Western health care systems into which Western biomedicine had been introduced as an alternate source of care. The decisions made by families and individuals regarding where to go for help were of intrinsic interest; there was also an applied dimension to this research, in that efforts were made in some cases to remove barriers to access to "modern" health care (Paul, 1955). One of the enduring contributions of these early studies of treatment choice was the demonstration that Western biomedicine did not quickly and completely supplant traditional forms of health care. Rather, non-Western peoples very quickly and easily developed complicated patterns of treatment choice that incorporated both traditional forms of medical care and modern biomedicine (Romanucci-Ross, 1969).

Furthermore, these two broad categories—traditional and modern—were too coarse to describe accurately what was going on. Instead, research demonstrated rich differentiation within each of these general categories. In many places, biomedicine includes, in addition to trained physicians, pharmacists who diagnose and treat using modern pharmacopeia. Then

there are the so-called "practical" physicians (*practicantes* in Central and South America), who sometimes have training in public health and treatment and who use syringes and antibiotics in treating acute cases of disease, yet are not a part of the formal system of biomedicine. Similarly, traditional forms of medical care can also be differentiated by practitioner. Many systems are divided into specialists who deal primarily with grave illnesses that are the result of witchcraft and sorcery, while others are herbalists skilled in diagnosis and the preparation of herbal infusions for treating illnesses that result from conditions such as an imbalance of humors that is widely believed in Latin America to lead to illness. There are also often specialists in massage or bone setting, who limit their treatment to conditions resulting from mechanical causes. In short, within any setting, there is a wide variety of specialists to choose from, not merely the single decision of traditional versus modern (Colson, 1970; Oths, 1994a; Romanucci-Ross, 1969; J. C. Young, 1981).

The diversity of treatment choice in the United States is coming to resemble that in traditional societies in the process of modernization more, not less, and for a variety of reasons. First, the growing populations of ethnic minorities in the United States, stemming in part from the steady immigration of people from Central and South America and the Caribbean, as well as from Southeast Asia, has had the effect of differentiating health care options. For example, the *botanicas* in New York City or Hartford are clear indicators of this diversity. These shops function much like the local pharmacy for *espiritistas* in the Puerto Rican community, specialized practitioners who can treat a variety of illnesses resulting from natural and supernatural causes, but who are especially skilled in dealing with supernatural problems (Garrison, 1977; Harwood, 1977). The process of medical pluralism accompanying the movement of Puerto Ricans to the urban Northeast is hardly unique, as the papers on cross-cultural medicine in a special issue of the *Western Journal of Medicine* showed. These papers demonstrated the integration of traditional and Western health beliefs and practices in the United States among groups as diverse as the Mien of Laos and Afghan migrants (Barker, 1992).

Second, there is an increasing diversity in the health care practices of European-Americans (our term for the majority population) in the United States. As a 1993 paper showed, "unconventional" health care practices are utilized widely in the general population of the United States (Eisenberg et al., 1993). The investigators in this study defined the notion of unconventional health care practices rather widely, to include the relaxation therapies and biofeedback that are used commonly by some biomedical practitioners; even excluding those treatment techniques, however, a substantial proportion of this general population sample reported the use of a variety of alternatives to traditional biomedicine. Some of these alternative forms of therapy are prescribed by a growing number of quasi-specialists, such as herbalists, while others are added to the list of self-care alternatives.

Third, despite the energies of organized biomedicine to achieve dominance in the delivery of health care, there is a tradition of alternative sources of care in the United States that shows no signs of declining. Most prominent among these is, of course, chiropractic (Oths, 1994b). Despite the enduring hostility of the biomedical establishment, chiropractic has continued to function as an alternative and at times as a complement to biomedicine.

Finally, in some senses, the growing diversity of the organization of health care in the United States has contributed to the complexity of treatment choice. In recent years, there has been an increase in the availability of alternatives to the traditional fee-for-service private practitioner, including health maintenance organizations, one-day surgical centers, birthing centers, women's clinics, and the free-standing emergency center, sometimes referred to in the biomedical establishment as the "doc-in-the-box" (Rylko-Bauer, 1988). While these institutions may not be alternatives in the same sense that a chiropractor is, they do represent another point at which individuals, in interaction with others, can make choices about how to handle a particular problem—choices that, in the long run, can have significant influence on outcomes.

Were not the range of choices complicating enough, it is clear that individuals do not simply settle on a single treatment alternative to the exclusion of other alternatives. Rather, the use of multiple alternatives, as described in developing societies (Oths, 1994a), is also commonplace in the United States. These multiple use patterns may mix traditional medicine and biomedicine within a particular ethnic minority, or multiple use may combine a free-standing emergency center with a private practitioner with a chiropractor. These patterns of resort to health care, the way people pick and choose their way through the maze of care options, may be sequential, in that they go from one to another, or they may be simultaneous, in that more than one practitioner (formal or informal) is consulted at the same time (A. Young, 1983). These practices are often not reported to the practitioners themselves, especially Western physicians, for fear of ridicule (Stafford, 1978). The result is that treatment consists of a variety of conflicting opinions, advice, and, sometimes, drugs.

The complexity of health care options in any society, including the United States, points to the importance of the sociocultural processes we have described as preceding treatment choice. For instance, the lay consultation social network, whatever its composition, plays a key role in the decision as to which of the existing treatment options a sick person should choose. Given the wide range of choices available, a detailed understanding of how cultural knowledge of health and sickness leads to a particular pattern of behaviors is essential from both a theoretical and an applied perspective.

PROVIDER–PATIENT INTERACTION AND TREATMENT OUTCOME

In Chrisman's (1977) model, the last stage in the episode of sickness is characterized by a final shift in behavior; namely, adopting the therapeutic regimen as recommended by the health provider of choice, a process he termed simply "adherence." If appropriate changes in behavior are made, such as adhering to a drug regimen or adopting a new diet, then a satisfactory outcome to the episode can be anticipated.

Again, this characterization of this stage in the process does little justice to the social relational and cultural processes involved. Here it is useful to return to Kleinman's (Kleinman et al., 1978) concept of the explanatory model (EM). As noted earlier, Kleinman introduced the EM explicitly as a way of providing the physician with a simple and straightforward means of eliciting patients' beliefs about their own diseases. These beliefs, if they structure the patient's understanding of his or her illness in a way that differs substantially from the way in which the physician understands the illness, may lead to considerable conflict. There may be sharp disagreement and substantial misunderstanding of the goals and motives of one or the other member in the interaction because of differences in the very definition of illness or disease or in the aims of therapy. A very simple example of such misunderstanding would be in the case of a chronic condition such as hypertension or diabetes, in which a patient's understanding of the disease is that it should be curable by medical intervention, while the physician's understanding is that it is a chronic condition that can only be managed and controlled, rather than cured.

An interesting example of this dimension of provider–patient interaction, and the importance of a congruence in EMs between them, is provided by Oths's (1994b) study of healing in a chiropractor's office. On the basis of direct observation and coding of interactions between the chiropractor and his patients, Oths concluded that part of the chiropractor's therapeutic effectiveness was attributable to his skills in socializing patients in the world view of chiropractic. That is, patients were taught to interpret their symptoms in terms of theories of chiropractic, to understand the treatment in terms of these theories, and to anticipate symptomatic and functional improvement in those terms. The patients' learning was accomplished gradually over the course of the several office visits and treatments required for any given episode, and it was facilitated by the efforts the chiropractor invested in building rapport with and understanding his patients. In the process, patients learned how to think about their illness episodes and what to anticipate at the end of treatment. Not surprisingly, patients who remained in treatment for a longer period of time achieved a high level of patient satisfaction. In part, we would argue, they did so because they adopted an EM that was congruent with that of the provider. Helman (1988) observed this same phenomenon at work between patients suffering from gastrointestinal complaints and their gastroenterologists.

At the other end of the continuum, of course, are those situations in which no attempt is made to bridge the gulf that can exist between patient and provider—a gulf that can be substantial. A worst-case scenario in such a situation can be illustrated by the case reported by Katon and Kleinman (1980) of a Native American woman admitted to the hospital in the late stages of pregnancy. The woman had suffered a previous miscarriage and was admitted because of conditions developing during her pregnancy that placed her at risk of preterm delivery. She did indeed deliver a nonviable preterm infant. During her recovery, she reported to staff that she "heard the baby cry" two days after its death. Alarmed, the hospital staff requested a psychiatric consultation. The psychiatrist interviewed the patient and determined that communication with a dead relative was in fact a culturally valued experience in the woman's ethnic group, that the experience helped to maintain the bonds of kinship that extend into the afterlife in this culture. It was recommended that the woman not receive psychiatric care, but rather be assisted by hospital staff in discussing her feelings and in carrying out a small ritual associated with death. The woman in turn made an uncomplicated recovery both physically and emotionally.

The danger here, of course, was that the patient's culturally valued experience, because it differed so dramatically from the cultural expectations of the staff, might have been interpreted as pathology by the staff and responded to accordingly. Fortunately, the consulting psychiatrist possessed the acumen to investigate the possibility; in less fortunate situations, however, such a gulf in culture between patient and providers has resulted in patients being mislabeled mentally ill and being given unnecessary treatment (Gaines, 1982).

It would seem obvious that this situation is one in which enhancing the cultural sensitivity of the health care providers would lead to better outcomes. In the clinical encounter, unrecognized expectations regarding the interaction between patient and healer may hinder communication, and hence chances for a successful clinical outcome, as when an Arizona physician's manner seems cold and distant to a Mexican-American mother (Stafford, 1978) or a California doctor's eye contact with a Native-American patient seems disrespectful (Kramer, 1992). There have been controlled intervention studies in which instructing the providers of care about issues of health beliefs has led to measurably increased adherence to treatment regimens (Inui, Yourtee, & Williamson, 1976). Kaplan, Greenfield, and Ware (1989) provided quite a different model. In controlled intervention studies, these researchers taught patients, rather than providers, how to influence physician–patient interaction. Essentially, patients were taught to be more assertive in interactions, to have their concerns heard and their questions answered. Furthermore, the patients studied in these trials were low-income Hispanic and African-American patients with chronic diseases (primarily diabetes and hypertension). In follow-up observations, those patients who were more assertive in their approach to the patient–provider relationship not only were more satisfied with their treatment, but also achieved better glycemic and blood pressure control. Unfortunately missing from these studies is a careful analysis of how the content of belief

systems on the part of both patients and providers entered into the interactions.

RESEARCH AND METHODOLOGICAL ISSUES

Research on cultural influences on health behaviors continues to be plagued by two substantial problems. First, much of the research either is anecdotal or comes in the form of case studies. While both the anecdote and the in-depth case study provide important insight into the processes that are operating, each is problematic in that neither the distributive reliability of the processes involved (i.e., how widely they generalize for a group) nor their explanatory efficacy relative to other influences can be assessed. Second, culture is far too often confounded with social class, ethnicity, language use, national origin, or even, in some cases, personality. The shared and learned knowledge that is constitutive of experience cannot be reduced to these overt indicators, which in any event usually measure other sorts of things (e.g., economic access or, in the case of personality, idiosyncratic beliefs).

Fortunately, there have been some substantial steps in formulating systematic models for studying culture, culminating most notably in the cultural consensus model developed by Romney, Weller, and Batchelder (1986). Drawing on the same sort of theoretical orientation as offered by D'Andrade (1984), Romney et al. (1986) argued that the fundamental issue in studying the knowledge that individuals use in any given domain of life is whether or not it is shared; it is this quality that distinguishes culture from idiosyncratic sorts of knowledge (i.e., personal beliefs). They then developed a mathematical model in which between-person variability in knowledge of, for example, illnesses can be seen as generated from a single underlying cultural model of illness. This formal model of cultural knowledge can then be tested statistically using the consensus model they developed (Romney et al., 1986). Basically, the model involves treating individuals as though they were the variables of interest, to test for an underlying dimension of culture that can reproduce their responses to a wide variety of questions about some domain of life.

The cultural consensus model does three things. First, it tests the "one-culture" model, or the notion that there is a body of shared cultural information. Second, it provides estimates of "cultural competence" for each individual. Deriving such estimates of the differing levels of cultural competence for individuals stems from the observation that all members of a single society or social group do not command equal knowledge or understanding of the culture of that group. Rather, there simply are some people who know their own culture better than others; these people were always the so-called "key informants" of traditional ethnography. The cultural consensus model provides a quantitative estimate of just how good an understanding of a domain of cultural knowledge an individual commands. Third, the consensus model provides estimates, based on the cultural competence of different individuals, of the content of the cultural domain being studied (Romney et al., 1986).

Garro (1989) used the consensus model to study beliefs about essential hypertension among a group of Ojibway Indians in western Canada. Following a series of in-depth interviews to establish the range of variability of the cultural information pool dealing with blood pressure, Garro developed a set of 67 true–false questions (e.g., "Do you think that before the white man came, Indians had high blood pressure") that were administered to 26 respondents. She found that indeed there was sufficient consistency in responses to justify the "one-culture" assumption. Cultural competence estimates that theoretically range from 0.00 to 1.00 ranged from a low of 0.00 to a high of 0.81, indicating that consensus can be achieved even when some individuals present extremely idiosyncratic responses. Finally, she generated a set of responses, weighted more heavily by the more culturally competent respondents, that represents a best estimate of the Ojibway cultural beliefs surrounding hypertension.

One important element of this approach is that these cultural models generalize well, even using relatively small samples of respondents. Of course, any such small sample must be selected carefully. It is perhaps even more important to have a good sampling of *information*, because this information will affect both the testing of the one-culture hypothesis and the resulting estimates of the content of knowledge.

There are several applications of this model that exemplify how it will be useful. For example, Pachter (1994) suggested using the same set of questions about illness causation and treatment for both patients and providers. It is almost a truism to say that patients and providers, especially Western-trained physicians, have different models of illness and disease, but the application of the consensus model could show rather precisely how and where those models differ most dramatically, a step that could be helpful in avoiding the kinds of problems alluded to above with respect to patient–provider interactions.

Oths (1994c) provided a different example of the application of the model, one that takes into account the issue of intracultural diversity. She was interested in cultural models of food and food use in an affluent Brazilian city, in order to understand the knowledge that might influence the adoption of a diet associated with increased risk of cardiovascular disease. Specifically, she wanted to determine whether there was higher prestige attached to foods that were high in saturated fat and cholesterol. Again, after a period of intensive interviewing, she developed an interview schedule in which respondents would rank the prestige value of foods and applied it in a sample of 18 respondents, ranging from poor *faveladas* (women living in squatter settlements) to elite women educated at the graduate level in United States institutions. She found no consensus among the entire group, which had been anticipated. When the women were broken into four groups based on socioeconomic status, however, except for the poorest group, she found within-group consensus. The middle groups indeed rated the food items with the highest fat content to be highest in social status; the elite group, on the other hand, was in the process of adopting a view consistent with upper-middle-class North American food culture, emphasizing the value of "light" foods such as fish and chicken. For the poorest group, there was still no consensus, since many of the food items were unfamiliar to them, their idea of a prestigious diet being the traditional (and healthful) one of rice and beans and fruits.

These examples illustrate the potential use of the cultural consensus model. It can provide, with a level of precision previously unavailable, an estimate of the degree of sharing and salience of cultural knowledge. It can also be used to study cultural diversity within a social group. The latter use of the model is particularly important, given the argument that culture is shared in particular social contexts within which social interaction is especially dense. The examination of cultural models in relation to specific social contexts is an important step in its own right. Beyond this step, however, the consensus model needs to be refined in such a way that measures can be developed for individuals that assess their degree of acceptance of the group-level consensus model. Measures of both group-level models and individual acceptance of such models would permit systematic testing of the predictive efficacy of cultural knowledge relative to other sorts of influences (detailed in other chapters of this volume) on the variety of health behaviors discussed.

This discussion has emphasized the necessity to examine cultural models in social context; to examine cultural models without also examining the immediate social relational contexts within which those models "work" would be to study disembodied knowledge. This consideration raises the question as does Pescosolido (1992), of just what the appropriate unit of analysis is in studies of health behavior. Given the thrust of Western culture, it is hardly surprising that social science conventionally treats the individual as the unit of analysis of ultimate importance. Rather than studying individuals, however, researchers should be studying individuals *in interaction*, bearing in mind that what is important is

some unit of analysis that identifies the critical participants in social interaction and the negotiation of strategies. Following the lead of Pescosolido (1992), Dressler (1994b) found this to be a useful strategy in examining the family correlates of chronic illness labels. More research in this area should help improve understanding of culture and action.

Finally, with respect to the study of health behaviors, there has been far more effort devoted to studying cultural influences on the treatment of disease than to studying those influences on behaviors that are adopted to remain healthy. Given the tremendous boom in the "wellness" industry in the United States this area seems ripe for investigation. With respect to cultural influences on wellness, Conrad (1994) found that participants in wellness programs structure discourse about such programs in profoundly moral terms. It is almost as though the programs are a secular version of the Reformation view of humans as ultimately perfectible. More research needs to be devoted to the cultural meaning systems that influence individuals' and families' decisions to become involved in these sorts of activities.

CONCLUSION

This discussion of health behaviors has emphasized how cultural influences come into play at all stages in the natural history of an episode of sickness, whether it be an episode of disease or an episode of illness. The discussion differed somewhat from past discussions in that it emphasized a formal model of cultural meaning systems and how that model of cultural systems cannot be divorced from the immediate social interactional context in which knowledge is shared, exchanged, and changed. It attempted to maintain a steady focus on the wider context of health behaviors, stressing the way in which these health behaviors are embedded firmly in the ongoing adjustments that individuals make as members of sociocultural groups in their everyday lives.

It is important to keep in mind, however, how much is left undone. There is continuing tension, sometimes creative and sometimes not, within the anthropological enterprise between those who attempt to systematize and quantify the study of culture and those who see their mission as more humanistic in the sense of simply documenting cultural differences. While this latter endeavor is important, at some point it must give way to the detailed and precise quantification of the influence of culture if that knowledge is to be translated into information that can be effectively applied to alter health behaviors. The importance of this effort is clear from two basic epidemiological facts. First, the growth in the United States population of ethnic minorities is and will continue to be substantial (Barker, 1992). Second, there is substantial variation among ethnic groups in the risk of disease, especially the chronic diseases that are major contributors to mortality in the United States (Dressler, 1993; Nickens, 1986; Harwood, 1981). There is a need to understand how ethnicity and disease are linked. In part, the link may be distinctive cultural practices with respect to health behaviors; in part, it is certainly the effect of structured inequality within American society. It is essential to learn more about how these factors interact to generate the natural history of sickness.

ACKNOWLEDGMENTS. Preparation of this chapter was supported in part by a research grant from the National Heart, Lung and Blood Institute (HL45663) to W. W. Dressler and an NIH FIRST award (HD29559) to K. S. Oths.

REFERENCES

Barker, J. C. (1992). Cultural diversity: Changing the context of medical practice. Cross-cultural medicine—A decade later [Special Issue]. *Western Journal of Medicine, 157,* 248–254.

Berkman, L. F., & Syme, S. L. (1979). Social networks, host resistance, and mortality. *American Journal of Epidemiology, 109,* 186–204.

Blumhagen, D. (1980). Hyper-tension: A folk illness with a medical name. *Culture, Medicine and Psychiatry, 4,* 197–227.

Blumhagen, D. (1982). The meaning of hyper-tension. In N. J. Chrisman & T. W. Maretzki (Eds.), *Clinically applied anthropology* (pp. 297–323). Dordrecht, Holland: D. Reidel.

Bohannon, P., & Glazer, M. (1973). *High points in anthropology.* New York: Alfred A. Knopf.

Boster, J. S. (1987). Introduction: Intra-cultural diversity. *American Behavioral Scientist, 31,* 150–162.

Burkett, G. L. (1991). Culture, illness, and the biopsychosocial model. *Family Medicine, 23,* 287–291.

Chrisman, N. J. (1977). The health seeking process: An approach to the natural history of illness. *Culture, Medicine and Psychiatry, 1,* 351–377.

Colson, A. (1970). The differential use of medical resources in developing countries. *Journal of Health and Social Behavior, 12,* 226–237.

Conrad, P. (1994). Wellness as virtue: Morality and the pursuit of health. *Culture, Medicine and Psychiatry, 18,* 385–401.

Crandon-Malamud, L. (1991). Phantoms and physicians: Social change through medical pluralism. In L. Romanucci-Ross, D. Moerman, & L. Tancredi (Eds.), *The anthropology of medicine* (pp. 85–112). New York: Bergin & Garvey.

D'Andrade, R. G. (1984). Cultural meaning systems. In R. A. Schweder & R. A. LeVine (Eds.), *Cultural theory: Essays on mind, self, and emotion* (pp. 88–119). Cambridge, England: Cambridge University Press.

Dressler, W. W. (1989). Type A behavior and the social production of cardiovascular disease. *Journal of Nervous and Mental Disease, 177,* 181–190.

Dressler, W. W. (1991). *Stress and adaptation in the context of culture: Depression in a southern black community.* Albany: State University of New York Press.

Dressler, W. W. (1993). Health in the African-American community: Accounting for health inequalities. *Medical Anthropology Quarterly, 7,* 325–345.

Dressler, W. W. (1994a). Cross-cultural differences and social influences in social support and cardiovascular disease. In S. A. Shumaker & S. M. Czajkowski (Eds.), *Social support and cardiovascular disease* (pp. 167–192). New York: Plenum Press.

Dressler, W. W. (1994b). Social status and the health of families: A model. *Social Science and Medicine, 39,* 1605–1613.

Eisenberg, D. M., Kessler, R. C., Foster, C., Norlock, F. E., Calkins, D. R., & Delbanco, T. L. (1993). Unconventional medicine in the United States. *New England Journal of Medicine, 328,* 246–252.

Engel, G. L. (1977). The need for a new medical model. *Science, 196,* 129–136.

Fisher, L., Terry, H. E., & Ranson, D. C. (1990). Advancing a family perspective in health research: Models and methods. *Family Process, 29,* 177–189.

Gaines, A. D. (1982). Knowledge and practice: Anthropological ideas and psychiatric practice. In N. Chrisman & T. Maretzki (Eds.), *Clinically applied anthropology: Anthro-*

pologists in health science settings (pp. 243-273). Dordrecht, Holland: D. Reidel.

Gaines, A. D. (Ed.). (1992). Ethnopsychiatry: The cultural construction of professional and folk psychiatries. Albany: State University of New York Press.

Garrison, V. (1977). Doctor, espiritista, or psychiatrist: Health-seeking behavior in a Puerto-Rican neighborhood of New York City. Medical Anthropology, 1, 65-190.

Garro, L. C. (1988). Explaining high blood pressure: Variation in knowledge about illness. American Ethnologist, 15, 98-119.

Geertz, C. (1973). The interpretation of cultures. New York: Basic Books.

Harwood, A. (1977). RX: Spiritist as needed. New York: Wiley.

Harwood, A. (1981). Ethnicity and medical care. Cambridge, MA: Harvard University Press.

Helman, C. (1988). Psyche, soma, and society: The social construction of psychosomatic disorders. In M. Lock & D. Gordon (Eds.), Biomedicine examined (pp. 95-122). Dordrecht, Holland: Kluwer Academic.

Holland, D. (1987). Culture sharing across gender lives: An interactionist corrective to the status-centered model. American Behavioral Scientist, 31, 234-239.

Inui, J. F., Yourtee, E. L., & Williamson, J. W. (1976). Improved outcomes in hypertension after physician tutorials. Annals of Internal Medicine, 84, 649-651.

Janes, C. R. (1990). Migration, social change, and health: A Samoan community in urban California. Stanford: Stanford University Press.

Janzen, J. M. (1978). The quest for therapy in lower Zaire. Berkeley: University of California Press.

Kaplan, S. H., Greenfield, S., & Ware, J. E. (1989). Assessing the effects of physician-patient interactions on the outcomes of chronic disease. Medical Care, 27 (Supplement), 5110-5127.

Kasl, S. U., & Cobb, S. (1966). Health behavior, illness behavior, and the sick role. Archives of Environmental Health, 12, 246-266.

Katon, W., & Kleinman, A. (1980). Doctor-patient negotiation and other social science strategies in patient care. In L. Eisenberg & A. Kleinman (Eds.), The relevance of social science for medicine (pp. 253-279). Dordrecht, Holland: D. Reidel.

Keefe, S. E., Padilla, A. M., & Carlos, M. L. (1979). The Mexican-American family as an emotional support system. Human Organization, 38, 144-152.

Keesing, R. H. (1994). Theories of culture revisited. In R. Borofsky (Ed.), Assessing cultural anthropology (pp. 301-310). New York: McGraw-Hill.

Kirmayer, L. J. (1994). Improvisation and authority in illness meaning. Culture, Medicine and Psychiatry, 18, 183-214.

Kleinman, A. (1980). Patients and healers in the context of culture. Berkeley: University of California Press.

Kleinman, A., Eisenberg, L., & Good, B. (1978). Culture,

illness, and care. Annals of Internal Medicine, 88, 251-258.

Kliger, R. (1994). Somatization: Social control and illness production in a religious cult. Culture, Medicine and Psychiatry, 18, 215-245.

Kramer, B. J. (1992). Health and aging of urban American Indians. Western Journal of Medicine, 157, 281-285.

Lin, N., Ensel, W. M., Simeone, R. S., & Kuo, W. (1979). Social support, stressful life events, and illness: A model and empirical test. Journal of Health and Social Behavior, 20, 108-119.

Lock, M. (1985). Models and practice in medicine: Menopause as syndrome or life transition? In R. A. Hahn & A. D. Gaines (Eds.), Physicians of western medicine (pp. 115-139). Dordrecht, Holland: D. Reidel.

McKinlay, J. B. (1981). Social network influences on morbid episodes and the career of help seeking. In L. Eisenberg & A. Kleinman (Eds.), The relevance of social science for medicine (pp. 77-110). Dordrecht, Holland: D. Reidel.

Mishler, E. G. (1981a). The social construction of illness. In E. G. Mishler, L. R. Amarasingham, S. T. Hauser, R. Liem, S. D. Osherson, & N. E. Waxter (Eds.), Social contexts of health, illness, and patient care (pp. 141-168). Cambridge, England: Cambridge University Press.

Mishler, E. G. (1981b). Patients in social context. In E. G. Mishler, L. R. Amarasingham, S. T. Hauser, R. Liem, S. D. Osherson, & N. E. Waxler (Eds.), Social contexts of health, illness, and patient care (pp. 24-53). Cambridge, England: Cambridge University Press.

Nickens, H. (1986). Health problems of minority groups: Public health's unfinished agenda. Public Health Reports, 101, 230-231.

Oths, K. S. (1994a). Health care decisions of households in economic crisis: An example from the Peruvian highlands. Human Organization, 53, 245-254.

Oths, K. S. (1994b). Communication in a chiropractic clinic: How a D.C. treats his patients. Culture, Medicine and Psychiatry, 18, 83-113.

Oths, K. S. (1994c). Social status and food preference in southeast Brazil. Abstracts of the annual meeting of the Society for Applied Anthropology, Cancun, Mexico, April 13-17. Oklahoma City, OK: Society for Applied Anthropology.

Pachter, L. M. (1994). Asthma beliefs and behaviors in four Latino groups. Abstracts of the annual meeting of the Society for Applied Anthropology, Cancun, Mexico, April 13-17. Oklahoma City, OK: Society for Applied Anthropology.

Parsons, T. (1951). The social system. Glencoe, IL: Free Press.

Paul, B. D. (Ed.). (1955). Health, culture, and community. New York: Russell Sage Foundation.

Pelto, P. J., & Pelto, G. H. (1975). Intra-cultural diversity: Some theoretical issues. American Ethnologist, 2, 1-18.

Pescosolido, B. A. (1992). Beyond rational choice: The social dynamics of how people seek help. American Journal of Sociology, 97, 1096-1138.

Romanucci-Ross, L. (1969). The hierarchy of resort in curative practices: The Admiralty Islands, Melanesia. *Journal of Health and Social Behavior, 10*, 201–208.

Romney, K. A., Weller, S. C., & Batchelder, W. H. (1986). Culture as consensus: A theory of culture and informant accuracy. *American Anthropologist, 88*, 313–338.

Rubel, A. J. (1964). The epidemiology of a folk illness: *Susto* in Hispanic America. *Ethnology, 3*, 268–283.

Rubel, A. J., O'Nell, C. W., & Ardon, R. C. (1984). *Susto, a folk illness*. Berkeley: University of California Press.

Rylko-Bauer, B. (1988). The development and use of free-standing emergency centers: A review of the literature. *Medical Care Review, 45*, 129–163.

Snow, L. F. (1993). *Walkin' over medicine*. Boulder, CO: Westview Press.

Spiro, M. E. (1986). Cultural relativism and the future of anthropology. *Cultural Anthropology, 1*, 259–286.

Stack, C. (1974). *All our kin: Strategies for survival in the black community*. New York: Harper & Row.

Stafford, A. M. (1978). The application of clinical anthropology to medical practice: Case study of recurrent abdominal pain in a preadolescent Mexican-American female. In E. E. Bauwens (Ed.), *The anthropology of health* (pp. 12–22). St. Louis, MO: C. V. Mosby.

Suchman, E. A. (1965). Stages of illness and medical care. *Journal of Health and Human Behavior, 6*, 114–128.

Swartz, M. (1991). *The way the world is*. Berkeley: University of California Press.

Ware, N. C., & Kleinman, A. (1992). Culture and somatic experience. *Psychosomatic Medicine, 54*, 546–560.

Young, A. (1982). The anthropologies of illness and sickness. *Annual Review of Anthropology, 11*, 257–285.

Young, A. (1983). The relevance of traditional medical cultures to modern primary health care. *Social Science and Medicine, 17*, 1205–1211.

Young, J. C. (1981). *Medical choice in a Mexican Village*. New Brunswick, NJ: Rutgers University Press.

VI
INTEGRATION

18

Personal and Social Determinants of Health Behavior

An Integration

David S. Gochman

This chapter provides an integration of major points and findings presented in this volume. Although its contents primarily reflect the contributions to this volume, rather than the larger body of scholarship about personal and social determinants of health behavior, they are consistent with this knowledge. An exception to this focus is the section on future directions, which includes additional perspectives.

Authors of individual chapters focused on specific single levels or components of personal or social systems and were free to select from the very broad range of health beliefs or actions embraced in the definition of health behavior that frames this *Handbook*. In contrast with and complementary to the basic organization of this volume, a major portion of this integration is organized around the following six broad categories of health behaviors: health cognitions, such as

definitions of health and illness, health beliefs, and attitudes; care seeking; preventive, protective, and safety behaviors; risk behaviors; responses to illness, including adherence and sick role; and lifestyle behaviors. The chapter will show how personal, family, social, institutional, community, and cultural factors serve as determinants of behaviors in each of these categories.

A brief overview of relevant conceptual models introduces the chapter. Each of the six categories of health behaviors is then examined in terms of relevant personal and social determinants. (Determinants not linked to a category in this volume are not discussed. Their omission does not mean that the determinants are not relevant to the behavior category; it means only that their relevance was not introduced in these chapters.) This is the chapter's major organizing principle and is the foundation of a "work-in-progress matrix-type framework" for organizing the larger body of health behavior knowledge; the framework is discussed in greater detail in Chapter 20 of Volume IV. The chapter continues with an analysis of some common themes and concludes with some directions for future research.

David S. Gochman • Kent School of Social Work, University of Louisville, Louisville, Kentucky 40292.

Handbook of Health Behavior Research I: Personal and Social Determinants, edited by David S. Gochman. Plenum Press, New York, 1997.

MAJOR CONCEPTUAL MODELS

The following synoptic presentation serves solely as background for this integration. Comprehensive, critical discussion of major conceptual models is provided in the chapters indicated.

Cognitive Representation Models

Cognitive representation models (Lau, Chapter 3) propose that persons have their own images or schemata of illnesses and health that are often at variance with the biomedical disease model. Important components of such cognitive images are the beliefs that comprise the identity given to symptoms, beliefs about the consequences of these symptoms, a time line for their duration, beliefs about their cause, and beliefs about their cure or control.

Health Belief Model

The health belief model (Strecher, Champion, & Rosenstock, Chapter 4) was the earliest cognitive conceptual framework designed to explain and predict health-related behaviors. The initial components of the model were perceived susceptibility, beliefs about being at risk for some health threat or condition; perceived seriousness or severity, beliefs that the health threat or condition would have appreciable negative consequences; perceived benefits, belief that there were net gains in taking a specified health action; and perceived barriers, beliefs that there were obstacles and costs involved in taking such actions.

Locus of Control

Locus of control (Reich, Erdal, & Zautra, Chapter 5) refers to the degree to which persons believe that things that happen to them are the result of their own ability to influence events as opposed to being the result of chance, fate, or powerful external forces. Locus of control models suggest that persons who have relatively strong

beliefs in their own "agency" or control over events will behave differently in a wide range of health or illness situations than persons who have low levels of such beliefs.

Protection Motivation Theory

Protection motivation theory (Rogers & Prentice-Dunn, Chapter 6) emphasizes threat and the effects of threatening health information as an impetus to initiating behavioral change. The major components of the theory are sources of information, the cognitive mediating processes of threat appraisals and coping appraisals, and modes of coping, i.e., adaptive coping behaviors that reduce the threat or maladaptive coping behaviors that do not manage the threat effectively. According to protection motivation models, information about a health threat initiates threat appraisal factors, some of which—such as intrinsic or extrinsic pleasures resulting from the risk behavior—increase the likelihood of a maladaptive response and some of which—such as the severity and likelihood of the threat—decrease the likelihood of a maladaptive response. The joint operation of these appraisal factors results in the final appraisal of threat. (There is some parallel between severity and likelihood of threat to perceived severity and perceived susceptibility components of the original health belief model.)

Behavioral Intention Models

A person's intention to engage in a specific behavior is the major theoretical outcome of the theory of reasoned action (TRA)/theory of planned behavior (TPB) (Maddux & DuCharme, Chapter 7). Critical components in these theories are attitudes toward a specific behavior, the evaluation of the behavior based on expectations about the behavior's outcome; perceived social norms, beliefs about other persons' support of the behavior; and perceived behavioral control, beliefs that the behavior can be enacted or changed. Perceived behavioral control is closely related to self-efficacy. Together, these factors predict a person's behavioral intention. More important, perceived behavioral control interacts with level of intention in predicting actual behavior or behavior change.

Social Cognitive and Social Learning Theories

Critical concepts in social cognitive theories (Baranowski, Chapter 9; Tinsley, Chapter 11) are outcome expectations, a person's beliefs that a specific result will occur if a behavior is undertaken; self-efficacy, a person's confidence that a behavior can be successfully enacted; and skills, the person's ability to perform the behavior. Closely linked are concepts from social learning theory, which include role modeling, the demonstration by someone of a particular behavior, and reinforcement, the reward or punishment of the behavior in social contexts.

Health Services Utilization Models

Health services utilization models (Aday & Awe, Chapter 8) are based on path analyses of personal/family, societal, and institutional factors that predict use of professional health services. Major components of the model at the personal/family level include need variables, such as illness or health status; predisposing variables, such as individual and family health beliefs and social status; and enabling variables, such as financial resources and insurance. Health technology and social norms are important components at the societal level, and the manner in which health care is organized and the degree to which it is available are important institutional components of these models.

Sick Role Models

Sick role, a conceptual framework proposed and developed by Parsons (1951), specified that persons who are ill have rights to be exempted from task and role responsibilities, as well as from the responsibility for their condition, and have duties to seek medical care as well as to adhere to medical advice and to recover. An expanded alternative model (Segall, Chapter 14) specifies that persons have rights to make decisions about health care and to be dependent on other laypersons for care and social support, contingent upon these others agreeing to do so, and have duties to maintain health and overcome illness, to engage in routine self-management, and to make use of a range of resources.

Cultural Consensus Models

The cultural consensus model (Dressler & Oths, Chapter 17) is a conceptual framework to assess the degree to which a body of information is shared within a social group. It provides an estimate of shared beliefs related to health and illness.

SELECTED HEALTH BEHAVIORS

Health Cognitions

Personal Determinants. Definitions of personal determinants of health and illness are provided by Gochman (Chapter 1) and highlighted in the discussion of cognitive representations (Lau, Chapter 3). Data demonstrate that most people define being healthy as embodying a combination of physical, emotional, and social functioning. In addition, they define being healthy as being more than free of disease. A person's observation that some somatic experiences deviate from cognitively represented baseline images for symptoms and for being healthy becomes the first step in the process of defining, or self-diagnosing, "being sick" (Lau). Moreover, developmental stages contribute to what is defined as health or illness, persons may maintain several different definitions of health simultaneously, and personal equilibrium and breakdown concepts both have relevance to definitions of health and illness (Gochman).

Family Determinants. The concept of "family coding," which refers to a system of shared norms that are used as guidelines for the family's behavior, has implications for health cognitions. Family coding would apply to how a family defines health, illness, and sickness, as well as to family stories about health-related experiences and the way the family interpreted and responded to those experiences (Tinsley, Chapter 11).

Cultural factors also influence the importance of the family in the process of labeling symptoms. The family, expressing its own interpretation of the culture in which it lives, may at times "negotiate" a label for a condition to avoid the labeling of one of its members as having a stigmatized condition that would reflect poorly on the family's status and prestige (Dressler & Oths, Chapter 17).

Social Determinants. Factors that contribute to social constructions of health and illness include the degree of social functioning and equilibrium. To the degree that a person's social functioning is inconsistent with or deviates from social expectations, there is disequilibrium in the social system, and the person may be defined, perceived, or labeled as being sick (Gochman, Chapter 10). Social systems vary greatly in the degree to which they allow behavioral flexibility or ease of masking or containing the unsatisfactory or deviant behavior. When such behaviors can no longer be masked or contained, the person is labeled as sick (Alonzo, 1984, cited in Gochman, Chapter 1).

Labeling persons as sick is also a way of preventing or reducing societal breakdown. By defining persons as sick, society allows those persons to be excused from performance of roles and tasks, with the understanding that they will seek care and recover and resume their role and task performance (Gochman).

Institutional Determinants. The historical evolution of the role of economic and political processes in the health care institutions of any

society is discussed at length by Fabrega (Chapter 2). Such institutions, whether they be practitioners themselves, settings of care, societal norms, or governmental policies related to access to care and treatment, acquire the power to define what is healthy and what is not and who is sick and who is not.

Cultural Determinants. Using the concept of the *healmeme*, a basic unit of cultural information about health and illness, Fabrega (Chapter 2) additionally demonstrates the relationship between cultural changes and changes in definitions and connotations of health and illness and shows how different types of cultural and societal organization, with different types of political and economic structures, vary in the patterns by which health and illness are defined. As societies developed from early family-level organizations to late-20th-century postindustrial cultures, definitions of health and illness moved from "holistic" conceptions embodying linkages between the sick person, the family, the social group, and the spiritual world to biomedical, physical definitions that isolated sickness and health from the larger social fabric. Illness became secularized, more "objectified," and the social and spiritual linkages became lost.

Cultural determinants of how information is learned, transmitted, and shared are also important determinants of health cognitions (Dressler & Oths, Chapter 17). Different cultural and ethnic groups within a society share different sets of information and have different patterns of information exchange with the larger society. Such differences in information sharing lead to different definitions of disease and different labels for similar clusters of symptoms. The same symptoms of fatigue, listlessness, loss of interest in everyday activities, and a sense of helplessness can be interpreted biomedically as being consistent with depression, chronic fatigue syndrome, or even poor nutrition. Yet in the Hispanic community, they could be interpreted as manifestations of *susto* ("magical fright").

The interplay of cultural values and personal

experiences results in the emergence of "cultural themes" that differentially value health and illness. Illness is not necessarily perceived negatively, but may be viewed as a liberating experience (Herzlich, 1973, cited in Gochman, Chapter 1). Cultural values also dominate prevailing "scientific" and professional definitions of health and illness (Herzlich, 1973, cited in Gochman, Chapter 1).

Care Seeking

Personal Determinants. From the data presented by Lau (Chapter 3), care seeking begins when a person experiences symptoms that deviate from the person's cognitive representations of illness and health. Within a context of self-regulatory and problem-solving models, such experiences initiate a process of interpretation, i.e., an attempt to understand the unusual event through use of cognitive representations; coping, i.e., planning and executing a course of action to return to equilibrium; and appraisal, i.e., assessing whether the coping strategy was successful and, if it was not, developing a new interpretation.

At the same time, interpretation and evaluation of symptoms, i.e., self-diagnosis, and decision to engage in some form of self-care are often symptom-specific. A majority of persons might seek a physician's care if they experienced unexplained weight loss or shortness of breath, although they would routinely resort to self-care for other conditions such as an upset stomach (Dressler & Oths, Chapter 17).

Aday and Awe's discussion of health services utilization models (Chapter 8) identifies three determinants of care seeking that have strong personal components: predisposing, enabling, and need factors. Predisposing factors include age and marital status and beliefs about health, illness, and health services. Enabling factors include financial resources such as insurance and savings. Need factors include health status as well as the person's response to illness.

The alternative, expanded sick role concept allows for individual "lay" initiatives in care seeking as well as illness management strategies (Segall, Chapter 14). Care seeking is thus seen as under the person's own control, rather than as being determined by others or defined by physicians, and includes self-care. Data demonstrate that laypersons are the primary providers of health care for themselves, that they routinely self-evaluate and self-treat.

Family Determinants. The role of extended kinship systems in care-seeking behavior in diverse ethnic and immigrant groups is demonstrated by Dressler and Oths (Chapter 17). Such kinship systems vary in resources—both material and informational—as well as in their interaction with the larger community.

Aday and Awe (Chapter 8) emphasize that predisposing, enabling, and need factors in care seeking operate within a family context and have family-level components. For example, family size is a predisposing factor and family financial status an enabling factor in care seeking.

Within the family, mothers have the primary responsibility for assessing the need for care and for obtaining it (Tinsley, Chapter 11). Moreover, factors such as family cohesiveness affect care seeking: More cohesive families tend to use prenatal and pediatric health services less frequently than less cohesive families (Geertsen, Chapter 13). Geertsen refers to the concept of "familism," the degree of importance of family and relatives in an individual's life, and shows that it can often encourage use of health services.

Social Determinants. Social factors such as the size of a person's social networks influence care-seeking behavior, although the direction of such influence is often mediated by larger cultural variables (Geertsen, Chapter 13). Some social networks encourage use of biomedical practitioners; others discourage it or encourage delay of such use or endorse the use of alternative practitioners. Moreover, membership in different social networks might result in conflicting influences. Geertsen distinguishes between social networks and social support, noting that lack of social support is often associated with greater care-seeking behavior.

Social roles related to gender influence differential rates of care-seeking behavior in women and men (Waldron, Chapter 15). Women have typically—but not always—shown a higher level of health service use than men.

An expanded sick role model is based on the social reciprocity between a person and others. One's ability to engage in self-care behavior, to be one's own primary caregiver, is dependent on the ability and inclination of others to accept responsibility for the sick person's ordinary task and role obligations and for helping in the caregiving process (Segall, Chapter 14).

Institutional Determinants. Larger system determinants of care seeking have increasingly assumed a greater importance in the evolution of health services utilization models. Aday and Awe (Chapter 8) point to the critical role of availability and accessibility of services in determining their use by individuals as well as the role of governmental and health care organization policies regarding the financing and arrangement of health care delivery. In addition, Aday and Awe point to societal products such as technology as important determinants of care-seeking behavior.

Cultural Determinants. A culture's political and economic structure strongly determines the hierarchies of healers and health care practitioners and the bases on which these hierarchies are established (Fabrega, Chapter 2). Such cultural hierarchies are important determinants of what types of care will be sought and which professionals will be sanctioned.

Cultural determinants involved in choosing between traditional and biomedical practitioners, and from among alternatives within these categories (e.g., seeking herbalists, or sorcerers, or bone-setters), are further emphasized by Dressler and Oths (Chapter 17). Dressler and Oths point to two contrasting components of ethnic group networks: those parts of the network that enable the group to exist separately from the majority culture and those parts that help the group to master the barriers it faces. The first component supports the existence of alternatives to the larger culture's health care professionals (e.g., *santería*, herbalists); the second component enables the group's members to cope effectively with the bureaucracies and institutions of the larger culture in the care-seeking process.

Preventive, Protective, and Safety Behaviors

Personal Determinants. The health belief model enjoyed a measure of success in predicting simple one-shot, non-habit-related behaviors such as attending preventive screenings for tuberculosis, high blood pressure, and Tay-Sachs status, and programs designed to inform about breast self-examination (BSE), seat belt use, exercise, nutrition, smoking, and making preventive visits to physicians (Strecher, Champion, & Rosenstock, Chapter 4). The model was extended to predict sick role behaviors such as accepting medical advice and has also been used to predict safe (or safer) sex behavior. Perceived barriers has proven to be the strongest single predictor across all behaviors and all studies. Of particular note was its value in predicting BSE, although direct effects for BSE were also found for perceived susceptibility and perceived benefits. In addition, in a variety of studies, perceived susceptibility proved an important predictor of preventive behaviors. Perceived barriers and susceptibility were also the most important predictors of intention to participate in mammography screening. Perceived severity seems not to play a critical role in such predictions.

Locus of control beliefs also predict preventive behaviors. Persons who perceive a locus of control within themselves (internals) engage in more health-related information seeking, assume greater responsibility for their health, and take greater precautions than persons who perceive control as lying outside themselves (externals).

The results, however, have not always been consistent or generalizable (Reich, Erdal, & Zautra, Chapter 5). Adding beliefs about self-efficacy improved the predictive value of control beliefs for exercise behavior: Persons with beliefs in internal control who also had higher levels of self-efficacy exhibited more exercise behaviors than persons with lower levels of self-efficacy. Other interactions, however, preclude further generalizations.

Finally, appearance motivation was found to be negatively related to some protective intentions. Persons with high levels of appearance motivation were less likely to intend to reduce their risk for skin cancers (Rogers & Prentice-Dunn, Chapter 6).

Family Determinants. Family socialization processes affect a variety of preventive and adaptive behaviors. Children growing up in families that use more strongly punitive and disciplinary methods were likely to show less independence in their use of seat belts, tooth brushing, exercising, regularity of bedtime, and hand washing than children in families that were more warmly nurturing (Tinsley, Chapter 11). The mother's role as a gatekeeper and supervisor of television viewing has implications for the child's initiation of risk behaviors as well as engaging in appropriate diet, exercise, and safety behaviors.

Institutional Determinants. Physician communication was found to be an important predictor of intentions to have a mammogram (Strecher, Champion, & Rosenstock, Chapter 4), as well as a correlate of prior mammography history.

Risk Behaviors

Personal Determinants. Contrary to the success of the health belief model in predicting preventive behaviors, the basic components of the model are less adequate, in themselves, in predicting changes in risk behaviors, particularly if these behaviors involve well-ingrained habitual actions such as smoking, eating, consumption of alcohol, and sexual practices (Strecher, Champion, & Rosenstock, Chapter 4). Findings linking perceived susceptibility to reductions in risky sexual behaviors are equivocal. Strecher et al. note that the concept of self-efficacy—the belief that one can execute a required behavior—has become an important component in health belief model research and has increased the value of the model in predicting selected safer sex practices and in changing patterns of substance abuse.

Data generated by protection motivation theory reveal something of a boomerang effect: High levels of threat coupled with low levels of coping skills led to an increase in risky behavior. If persons do not believe that threat can be successfully avoided, then they apparently have no reason to restrain their behaviors (Rogers & Prentice-Dunn, Chapter 6).

Family Determinants. Tinsley (Chapter 11) reveals the importance of maternal role modeling for the emergence of risk behaviors such as smoking. Maternal smoking was clearly related to the likelihood that the child would smoke.

Social Determinants. Waldron (Chapter 15) provides ample discussion of gender differences in, and determinants of, a representative variety of risk behaviors. For example, women smoke and consume alcohol to appreciably lesser degrees than men, but also show greater risks, for example, in excessive weight loss behaviors. Waldron discusses the components of gender roles that might account for such differences; e.g., dieting behaviors are seen as part of the female gender role, and competitive sports, with their attendant risks, are seen as part of the male gender role.

Theories of planned behavior/reasoned action suggest that social norms—as they are interpreted or perceived by an individual—play a role in supporting or discouraging risky behaviors, as well as in predicting whether the person intends to change the behavior (Maddux & DuCharme, Chapter 7).

Institutional Determinants. Occupational and work-related factors such as job stress and perceived lack of job control are related to risk behaviors such as smoking and alcohol use (Eakin, Chapter 16). In addition, workplace norms—or the workplace culture—may influence rates of alcohol consumption. Inadequacies in workplace supervision may also increase the likelihood that employees will smoke and drink, as well as disregard occupational safety regulations. Eakin further notes that perceived lack of supervisory supportiveness may be related to greater use of sleeping pills and tranquilizers. Characteristics of institutional, organizational, or occupational "culture" also have effects on perceptions of risk behaviors. Medical specialists in a "competitive–individualistic" work culture viewed the risk of radiological harm as a legitimate one to be accepted in return for both tangible rewards (money) and intangible rewards (autonomy, status). They derived their perceptions of their ability to deal with the risks from their own sense of control. In contrast, administrators and technicians in a "bureaucratic" work culture developed their perceptions from the routinization of risk and from adhering carefully to safety procedures (Eakin).

Cultural Determinants. Cultural values and norms that underlie the differential socialization of men and women affect risk behaviors (Waldron, Chapter 15). The norms of Eurocentric cultures encourage men to be bold and to take more risks and women to be more cautious. Men are additionally encouraged to be more competitive, and thus are at greater risk for athletic accidents and injuries.

Responses to Illness, Adherence, and Sick Role

Personal Determinants. Lau's analysis (Chapter 3) of cognitive representations of illness suggests that a discrepancy between experienced symptoms, one's baseline for such symptoms, and one's definition of health is the first step in illness behavior. A self-regulatory mecha-

nism interprets social messages, either from experienced symptoms or from others, including physicians as well as members of social networks, and initiates behaviors that help a person to define the meaning of somatic problems, to act to remove the risk, and to return to some "healthy" equilibrium. According to Lau, persons integrate elements of stored knowledge and devise some means of coping with the disequilibrium, then appraise the outcome of this coping in terms of symptom reduction. If symptoms persist or worsen, then the person engages in additional self-regulatory behavior. This self-regulatory model pairs cognitive representation with an emotional reaction, triggered by the deviation from equilibrium.

The health belief model has generated much research on acceptance of medical regimens, a critical component of response to illness or sick role behavior. For example, in a sample of adolescents with insulin-dependent diabetes, perceived susceptibility (threat) and perceived barriers/benefits proved to be strong predictors of regimen acceptance (Strecher, Champion, & Rosenstock, Chapter 4).

Social Determinants. How social relationships predict responses to illness can be seen in the way that positive social support—defined as instrumental or emotional support—was negatively related to taking medication and to perceiving health problems and in the way that negative social support—defined as the presence of persons who cause problems—was positively related to taking medication and to perceptions of health problems (Reich, Erdal, & Zautra, Chapter 5).

Institutional Determinants. Institutional determinants of sick role and illness behavior can be readily seen in the differences or discrepancies between physician and patient belief systems. These differences, strongly affected by cultural factors, may lead to inappropriate diagnoses and treatment responses, which in turn can have negative effects on adherence and other sick role behaviors (Dressler & Oths, Chapter 17).

Cultural Determinants. Cultural factors have an impact on sick role behaviors and responses to illness by their determination of patterns of information exchange through social interaction (Dressler & Oths, Chapter 17).

Lifestyle Behaviors

Personal Determinants. The concept of lifestyle, often only fuzzily understood, is given a clear definition by Cockerham (Chapter 12). Healthful lifestyles involve decisions to live in a healthful manner, including decisions about food, exercise, coping with stress, and physical appearance. (They also involve eliminating risk behaviors, discussed earlier in this chapter.) Cockerham also notes that education is a more powerful predictor of lifestyle than either occupation or income. Among the cognitive models, protection motivation theory, the theories based on behavioral intentions (TRA, TPB), and the stages of change model focus more than other models on personal determinants of lifestyle changes.

Research using protection motivation theory has covered a wide range of behaviors, including exercise and diet. Although the model has been used primarily to predict the *intention* to engage in the lifestyle behavior, it has also had success in predicting the behavior itself (Rogers & Prentice-Dunn, Chapter 6).

TRA/TPB has also been used in predicting a large number of behavioral/lifestyle changes. Maddux and DuCharme (Chapter 7) report that perceived behavioral control increased the intention to engage in weight loss behaviors. The attitudinal component of the theory predicted a considerable amount of the variance in exercise intentions and was apparently a more stable and significant predictor of intentions to change than was perceived social norms. Findings, however, were not always consistent. Moreover, Maddux and DuCharme point out, persons trying to change lifestyle behaviors continually face having to balance engaging in a simple behavior, such as putting on a condom or putting down a cigarette, and powerful urges such as sex and cravings for nicotine.

Finally, persons with beliefs in internal control who also placed a high value on health were more successful at quitting smoking than those for whom health was less valued (Reich, Erdal, & Zautra, Chapter 5).

Family Determinants. Family factors that affect eating behavior include patterns of grocery shopping and food preparation, and financial resources (Baranowski, Chapter 9). Such factors together with strongly ingrained food preferences also present barriers to dietary change. The primary determinant of whether a child eats a food is whether a parent serves it at the dining table. Parental failure to keep fruits and vegetables in the house accounts for children's low consumption of these foods. Baranowski also observes an increase in the impact of children's own food preferences on the family's diet, particularly on breakfast foods.

Social Determinants. The impact of social norms and values on lifestyle is discussed extensively by Cockerham (Chapter 12), who observes their linkage to status groups and to social patterns of consumption. The social norm component of TRA/TPB was also shown to have some impact on intentions to engage in exercise behaviors (Maddux & DuCharme, Chapter 7). Social norms within the workplace have affects on maintenance of the behavior change in using ear protectors (Eakin, Chapter 16).

Gender roles also play an important part in maintaining or changing diet and exercise patterns. Female concern for being thin may account for restricted dietary intake, and male concern for fitness may account for participation in and continuation of exercise and fitness programs (Waldron, Chapter 15).

Institutional Determinants. The distribution of food stores in a community has an impact on the differential availability of nutritional foods (Baranowski, Chapter 9). Larger supermarkets, which are more likely than small neighborhood groceries or convenience stores to carry a selection of nutritious foods, are also more likely to be accessible to middle-class families than to families living on more limited financial resources.

Cultural Determinants. Data generated by the cultural consensus model (Dressler & Oths, Chapter 17) show that contrary to assumptions about cultural uniformity, different social strata within a culture may share different bodies of information about food. Moreover, women in the middle social strata of Brazilian culture rated food with the highest fat content to be the highest in social status; women in the very highest stratum, in contrast, attributed higher social status to foods lighter in fat, consistent with their adopting more of the food culture of the North American upper middle class. The degree to which subcultural groups within a population have different preferences for fatty foods, for example, has implications for population-based interventions attempting to change their diets.

COMMON THEMES

Five themes underlie a number of aspects of health behavior research throughout this volume: conceptual issues, methodological issues, professional versus phenomenological perspectives, the role of affect, and the size of the focal system.

Conceptual Issues

Conceptual issues include conceptual development, clarity, and confusion. Though these issues overlap considerably, issues of clarity can be seen as complements to issues of confusion.

Conceptual Development. Conceptual development over nearly half a century (1950s to mid-1990s) can be seen in several of the major frames of reference dealt with in this volume, particularly in cognitive models, the health services utilization model, and the concept of sick role. Since the emergence of the health belief model in the late 1950s (e.g., Rosenstock, Der-

ryberry, & Carriger, 1959), all of the cognitive frameworks for understanding health behavior have evolved from fairly simple ones with a few belief/perceptual variables to far more complex schemata composed of and integrating cognitive, affective, and social variables, such as the most recent revisions of behavioral intention theory (Maddux & DuCharme, Chapter 7).

In similar fashion, the health services utilization model, which initially dealt almost entirely with demographic, perceptual, and health status characteristics of individuals, has evolved into a far more complex framework, incorporating and systematically elaborating, in a more explicit way, characteristics of families, communities, and governmental policy. Moreover, the ethical issue of social equity has become an integral component of the model in relation to its use in the planning of health services (Aday & Awe, Chapter 8).

The Parsonian conceptualization of sick role (Parsons, 1951) initially dealt exclusively with patient and physician interaction, particularly in relation to acceptance of medical advice. It has evolved into a model that includes social interactions and reciprocity and the rights of lay caregivers (Segall, Chapter 14).

Conceptual Clarity. Important conceptual clarifications include refinements made in thinking about risk behaviors, habitual and volitional behaviors, and "outcomes." Risk and risk reduction behaviors are seen as having considerable commonality; they are generally simple to perform, yet they are usually associated with powerful human urges or pleasures that are hard to resist, such as sex drives, hunger and thirst, and the desire to avoid pain and discomfort (Maddux & DuCharme, Chapter 7).

The distinction between volitional and habitual behaviors has assumed special importance in attempts to change risk behaviors. Initial assumptions—consistent with cognitive, rational models—that target behaviors are under volitional control have been appropriately questioned (e.g., Kirscht, 1988; Maddux & DuCharme,

Chapter 7); most risk behaviors are habitual, rather than volitional. The theory of planned behavior accommodates this difference by incorporating the concept of *perceived behavioral control*, which denotes the belief about how easy or difficult it is to perform the behavior.

Increased clarity can also be seen in the elaboration of the concept of situational cues. Maddux and DuCharme note the important distinction that needs to be made between situational events that serve as cues to the decision process—driving the intention to change behavior—and those that serve as cues to action—driving habitual behavior.

A final example of increased clarity is the conceptualization of health status. In the original health services utilization model, health status had been thought of solely as a determinant of care-seeking behaviors, or the use of services. It has been reconceptualized as both an outcome and a determinant of health behaviors. Aday and Awe (Chapter 8) point out that not only do personal need factors, including health status, serve as predictors of use of services, but also use of services, as one would expect, has a reciprocal effect on health status.

Conceptual Confusion. At the same time that considerable progress has been made in theoretical development and elaboration, problems with conceptual clarity continue to plague health behavior research, as they probably do any other area of scholarly inquiry. A number of the cognitive models in particular manifest problems in clear specification of variables. For example, research driven by behavioral intention theory has sometimes confounded "goals" and "behavior" (Maddux & DuCharme, Chapter 7); e.g., intending to lose weight has been confounded with intending to engage in specific eating behaviors. Thus, there is confusion about whether measures of perceived behavioral control reflect control over the behaviors or control over goal attainment.

Strecher, Champion, and Rosenstock (Chapter 4) further note that operational definitions are not always logical derivations of concepts. Additional lack of clarity can be seen in the differences between the original definition of "intention" as one's estimate of the likelihood that one will perform a specific behavior (Fishbein & Ajzen, 1975, cited in Maddux & DuCharme, Chapter 7) and the way in which others have defined it, e.g., as what one intends or plans to do.

Increased clarity is also needed in the area of "social ties" (Geertsen, Chapter 13). Does the concept of having an abundance of social ties mean having numerous connections with the larger community or society? Or does it mean having more intense linkages with smaller groups?

Contributing to this confusion is the use of different labels or variable names for measures of the same construct. Maddux and DuCharme point out that exceptionally high statistical correlations between "self-efficacy" and "intention" may mask their essential identity. Considerable variability also exists in measures of self-efficacy (Strecher et al.). Cockerham (Chapter 12) observes the lack of clarity in defining lifestyle concepts and asks for greater explicitness in expressing what lifestyle concepts are supposed to measure.

Finally, moving away from personal or psychological variables, there is substantial confusion in the use of larger system concepts such as family (noted by Baranowski, Chapter 9), race, or culture. Health behavior research purporting to deal with family factors in fact often deals with *individual* characteristics of a single family member, e.g., mother's education, rather than with a *family* characteristic, e.g., patterns of interaction among members (e.g., Gochman, Chapter 10).

Similarly, terms such as "race" and "ethnicity" are used very loosely to refer to assumed similarities and differences in "cultural" orientations unsupported by any empirical evidence (Geertsen). Moreover, the term "culture" is often confounded with social class, ethnicity, language grouping, and nativity (Dressler & Oths, Chapter 17). Finally, the term "culture" needs to be reconceptualized as something dynamic rather than static, to allow for the slow but regular changes that take place in many cultures, particularly the cultures of ethnic and immigrant minority groups as they experience increasing encounters with the larger society, the culture of which is itself changing (Geertsen).

Methodological Issues

Methodological issues include those of measurement, sampling, and procedure. These are "boilerplate" concerns: Their problematic nature, and the criticisms of them made by the contributors to this volume, can be repeated for nearly any corpus of research on any topic.

Measurement. A major measurement issue is closely related to conceptual definitions and confusion. There is often little consensus about what variable is being measured and how it should be measured. There are few standardized measures of important health behavior concepts. Champion's work on measuring health belief variables (e.g., Champion, 1984, 1993, cited in Strecher, Champion, & Rosenstock, Chapter 4), Bush and Iannotti's (1988) work on measuring health belief model variables in children, and Parcel and Meyer's (1978) work on measuring locus of control beliefs in children represent some of the few attempts to focus on and continually refine a standardized instrument related to a theoretical model, but these measures have not yet been widely used, and little uniformity exists. For example, "use of service" can be defined and measured variously in terms of sources of care, total number of physician visits, number of acute episode visits, length of delay in seeking care, or participation in a specific treatment program (Geertsen, Chapter 13).

Similarly, some variables are measured in ways that may not be what the researcher intends. For example, Maddux and DuCharme (Chapter 7) note the confounding of attitudinal characteristics, such as identifying a lack of interest in engaging in a behavior as a barrier to engaging in the behavior. Attitudes and barriers are conceptually distinct and should not be con-

founded. The larger point is that measurement should be more logically derived from concepts. Failure to derive measures logically hinders the systemic development of health behavior knowledge.

Measurement issues also include the lack of clarity inherent in instruments. Geertsen points out that questions about family contact may be differentially interpreted to mean nuclear or extended family and thus leave the results open to misinterpretation. Geertsen, among others, argues for the need to increase the precision with which questions are expressed. Cockerham (Chapter 12) links his hope for greater conceptual explicitness in lifestyle concepts with a call for an increase in the validity of their measures.

Finally, the technology of measurement—as opposed to the substance—merits critical comment. Much health behavior research relies on recall, with the inherent problems presented by fading memory and distortion. There may be appreciable underreporting of social contacts and medical visits (Geertsen). Use of health care diaries may be a way of reducing errors attributable to memory bias and may increase information about the way in which people arrive at a definition of illness and about their care-seeking responses for specific symptoms. Such diaries, on the other hand, require a great deal of effort from the respondents and present problems in getting people to complete them for extended periods of time; they have relatively low completion rates compared to health surveys (Geertsen).

Sampling. One major sampling problem in health behavior research is the difficulty of incorporating "nonusers" of health services, members of minority ethnic or cultural groups, and socially isolated persons in sampling frames. Socially isolated persons have low participation rates in research, especially in studies on the impact of social linkages on health behavior (Geertsen, Chapter 13), raising serious questions about the generalizability of findings. There are also relatively low rates of representation of persons with strong in-group ties to immigrant subcultures and of members of "parochial" social groups who may be reluctant to answer survey questions (Geertsen).

Convenience sampling, although less appropriate, is more often the norm in health behavior research than is population sampling. For example, use of members of prepaid plans or users of specific clinics as a basis for making generalizations about a range of health behaviors automatically excludes both persons who do not use services at all and persons who do not use the programs or services from which the sample is drawn (Geertsen). It may also exclude appreciable socioeconomic and ethnic population segments.

Although some health behavior research reaches out to specific ethnic, religious, or cultural groups, these groups are often incorrectly assumed to be homogeneous with references to ethnic, religious, or cultural characteristics. For example, identifying a group as Protestant or Catholic and treating its members identically glosses over the diversity in health-related beliefs and behaviors manifested by these denominations (Geertsen). Important subcultural differences may thus be hidden.

While a sound argument is consistently made for increased cross-cultural research (e.g., Lau, Chapter 3; Geertsen) to increase the generalizability of health behavior research findings, equally cogent arguments can be made for highly selective and sensitive sampling within a single culture. In complementary fashion, in relation to assessing cultural effects within small groups, there is a need for systematic sampling of "key informants," those persons in a small group shown by the cultural consensus model to know their culture well, as well as of "information" and how it is processed and transmitted within small cultural groups (Dressler & Oths, Chapter 17).

Procedure. As would be expected, studies conducted by psychologists have used experimental or quasi-experimental designs; those conducted by sociologists have typically used surveys; those conducted by anthropologists have used ethnological methods including anecdotal and observational materials. This diversity in design has been a strength in the development of health behavior knowledge, but there are limitations inherent in many of the method.

Most health behavior research has been nonlongitudinal, a practice that limits understanding and precludes the establishment of causality. For example, the presumed linkage between perceptions of the magnitude of health threats such as hypertension and their demonstrated magnitudes can be established only through longitudinal studies (Rogers & Prentice-Dunn, Chapter 6). Moreover, only longitudinal research can establish the differential impact of protection motivation theory variables in an adherence setting, in which a health condition or threat has already been identified, from their impact at a stage at which the health threat is not yet manifest (Rogers & Prentice-Dunn).

Nonlongitudinal studies also preclude establishing causality between social factors and health behaviors. Inferring from Reich, Erdal, and Zautra (Chapter 5), observed correlations between health behaviors and social linkage might be reciprocal or might reflect the unidirectional impact of either the health behaviors or health status. Finding that persons with diminished health status had reduced social linkages could as well reflect the negative impact of poor health on maintaining social contacts (Reich et al.) as the usually presumed impact of social interaction on health.

Professional versus Phenomenological Perspectives

Health behavior research shows a systematic movement away from medical and other professional or "objective" models toward increasing inclusion of phenomenological, layperson, or "subjective" models. Three concepts discussed in this volume show this movement particularly well: health cognitions, sick role, and lay caregiving.

Health Cognitions.   Fabrega's (Chapter 2) delineation of the historical evolution of cultural beliefs about health and illness, with their implications for a range of health behaviors—particularly for attributions of disease, legitimating care seeking, and the social control of responses to illness—places industrial-age, 20th-century beliefs about biomedicine in a larger social, economic, and political context. Each society or type of society, as it evolved, developed *heal-memes*, or normative beliefs about health, illness, and treatment. The biomedical (medical) model that is preponderant in Eurocentric, industrial societies is only one of several possible patterns of healmemes that could be valid within any specific social, cultural, and economic context. The often low reliability levels of diagnoses based on the medical model make it apparent that cultural and other nonmedical factors are at work in defining illness (Dressler & Oths, Chapter 17) and responses to illness.

The cultural construction of healmemes has its parallel in cognitive representations of illness (Lau, Chapter 3). These representations can be considered as the personal side of healmemes. Cognitive representation models emphasize the importance of personal, phenomenological, lay beliefs in the definition of illness and in the decision to seek care.

Other cognitive models have also shown a movement away from uncritical acceptance of a medicocentric perspective. Early research generated by the health belief model assumed the correctness of medical/professional advice and information and the axiomatic appropriateness of adherence to it. Research conducted during the 1960s and 1970s failed to recognize the considerable discrepancy between lay and professional perceptions of benefits. Later research showed the importance, as predictors of behaviors, of lay perceptions and benefits and barriers, which were often at variance with professional perspectives. New emphasis on lay perceptions (Strecher, Champion, & Rosenstock, Chapter 4) reflects a reframing of the original medical contextualization.

The literature on occupational determinants provides evidence of analogous change. Eakin (Chapter 16) points out the movement away from uncritical acceptance of professional perspectives—those of organizational management—toward acceptance and inclusion of workers' own views of health, safety, and injury issues.

Finally, there is a need to recognize the extensive documentation of differences in physician and patient perspectives. Patients and providers often have very different disease models (Dressler & Oths; Fabrega; Lau).

Sick Role.   The demedicalization of the sick role (Segall, Chapter 14) transforms the concept from one reflecting a hierarchy focused on the physician's power, authority, and control over a passive patient into one more reflective of egalitarianism. This modified sick role concept embraces an appreciation of self-care—the predominant mode of primary care—in which the person with a condition or illness is viewed as an active participant in the treatment process, along with similarly active roles for other laypersons involved in the primary caregiving process. This reconceptualization stresses the importance of lay beliefs and separates the sick role from the patient role.

While the original Parsonian conceptualization emphasized patient rights and responsibilities in the context of interaction with physicians (and possibly other health care professionals), this reconceptualization recognizes that others who are part of the sick person's life also have rights and that the sick person's rights exist within a social context. Accordingly, the legitimation of the sick role often lies within informal social networks, in the willingness of others to be active caregivers or to assume the necessary role and task obligations of the sick person, rather than within formal interaction with physicians and other professionals and adhering to their advice.

Segall recognizes, moreover, that the discipline of sociology, particularly what has been termed a "sociology of medicine," has begun to move away from a medicocentric perspective toward one that views biomedicine as but one of a range of elements associated with health, health behaviors, and health care. Segall also notes the political struggles within sociology that accompany this transformation and affirms that such a change is part of the evolution of medical sociology, rather than a reflection of this end.

Lay and Nonmedical Caregiving. Another movement away from medicocentrism is explicit in the concept of self-regulation, especially noted by Lau (Chapter 3). Self-regulatory models give primacy to the individual's attempts to reestablish equilibrium after it has been disrupted through a perceived discrepancy between experienced symptoms and the baseline cognitive representations for somatic experiences and illness (Lau).

In addition to self-regulation models, health behavior research is paying increasing attention to lay care in contrast to "official" or professional health care (Geertsen, Chapter 13). Moreover, the revised health services utilization model includes nonmedical care providers such as pharmacists and care provided in the person's home.

Role of Affect

The early psychological models for understanding health behaviors (e.g., health belief model, locus of control) emphasized cognitive, rational components, consistent with their derivation from Lewinian theory, with its emphasis on meaning and making sense of experiences. Although various combinations of perceived susceptibility and perceived severity were assumed to have motivational, threat, or other affective value in early research derived from the health belief model, affect or emotional responses were accorded little explicit attention.

In protection motivation theory, on the other hand, affect or emotionality occupies a prominent position. Protection motivation theory was developed to explain the effects of fear appeals on persuasion (Rogers & Prentice-Dunn, Chapter 6) and gives primacy to the concepts of threat and threat appraisal, explicitly linking these concepts with perceived susceptibility (perceived vulnerability), which in the terms of the theory refers to the belief in the likelihood that some event will occur if there is no adaptive response or no modification of an existing behavior, and with perceived severity, which the theory defines as the degree of harm believed to be inherent in the event's occurrence. Research generated by the theory has shown that the effects of threat on behavioral change are complex and that threat interacts in appreciable ways with how people evaluate their coping abilities (coping appraisal). Where threat is especially strong and people do not believe they can cope effectively with it, increases in threat produce seemingly paradoxical greater intentions to engage in risk behavior because those threatened see no point in trying to cope.

At the same time, questions about the specific role of threat arise in the context of the revisions of the health belief model. The threat construct adds little value for respondents such as smokers, who already perceive themselves at risk (Strecher, Champion, & Rosenstock, Chapter 4). Their risk perceptions may be "unrealistic," however, since a larger proportion of smokers, compared to nonsmokers, underestimate their actual (statistical) risk. They perceive risk but misjudge its magnitude. The underlying role of emotions in risk behavior mentioned earlier bears repeating. Risk behaviors are nearly always embedded in, or reflecting of, powerful human urges.

Finally, affect is also a component in social interactions related to care seeking and acceptance of treatments. The importance of close relationships as sources of emotional support in these behaviors is especially noted by Geertsen (Chapter 13).

Size of the Focal System

There is an emerging consensus that health behaviors can best be understood and predicted through models that include a range of social systems of varying sizes. Models that deal only with the individual or only with a single social system are doomed to predict minimal variance and are inappropriate foundations for successful applications and interventions to improve health status through changing behavior.

Societal and Institutional Determinants. Although the health behavior literature has historically alluded to social, cultural, and "sociocultural" factors, detailed and careful consideration of "macro" factors has been lacking. Since the late 1970s, there has been increased attention to such factors. Macrosociological theory (e.g., Blau, 1977, referred to by Geertsen, Chapter 13), derived from 19th-century sociology, suggests that increased diversity in the larger society leads to increased heterogeneity in patterns of social ties. This heterogeneity in turn, while it creates conflicting normative pressures, erodes the effects of interlocking traditional parochial influences. This social change has the potential for affecting a range of health behaviors, e.g., decisions to seek care and what type of care to choose.

The health services utilization model has continued to expand its focus from the individual to embrace a range of factors as predictors of use of services: familial; social, including lay referral systems; institutional; community; and governmental factors, including policies. Its most recent version provides an excellent example of appropriate integration of macro factors (Aday & Awe, Chapter 8).

The role of the economic system—as opposed to individual economic resources—in determining health behaviors is also being recognized. Eakin (Chapter 16) points out how the macroeconomic system subordinates health to corporate profit, which in turn threatens the legitimacy of being sick and discourages appropriate sick role and safety behaviors. Fabrega (Chapter 2) also argues cogently that distal economic and political factors, mediated by social and cultural norms, determine a range of health behav-

iors, including definitions and care-seeking behaviors.

Dressler and Oths (Chapter 17) also argue that health behavior needs to be seen less as a function of decision making and more as a social group process beginning with symptom definition and continuing through evaluation of treatment outcomes. Health behavior thus reflects individuals being continually involved in social interactions, rather than individuals by themselves acting on their own. One important instance of this interaction can be seen in the expanded conception of the sick role. Within this model, enacting the sick role involves the rights of others (Segall, Chapter 14).

FUTURE RESEARCH DIRECTIONS

Methodology

The "Boilerplate." A discussion of future directions for research on the personal and social determinants of health behavior would be remiss if it did not include a restatement of "boilerplate" themes, although many of these themes are the mirror images of the earlier discussion of methodological issues. Future research in health behavior (as in any of the dimensions of social/behavioral science) must change in the following ways, among others: be increasingly longitudinal; embrace more diverse samples, including hard-to-reach "nonuser" populations; include more appropriate, valid, and reliable measures and employ consensually agreed-upon identical or comparable measures across diverse studies; eliminate or reduce measurement errors, such as those attributable to subject recall; and avoid uncritical acceptance of medical/professional perspectives. The specific points already made need not be repeated, but some areas especially in need of longitudinal study should be mentioned.

Specific Areas for Longitudinal Study. Three issues particularly in need of careful longitudinal study relate to timing or temporality: the relationship between information, threat, and coping; the impact of long-term coping on cognitive mediating processes; and the sequential impact of health beliefs.

Research generated by protection motivation theory raises important questions about information, threat, and coping. Typically, studies have presented information about coping with threat *after* the threat itself is either induced or experienced. Rogers and Prentice-Dunn (Chapter 6) raise the question of what the effects would be if the order were reversed and such information were presented prior to the threat experience. Such effects can be determined only through systematic longitudinal study.

Rogers and Prentice-Dunn also raise a question about the impact of long-term coping behaviors upon cognitive mediating processes: Do such behaviors, in persons who acquire and demonstrate them, have a subsequent impact on cognitive mediating processes such as perceptions of response efficacy, self-efficacy, intrinsic and extrinsic rewards, severity, vulnerability, and appraisals of threat and coping abilities? Again, only longitudinal study can answer these questions.

In research derived from the health belief model, questions arise about the possible differential importance of model components (Strecher, Champion, & Rosenstock, Chapter 4). Beliefs about susceptibility and severity might be important in the establishment of threat. Once threat exists, their importance may be diminished while beliefs about benefits and barriers assume greater predictive value. Only through longitudinal study can such sequential differences in the importance of beliefs be established.

Primate Study. One important point that was not considered in the discussion of methodological issues must be introduced here: the use of data generated by observation of nonhuman primate groups. Fabrega (Chapter 2), noting that it is impossible to know and understand sickness and healing in early human groups prior to the emergence of modern *Homo sapiens*,

thoughtfully suggests that medical and healing themes be examined in primate groups closely related to humans. Knowledge about social and affective communication, social and family organization, bonding, and so forth in such primates is accumulating through the observations of ethologists and comparative psychologists. Controlled and naturalistic investigations of how these species respond to illness, debility, and disability can provide some insights into how such states were expressed, communicated, and dealt with in prehuman society. Such knowledge would enrich understanding of the evolution of human health behavior and "healmemes" throughout human history.

Content Areas

The individual chapters identify a number of specific directions for future health behavior research. The following discussion moves beyond these specifics. Two areas that transcend specific levels of analysis seem particularly important focal points for future health behavior research: health-relevant motivation and the search for meaning. A third area is one that is nearly absent from this volume, and in the health behavior literature as well: community and institutional factors.

Health-Relevant Motivation. A critical area for future research is health-relevant motivation. Few studies have been conducted on "health" or the "desire for health" or "the wish to possess good health" as motives, or on the relationship of these motives to overt health behaviors. Possibly, health in itself may not be a potent motive for eliciting health behaviors. It has not been observed to be a potent motive in young populations (Gochman, 1975, 1986), and little research has been done to demonstrate its potency in adults, although Lau, Hartman, and Ware (1986) have begun important research in this area.

Moreover, it may be increasingly important to differentiate between health as a motive and other motives that can effectively be drawn upon to generate health behavior—what might be termed *health-relevant*, or *health-germane*, motivation. Thus, a more basic question for future health behavior research might be: What are the motives that can be used to generate health behavior? The desires to be physically or socially active, occupationally and professionally useful or successful, or responsible to family and friends may turn out to be more relevant to health behavior than "health" itself.

In this context, health behavior research must address issues, such as those raised by Burt (1984), of whether health is perceived as juxtaposed with pleasure, indicating that actions considered to be healthful are often thought to be unappealing, distasteful, and otherwise noxious; and those raised by Bruhn (1988) about the conflict between personal risk and other motives and values and about the "trade-offs" involved in changing behavior. Maddux and DuCharme (Chapter 7) make the cogent point that many health-promoting behaviors involve giving up some pleasure and comfort for the sake of future benefits that are less tangible. Few instruments exist to measure health as a motive. Future research will require methodological advancement in this area.

The Search for Meaning.   Health as a motive and motives relevant to health lead to questions about the salience or meaning of health and of terms related to it: the meaning of illness, the meaning of treatment, and the meaning of the health care environment. The profession of social work has a tradition of borrowing from a variety of disciplines (e.g., Bartlett, 1961), yet in one very critical area, it can claim proper "ownership." In health settings, particularly hospitals and clinics, it is the particular responsibility of the professional social worker on the interdisciplinary care team to explore, understand, and work with the "meaning" of an illness or a condition for the patient and the patient's family (Bartlett, 1961, pp. 134–135). In such a context, "meaning" differs from what illness means in

general (and as it is treated by Gochman, Chapter 1). In such a context, meaning assumes a phenomenological dimension; the "meaning" of illness represents its salience and implications for the patient and the patient's family and significant others. What the illness experience means in these terms has important implications for health behavior—for preventive activities, for acceptance of a regimen, for giving up the sick role, for rehabilitation, and the like.

Ben-Sira (1977) addressed the meaning of illness in his study of the person's "image" of an illness, or "involvement" with a disease, and devised a way of incorporating elements of the health belief model into a single measure of the "salience" of an illness to the patient. He further related such meaning, or salience, to preventive behavior. Building upon the meanings attached to cognitive representations (Lau, Chapter 3), family coding (Tinsley, Chapter 11), social attachments (Geertsen, Chapter 13), being sick (Segall, Chapter 14), work (Eakin, Chapter 16), and socially and culturally exchanged information (Dressler & Oths, Chapter 17), future health behavior research should pursue research on the phenomenological "meanings" or personal processing of health, illness, and treatment.

Community and Institutional Determinants. Literature searches reveal very few studies that attempted to link health behaviors with characteristics of communities and their institutions. Although some attempts have been made to relate selected demographic characteristics of communities to risk and lifestyle behaviors (e.g., Duncan, Jones, & Moon, 1993) or to show community variability in these behaviors (e.g., Diehr et al., 1993), there is no body of knowledge about the impact on diverse health behaviors of community characteristics. Future research should determine whether community variability in health behaviors exists and how such variability is accounted for by community characteristics. Analyses of communities (e.g., Longres, 1995; Poplin, 1979) suggest that such characteristics include size; economic development and opportunities; rural or urban location; use of space, including the esthetics of structures and of open green areas; ethnic, religious, and sexual diversity; political and power structures and stratification patterns; norms and public policies; cultural, social, recreational, health, and educational resources; minority–majority relations; and levels of competition, conflict, and harmony.

Similarly, there is no body of knowledge about the impact of institutional characteristics on health behaviors. People live much of their lives within institutions such as schools, workplaces, and religious and social organizations. Future research is needed to determine how much of the variance in health behaviors is accounted for by institutional characteristics. Analyses of institutions and organizations (e.g., Etzioni, 1964; Scott, 1981) suggest that such relevant characteristics appear similar to those for communities and include size and growth patterns; location; the esthetics of the institutional's physical environment; ethnic, religious, and sexual diversity of members/participants; leadership and decision-making structures; norms and policies; the institutional culture; and levels of competition, conflict, and harmony.

SUMMARY

A wide range of health behaviors can readily be seen to be influenced by a broad spectrum of factors in personal and social systems. From the chapters written for this volume, health cognitions, care seeking, preventive, protective, and safety behaviors, risk behaviors, and lifestyles can be seen to be affected by nearly all—if not all—of the personal, family, social, institutional, and cultural determinants considered.

Despite problems in clarity in a number of conceptual frameworks, health behavior research has made appreciable strides in increasing the complexity of its conceptual models and in the range of behaviors it observes. Standardized measuring instruments; improved sampling of nonusers, isolated persons, and members of un-

assimilated subcultures; and more longitudinal studies remain methodological challenges. Health behavior research has become increasingly demedicalized, more acceptant of affective, noncognitive variables, and more likely to focus on larger social systems rather than solely on the person. Primate study; health-relevant motivation; the larger issues of the phenomenological meanings of health, illness, and treatment; and the impact of community and institutional characteristics constitute a critical agendas for future health behavior research.

REFERENCES

Bartlett, H. M. (1961). *Social work practice in the health field*. New York: National Association of Social Workers.

Ben-Sira, Z. (1977). Involvement with a disease and health-promoting behavior. *Social Science and Medicine, 11*, 165–173.

Bruhn, J. G. (1988). Life-style and health behavior. In D. S. Gochman (Ed.), *Health behavior: Emerging research perspectives* (pp. 71–86). New York: Plenum Press.

Burt, J. J. (1984). Metahealth: A challenge for the future. In J. D. Matarazzo, S. M. Weiss, J. A. Herd, N. E. Miller, & S. M. Weiss (Eds.), *Behavioral health: A handbook of health enhancement and disease prevention* (pp. 1239–1248). New York: Wiley.

Bush, P. J., & Iannotti, R. J. (1988). Origins and stability of children's health beliefs relative to medicine use. *Social Science and Medicine, 27*, 345–352.

Diehr, P., Koepsell, T., Cheadle, A., Psaty, B. M., Wagner, E., & Curry, S. (1993). Do communities differ in health behaviors? *Journal of Clinical Epidemiology, 46*, 1141–1149.

Duncan, C., Jones, K., & Moon, G. (1993). Do places matter? A multi-level analysis of regional variations in health-related behaviour in Britain. *Social Science and Medicine, 37*, 725–733.

Etzioni, A. (1964). *Modern organizations*. Englewood Cliffs, NJ: Prentice-Hall.

Gochman, D. S. (1975). The measurement and development of dentally relevant motives. *Journal of Public Health Dentistry, 35*, 160–164.

Gochman, D. S. (1986). *Youngsters' health cognitions: Cross-section and longitudinal analyses*. Louisville, KY: Health Behavior Systems.

Kirscht, J. P. (1988). The health belief model and predictions of health actions. In D. S. Gochman (Ed.), *Health behavior: Emerging research perspectives*. New York: Plenum Press.

Lau, R. R., Hartman, K. A., & Ware, J. E., Jr. (1986). Health as a value: Methodological and theoretical considerations. *Health Psychology, 5*, 25–43.

Longres, J. F. (1995). *Human behavior in the social environment* (2nd ed.), Itasca, IL: Peacock.

Parcel, G. S., & Meyer, M. P. (1978). Development of an instrument to measure children's health locus of control.In K. A. Wallston & B. S. Wallston (Eds.), Health locus of control [Special issue]. *Health Education Monographs, 6*, 149–159.

Parsons, T. (1951). *The social system*. Glencoe, IL: Free Press.

Poplin, D. E. (1979). *Communities: A survey of theories and methods of research* (2nd ed.). New York: Macmillan.

Rosenstock, I. M., Derryberry, M., & Carriger, C. K. (1959). Why people fail to seek poliomyelitis vaccination. *Public Health Reports, 74*, 98–103.

Scott, W. R. (1981). *Organizations: Rational, natural and open systems* (2nd ed.). Englewood Cliffs, NJ: Prentice-Hall.

Concepts and Definitions

A Glossary for Health Behavior Research

With few exceptions, the definitions in this Glossary are either taken verbatim, paraphrased, or abstracted from this *Handbook*. Specific chapters and, where appropriate, sources cited herein are identified. Italicized terms within a definition denote additional Glossary entries.

Consistent with the focus of this *Handbook* on health *behavior*, the Glossary does not routinely define diseases or medical treatments. Space limitations preclude defining every "named" intervention or program, or every social or behavioral science model that is not especially focused on health behavior. A number of these programs and models, however, are listed in the Index.

acceptance See *adherence; compliance.*

access framework A conceptual refinement of the *health services utilization model* that predicts the use of and satisfaction with health care; basic components are health policy, the organizational and accessibility characteristics of the delivery system, and *predisposing, enabling,* and *need factors* (Aday & Andersen, 1974, in Aday & Awe, I, 8). See *utilization framework.*

action stage In the *transtheoretical model,* the phase in which persons have modified their behavior and are participating in the appropriate health practice (Prohaska & Clark, III, 2).

active coping In health contexts, a tendency or motivation to exercise personal control, reflecting preference for decision making in health care, preference for behavioral involvement, and low expectations that health care professionals can control one's health (Christensen, Benotsch, & Smith, II, 12).

active patient orientation See *mutual participation model.*

active prevention See *prevention, active.*

activities of daily living (ADL) Instrumental and basic behaviors necessary for everyday life (Prohaska & Clark, III, 2).

adherence Practice of following health care provider recommendations (Clark, II, 8; Chrisler, II, 17); "an interdependent network of regimen behaviors rather than a single behavior" (Wysocki & Greco, II, 9); following recommended screening procedures (Rimer, Demark-Wahnefried, & Egert, II, 15); congruence between patient behaviors and advice or instructions provided by health care providers; medical adherence: how closely a patient's medication-taking behaviors match instructions prescribed by a physician (Creer & Levstek, II, 7). The concept embraces total adherence and acceptance, as well as degrees thereof; in relation to smoking, it includes not only total cessation, but also participation in cessation activities, as well as the actions of change agents (Glasgow & Orleans, II, 19). It connotes active, voluntary behavior designed to produce a therapeutic effect (Chrisler, II, 17). See *compliance.*

ADL See *activities of daily living.*

affective behavior, physician's Comprises acts aimed at establishing a relationship with patients in which the physician accepts the patient as a human being whose anxiety-arousing problems cannot be alleviated by technical procedures; it involves the physician attributing therapeutic importance to, and engaging in warm, open relations with the patient; being attentive to problems that may not be related to disease; gathering information about personal and family problems and social relations; and explaining the rationale of the diagnosis and treatment (Ben-Sira, II, 2).

AIDS Acquired immunodeficiency syndrome: a condition in which exposure to the *HIV* (human immunodeficiency virus) leads to the destruction of the body's natural defenses against infection (Thomason & Campos, III, 8).

analytical framework for the study of child survival A conceptual model designed to understand morbidity and mortality in children in developing countries; basic components are maternal factors, environmental contamination, nutrient deficiency, and injury and personal illness control (Mosley & Chen, 1984, in Coreil, III, 9).

anthropology of medicine See *medical anthropology*.

appropriate interventions/care Lists of indications for use of procedures consensually generated by nationally recognized experts (Rand Corporation/McGlynn, Kosecoff, & Brook, 1990, in DiMatteo, II, 1). Compare *inappropriate/unnecessary care*.

attributable risk Amount of disease (disability or mortality) in a population group that could be eliminated if a risk factor were eliminated (Prohaska & Clark, III, 2).

authority, physician The physician's power over others (Haug, II, 3).

autonomy, physician The physician's power or ability to resist or withstand being compelled by others (Haug, II, 3).

autonomy, principle of A moral standard stressing the obligation to respect rights to self-determination (Nilstun, IV, 11).

autonomy, self-care See *self-care autonomy*.

availability bias A concept that explains safety and risk avoidance behaviors, denoting the inclination to be inordinately influenced by dramatic events that have low probabilities of happening but are vivid in memory; ease of recall being a function of saliency, recency, and emotional impact (Slovic, 1978, in Cohen & Colligan, II, 20).

behavioral epidemiology The study of the relationships between lifestyles and mortality and morbidity patterns in a population (Rakowski, III, 5).

behavioral model See *health services utilization model*.

beneficence, principle of A moral standard stressing the obligation to benefit others, especially not to harm them (Nilstun, IV, 11).

bruxism Spasmodic grinding of the teeth in other than chewing movements (Gift & White, IV, 7).

caregiver, informal Layperson who provides personal care to an older, ill family member or close friend (Wright, III, 13).

care-seeking behavior, theory of A conceptual framework in nursing, incorporating components of the *health belief model*, *theory of reasoned action*, and Triandis's theory of interpersonal behavior; designed to predict preventive rather than illness-related behaviors; basic components are affective arousal, perceived utility, *social norms*, and habits (Lauver, 1992a, in Blue & Brooks, IV, 5).

central place theory A conceptual framework based on land economics that is used to relate a hierarchy of levels of health care services to concentrations of population and distances (Scarpaci & Kearns, II, 5).

children's health belief model A conceptual framework for understanding children's health behaviors, incorporating components of the *health belief model*, environmental variables, and readiness factors (O'Brien & Bush, III, 3).

chronic Referring to an illness or condition that is incurable and lasts through a person's lifetime (Gallagher & Stratton, III, 11).

cognitive appraisal The process of intellectually evaluating and deciding on available options to engage in a particular behavior (Cowell & Marks, III, 4).

cognitive developmental theory A conceptual framework for understanding the development of children's thinking; assumes that children take an active rather than a passive role in constructing their own knowledge and understanding of health and illness and that they move through universally recognized sequences in doing so (O'Brien & Bush, III, 3).

cognitive representations Personal images or schemata of illness, disease, and being healthy, and the meanings attached to these images; persons develop their own individualized images or schemata in relation to symptoms and illness that are often different from the representations of physicians and the medical community (Lau, I, 3).

coming out Disclosure of nonheterosexual identity by a lesbian or a gay man (VanScoy, III, 7); can also mean self-recognition of such identity.

commonsense representation of illness The images or schemata of illness, disease, or symptoms held by a layperson; the images include an identity, a set of consequences, a time-line, a cause, and a cure or control (Lau, I, 3).

communication Exchange of meaning, either verbally or nonverbally, between people to establish a commonality of thought, attitude, feeling, and ideas (DiMatteo, II, 1).

communication campaign Use of mass media on a health topic, typically involving television, radio, newspaper, magazines, and other channels to convey health information or to provide motivation for health actions (Swinehart, IV, 18).

community A social entity or system made up of individuals together with formal organizations, such as local government, businesses, and educational institutions, and voluntary organizations, such as religious, fraternal, or service groups; informal social networks; and families. Critical to the concept is the premise that various components are related to each other and have the potential for being mobilized in relation to health promotion programs (Schooler & Flora, IV, 15).

community health promotion Interventions for effecting change in communities that involve social planning, social action, and locality development (Rothman, 1979, in Schooler & Flora, IV, 15).

community organization An intervention strategy designed to empower a community and to enhance its competence and problem-solving ability; of particular importance for increasing the success of a *health promotion* program (Schooler & Flora, IV, 15).

compadrazgo A system of selecting *comadres* (female friends) and *copadres* (male friends) for one's children; levels of perceived support from these friends are related to health status and health behavior (Dressler & Oths, I, 17).

competence gap The difference in health-related knowledge and skill between physicians and other health professionals and their patients or clients (Haug, II, 3).

compliance Degree of correspondence between the physician's prescription and the patient's behavior (Sackett & Haynes, 1976, in DiIorio, II, 11; Morisky & Cabrera, II, 14); congruence between medical recommendations and the degree to which a patient takes medicine, follows a diet, or changes lifestyle behaviors (Trostle, II, 6); an ideology that transforms a physician's theories about patients' behavior into research strategies and potentially coercive interventions that strengthen physicians' authority (Trostle, II, 6). See also *adherence*.

conscientiousness factor A theoretical personality dimension reflecting "will to achieve," "dependability," and "self-control" thought to be related to medication adherence in renal dialysis patients (Christensen et al., II, 12).

consciousness raising A component of the *transtheoretical model*, denoting a process by which people move from not being ready to initiate a behavior to being ready to initiate it (Rakowski, III, 5).

consumerism A framework for viewing physician–patient interactions that argues for patient autonomy and sole decision making as essential in combating physician paternalism (DiMatteo, II, 1), or in which an "activist" patient approaches health care as a problem-solving endeavor that requires active coping (Pratt, 1978, in Wiese & Gallagher, IV, 4).

contemplation In the *transtheoretical model*, the stage in which people are aware that a problem exists and are seriously thinking about overcoming it (Prohaska & Clark, III, 2).

contracting Use of a written document, resulting from the negotiation of a treatment plan between a patient and medical personnel, that identifies the reinforcements the patient will receive contingent on performing the behaviors stipulated in the treatment plan (Creer & Levstek, II, 7).

control beliefs See *locus of control*.

control demand model A conceptual framework developed to understand how workplace characteristics are related to health behaviors such as smoking, alcohol use, exercise, and self-protective behavior; basic components are levels of control over work, psychological demands, and social support (Eakin, I, 16).

control, perceived behavioral See *perceived behavioral control*.

convergence hypothesis A proposition that suggests that as gender roles become more similar, gender differences in health behavior decrease or disappear (Waldron, I, 15).

conversation model A conceptual framework for viewing physician–patient interactions in which the patient continually provides the physician information about values, preferences, and constraints and the physician engages in "thinking out loud" about possible courses of action, recommended interventions, and their implications, using language that is understood by the patient (DiMatteo, II, 1).

coping appraisal Evaluation of adaptive responses to threat; a component of the *protection motivation theory* (Rogers & Prentice-Dunn, I, 6).

coping mode Way of responding to threat messages (Rogers & Prentice-Dunn, I, 6). See *protection motivation theory*.

cue to action A stimulus, either internal or external, that can trigger health-related cognitive processes or health actions (Strecher, Champion, & Rosenstock, I, 4).

cultural consensus model A conceptual framework to assess the degree to which a body of information is shared within a social group; provides an estimate of shared beliefs related to health and illness (Dressler & Oths, I, 17).

culture A set of interlocking cognitive schemata that literally construct much of what people do on a daily basis; the manner in which a social group stores and transmits information; a system of symbols or abstract elements that are learned and patterned socially (Dressler & Oths, I, 17).

damaging cycle A chain of events in which a somatic disturbance leads to a detrimental appraisal of health, which then precipitates stress, which then increases the risk of further somatic disturbance (Ben-Sira, II, 2).

decisional balance theory A conceptual framework for understanding how persons make specific choices, based on comparisons of perceived positive and negative aspects of a behavior, and including gains and losses to self and others and approval or disapproval of self and others (Janis & Mann, 1977, in Marcus, Bock, & Pinto, II, 18).

demography, health See *health demography*.

deskilling Transference of work functions once controlled exclusively by physicians or nurses to positions lower down on the occupational hierarchy (Salloway, Hafferty, & Vissing, II, 4).

developing country A designation based on economic, demographic, and social/health indicators, given to a nation that is relatively poor, with a relatively young and fertile population and relatively scarce health and social resources (Coreil, III, 9).

developmental model of diabetes self-management A conceptual framework for understanding

the responsibilities that patients and families can assume in monitoring, evaluating, and adjusting treatment for insulin-dependent diabetes mellitus; basic components include demographic factors, family functioning, psychological stress, and interactions with providers to acquire necessary skills (Wysocki & Greco, II, 9). See *self-management, childhood diabetes; self-regulation/self-regulatory skills*.

diagnosis Naming of a condition by medical professionals; represents the interplay of social, institutional, and cultural factors together with personal symptoms through which time and location at which medical professionals and other parties determine the existence and legitimacy of a condition (Brown, 1995, in Gochman, IV, 20).

diagnosis related group/diagnostic related group (DRG) One of 438 groupings of patient conditions that have been the basis for federal reimbursements to hospitals for Medicare patients since 1983 (Daugherty, IV, 10); hospitals are paid a fixed amount for a given DRG regardless of length of stay and services provided.

disease A biological/organic abnormality; not identical to illness (Lau, I, 3); the measurable deviation of an organic system from some independently defined optimum (Dressler & Oths, I, 17).

doctrine of specific etiology See *specific etiology, doctrine of*.

DRG See *diagnosis related group*.

drinking culture Group norms, particularly within work settings, that encourage and support consumption of alcohol; closely related to *occupational culture* (Eakin, I, 16).

ecological model A conceptual framework that integrates five levels of personal and social systems: intrapersonal, interpersonal, organizational, community, and public policy in public health efforts (Buchanan, IV, 9).

edentulous Without teeth; toothless (Gift & White, IV, 7).

effectiveness Benefits of medical care measured by improvements in health (Aday & Awe, I, 8).

efficiency A relationship between improvements in health and the resources required to produce them (Aday & Awe, I, 8).

elaboration likelihood model A conceptual framework to predict attitude change; persuasion is proposed to be a function of the audience's active involvement in processing a message and the importance of the message's topic to the audience (Petty &

Cacioppo, 1986, in Rogers & Prentice-Dunn, I, 6; Wiese & Gallagher, IV, 4).

emic Denotes a way of knowing reflecting an internal or cultural "insider" perspective (Weidman, 1988, in Gochman, I, Part V); emic behavior is behavior that a person believes to be related to health, regardless of whether it is externally validated (Eakin, I, 16). Compare *etic*.

empowerment Enabling individuals, families, and communities to take control over their lives and their environment (e.g., Rappaport, 1984, in Schooler & Flora, IV, 15).

enabling factor A resource characteristic, such as family income or community availability, that predicts use of health services; a component of the *health services utilization model* (Aday & Awe, I, 8).

energized family A conceptual framework for understanding the family as a social system; basic components are regularity of interaction among members, contacts with the larger community, working together to advance members' interests, and coping with and mastering their lives. Energized families tend to encourage autonomy, rather than use "autocratic" parenting, and to socialization methods, resulting in children with better levels of health behaviors (Pratt, 1976, in Gochman, I, 10; Tinsley, I, 11).

epidemiology "Study of the distribution and determinants of diseases and injuries in human populations" (Inhorn, 1995, in Gochman, IV, 20).

epidemiology, behavioral See *behavioral epidemiology*.

epidemiology, psychosocial See *psychosocial epidemiology*.

equity The degree to which the benefits and burdens of medical care are fairly distributed in a population (Aday & Awe, I, 8); the degree to which participants (either patients or professionals) believe that the ratio of benefits received to their efforts and resources expended is equal or skewed in their favor (Daugherty, IV, 10).

etic Denotes a way of knowing reflecting an external or cultural "outsider" perspective (Weidman, 1988, in Gochman, I, Part V). Etic behavior is behavior that external observers believe to be related to health, independent of the behaving individual's beliefs (Eakin, I, 16). Compare *emic*.

eudaimonistic health A state of exuberant well-being (Lau, I, 3).

exercise Physical activity of moderate intensity (Marcus et al., II, 18).

explanatory model A cognitive framework of health processes based on both cultural knowledge and idiosyncratic experience that is used to understand health status, illness, and sickness; basic components include etiology, timing of onset of symptoms, pathophysiology, course of sickness, and treatment. Explanatory models exist at both lay and professional levels (Kleinman, 1980, & Kleinman, Eisenberg, & Good, 1978, in Dressler & Oths, I, 17).

facilitative environment An environment in which "nonsmoking cues and cessation information are persistent and inescapable" (Glynn, Boyd, & Gruman, 1990, in Glasgow & Orleans, II, 19).

familism Importance of family and relatives in a person's live, particularly in relation to care-seeking behavior (Geertsen, I, 13).

family aggregation A concept denoting intrafamilial similarities in health variables compared to nonfamilial similarities (Sallis & Nader, 1988, in Gochman, I, 10).

family code A system of norms for a family's behavior, including core assumptions, beliefs, family stories, myths, and rituals (Tinsley, I, 11).

family concordance Degree to which members of a family exhibit similarity in a specified health behavior (Baranowski, I, 9).

family, energized See *energized family*.

family health culture The unique combination of family experiences, beliefs, perceptions of symptoms, and reactions to the perceptions that influences the way in which families seek care or treatment (Black, 1986, in Gochman, I, 10).

fighting the illness A posture of gritty defiance as a way of dealing with a chronic illness (Gallagher & Stratton, III, 11).

fixed role hypothesis A proposition suggesting that men's more structured role obligations, compared with women's, may make it more difficult for men to engage in care-seeking behavior and thus accounts for women's greater use of health services (Marcus & Siegel, 1982, in Gochman, I, Part IV).

Flexner Report An analysis and recommendations relevant to United States medical education, prepared by Abraham Flexner in 1910, that became the basis for the reform of and standardization of medical training; remains a critical foundation for late 20th-century medical education (Weise & Gallagher, IV, 4).

folk illness A shared interpretation of a cluster of symptoms within a social group that is at variance with a biomedical framework (Dressler & Oths, I, 17).

framework of relationships model A conceptual scheme for understanding compliance behavior, especially for epilepsy; basic components are the *health services utilization model*, the *health belief model*, and health education, with an emphasis on adequate financial and community resources (Di Iorio, II, 11).

gay Without a gender qualifier, refers to a homosexual, a person who engages or desires to engage in sexual behavior with a person of the same gender (Kauth & Prejean, III, 6).

gay man A male who engages or desires to engage in sexual behavior with another male; a homosexual (Kauth & Prejean, III, 6).

gender role The social roles, behaviors, attitudes, and psychological characteristics that are more common, more expected, and more accepted for one sex or the other; includes a group of interrelated behaviors, attitudes, and psychological characteristics that influence a variety of risk and risk-taking behaviors as well as care-seeking behaviors (Waldron, I, 15).

GOBI Acronym for *G*rowth monitoring, *O*ral rehydration, *B*reast-feeding and *I*mmunization, the four cornerstone child survival interventions in developing countries (Coreil, III, 9).

grazing Snacking throughout the day (O'Brien & Bush, III, 3).

group ties See *social ties.*

habit A behavior that does not require conscious effort but is set in motion by situational cues (Schneider & Shiffrin, 1977, in Maddux & DuCharme, I, 7) and is less under the control of conscious cognitive processes and deliberate decisions.

healing The social processes and actions brought to bear to deal with a condition of disease or illess (Fabrega, I, 2).

healing culture The totality of institutions involved in treatment of disease, including biomedical and alternative approaches and the range of choices available, and the culture of medicine and its rituals and stresses (e.g., Foster & Anderson, 1978, in Gochman, IV, 20).

healmeme A unit of symbolic cultural information that gives meaning to the domain of health, well-being, sickness, and healing; underlies and constitutes a society's health-related beliefs and behaviors (Fabrega, I, 2).

health A state of being, almost impossible to define satisfactorily; includes components of physiological, psychological, and social functioning (Gochman I, 1; Lau, I, 3). What is considered to be health is appreciably determined by societal and cultural factors (Fabrega, I, 2). A continuous variable reflecting a capacity or ability to perform, as well as the use of that capacity to achieve expectations and to negotiate the demands of the social and physical environment (Tarlov, 1992, in Reed, Moore-West, Jernstedt, & O'Donell, IV, 2); "an individual or group capacity relative to potential to function fully in the social and physical environment" (Tarlov, 1992, in Flipse, IV, 3).

health behavior, formal Actions taken for the prevention or treatment of a condition or for the maintenance or enhancement of health that involve the use of institutionalized services such as physicians and hospitals (Pol & Thomas, III, 1).

health behavior, informal Actions taken for the prevention or treatment of a condition or for the maintenance or enhancement of health that do not involve the use of institutionalized services such as physicians and hospitals; these actions include self-care, tooth brushing, and use of over-the-counter medications (Pol & Thomas, III, 1).

health belief model A conceptual framework designed to predict preventive actions and eventually used to predict illness and sick role behaviors; basic components of the model are perceived susceptibility to some illness, perceived severity or seriousness of that condition, perceived benefits of taking a specified action, and perceived barriers to taking such action (Strecher, Champion, & Rosenstock, I, 4).

health care management See *management, health care.*

health care manager See *manager, health care.*

health culture A society's repertoire of patterns for cognition, affect, and behavior in relation to health, sickness, and well-being (Weidman, 1988, in Gochman, I, Part V).

health demography Application of the content and methods of demography to the study of health-related phenomena; analyzes the influence of demographic factors such as age, marital status, and income on the health status and health behavior of poplations and the differential impact of health-related phenomena on demographic groupings; focuses on the implications of population change for health care (Pol & Thomas, III, 1). See *behavioral epidemiology; psychosocial epidemiology.*

health education   Efforts to change behavior in order to improve health (Glanz & Oldenburg, IV, 8); "any combination of learning experiences designed to facilitate voluntary adaptations of behavior conducive to health" (Green, Kreuter, Deeds, & Partridge, 1980, p. 7, in Glanz & Oldenburg, IV, 8).

health input–output model   See *input-output model, health*.

health maintenance organization (HMO)   A prepaid group practice for delivering comprehensive health care from a specific set of providers. See *managed care*.

health policy   Aggregate of federal, state, and local laws, rules, and regulations that govern the financing, regulation, and organization of health care (Aday & Awe, I, 8).

health-promoting self-care system model   A conceptual framework for nursing, integrating self-care deficit nursing theory, the *interaction model of client health behavior*, and the *health promotion model of nursing*, designed to predict individual autonomy and responsibility for health-promoting behaviors (Simmons, 1990a, in Blue & Brooks, IV, 5).

health promotion   "any combination of health education and related organizational, economic, and environmental supports for behavior of individuals, groups, or communities conducive to health" (Green & Kreuter, 1991, in Glanz & Oldenburg, IV, 8); "the science and art of helping people change their lifestyle to move toward a state of optimal health ... by a combination of efforts to enhance awareness, change behavior, and create environments that support good health practices" (O'Donnell, 1989, in Glanz & Oldenburg, IV, 8); "the process of enabling people to increase control over, and to improve, their health ... a commitment to dealing with the challenges of reducing inequities, extending the scope of prevention, and helping people to cope with their circumstances ... creating environments conducive to health, in which people are better able to take care of themselves" (Epp, 1986, in Glanz & Oldenburg, IV, 8). The term was seldom used prior to 1980.

health promotion model, nursing   A conceptual framework for nursing, similar to the *health belief model*, used to predict engaging in behaviors that maintain or improve well-being, rather than prevent disease; basic components are importance of health, perceived control of health, perceived *self-efficacy*, definition of health, perceived health status, *perceived benefits* of health-promoting behaviors, and *perceived barriers* to health-promoting behaviors (Pender, 1982, in Blue & Brooks, IV, 5).

health psychology   "The aggregate of the specific educational, scientific, and professional contributions of the discipline of psychology to the promotion and maintenance of health, the prevention and treatment of illness, the identification of etiologic and diagnostic correlates of health, illness and related dysfunction" (Matarazzo, 1980, p. 815, in Gochman, IV, 20); "any aspect of psychology that bears upon the experience of health and illness, and the behavior that affects health status" (Rodin & Stone, 1987, pp. 15–16, in Gochman, IV, 20).

health-seeking process model   A conceptual framework for understanding people's experiences with sickness holistically as natural histories of illness; basic components are symptom definition, illness-related shifts in role behavior, lay referral, treatment actions, and adherence (Chrisman, 1977, in Dressler & Oths, I, 17).

health service system   Arrangements for the potential rendering of care to consumers, including the volume and distribution of services and their accessibility and organization (Aday & Awe, I, 8). See *health services utilization model*.

health services utilization model   A conceptual framework designed to predict use of health care, such as visits to physicians and dentists and use of medications and clinical facilities; basic components are *predisposing*, *enabling*, and *need factors* (Aday & Awe, I, 8); sometimes referred to as the *behavioral model*.

heterosexism   An assumption, especially among health providers and institutions, that heterosexuality, or male–female sexual expression, is normative and superior to others (VanScoy, III, 7).

HIV   See *AIDS*.

HMO   Acronym for *health maintenance organization* (Daugherty, IV, 10). See *managed care*.

homeless assistance act, Stewart B. McKinney   A 1987 federal law that extended the National Health Care for the Homeless Initiative to a total of 109 cities (Wright & Joyner, III, 10).

homeless, literally   Persons who spend their nights either in outdoor locations, in temporary overnight shelters, or in other places not intended for human habitation (Wright & Joyner, III, 10).

homelessness   No agreed-upon definition (Wright & Joyner, III, 10). See *homeless, literally; housed, marginally*.

homophobia   An irrational fear of homosexuality (Eliason, Donelan, & Rundall, 1992, in Vanscoy, III, 7).

housed, marginally   Persons with a claim to some minimal housing, but who are at high risk of being *homeless* (Wright & Joyner, III, 10).

illness   The subjective experience of some biological/organic/social/emotional abnormality; not identical to disease (e.g., Lau, I, 3); the social and psychological concomitants of putative physiological problems (Conrad, 1990, in Gochman, I, 1); incapacity for role performance (Gerhardt, 1989a, in Gochman, I, 1); motivated deviance (Segall, I, 14); the individual experience of suffering or distress, or disvalued states of being and functioning (Dressler & Oths, I, 17).

illusion of safety   Workers' practicing of safe behavior under supervision but of unsafe behavior, such as taking shortcuts and engaging in risky actions, in the absence of supervision; convinces management that it has done its job and that safety regimens are being followed when in reality they are not (Cohen & Colligan, II, 20).

image theory   A conceptual framework for decision making based on the fit between alternative choices and an individual's images, plans, or principles (Mitchell & Beach, 1990, in Rogers & Prentice-Dunn, I, 6).

inappropriate/unnecessary care   A medical intervention with risks that exceed the potential benefit to the patient (DiMatteo, II, 1). Compare *appropriate intervention/care*.

informal caregiver   See *caregiver, informal*.

information seeking   A generic process that underlies behavior change and comprises a cluster of behaviors including but not limited to reading articles about health, attending to media programs on health, and reading food package labels (Rakowski, III, 5; Swinehart, IV, 18).

information vigilance factor   A tendency or motivation to attend actively to threat-relevant information and sensory experiences related to health and treatment, reflecting *information seeking*, internal health *locus of control*, and monitoring of sensory information (Christensen et al., II, 12).

inoculation theory   A conceptual framework suggesting that providing persons in advance with information and counterarguments enables them to resist persuasive and pressuring appeals to engage in risk behaviors; sometimes termed "social inocula-

tion theory" (McGuire, 1968, in Kelder et al., IV, 14; Bruhn, IV, 1).

input–output model, health   A framework combining external factors such as the physical and community environments and the macrosocial structure with internal biological–genetic–psychic factors as predictors of role fulfillment and well-being (Tarlov, 1992, in Flipse, IV, 3).

inreach   Directing health promotion and prevention strategies at persons already in the health care system (Rimer et al., II, 15).

intention, behavioral   A person's subjective probability or prediction of performing a specified behavior; a basic component of the *theory of reasoned action*/theory of planned behavior. It has been inaccurately defined as what a person intends or plans to do and the degree to which a person has developed conscious plans to enact some behavior in the future (Maddux & DuCharme, I, 7). See *self-prediction*.

interaction model of client health behavior   A conceptual framework in nursing to explain and predict a range of health behaviors; basic components are elements of client singularity, such as background, motivation, cognitive appraisal, and affective responses, and elements of client–professional interactions, such as affective support, health information, decisional control, and professional competence (Cox, 1982, in Blue & Brooks, IV, 5).

interfamilial consensus   A concept denoting the degree of similarity in illness-related conceptions in randomly selected pairs of persons (Susman et al., 1982, in Gochman, I, 10).

intrafamilial transmission   A concept denoting the degree of similarity in illness-related conceptions found in parent–child pairs (Susman et al., 1982, in Gochman, I, 10).

justice as fairness   A conceptual framework applied to health issues that stipulates that each person has an equal right to liberty, that persons with similar abilities and skills should have equal access to services, and that social and economic institutions should be arranged to benefit maximally the least well off (Nilstun, IV, 11).

justice, principle of   A moral standard stressing the obligation to act fairly in the distribution of burdens and benefits, especially not to discriminate against anyone (Nilstun, IV, 11).

KAP (acronym for *K*nowledge, *A*ttitudes, and *Prac*tices)   A standardized measure to assess knowledge of disease risk factors, use of a health service, and perceptions of therapeutic efficacy; used extensively in *developing countries* (Coreil, III, 9).

landscape, therapeutic A combination of physical and humanly imposed environmental characteristics of treatment settings that facilitate the healing process (Gesler, 1992, in Gochman, IV, 20).

language of distress Terminology as well as non-verbal cues that patients use to present their conditions to health professionals (Helman, 1991, in Gochman, IV, 20).

lay-intelligible cues An action on the part of the physician that serves as a basis for the patient's understanding of a condition and its treatment and for the patient's evaluation of the physician's treatment and competence (Ben-Sira, II, 2).

lay referral system The informal network of family members, friends, and community contacts who provide information and advice about the care-seeking process prior to use of a professional (Geertsen, I, 13).

learned resourcefulness Tendency to apply self-control skills in solving behavioral problems, e.g., use of strategies to delay gratification or tolerate frustration (Rosenbaum, 1980, in Christensen et al., II, 12).

lesbian A woman who engages or desires to engage in sexual behavior with another female; the preferred term is "lesbian identity," denoting a woman whose identity is defined by other women (VanScoy, III, 7).

lesbian epistemology A way of knowing the world that reflects a lesbian's own identity and constructions of reality, including of health and illness, in contrast to patriarchal, heterosexist constructions (VanScoy, III, 7).

lesbian invisibility The degree to which lesbian health issues or lesbian identity are hidden or ignored in health services and in the lesbian's interactions with the health care system (VanScoy, III, 7).

libertarianism A conceptual framework applied to health issues that emphasizes the liberty of all individuals to do what they please with themselves and their property, provided they do not interfere with the like liberty of others (Nilstun, IV, 11).

lifespan A framework for individual development that includes chronological age as well as biological and social role transitions (Prohaska & Clark, III, 2).

lifestyle Utilitarian social practices and ways of living adopted by an individual that reflect personal, group, and socioeconomic identities. A health lifestyle involves decisions to live or not to live healthfully; decisions about food, exercise, coping with stress, smoking, alcohol and drug use, risk of accidents, and physical appearance; and reflects social norms and values (Cockerham, I, 12).

lifestyle changes Modifications of behavior resulting from negotiated agreements rather than physician's orders (Chrisler, II, 17).

locality development A cooperative, broadly based approach to community health promotion interventions involving wide discussion and joint problem solving among many diverse groups (Rothman, 1979, in Schooler & Flora, IV, 15).

locational attributes Proximity, centrality, and convenience of health care facilities (Scarpaci & Kearns, II, 5).

locus of control, internal Beliefs that things that happen are a result of one's own ability to influence events as opposed to being the result of chance or fate or of powerful other forces; has been used to predict varied health behaviors (Reich, Zautra, & Erdal, I, 5).

managed care A form of delivering health services in which an organization assumes total responsibility and financial risk for its participants' health, providing all needed services and treatments on a prepaid, capitation basis; an outgrowth of *health maintenance organizations (HMOs)* (Daughtery, IV, 10).

management, health care Tasks of planning, organizing, directing, communicating, coordinating, and monitoring organizational functions in health settings by persons specifically designated and empowered to do so; execution of these tasks through an orderly institutional process carried out by persons designated as managers, regardless of their specific titles (Daugherty, IV, 10).

manager, health care An administrator, executive, director, or chief; anyone who has, or shares in, the legal authority and responsibility for the functions, direction, and achievements of a health organization (Daugherty, IV, 10).

media advocacy Use of mass media to advance a social or public policy objective (Pertschuk, 1988, in Schooler & Flora, IV, 15).

medical anthropology The study of cultural factors related to disease and its explanations, and to healing, treatment, responses to illness and interactions between healers and persons who are sick (Gochman, IV, 20).

medical geography   The study of physical, climatic, and locational factors related to disease and its explanations and to healing, treatment, responses to illness, and interactions between healers and persons who are sick (Barrett, 1993, in Gochman, IV, 20).

medical model   A framework for looking at illness that is based largely on the 19th-century linkages of germ theory and acute diseases and that accords physicians and medical institutions primacy in diagnosis and treatment; an overdependence on medical metaphors in dealing with behavioral variability and problems in living.

medical pluralism   Existence of a multiplicity of medical systems, usually biomedical plus varied indigenous ones, within a society; alternatively, a multiplicity of healing techniques, rather than of medical systems (Durkin-Longley, 1984, in Gochman, I, Part V; Stoner, 1986, in Gochman, IV, 20).

medical sociology   The study of social and societal factors related to disease and its explanations and to healing, treatment, responses to illness, and interactions between healers and persons who are sick (Gochman, IV, 20).

medicalization   Expansion of the jurisdiction of the profession of medicine to include many problems not previously defined as medical entities (Gabe & Calnan, 1989, in Gochman, I, Part IV).

medication event monitor system   A device attached to a medication bottle that records the date and time of every opening, for use in studying adherence (Di Iorio, II, 11).

medicocentrism   Practice of viewing health- and illness-related phenomena solely from the point of view of the physician, particularly in reference to *sick role* (Segall, I, 14).

meme   A unit of symbolic cultural information (Fabrega, I, 2). See *healmeme*.

mental illness, severe (SMI)   A diagnosis in the family of schizophrenic or any other psychotic disorders, or any bipolar disorder, as well as any other medical disorder that is of at least 2 years' duration and disables the patient in at least two major areas of life (Hawley, III, 12).

mutual participation model   A framework for physician–patient interaction in which the patient takes an active role in care and both parties share the goal of the patient's well-being (Szasz & Hollender, 1956, in DiMatteo, II, 1).

narrative representation   Presentation of materials in the context of a story about someone doing something, for some purpose, that results in specific consequences; used in interventions to increase safety and reduce injury (Cole, IV, 17).

narrative thinking   Translation of personal experiences into stories that integrate facts, perceptions, emotions, intentions, actions, and consequences into coherent meaning; involves knowing through stories lived and stories heard and told; contrasted with *paradigmatic thinking* (Howard, 1991, in Cole, IV, 17).

National Health Care for the Homeless   An initiative take in 1984 by the Robert Wood Johnson Foundation and the Pew Charitable Trusts to establish health care clinics for the homeless in 19 United States cities (Wright & Joyner, III, 10).

need factor   A characteristic such as health status or illness that predicts use of health services; a component of the *health services utilization model* (Aday & Awe, I, 8).

negotiating   An intervention to increase adherence that involves medical personnel and the patient jointly discussing and agreeing upon the treatment plan (Creer & Levstek, II, 7).

negotiating model of decision making   A framework for physician–patient interaction in which physician and patient belief systems and expectations are given equal value (Reed et al., IV, 2).

occupational culture   Group norms and practices within work settings that often shape the discourse on health, including how workers define situations of threat and danger, and influence risk behaviors such as smoking and alcohol use (Eakin, I, 16).

operational research model   A way of conducting investigations that begins with a practical, problem-focused question rather than with a conceptual framework; characteristic of research in international health (Coreil, III, 9).

oral rehydration therapy (ORT)   An intervention to treat diarrheal conditions in *developing countries* (Coreil, III, 9).

organizational barrier   A structural problem within the health care system that hampers a patient's perceptions of availability and accessibility of care; organizational barriers may include compromised quality of care, patient's perceptions of inhospitable facilities, distance and transportation problems, waiting time, inflexible hours, dearth or lack of bilingual or bicultural staff, and exclusionary policies (Morisky & Cabrera, II, 14).

organizational culture See *occupational culture*.

outcome expectancy A person's beliefs about the consequences of some behavior (e.g., Maddux & DuCharme, I, 7; Baranowski, I, 9); perceived value of the consequence of a given behavior (Di Iorio, II, 11).

pain A multifaceted noxious experience involving sensory, cognitive, and emotional dimensions (Gift & White, IV, 7).

paradigmatic thinking Cognitive processes concerned with the construction of context-free and abstract formal concepts and principles; both the goal and method of science, logic, and mathematics, in contrast to *narrative thinking* (Cole, IV, 17).

parochialism/cosmopolitanism A conceptual framework for understanding social ties within families and families' relationships to the larger community. Parochial families are presumed to demonstrate strong commitment to family (usually paternal) tradition and authority and to have enduring friendships primarily with persons whose backgrounds are similar to their own; cosmopolitan families demonstrate less commitment to family authority and expand their friendships over time, including persons with diverse backgrounds. This typology has guided some research into use of health services and attitudes toward health professionals, but its value has been limited (Suchman, 1965, in Geertsen, I, 13).

passive prevention See *prevention, passive*.

paternalism Characterizing an act by a person or a group, *P*, intended to avert some harm or promote some good for a person or a group, *Q*, where *P* has no reason to believe that the act agrees with the current preferences, desires, or dispositions of *Q*, and *P*'s act is a limitation of *Q*'s right to self-determination (Nilstun, IV, 11).

patient role The component of the sick role that involves interaction with health professionals and/or the formal health care system, in contrast to *self-care* and informal care behaviors (Segall, I, 14).

perceived barriers A person's belief that a specified health action has negative value, particularly in terms of impediments or costs; a component of the *health belief model* (Strecher et al., I, 4).

perceived behavioral control A person's belief in the relative ease or difficulty of performing a specified health action; importance increases as volitional control decreases (Maddux & DuCharme, I, 7); similar to *self-efficacy*.

perceived benefits A person's belief that a specified health action has positive value, particularly in reducing the threat of an illness or health condition; a component of the *health belief model* (Strecher et al., I, 4).

perceived health competence Belief in one's ability to influence one's personal health outcomes effectively (Christensen et al., II, 12).

perceived severity/seriousness A person's belief that an illness or health condition would have negative consequences; a component of the *health belief model* (Strecher et al., I, 4).

perceived social norm A person's belief about how other people view and evaluate a behavior (e.g., Maddux & DuCharme, I, 7).

perceived susceptibility A person's belief about risk for an illness or health condition; a component of the *health belief model* (Strecher et al., I, 4).

perceived threat A function of perceived susceptibility and perceived seriousness providing an impetus for taking some action; a component of the *health belief model* (Strecher et al., I, 4); also a component of *protection motivation theory*.

physician authority See *authority, physician*.

physician autonomy See *autonomy, physician*.

poverty An exceptionally low standard of living officially defined by the U.S. Bureau of the Census, based ultimately on cost of food and adjusted annually for inflation (Wright & Joyner, III, 10).

power, patient The degree to which patients exert control over encounters with physicians and other health care professionals; basic factors are the patient's age, gender, race, education and knowledge, and health status (Haug, II, 3).

power, physician Dominance of and control by the physician over patients and other health professionals; basic factors are the physician's age, gender, race, practice style, and social status (Haug, II, 3).

precaution adoption process model A conceptual framework to predict protective or risk-reducing behavior; identifies five basic stages—unaware, aware but not personally engaged, engaged but deciding on a course of action, planning to act but not yet doing so, and acting—plus a maintenance stage (Weinstein & Sandman, 1992, in Gochman, I, Part II). See *transtheoretical model*.

PRECEDE Acronym for part of a conceptual framework for developing and evaluating health education programs, denoting the basic terms: *Predisposing, Reinforcing,* and *Enabling Causes in Educational Di-*

agnosis and *Evaluation* (Green, Kreuter, Deeds, & Partridge, 1980, in Glanz & Oldenberg, IV, 8). See *PROCEED*.

precontemplation In the *transtheoretical model*, the stage at which there is no apparent intention to change behavior (Prohaska & Clark, III, 2).

predisposing factor A characteristic such as a health belief, family composition, or social position of family that predicts use of health services; a component of the *health services utilization model* (Aday & Awe, I, 8).

preparation In the *transtheoretical model*, the stage at which a person has taken small steps to engage in some behavior but has not yet taken effective action (Prohaska & Clark, III, 2).

PREPARED™ Acronymic name of a system of improving provider–patient communication and patient self-efficacy and satisfaction; denotes the basic components: recommended *Procedure*, *Reason* for it, patient's *Expectations*, *Probability* of achieving them, *Alternative* treatments, *Risks*, *Expenses*, prior to making a *Decision* (DiMatteo, II, 1).

prevention, active Individual actions to eliminate or reduce the likelihood of a negative health outcome, in contrast to *passive prevention* (Gauff & Miller, 1986, in Gochman, I, 1).

prevention, passive Societal, institutional, or governmental activities to eliminate or reduce the likelihood of a negative health outcome, in contrast to *active prevention* (Gauff & Miller, 1986, in Gochman, I, 1).

prevention/preventive behavior Any activity (medically recommended or not) undertaken to eliminate or reduce the likelihood of contracting a disease or incurring a negative health outcome, or of detecting a disease at an early, asymptomatic stage (Gochman, I, 1).

prevention, primary Reduction or elimination of risk factors (Last, 1987, in Buchanan, IV, 9).

prevention, secondary Asymptomatic detection of a disease in its early stages (Gochman, I, 1).

principle of justice See *justice, principle of.*

problem-based learning An approach to professional education in which curricular materials resemble problems that students will face as practitioners (Bruhn, IV, 1).

PROCEED Acronym for part of a conceptual framework for developing and evaluating health education programs, denoting the basic terms: *Policy, Regulatory,* and *Organizational Constructs* for *Edu-*cational and *Environmental Development* (Green et al., 1980, in Glanz & Oldenburg, IV, 8). See *PRECEDE*.

professional role See *role, physician/provider.*

protection motivation theory A conceptual framework to determine the effects of threatening health information on attitude and behavior change; basic components are internal and external sources of information, cognitive mediating processes of *threat appraisal* and *coping appraisal*, and adaptive or maladaptive coping modes (Rogers & Prentice-Dunn, I, 6).

psychosocial epidemiology Application of epidemiological methods to determine health-related personal and social characteristics in a population, e.g., people's perceptions of social support, religiosity, and health (Rakowski, III, 5).

public health Collective actions of society to assure the conditions for people to be healthy (Institute of Medicine, 1988, in Buchanan, IV, 9).

reactance Workers' tendency to be defiant about safety and risk behaviors as a way of maintaining their control when they believe their behavior is being manipulated (Cohen & Colligan, II, 20). See *illusion of safety.*

reciprocal determinism A concept expressing the constant interaction between a person, the person's behavior, and the person's family and social environment in the development and maintenance of health behaviors (Baranowski, I, 9; Baranowski & Hearn, IV, 16).

relapse In the *transtheoretical model*, the movement from one stage to a previous stage (Prohaska & Clark, III, 2); in the context of regimens of dental flossing and brushing for plaque removal, defined as *adherence* at less than 43% (McCaul, II, 16).

relapse prevention model A conceptual framework, derived from *social learning theory*, for understanding how and why people backslide from a path of behavior change (Marlatt & Gordon, 1985, in Marcus et al., II, 18).

relative risk Ratio of adverse health consequences of a specified behavior accruing to groups who do and do not perform that behavior (Prohaska & Clark, III, 2).

resource model of preventive health behavior A conceptual framework in nursing to predict health actions; basic components are health resources, including perceived health status, energy level, concern about health, feelings about taking care of one's health; and social resources, such as educational level and income (Kulbok, 1985, in Blue & Brooks, IV, 5).

response efficacy Belief that adopting a behavior will reduce some threat (Strecher et al., I, 4).

risk behavior, sexual Any behavior that increases the likelihood of a sexually transmitted disease (STD), including *AIDS*; such behaviors include sexual intercourse without latex protection, actions that expose open sores or cuts to infected bodily fluids, and sharing intravenous drug use apparatus (Thomason & Campos, III, 8).

risk, relative See *relative risk*.

role, physician/provider A set of normative expectations for the full-time professional activity of caring for the sick, involving the development of technical proficiency, affective neutrality, and objectivity and placing the welfare of the patient above that of the professional's personal interests (Parsons, 1951, 1975, in Salloway et al., II, 4).

role, sick See *patient role*; *sick role*.

safe sex Sexual behavior in which there is no chance of direct bloodstream access to infected blood, blood products, seminal fluid, vaginal fluid, or breast milk (Thomason & Campos, III, 8).

safer sex Sexual behavior that reduces the likelihood of exchange of bodily fluids (Thomason & Campos, III, 8).

secular trend Health behavioral changes in a community that are not attributable to health education or health promotion intervention (Glanz & Oldenburg, IV, 8).

selective survival Changes in the composition of a population due to the higher mortality rates at advancing age of individuals participating in risk behaviors (Prohaska & Clark, III, 2).

self-care A process whereby laypersons can function effectively on their own behalf in health promotion and prevention and in detecting and treating disease (Levin, 1976, in Gochman, I, Part IV); often used interchangeably with *self-management, self-regulation* (Di Iorio, II, 11). See *self health management*.

self-care agency An individual's capacity to gather information, make decisions, and perform skillfully the behaviors necessary to assume personal control in health promotion and maintenance as well as in the prevention and treatment of illness (e.g., Orem, 1985, in Blue & Brooks, IV, 5).

self-care autonomy Demonstrating the ability and skills necessary to self-manage a condition (Wysocki & Greco, II, 9).

self-care autonomy, appropriate Expecting a child to have the requisite ability and skills to manage a condition at a level appropriate to the child's maturity (Wysocki & Greco, II, 9).

self-care autonomy, constrained Expecting a child to have the requisite ability and skills to manage a condition at a level less than appropriate to the child's maturity (Wysocki & Greco, II, 9).

self-care autonomy, excessive Expecting a child to have the requisite ability and skills to manage a condition at a level greater than appropriate to the child's maturity (Wysocki, II, 9).

self-efficacy Belief or judgment about one's ability to execute some action successfully (Strecher et al., I, 4; Maddux & DuCharme, I, 7); confidence in one's ability to perform a particular behavior (Baranowski, I, 9). See *health belief model*; *perceived behavioral control*; *protection motivation theory*; *theory of reasoned action*.

self health management Undertaking of lay activities to promote health, to prevent illness, and to detect and treat illness when it occurs; includes a range of behaviors such as: health maintenance activities, illness prevention, symptom evaluation, self-treatment, and use of a variety of health resources such as lay network members as well as diverse health professionals (Segall, I, 14).

self-management, childhood diabetes Assumption of responsibility by a patient and the patient's family for monitoring, evaluating, and adjusting treatment; basic components include demographic factors, family functioning, psychological stress, and interactions with providers to acquire necessary skills (Wysocki & Greco, II, 9). See *self-regulation/self-regulatory skills*.

self-management, epilepsy Sum total of steps a person takes to control seizures and to control the effects of having a seizure disorder; common practices include taking medications at prescribed times, avoiding factors that trigger seizures, following safety precautions such as not driving when seizures are not under control, avoiding running out of medications, consulting with professionals about treatment or unexpected problems, and monitoring seizure frequency; often used interchangeably with *self-care, self-regulation* (Di Iorio, II, 11).

self-prediction What one states one will do in contrast to *behavioral intention*: what one predicts one will do (Maddux & DuCharme, I, 7). See *intention*, *behavioral*; *theory of reasoned action*.

self-regulation/self-regulatory skills   Ability to control or change one's health behavior, including goal setting, monitoring movement toward goals, exerting effort and skill to reach goals, and rewarding self for attaining goals (Baranowski, I, 9); used interchangeably with *self-care*, *self-management* (Di Iorio, II, 11); a conceptual framework designed to understand behavior change, particularly in relation to disease management; basic components include *self-efficacy*, *outcome expectancy*, monitoring feedback, role modeling, social support, and learning of necessary skills (Clark, II, 8).

sense of place   Personal and social meanings or particular significance that people attach to physical locations or settings, as distinct from the objective or physical space dimensions (Tuan, 1974, in Scarpaci & Kearns, II, 5; Gochman, IV, 20).

setting   The conventional "bricks and mortar" facilities in which health care takes place as well as the psychosocial implications of such places for provider–patient encounters (Scarpaci & Kearns, II, 5).

sex, safe   See *safe sex*.

sexism   In health care, a focus primarily on male health issues and on health roles for women that are subordinate to those of men (Elder, Humphreys, & Lakowski, 1988, in VanScoy, III, 7).

shared decision making model   A framework for physician–patient interaction in which the physician is obliged to present the patient with all available information without filtering it, and without giving advice, in order for the patient to be able to make the most informed decision about care (Wennberg, 1990, in Reed et al., IV, 2).

sick call   The processing of health complaints in correctional facilities, which requires that inmates sign up, have their requests reviewed and triaged, and then be seen by a provider; inmates have no choice of providers or of appointment time (Anno, III, 14).

sick role   A conceptual framework developed by Parsons (1951, in Segall, I, 14) for analyzing the behavior of a person who has been diagnosed as ill; basic components are the person's rights to be exempt from responsibility for the incapacity and from normal role and task obligations and the person's duties to seek professional care and to abide by professional advice and recover (Segall, I, 14).

sick role, alternative   Elaboration of the Parsonian *sick role* model, adding the person's rights to make decisions about health care and to be dependent on lay others for care and social support and the person's duties to maintain health and overcome illness and to engage in routine self-management; assumes that members of the person's social network are prepared to take on added responsibilities and to function as caregivers as needed (Segall, I, 14).

sickness   A departure from being healthy, often defined through a combination of symptoms experienced, not feeling "right" or "normal," and consequences such as restricted activity (Lau, I, 3); the social side of illness (Gochman, I, 1); the social construction of an episode of illness, the way illness is dealt with in society (Fabrega, I, 2); a form of deviance (Segall, I, 14); the contextualized definition of dysfunction, a process by which signs and symptoms are given socially recognizable meanings (Dressler & Oths, I, 17).

social action   An approach to community health promotion interventions involving advocacy or conflict strategy that entails mass mobilization of low-power components and use of political pressure (Rothman, 1979, in Schooler & Flora, IV, 15).

social cognitive theory   A general social psychological conceptual framework adapted to understand the acquisition or health behaviors; basic components are *outcome expectancy*, *self-efficacy*, skills, and social evaluation of and feedback on behavior (Baranowski, I, 9; Di Iorio, II, 11; Marcus et al., II, 18).

social epidemiology   See *psychosocial epidemiology*.

social learning theory   A conceptual framework for understanding the acquisition of health behaviors; basic components are observation, modeling, and reinforcement in interpersonal contexts (Tinsley, I, 11; Marcus et al., II, 18).

social marketing   Use of merchandising and advertising techniques to increase the effectiveness of health-related campaigns, e.g., for immunizations and family planning; basic components are lowering the price; responding to market demands, such as needs; emphasizing relative advantages of the service or product; making the service or product accessible to the population; and using a full range of mass media to promote the service or product (Buchanan, IV, 9).

social network   A broad conceptual framework for examining social ties and social support; includes dimensions of structure (e.g., number and density of linkages, interaction (e.g., nature and quality), and function (e.g., provision of information, resources, and emotional support). Not identical to *social support*; networks may be unsupportive (Ritter, 1988, in Gochman, I, Part IV).

social norms   Generally held beliefs about the appropriateness or desirability of some behavior.

social planning   A technical approach to community health promotion interventions using rational empirical processes of data accumulation, and persuasion involving experts (Rothman, 1979, in Schooler & Flora, IV, 15).

social structure   The organization or patterning of social ties; regularities in interpersonal linkages. *Parochialism/cosmpolitanism* has been a major typology of social structure relevant to health behavior research (Geertsen, I, 13).

social support   Aggregate of social ties involving interpersonal relationships that protect people from negative experiences, including both structural (e.g., living arrangements, participation in social activities) and functional (e.g., emotional support, encouraging expression of feelings, provision of advice) dimensions (e.g., Ritter, 1988, in Gochman, I, Part IV); a range of interpersonal exchanges that include not only the provision of physical, social, and emotional assistance, but also the subjective consequences of making individuals feel that they are the subject of enduring concern by others (Pilisuk & Parks, 1981, in Morisky & Cabrera, II, 14).

social support, directive   Assumption by others of responsibility for tasks or decisions in relation to *adherence* (Fisher et al., II, 10).

social support, nondirective   Participation by others in cooperating, sharing, and expressing understanding of feelings in relation to *adherence* without attempts to control or alter tasks or decisions (Fisher et al., II, 10).

social ties   Interpersonal linkages, including those with household members, relatives, and friends (Geertsen, I, 13).

sociology of medicine   See *medical sociology*.

specific etiology, doctrine of   An essentially mechanistic medical model that specified that for each illness there was a single, necessary, and sufficient causal agent or pathogen (Pasteur, 1873 [cited in Hamann, 1994], in Wiese & Gallagher, IV, 4).

stage models of adoption   See *transtheoretical model*.

stages of change models   See *transtheoretical model*.

stepped-care model   A conceptual framework for increasing smoking cessation that matches intensity of treatment to stages of change (Glasglow & Orleans, II, 19).

stereotyping   Physician's categorization of a patient as bad or undesirable, using the patient's behavior as a clue indicative of potential challenge to the physician's authority (Ben-Sira, II, 2).

support-mobilizing hypothesis   A conceptual framework for understanding caregiver behavior, based on the assumption that stress will motivate the caregiver to elicit support (Bass, Tausig, & Noelker, 1988/1989, in Wright, III, 13).

t'ai chi   An ancient Chinese system of exercise and meditation being introduced in selected religious communities as a health behavior intervention (Duckro, Magaletta, & Wolf, III, 15).

theory of planned behavior   See *theory of reasoned action*.

theory of reasoned action   A conceptual framework designed to predict intentions to engage in or change specified health behaviors (Maddux & DuCharme, I, 7); basic components are a person's attitudes toward a specified behavior and a person's perceptions of the social norms regarding the behavior. See *intention, behavioral*; *self-prediction*.

therapeutic landscape   See *landscape, therapeutic*.

threat appraisal   Evaluation of maladaptive responses (Rogers & Prentice-Dunn, I, 6). See *protection motivation theory*.

transtheoretical model   A conceptual framework for predicting behavior change that assumes a progression of stages from *precontemplation* of change through *contemplation, preparation, action*, maintenance, and *relapse*, with different intervention approaches appropriate for each stage (Prohaska & Di Clemente, 1992, in Gochman, I, Part II; Rimer et al., II, 15; Glasgow & Orleans, II, 19); incorporates behavioral intentions, *decisional balance theory, self-efficacy*, and individual processes of behavioral change (Marcus et al., II, 18).

utilitarianism   A conceptual framework applied to health issues that emphasizes the maximization of some desired state (Nilstun, IV, 11).

utilization framework   A refinement of the *health services utilization model* designed to predict type and purpose of health care use; basic components are societal determinants such as technology and social norms, health service system resources and organizations, and *predisposing*, *enabling*, and *need factors* (Andersen & Newman, 1973, in Aday & Awe, I, 8).

value-based learning   An approach to professional education that places values, ethics, and moral issues at the curricular core (Bruhn, IV, 1).

wellness   Realization of the optimum health potential of an individual, family, or community; achieved by enhancing physical, psychological, and sociological well-being through activities aimed at the promotion of health (Blue & Brooks, IV, 5).

window of vulnerability   A period in the family life cycle when the strength of the family's influence on health behaviors has the potential for diminishing (Lau, Quadrel, & Hartman, 1990, in Gochman, I, 10).

worksite program   One or more health promotion activities conducted in an occupational setting (Schooler & Flora, IV, 15).

Contents of Volumes I–IV

VOLUME II.   PROVIDER DETERMINANTS

I.   Overview

II.   Interactional and Structural Determinants

III.   Adherence to and Acceptance of Regimens

A.   General Perspectives

B.   Disease-Focused Regimens

VOLUME III.   DEMOGRAPHY, DEVELOPMENT, AND DIVERSITY

VOLUME IV.   RELEVANCE FOR PROFESSIONALS AND ISSUES
FOR THE FUTURE

Index to Volumes I–IV

In addition to the entries in this Index, the reader is encouraged to look at the Contents of each volume and the Contents of Volumes I–IV that appears at the end of each volume, as well as at the Glossary contained in each volume. Space limitations precluded listing *every* intervention or program, government document, or disease or condition identified in the chapters. Similarly, passages dealing *solely* with etiologies, morbidity, mortality, and demographic correlates of diseases with no relevance for health behavior were not indexed.

ISBN 0-306-45443-2

90000